Neural Plasticity: An Updated Review

Neural Plasticity: An Updated Review

Editor: Christopher Mosley

FOSTER
ACADEMICS
www.fosteracademics.com

www.fosteracademics.com

FOSTER ACADEMICS

Cataloging-in-Publication Data

Neural plasticity : an updated review / edited by Christopher Mosley.
p. cm.
Includes bibliographical references and index.
ISBN 978-1-63242-905-6
1. Neuroplasticity. 2. Neurophysiology. 3. Adaptation (Physiology).
4. Developmental neurobiology. I. Mosley, Christopher.
QP363.3 .N48 2020
612.82--dc23

Foster Academics,
118-35 Queens Blvd., Suite 400,
Forest Hills, NY 11375, USA

ISBN 978-1-63242-905-6 (Hardback)

Contents

Preface

Neural plasticity or neuroplasticity refers to the brain's ability to change throughout an individual's life. It can be expressed at the level of individual neurons to cortical remapping in response to injury. Synaptic plasticity is expressed at the single cell level in terms of changes in the connections between neurons, while changes in their intrinsic excitability is due to non-synaptic plasticity. Environmental stimuli, behavior, thought and emotions can cause neuroplastic changes. Neurogenesis can occur in the adult brain and persist into old age. Such changes are mostly restricted to the olfactory bulb and hippocampus, but can occur in other parts of the brain as well. Neural plasticity can have implications in the treatment of brain damage, vision correction, brain training especially in case of learning disabilities, etc. The association of neural plasticity with the phenomenon of phantom limb sensation, the effect of meditation on the brain, the neurobiological effects of physical exercise, etc. are some of the areas that are being actively researched. This book includes some of the vital pieces of work being conducted across the world, on various topics related to neural plasticity. It presents this complex subject in the most comprehensible language. It is meant for students who are looking for an elaborate reference text on neuroplasticity.

The researches compiled throughout the book are authentic and of high quality, combining several disciplines and from very diverse regions from around the world. Drawing on the contributions of many researchers from diverse countries, the book's objective is to provide the readers with the latest achievements in the area of research. This book will surely be a source of knowledge to all interested and researching the field.

In the end, I would like to express my deep sense of gratitude to all the authors for meeting the set deadlines in completing and submitting their research chapters. I would also like to thank the publisher for the support offered to us throughout the course of the book. Finally, I extend my sincere thanks to my family for being a constant source of inspiration and encouragement.

Editor

1

Relationship between Insulin Levels and Nonpsychotic Dementia

Qiu-xia Pan, Xiao-juan Li, Yue-yun Liu, Fang-fang Wang, Ya-jing Hou, Qing-lai Bian, Wen-qi Qiu, Zhi-yi Yan, You-ming Jiang, and Jia-xu Chen

School of Basic Medical Science, Beijing University of Chinese Medicine, No. 11 North Third Ring Road, Chaoyang, Beijing 100029, China

Correspondence should be addressed to Jia-xu Chen; chenjiaxu@hotmail.com

Academic Editor: Fushun Wang

Objectives. To explore the relationship between insulin levels and nonpsychotic dementia. *Methods.* Six electronic databases (PubMed, Cochrane, SCI, CNKI, VIP, and Wanfang) were searched from January 1, 2007, to March 1, 2017. Experimental or observational studies that enrolled people with nonpsychotic dementia or abnormal insulin levels in which insulin levels or MMSE scores (events in nonpsychotic dementia) were the outcome measures. Random-effects models were chosen for this meta-analysis. Sample size, mean, s.d., and events were primarily used to generate effect sizes (with the PRIMA registration number CRD42017069860). *Results.* 50 articles met the final inclusion criteria. Insulin levels in cerebrospinal fluid were lower (Hedges' $g = 1.196$, 95% CI = 0.238 to 2.514, and $P = 0.014$), while the levels in peripheral blood were higher in nonpsychotic dementia patients (Hedges' $g = 0.853$ and 95% CI = 0.579 to 1.127), and MMSE scores were significantly lower in the high insulin group than in the healthy control group (Hedges' $g = 0.334$, 95% CI = 0.249 to 0.419, and $P = 0.000$). *Conclusions.* Our comprehensive results indicate that blood insulin levels may increase in patients with nonpsychotic dementia.

1. Introduction

Dementia is a general term for a decline in mental ability severe enough to interfere with daily life, and it is a common clinical syndrome that is not only a leading cause of death globally but also a burden on families and society. There is no one test to determine if someone has dementia. Doctors diagnose Alzheimer's and other types of dementia based on a careful medical history, a physical examination, laboratory tests, and the characteristic changes in thinking, day-to-day function, and behavior associated with each type. At present, all of the Mini-Mental State Examination (MMSE), Hasegawa's dementia scale, clinical dementia rating, cognitive abilities screening instrument, Alzheimer's disease assessment scale-cognitive section, activity of living, Functional Activities Questionnaire, and clock-drawing test can be used in the diagnosis of dementia, among which, the MMSE is widely used.

As it is harder to determine the exact type of dementia because the symptoms and brain changes of different dementias can overlap, and in some cases, a doctor may diagnose "dementia" and not specify a type. In these cases, we divided the dementia into two aspects (psychotic dementia and nonpsychotic dementia) according to the day-to-day functions, behaviors, and medical history of the patients. Psychotic dementia is caused by mental illness, which means that dementia is caused by depression, schizophrenia, and other mental disorders, while nonpsychotic dementia excludes the dementia caused by mental illness (psychotic dementia) [1], for example, Alzheimer's disease (AD), vascular dementia (VD), and brain lesions. In addition, mild cognitive impairment (MCI) is a "clinical" diagnosis representing a doctor's best professional judgment about the reason for a person's symptoms. MCI causes a slight but noticeable and measurable decline in cognitive abilities, including memory and thinking skills. A person with MCI is at an increased risk of developing Alzheimer's or another dementia. Medical history, assessment of independent function and daily activities, input from a family member or trusted friend, assessment of mental status, in-office neurological examination, evaluation of mood, and laboratory tests were the primary diagnostic route.

Many risk factors are associated with nonpsychotic dementia. These include older age, gender (i.e., female), a low educational level, a low socioeconomic level, certain physical diseases, and a family genetic history. Recently, abnormal insulin levels were shown to be an important factor that influences the occurrence of nonpsychotic dementia. Umegaki et al. [2] performed a prospective study in which cognitive function scores were assessed at baseline and after 3 years in the same patient group. The results suggested that higher insulin and glycol-hemoglobin levels were associated with diabetes-related cognitive dysfunction.

Insulin is an active substance with a variety of biological functions that affect growth and apoptosis in neurons by participating in blood glucose metabolism [3–8]. The discovery of insulin in the brain suggested that insulin not only participates in metabolism and growth but is also involved in higher cognitive functions, such as learning and memory [3–5]. Insulin has been shown to increase the expression of amyloid precursor protein (APP), beta-amyloid 42 (Aβ42), and hyperphosphorylated tau in the hippocampus and frontal cortex in rats [6, 9]. Thus, there may be mechanistic and sequential associations among insulin, impaired cognitive function, and structural AD-like changes.

In humans, aging is associated with decreased metabolic turnover, decreased glucose utilization, and decreased insulin levels because of effects on the regulation of the insulin signaling pathway. Some authors have argued that abnormal insulin metabolism is caused by aging and does not share a causal relationship with nonpsychotic dementia. For example, Burns et al. [8] assessed the relationship between insulin resistance and conditions including cognitive decline and brain atrophy for two years in patients with early AD and nondemented controls. The authors found that insulin was differentially associated with cognitive decline and atrophy in AD and elderly patients. Furthermore, higher levels of peripheral insulin may exert AD-specific benefits, and insulin signaling may be affected by AD-associated systemic physiological changes. Finally, Dorrance et al. [10] supported the notion that insulin resistance exerts positive effects on cerebral vasculature dementia.

Furthermore, exogenous insulin interventions or treatments have been shown to alleviate nonpsychotic dementia symptoms in patients with insulin resistance and improve their Mini-Mental State Examination (MMSE) scores [11, 12]. However, other studies have demonstrated that insulin levels are negatively correlated with nonpsychotic dementia [13]. In addition, some studies have found no relationship between the occurrence of nonpsychotic dementia and insulin levels when patients were compared with healthy control subjects (HCs) [14, 15]. Therefore, both negative and positive correlations have been observed, resulting in controversy regarding whether high insulin levels or low insulin levels cause nonpsychotic dementia. Thus, a meta-analysis of this subject is warranted.

The present meta-analysis was aimed at determining whether nonpsychotic dementia is associated with altered levels of insulin in the blood or cerebrospinal fluid (CSF). We used meta-analytical techniques because they allow data from individual studies to be quantitatively combined to improve the strength of preclinical and clinical evidence.

2. Materials and Methods

The meta-analyses performed in this study adhered to the guidelines recommended by the Preferred Reporting Items for Systematic Reviews and Meta-Analysis (PRISMA) statement [16] and are registered with the international prospective register of systematic reviews (PROSPERO). Its PRISMA registration number is CRD42017069860.

2.1. Literature Search. Two investigators (Qiu-xia Pan and Xiao-juan Li) independently performed a systematic review of English language publications using the PubMed, SCI, and Cochrane Library databases and Chinese language publications using the CNKI, VIP, and Wanfang databases.

The following search terms were used in the database search: (Dementia or Alzheimer's disease/AD or Mild cognitive impairment/MCI) and (Insulin or insulin signaling pathway). The search was performed to obtain articles published from January 1, 2007, to March 1, 2017. The initial search generated 1287 records, including 474 English and 813 Chinese records. After we screened the titles and abstracts, 263 appropriate articles, including 120 English and 143 Chinese papers, that were related to the present subject were selected for full-text scrutiny. Original studies that reported data on peripheral blood and CSF insulin concentrations in at least two groups of subjects (i.e., dementia or AD and MCI) were included.

2.2. Quality Assessment. Studies were appraised for methodological quality using the Newcastle-Ottawa Scale (NOS). The NOS defines the study quality of observational studies (i.e., case-control studies and cross-sectional studies) using an 8-item scale (scored 0–9 points). Two investigators (Qiu-xia Pan and Xiao-juan Li) independently assessed the quality of each paper, and any disagreements were resolved by consensus in a group meeting.

2.3. Study Selection. After further evaluating the 135 originally selected articles, 50 high-quality (i.e., had 5–9 points on the NOS, Table 1) [17] articles describing observational studies were included in this study. The remaining 85 articles were excluded for the following reasons: there were no necessary data on insulin concentrations [13, 18–27]; related genes and insulin signaling pathway proteins were the main study outcomes [28–36]; there was no clear description or record of a cognitive function evaluation [37–42]; the design of the experiments was unreasonable for the purpose of this study [43–52]; the experimental methods were incomplete [53–60]; the papers did not provide completely related data [61–66]; data from only one group were reported [2, 67–74]; the papers reported data from the same cohort of

Table 1: Quality assessment of the included studies according to the Newcastle-Ottawa Scale (NOS)*.

Study names	S1	S2	S3	S4	C1a	C1b	E1a	E1b	E2	E3	Total points
Si-ling Liu, 2011	1	1	1	1	0	1	1	0	0	0	6
Qin-yun Li, 2015	1	1	1	1	0	1	1	0	1	0	7
Zong-yuan Wang, 2008	1	1	1	1	0	1	1	0	1	0	7
Abimbola A. Akintola, 2015	0	1	1	0	0	1	1	0	1	0	5
Angela J. Hanson, 2016	1	1	0	0	1	0	1	0	1	0	5
J.K. Morris, 2016	1	1	0	0	0	1	1	0	1	0	5
G. Stennis Watson, 2009	1	1	1	1	0	1	1	0	1	0	7
Robert Krikorian, 2012	1	1	0	0	0	1	1	0	1	0	5
E. Rönnemaa, B. Zethelius, and J. Sundelöf, 2009	1	1	0	1	1	0	0	1	1	0	6
Galit Weinstein, 2015	0	1	1	1	0	1	1	0	1	0	6
Jeffrey M. Burns, 2012	0	1	1	1	0	1	1	0	1	0	6
Auriel A. Willette, 2015	0	1	1	1	0	1	1	0	1	0	6
Amber S. Watts, 2013	1	1	1	1	1	1	1	0	1	1	9
Josh D. Woolley, 2014	1	1	0	0	1	0	1	0	1	1	6
Xiao-hong Sun, 2010	1	1	0	1	1	0	1	0	1	0	6
Lu Zhang, 2011	1	1	0	1	1	0	1	0	1	0	6
Wei-gang Liu, 2009	1	1	0	0	1	0	1	0	1	0	5
Gui-qing Chen, 2015	1	1	0	1	1	0	1	0	1	1	7
Zhi-juan Wang, 2014a	1	1	0	1	1	0	1	0	1	0	6
Jun-shi Zhang, 2016	1	0	0	1	1	1	1	0	1	1	7
Jin-geng Li, 2013	1	1	0	1	1	1	1	0	1	1	8
Zhi-dong Yang, 2007	1	0	1	1	0	1	1	0	1	0	6
Hong-mei Yue, 2014	1	1	0	1	1	1	1	0	1	0	7
Liang-mi Li, 2015	1	1	1	1	1	1	1	0	1	0	8
Qing-chun Xia, 2015	1	1	0	1	1	1	1	1	1	0	8
Ran Song, 2015	1	1	0	1	1	1	1	0	1	1	8
Yu-mei Yang, 2009	1	0	0	1	1	1	1	0	1	0	6
Xiao-lan Liu, 2008	1	1	0	1	1	1	1	0	1	1	8
Rong-wei Zhang, 2008	1	1	0	0	1	0	1	0	1	0	5
Bin-bin Zang, 2011	1	1	0	1	1	1	1	0	1	0	7
Zhi-juan Wang, 2014b	1	1	1	1	1	0	1	0	1	0	7
Hong-shan Pan, 2016	1	1	0	1	1	0	1	0	1	0	6
Nan Mu, 2010	1	1	1	1	1	0	1	0	1	0	7
Yan-Wu, 2008	1	1	0	1	1	0	1	0	1	0	6
Hong-li Li, 2013	1	1	0	1	1	0	1	0	1	0	6
Jill K. Morris, 2014	1	0	0	0	1	1	1	0	1	1	6
Wen-qing Xia, 2016	1	1	1	1	1	0	1	0	1	0	7
Chin-Chou Huang, 2014	1	1	1	1	0	1	1	0	1	0	7
Rosebud O. Roberts, 2014	1	1	1	0	0	1	1	0	1	0	6
Mkaya Mwamburi, 2016*	1	1	0	1	0	0	1	1	1	0	6
Heather Kenna, 2013	1	1	1	1	1	0	1	0	1	0	7
Yen-Chun Fan, 2017	1	1	1	1	0	1	1	0	1	0	7
Laura D. Baker, 2011	0	1	1	1	0	1	1	0	1	0	6
M.S. Beeri, 2008	0	1	1	1	0	1	1	0	1	0	6
Hannah Bruehl, 2009	1	1	1	1	1	1	1	1	1	0	9
Xiao-bing Zhou, 2012	0	1	0	1	1	0	1	0	1	0	5
Qiong-yu Zhang, 2012	1	1	0	0	1	1	1	0	1	0	6

Table 1: Continued.

Study names	S1	S2	S3	S4	C1a	C1b	E1a	E1b	E2	E3	Total points
Xiao-hong, Zhao, 2009	1	1	0	1	1	1	1	0	1	0	7
Jun-yi Wu, 2013	1	1	0	1	1	1	1	0	1	0	7
Sheng Huang, 2015	1	1	0	1	1	1	1	0	1	0	7

Note. S1: eligibility criteria; S2: representativeness of the cases; S3: community controls; S4: the controls had no history of disease (endpoint); C1a: important factor basis between two groups; C1b: study controls for additional factor basis between two groups; E1a: secure record of exposure; E1b: structured interview where blind to case about the exposure; E2: same method of ascertainment for cases and controls; E3: nonresponse rate. *Cross-sectional study.

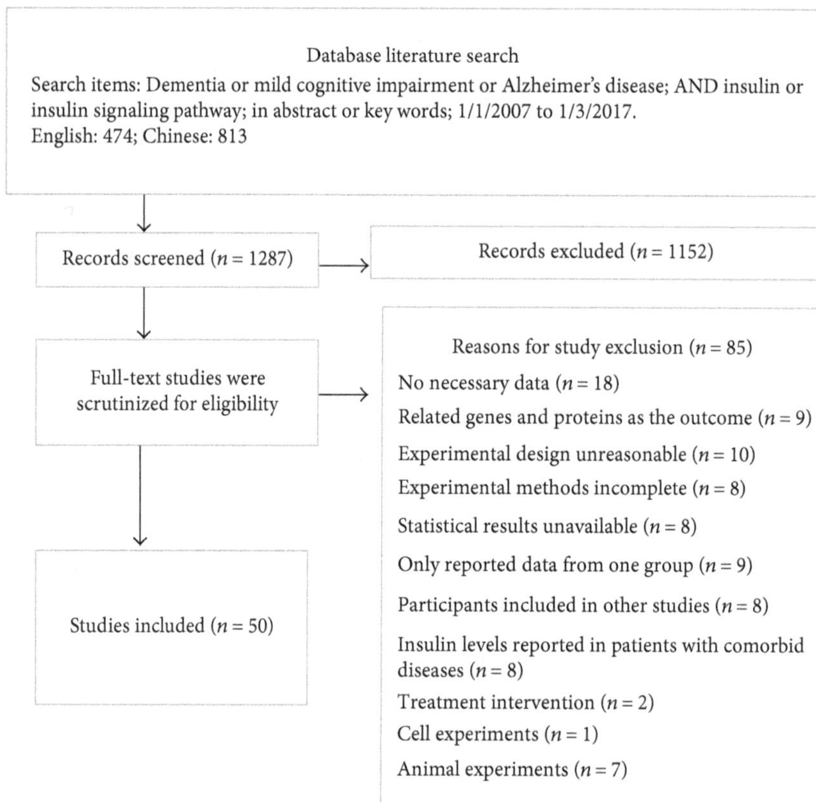

Figure 1: Preferred Reporting Items for Systematic Reviews and Meta-Analysis flowchart of the literature search.

patients who were used in another study [75–81]; insulin levels were reported in patients with comorbid diseases (in addition to diabetes, metabolic syndrome and related diseases can also lead to nonpsychotic dementia [82–89]), such as cognitive dysfunction caused by depression or anxiety [85]; serum insulin was measured before and after insulin treatment or other treatments that could influence insulin metabolism in patients with nonpsychotic dementia; only changes in the MMSE scores before and after the treatment were analyzed, while differences between the observation group and the control group were not analyzed [11, 12]; and the studies involved cell experiments [90] or animal experiments [6, 91–96] (for the flowchart, see Figure 1).

2.4. Data Extraction. Data regarding sample size, mean, standard deviation (s.d.), events, and P values were extracted as the primary outcomes. Two investigators (Qiu-xia Pan and Xiao-juan Li) independently extracted the data, and the results were verified by another team member (Zhi-yi Yan). Any inconsistencies were resolved by consensus. Tables 2 and 3 summarized the included studies and present the demographic and clinical characteristics of the included patients.

2.5. Statistical Analysis. Comprehensive Meta-Analysis Version 2 software (Biostat, Englewood, NJ, USA) was used for all statistical analyses. The sample size, mean, s.d., and events were primarily used to generate effect sizes (ESs) (the sample size and P value were used in some studies in which the mean, s.d., and events were not available). The ESs were calculated as the standardized mean difference in insulin levels or MMSE scores between groups and converted to Hedges' g, which provides an unbiased ES that is adjusted for the sample size. In pooled ESs, 95% confidence intervals (95% CIs) were used to assess significant differences. Random-effects models were chosen for this meta-analysis because we hypothesized that within-study and

TABLE 2: Baseline subject characteristics (nonpsychotic dementia and HCs).

Names (IN) mmol/l	Age		Edu	Sex		Number		Nonpsychotic dementia		HC		Sample	State	Drug	P value
	Ex	HC		Men	Women	Ex	HC	Mean	s.d.	Mean	s.d.				
Si-ling Liu, 2011 AD	72	72	11.2	34	19	23	30	—	—	—	—	Serum	Fast	—	$P < 0.05$ H
Qin-yun Li, 2015 AD	77	75	10.1	126	120	126	120	11.78	6.6	6.28	3.36	Serum	Fast	No	$P = 0.04$ H
Zong-yuan Wang, 2008 a AD L	70	72	—	—	—	14	12	5.7	6.9	4.5	3.5	Plasma	Fast	No	$P < 0.05$ H
Zong-yuan Wang, 2008 b AD (MH)	70	72	—	—	—	9	12	10.3	9.8	4.5	3.5	Plasma	Fast	No	$P < 0.05$ H
Zong-yuan Wang, 2008 c AD L	70	72	—	—	—	14	12	3.4	0.3	3.3	0.4	CSF	Fast	No	$P > 0.05$
Zong-yuan Wang, 2008 d AD (MH)	70	72	—	—	—	9	12	2.4	0.2	3.3	0.4	CSF	Fast	No	$P < 0.05$ L
Abimbola A. Akintola, 2015 multi	66	66	—	62	70	75	57	—	—	—	—	Plasma	Fast	No	$P = 0.07$
Angela J. Hanson, 2016 AD	68	72	—	163	156	199	120	15.6	—	11.7	—	Plasma	Fast	—	$P = 0.0005$ H
J.K. Morris, 2016 AD L	71	72	17	22	29	14	37	8.73	7.8	4.19	3.8	Plasma	Fast	Yes	$P = 0.023$ H
G. Stennis Watson, 2009 AD	76	74	15	13	22	16	19	8.2	4.3	8.9	4.8	Plasma	Fast	No	$P > 0.05$
Robert Krikorian, 2012 MCI	71	68	15	—	—	11	12	14.4	6	16.9	6	—	Fast	No	$P = 0.40$
E. Rönnemaa, B. Zethelius, and J. Sundelöf, 2009 multi	71	71	—	—	—	257	868	—	1.0	—	0.96	Plasma	Fast	Yes	$P = 0.04$ H
Galit Weinstein, 2015 multi	47	47	—	2156	1782	215	3723	—	—	—	—	—	Fast	Yes	$P = 0.036$ H
Jeffrey M. Burns, 2012 AD	75	73	16	59	50	48	61	8.4	5.4	7.2	4.6	Serum	Fast	—	$P = 0.19$
Auriel A. Willette, 2015 a MCI	76	76	15	95	185	194	26	2.78	3.08	2.98	3.10	Plasma	Fast	—	$P = 0.589$
Auriel A. Willette, 2015 AD b	76	76	15	95	185	60	26	2.41	1.46	2.98	3.10	Plasma	Fast	—	$P = 0.589$
Amber S. Watts, 2013 AD	75	74	—	61	87	75	73	—	—	—	—	Serum	Fast	—	$P = 0.001^{*}$
Josh D. Woolley, 2014 a AD	59	57	15	16	19	17	18	—	—	—	—	Serum	-3 min	—	$P < 0.01$ H
Josh D. Woolley, 2014 b (bvFTD)	59	57	15	18	19	19	18	—	—	—	—	Serum	−30 min	—	$P < 0.05$ H
Xiao-hong Sun, 2010 AD	—	—	—	32	58	45	44	12.36	8.627	6.541	9.120	Serum	Fast	—	$P < 0.05$ H
Lu Zhang, 2011 a AD L	72	72	—	59	44	41	35	1.07	0.21	1.51	0.27	CSF	—	—	$P < 0.05$ L
Lu Zhang, 2011 b AD MH	72	72	—	59	44	27	35	0.68	0.11	1.51	0.27	CSF	—	—	$P < 0.01$ L
Wei-gang Liu, 2009 a AD L	71	71	—	66	59	31	70	7.9	2.0	6.8	2.5	—	Fast	—	$P < 0.01$ H
Wei-gang Liu, 2009 b AD MH	71	71	—	66	59	24	70	8.0	2.4	6.8	2.5	—	Fast	—	$P < 0.01$ H
Wei-gang Liu, 2009 c AD L	71	71	—	45	38	27	35	0.27	0.08	0.29	0.10	CSF	—	—	$P > 0.05$
Wei-gang Liu, 2009 d AD MH	71	71	—	45	38	21	35	0.22	0.12	0.29	0.10	CSF	—	—	$P < 0.05$ L
Gui-qing Chen, 2015 AD	78	78	7	94	31	95	80	9.758	7.42	6.384	5.89	Serum	Fast	—	$P = 0.023$ H
Zhi-juan Wang, 2014 a AD	67	67	—	28	22	30	20	7.94	6.81	9.25	5.51	Serum	Fast	—	$P > 0.05$
Zhi-juan Wang, 2014 b VD	67	67	—	29	23	30	20	7.89	6.55	9.25	5.51	Serum	Fast	—	$P > 0.05$
Jun-shi Zhang, 2016 AD	76	76	—	47	39	43	43	11.79	6.62	6.25	3.34	Serum	Fast	—	$P < 0.05$ H
Jin-geng Li, 2013 a AD L	73	73	7	39	46	18	30	10.667	10.51	6.793	14.75	—	Fast	—	$P < 0.01$ H
Jin-geng Li, 2013 b AD M	73	73	7	39	45	20	30	9.203	5.36	6.793	14.75	—	Fast	—	$P < 0.01$ H

Table 2: Continued.

Names (IN) mmol/l	Age		Edu	Sex		Number		Nonpsychotic dementia		HC		Sample	State	Drug	P value
	Ex	HC		Men	Women	Ex	HC	Mean	s.d.	Mean	s.d.				
Jin-geng Li, 2013 c AD H	73	73	7	39	46	17	30	9.324	7.48	6.793	14.75	—	Fast	—	$P < 0.01$ H
Jin-geng Li, 2013 d AD (total)	73	73	7	39	46	55	30	9.718	10.31	6.793	14.75	—	Fast	—	$P < 0.01$ H
Zhi-dong Yang, 2007a AD L	—	—	—	36	43	21	31	16.1	3.7	11.6	4.3	Plasma	Fast	—	$P < 0.05$ H
Zhi-dong Yang, 2007 b AD MH	—	—	—	36	43	27	31	22.1	5.2	11.6	4.3	Plasma	Fast	—	$P < 0.05$ H
Zhi-dong Yang, 2007 c AD L	—	—	—	36	43	21	31	0.98	0.33	1.12	0.31	CSF	Fast	—	$P > 0.05$
Zhi-dong Yang, 2007 d AD MH	—	—	—	36	43	27	31	0.63	0.17	1.12	0.31	CSF	Fast	—	$P < 0.05$ L
Hong-mei Yue, 2014 a MCI	72	72	10	—	—	116	76	19.90	1.62	11.15	1.60	Serum	Fast	—	$P < 0.05$ H
Hong-mei Yue, 2014 b AD L	72	72	10	—	—	81	76	17.90	5.6	11.15	1.6	Serum	Fast	—	$P < 0.05$ H
Hong-mei Yue, 2014 c AD M	72	72	10	—	—	72	76	27.08	1.6	11.15	1.6	Serum	Fast	—	$P < 0.05$ H
Hong-mei Yue, 2014 d AD H	72	72	10	—	—	34	76	34.10	1.61	11.15	1.6	Serum	Fast	—	$P < 0.05$ H
Liang-mi Li, 2015 a AD	73	73	—	117	103	80	70	7.94	0.83	8.23	1.04	Serum	Fast	—	$P > 0.05$
Liang-mi Li, 2015 b VD	73	73	—	117	103	70	70	7.89	0.89	8.23	1.04	Serum	Fast	—	$P > 0.05$
Qing-chun Xia, 2015 a AD L	70	70	—	27	63	34	30	30.29	20.00	20.15	20.50	Plasma	Fast	No	$P < 0.05$ H
Qing-chun Xia, 2015 b AD MH	70	70	—	27	63	26	30	40.29	21.10	20.15	20.50	Plasma	Fast	No	$P < 0.05$ H
Ran Song, 2015 VD	65	65	—	53	32	39	46	8.88	0.31	4.97	2.01	Serum	Fast	Yes	$P < 0.001$ H
Yu-mei Yang, 2009 MCI	63	63	—	81	114	51	144	10.50	—	8.10	—	—	Fast	—	$P = 0.001$ H
Xiao-lan Liu, 2008 VD	74	74	—	88	32	40	40	10.01	—	8.7	—	—	Fast	No	$P > 0.05$
Rong-wei Zhang, 2008 a MVCI	73	73	—	56	38	37	34	13.5	1.4	10.40	1.2	Serum	Fast	—	$P < 0.05$
Rong-wei Zhang, 2008 b VD	73	73	—	56	38	23	34	15.4	2.0	10.40	1.2	Serum	Fast	—	$P < 0.05$ H
Bin-bin Zang, 2011 multi	76	76	—	33	27	30	30	6.42	0.58	5.53	1.03	Serum	Fast	—	$P < 0.05$ H
Zhi-juan Wang, 2014 c AD	74	74	—	69	35	68	36	7.82	6.46	8.37	5.31	Serum	Fast	—	$P > 0.05$
Hong-shan Pan, 2016 AD	69	69	—	50	40	45	45	7.7	4.5	9.4	4.9	—	Fast	No	$P > 0.05$
Nan Mu 2010, a AD L	81	81	—	—	—	13	32	25.38	53.11	20.75	21.51	Serum	Fast	—	$P = 0.605$
Nan Mu, 2010 b AD M	81	81	—	—	—	12	32	17.38	14.89	20.75	21.51	Serum	Fast	—	$P = 0.605$
Nan Mu, 2010 c AD H	81	81	—	—	—	9	32	9.11	6.03	20.75	21.51	Serum	Fast	—	$P = 0.605$
Yan-Wu, 2008 a VD L	62	62	—	—	—	35	15	12.89	4.52	10.01	4.15	—	Fast	—	$P < 0.05$ H
Yan-Wu, 2008 b VD M	62	62	—	—	—	15	15	13.13	5.13	10.01	4.15	—	Fast	—	$P < 0.01$ H
Yan-Wu, 2008 c VD H	62	62	—	—	—	11	15	15.32	5.31	10.01	4.15	—	Fast	—	$P < 0.01$ H
Hong-li Li, 2013 AD	74	74	—	56	69	55	70	5.75	4.23	3.71	1.87	Serum	Fast	—	$P < 0.05$ H

Note. Ex: experimental group; HC: healthy control group; HCs: healthy control subjects; Edu: average years of education of all participants; state: sampling time; drug: participants received or did not receive medication interventions during the course of the study; AD: Alzheimer's disease; VD: vascular dementia; multi: nonpsychotic dementia caused by multiple diseases; MCI: mild cognitive impairment; L/M/H: different severities (light/mild, middle, and heavy) of nonpsychotic dementia, respectively; MVCI: mild cognitive impairment caused by vascular disease; H: high insulin levels in patients in the experimental group; L: low insulin levels in patients in the experimental group. *This study included a comparison of log values, and although the P value was <0.05, the actual analysis showed that insulin levels were not associated with events in nonpsychotic dementia.

TABLE 3: Baseline characteristics of the subjects (abnormal insulin levels and HCs).

Names (events/MMSEs)	Age		Edu	Sex		Number		Ex		HC		P value
	Ex	HC		Men	Women	Ex	HC	Mean Events	s.d.	Mean Events	s.d.	
Wen-qing Xia, 2016	59.5	56.2	10.3	32	38	38	32	28.8	1.1	29.1	1.2	$P < 0.001$ H
Chin-Chou Huang, 2014	79	79	—	73941	68803	71433	71311	8572		4992		$P < 0.001$ H
Rosebud O. Roberts, 2014	80	79	14	423	326	154	595	—	—	—	—	$P = 0.914$
Mkaya Mwamburi, 2016 a	75	80	12	—	—	70	67	25.3	3.4	25.4	4.2	$P = 0.914$
Mkaya Mwamburi, 2016 b	75	80	12	—	—	67	67	25.1	3.6	25.4	4.2	$P = 0.914$
Mkaya Mwamburi, 2016 c	75	80	12	—	—	83	67	25.4	3.2	25.4	4.2	$P > 0.05$
Heather Kenna, 2013	59	57	16	—	—	10	10	28.9	0.9	29.5	1.0	$P < 0.001$ H
Yen-Chun Fan, 2017	53	53	—	27360	24220	10316	41246	413		825		$P < 0.05$ H
Laura D. Baker, 2011	74	74	—	—	—	12	11	—	3.3	—	1.5	$P < 0.05$ H
M.S. Beeri, 2008	—	—	—	111	137	124	124	—	—	—	—	$P < 0.05$ H
Hannah Bruehl, 2009	59	60	15	42	46	41	47	—	—	—	—	—— H
Xiao-bing Zhou, 2012	73	73	—	252	280	162	370	81		66		$P < 0.05$ H
Qiong-yu Zhang, 2012	62	62	9	—	—	81	103	25.34	4.72	23.42	5.50	$P < 0.05$ H
Xiao-hong Zhao, 2009	65	65	—	—	—	31	71	17.46	9.51	10.19	6.09	$P < 0.001$ H
Jun-yi Wu, 2013	71	71	—	93	48	60	81	38		25		$P < 0.05$
Sheng Huang, 2015	65	65	—	49	51	58	42	41		18		$P < 0.05$
Jill K. Morris, 2014	76	74	16	165	99	97	167	—		—		$P = 0.009$ H

Note. Ex: experimental group; HC: healthy control group; HCs: healthy control subjects; Edu: average years of education of all participants; H: high insulin levels in patients in the experimental group; L: low insulin levels in patients in the experimental group.

between-study moderators would result in differences in the true ESs [97]. We excluded one study at a time to determine whether the results were unduly secondary to a particular study. Data regarding the average age and gender distribution of the patients and the classification and severity of cases of nonpsychotic dementia (i.e., MMSE) were also extracted.

Significant differences in heterogeneity across studies were assessed using Cochran's Q test [98], and statistical significance was set at $P < 0.1$. Using these parameters, we found that there was between-study heterogeneity. Inconsistencies across studies were identified using the I^2 index, which evaluates the impact of heterogeneity. I^2 values of 0.25, 0.50, and 0.75 indicate small, moderate, and high levels of heterogeneity, respectively. We then performed unrestricted maximum-likelihood random-effects metaregressions of the ESs [99] to determine whether covariates, including age, gender distribution (i.e., the proportion of males) and MMSE scores, represented moderators that influenced the ESs. We then performed unrestricted maximum-likelihood random-effects metaregressions of the ESs.

Funnel plots were generated by plotting the ESs against the precision (inverse of the standard error) of each study and used to visually inspect the studies for publication bias. The significance of any observed publication bias was determined using Egger's test [100], which assesses the degree of asymmetry in funnel plots. The classic fail-safe N method [101], which is an analysis that results in the number of missing (unpublished) studies that would increase the observed P value to >0.05, was also used to investigate publication bias. Statistical significance was set at a P value < 0.05 unless otherwise indicated. P values < 0.1 were reported as trends.

3. Results

3.1. Included Studies. In total, 50 high-quality studies (5–9 points) were included in this analysis. These included 206207 participants, and 77 sets of data were summarized for the subsequent analysis. The results were divided into the following three areas according to differences in study objectives: (1) the relationship between insulin levels in the CSF and the risk of nonpsychotic dementia; (2) variability in cognitive function scores (i.e., MMSE scores) and insulin levels in the peripheral blood; and (3) differences in insulin levels between nonpsychotic dementia and nondementia patients (assuming that high insulin levels and nonpsychotic dementia are positively correlated).

3.2. Main Associations between CSF Insulin Levels and Nonpsychotic Dementia. First, we compared the insulin levels (mU/L) in the CSF between patients with nonpsychotic dementia and HCs. Eight sets of data were extracted from 4 studies involving a total of 300 individuals. A random-effects meta-analysis was performed, and the results showed that the nonpsychotic dementia patients had significantly lower CSF insulin levels than were observed in the HCs (Hedges' $g = 1.196$, 95% CI = 0.238 to 2.514, and $P = 0.014$; Figure 2). A sensitivity analysis indicated that our results were significantly influenced by all studies (Additional File 1). In addition, significant heterogeneity

Meta-analysis

Study name	Hedges' *g*	Standard error	Variance	Lower limit	Upper limit	*Z* value	*P* value
	Statistics for each study						
Zong-yuan Wang, 2008 c	−0.277	0.383	0.147	−1.028	0.473	−0.724	0.469
Zong-yuan Wang, 2008 d	2.611	0.584	0.342	1.466	3.757	4.468	0.000
Wei-gang Liu, 2009 c	−0.215	0.254	0.064	−0.712	0.282	−0.847	0.397
Wei-gang Liu, 2009 d	0.640	0.279	0.078	0.094	1.187	2.296	0.022
Lu Zhang, 2011 a	1.819	0.271	0.074	1.287	2.351	6.702	0.000
Lu Zhang, 2011 b	3.799	0.425	0.180	2.966	4.631	8.945	0.000
Zhi-dong Yang, 2007 c	−0.433	0.282	0.079	−0.985	0.118	−1.539	0.124
Zhi-dong Yang, 2007 d	1.898	0.314	0.098	1.282	2.513	6.047	0.000
	1.196	0.489	0.239	0.238	2.154	2.446	0.014

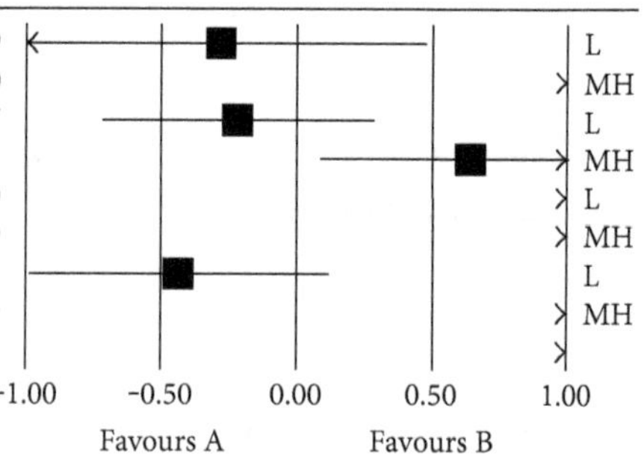

FIGURE 2: Forest plot of the random-effects meta-analysis of differences in CSF insulin levels between nonpsychotic dementia patients and healthy controls (HC). In all, 8 sets of data encompassing a total of 300 individuals were included. The sizes of the squares are proportional to study weight. CI, confidence interval.

Meta-analysis

Study name	Hedges' *g*	Standard error	Variance	Lower limit	Upper limit	*Z* value	*P* value
	Statistics for each study						
Wen-qing Xia, 2016	−0.259	0.238	0.057	−0.726	0.208	−1.086	0.278
Chin-Chou Huang, 2014	0.328	0.010	0.000	0.307	0.348	31.855	0.000
Rosebud O. Roberts, 2014	0.280	0.091	0.008	0.103	0.458	3.091	0.002
Laura D. Baker, 2011	0.692	0.415	0.172	−0.121	1.506	1.668	0.095
M.S. Beeri, 2008	0.209	0.127	0.016	−0.040	0.458	1.647	0.100
Mkaya Mwamburi, 2016 a	−0.026	0.170	0.029	−0.359	0.307	−0.153	0.878
Mkaya Mwamburi, 2016 b	−0.076	0.172	0.030	−0.413	0.261	−0.444	0.657
Mkaya Mwamburi, 2016 c	0.000	0.163	0.027	−0.320	0.320	0.000	1.000
Heather Kenna, 2013	−0.604	0.439	0.193	−1.464	0.256	−1.376	0.169
Yen-Chun Fan, 2017	0.394	0.034	0.001	0.328	0.460	11.655	0.000
Rachel A. Whitmer, 2009 L	0.319	0.041	0.002	0.239	0.400	7.783	0.000
Xioa-bing Zhou, 2012	0.841	0.114	0.013	0.617	1.065	7.354	0.000
Qiong-yu Zhang, 2012	0.370	0.149	0.022	0.077	0.662	2.479	0.013
Xiao-hong Zhao, 2009	0.990	0.225	0.050	0.550	1.430	4.408	0.000
Jun-yi Wu, 2013	0.742	0.197	0.039	0.355	1.129	3.758	0.000
Sheng Huang, 2015	0.639	0.232	0.054	0.184	1.095	2.750	0.006
Jill K. Morris	0.303	0.128	0.016	0.052	0.554	2.368	0.018
	0.334	0.043	0.002	0.249	0.419	7.691	0.000

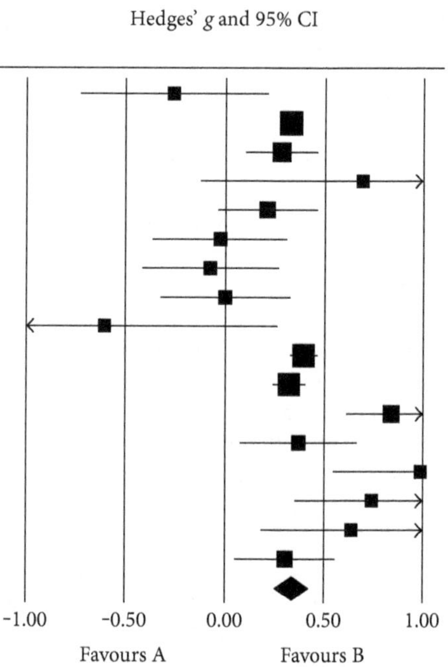

FIGURE 3: Forest plot of the random-effects meta-analysis of differences in MMSE scores between abnormal insulin levels and HC subjects. In all, 17 sets of data encompassing a total of 197114 individuals were included. The sizes of the squares are proportional to study weight. CI, confidence interval.

was observed among the studies in this meta-analysis (Q = 128.753, d.f. = 7, I^2 = 94.563, and P = 0.000).

3.3. Main Associations between MMSE Scores and Abnormal Insulin Levels in the Peripheral Blood. Second, we compared the MMSE scores and the incidence of nonpsychotic dementia between patients with abnormal levels of insulin and HCs. Sixteen sets of data were extracted from 15 studies involving a total of 197114 individuals. A random-effects meta-analysis was performed, and the results showed that high insulin levels were associated with a higher risk of nonpsychotic dementia than was observed in the HCs (Hedges' g = 0.334, 95% CI = 0.249 to 0.419, and P = 0.000; Figure 3). A sensitivity analysis indicated that our results were not unduly influenced by any particular study (Additional File 2). Furthermore, high heterogeneity was observed among the studies in this meta-analysis (Q = 65.130, d.f. = 16, I^2 = 75.434, and P = 0.000).

3.4. Main Associations between Insulin Levels and Nonpsychotic Dementia. Third, we compared the levels of insulin (mU/L) in the peripheral blood between patients with

Meta-analysis

Study name	Subgroup within study	Hedges' g	Standard error	Variance	Lower limit	Upper limit	Z value	P value
		Statistics for each study						
Si-ling Liu, 2011	AD	0.457	0.277	0.077	−0.085	1.000	1.654	0.098
Qin-yun Li, 2015	AD	1.040	0.136	0.018	0.774	1.305	7.670	0.000
Zong-yuan Wang, 2008 a	AD	0.207	0.382	0.146	−0.541	0.956	0.543	0.587
Zong-yuan Wang, 2008 b	AD	0.808	0.441	0.195	−0.057	1.673	1.830	0.067
Abimbola .A.Akintola, 2015	Multi	−0.319	0.176	0.031	−0.664	0.025	−1.816	0.069
Angela J .Hanson, 2016	AD	0.359	0.116	0.013	0.132	0.587	3.093	0.002
J.K. Morris, 2016	AD	0.864	0.321	0.103	0.236	1.493	2.696	0.007
G.Stennis Watson, 2009	AD	−0.149	0.332	0.110	−0.800	0.501	−0.450	0.653
Robert Krikorian, 2012	MCI	−0.402	0.407	0.165	−1.199	0.395	−0.988	0.323
E.Rönnemaa, B. Zethelius, and J. Sundelöf, 2009	Multi	0.124	0.071	0.005	−0.015	0.264	1.751	0.080
Galit. Weinstein, 2015	Multi	0.126	0.070	0.005	−0.011	0.264	1.799	0.072
Jeffrey M. Burns, 2012	AD	−0.240	0.192	0.037	−0.617	0.137	−1.248	0.212
Auriel A. Willette, 2015 a	MCI	−0.065	0.208	0.043	−0.473	0.343	−0.311	0.756
Auriel A.Willette, 2015 b	AD	−0.271	0.234	0.055	−0.728	0.187	−1.158	0.247
Amber S.Watts, 2013	AD	−0.549	0.167	0.028	−0.876	-0.223	−3.296	0.001
Josh D. oolley, 2014 a	AD	0.808	0.344	0.119	0.133	1.483	2.347	0.019
Josh D.Woolley, 2014 b	bvFTD	0.544	0.328	0.108	−0.099	1.187	1.658	0.097
Xiao-hong Sun, 2010	AD	0.650	0.216	0.047	0.227	1.073	3.013	0.003
Wei-gang Liu, 2009 a	AD	0.463	0.217	0.047	0.038	0.887	2.136	0.033
Wei-gang Liu, 2009 b	AD	0.481	0.237	0.056	0.016	0.946	2.027	0.043
Gui-qing Chen, 2015	AD	0.497	0.153	0.024	0.196	0.797	3.237	0.001
Zhi-juan Wang, 2014 a	AD	−0.204	0.285	0.081	−0.762	0.355	−0.715	0.474
Zhi-juan Wang, 2014 b	VD	−0.217	0.285	0.081	−0.776	0.341	−0.763	0.446
Jun-shi Zhang, 2016	AD	1.047	0.228	0.052	0.600	1.494	4.590	0.000
Jin-geng Li, 2013 a	AD	0.286	0.295	0.087	−0.292	0.863	0.969	0.332
Jin-geng Li, 2013 b	AD	0.198	0.285	0.081	−0.360	0.757	0.697	0.486
Jin-geng Li, 2013 c	AD	0.197	0.299	0.090	−0.390	0.783	0.657	0.511
Zhi-dong Yang, 2007 a	AD	1.089	0.298	0.089	0.504	1.673	3.652	0.000
Zhi-dong Yang, 2007 b	AD	2.186	0.330	0.109	1.540	2.832	6.632	0.000
Hong-mei Yue, 2014 a	MCI	5.406	0.313	0.098	4.793	6.019	17.294	0.000
Hong-mei Yue, 2014 b	AD	1.609	0.183	0.034	1.250	1.968	8.792	0.000
Hong-mei Yue, 2014 c	AD	9.905	0.599	0.358	8.732	11.078	16.549	0.000
Hong-mei Yue, 2014 d	AD	14.217	0.980	0.961	12.296	16.138	14.505	0.000
Liang-mi Li, 2015 a	AD	−0.309	0.164	0.027	−0.630	0.012	−1.886	0.059
Liang-mi Li, 2015 b	VD	−0.349	0.169	0.029	−0.681	-0.017	−2.062	0.039
Qing-chun Xia, 2015 a	AD	0.616	0.253	0.064	0.119	1.113	2.431	0.015
Qing-chun Xia, 2015 b	AD	0.956	0.279	0.078	0.408	1.503	3.423	0.001
Ran Song, 2015	VD	2.592	0.293	0.086	2.017	3.167	8.836	0.000
Yu-mei Yang, 2009	MCI	0.509	0.164	0.027	0.186	0.831	3.094	0.002
Xiao-lan Liu, 2008	VD	−0.441	0.224	0.050	−0.880	-0.001	−1.967	0.049
Rong-wei Zhang, 2008 a	VD MCI	2.344	0.306	0.094	1.743	2.944	7.649	0.000
Rong-wei Zhang, 2008 b	VD	3.142	0.397	0.157	2.364	3.919	7.917	0.000
Bin-bin Zang, 2011	Multi	1.051	0.272	0.074	0.517	1.585	3.859	0.000
Zhi-juan Wang, 2014 c	AD	−0.090	0.205	0.042	−0.491	0.312	−0.438	0.661
Hong-shan Pan, 2016	AD	−0.358	0.211	0.044	−0.771	0.055	−1.700	0.089
Nan Mu, 2010 a	AD	0.136	0.323	0.105	−0.498	0.770	0.420	0.674
Nan Mu, 2010 b	AD	−0.166	0.333	0.111	−0.818	0.487	−0.497	0.619
Nan Mu, 2010 c	AD	−0.589	0.376	0.141	−1.326	0.147	−1.569	0.117
Yan-Wu, 2008 a	VD	0.642	0.310	0.096	0.034	1.251	2.068	0.039
Yan-Wu, 2008 b	VD	0.651	0.365	0.133	0.065	1.366	1.782	0.075
Yan-Wu, 2008 c	VD	1.101	0.414	0.171	0.291	1.912	2.663	0.008
Hong-li Li, 2013	AD	0.647	0.184	0.034	0.287	1.007	3.523	0.000
		0.853	0.140	0.019	0.579	1.127	6.110	0.000

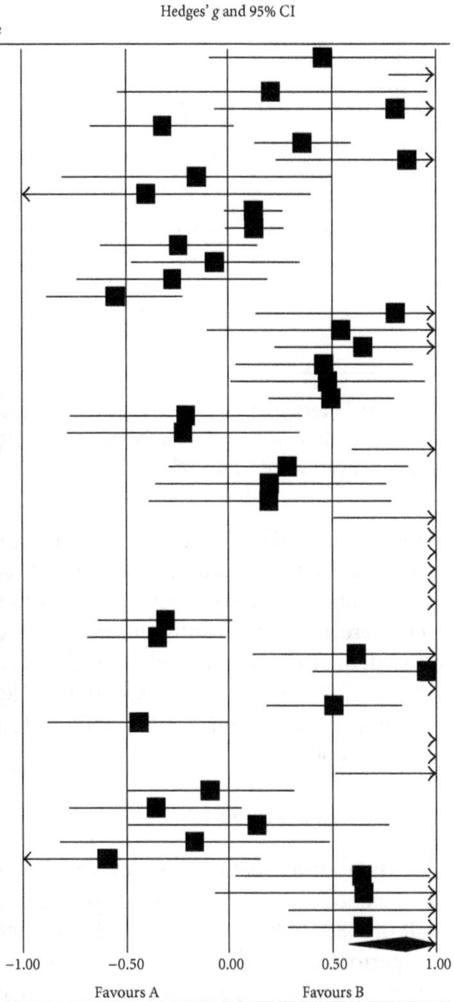

FIGURE 4: Forest plot of the random-effects meta-analysis of differences in blood insulin concentrations between nonpsychotic dementia patients and HCs. In all, 52 sets of data encompassing a total of 8931 individuals were included. The sizes of the squares are proportional to study weight. CI, confidence interval.

nonpsychotic dementia and HCs. Fifty-two sets of data were extracted from 36 studies involving a total of 8931 individuals. A random-effects meta-analysis was performed, and the results showed that the nonpsychotic dementia patients had significantly higher insulin levels than were observed in the HCs (Hedges' $g = 0.853$, 95% CI $= 0.579$ to 1.127, and $P = 0.000$; Figure 4). A sensitivity analysis indicated that our results were not unduly influenced by any particular study (Additional File 3). However, significant heterogeneity was observed among the studies in this meta-analysis ($Q = 1184.942$, d.f. $= 51$, $I^2 = 95.696$, and $P = 0.000$).

3.5. Investigation of Heterogeneity. Fourth, to identify the potential sources of the heterogeneity observed in this meta-analysis, we performed subgroup analyses primarily by considering the sources of the samples (i.e., serum or plasma) and the reported medications used in the patients. We then performed subgroup analyses according to the class of the samples (i.e., VD or AD) and the degree of nonpsychotic dementia in the patients.

The subgroup analysis showed that compared with the levels observed in the HCs, serum insulin levels were significantly higher in the patients with nonpsychotic dementia (25 sets of data were extracted from 17 studies; Hedges' $g = 1.482$, 95% CI $= 0.909$ to 2.056, and $P = 0.000$), and the same trend was observed in the plasma (13 sets of data were extracted from 9 studies; Hedges' $g = 0.445$, 95% CI $= 0.154$ to 0.736, and $P = 0.003$). Compared with the plasma group, the serum group had significantly greater ESs in the nonpsychotic dementia patients with higher insulin levels. High levels of heterogeneity were observed among studies that included serum ($Q = 1011.719$, d.f. $= 25$, $I^2 = 97.529$, and $P = 0.000$) or plasma ($Q = 79.543$, d.f. $= 12$, $I^2 = 84.914$, and $P = 0.000$) insulin levels. Subgroup analyses of studies involved patients who did not take any drugs, who took drugs without effect on glucose and lipid metabolism, and who are on drug withdrawal that lasted longer than

Meta-analysis

Study name	Subgroup within study	Hedges' g	Standard error	Variance	Lower limit	Upper limit	Z value	P value
		Statistics for each study						
Zhi-juan Wang, 2014 b	VD	−0.217	0.285	0.081	−0.776	0.341	−0.763	0.446
Liang-mi Li, 2015 b	VD	−0.349	0.169	0.029	−0.681	−0.017	−2.062	0.039
Ran Song, 2015	VD	2.592	0.293	0.086	2.017	3.167	8.836	0.000
Xiao-lan Liu, 2008	VD	−0.441	0.224	0.050	−0.880	−0.001	−1.967	0.049
Rong-wei Zhang, 2008 b	VD	3.142	0.397	0.157	2.364	3.919	7.917	0.000
Yan-Wu, 2008 a	VD	0.642	0.310	0.096	0.034	1.251	2.068	0.039
Yan-Wu, 2008 b	VD	0.651	0.365	0.133	−0.065	1.366	1.782	0.075
Yan-Wu, 2008 c	VD	1.101	0.414	0.171	0.291	1.912	2.663	0.008
		0.868	0.455	0.207	−0.024	1.760	1.907	0.056

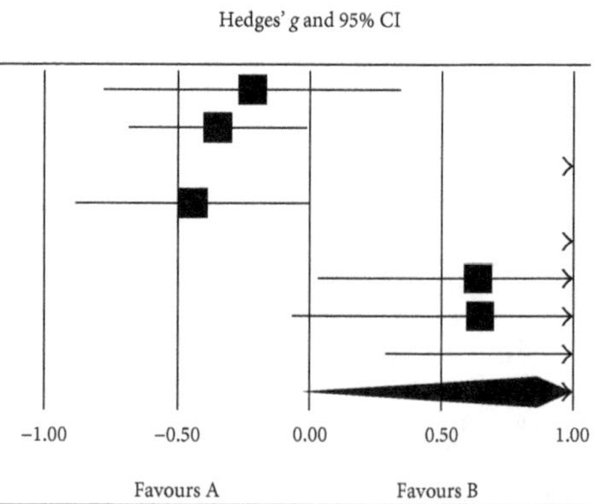

FIGURE 5: Forest plot of the random-effects meta-analysis of differences in blood insulin concentrations between VD patients and HC subjects. In all, 8 sets of data encompassing a total of 488 individuals were included. The sizes of the squares are proportional to study weight. CI, confidence interval.

2 weeks. The subjects were then grouped, and 10 sets of data were extracted from 8 studies involving a total of 731 individuals. A random-effects meta-analysis showed that insulin levels were not significantly different between the nonpsychotic dementia patients and HCs (Hedges' $g = 0.194$, 95% CI = −0.251 to 0.640, and $P = 0.393$). High levels of heterogeneity were also found ($Q = 76.093$, d.f. = 9, $I^2 = 88.172$, and $P = 0.000$).

3.6. Subgroup Analyses

3.6.1. Associations between Insulin Levels and the VD Group. Eight sets of data were extracted from 6 studies involving a total of 488 individuals. A random-effects meta-analysis was performed, and the results showed that the risk of VD was higher in patients with high insulin levels than in the HCs (Hedges' $g = 0.868$, 95% CI = −0.024 to 1.760, and $P = 0.056$; Figure 5). A sensitivity analysis indicated that two studies could have influenced this outcome (Additional File 4). This was not surprising because the P values of the meta-analysis outcomes were only slightly higher than 0.05. Significant heterogeneity was observed among the studies in this meta-analysis ($Q = 145.849$, d.f. = 8, $I^2 = 95.201$, and $P = 0.000$).

3.6.2. Associations between Insulin Levels and the AD Group. Thirty-four sets of data were extracted from 24 studies involving a total of 8407 individuals. A random-effects meta-analysis was performed, and the results showed that the nonpsychotic dementia patients had significantly higher insulin levels than were observed in the HCs (Hedges' $g = 0.852$, 95% CI = 0.494 to 1.209, and $P = 0.000$; Figure 6). A sensitivity analysis indicated that these results were not unduly influenced by any particular study (Additional File 5). However, high levels of heterogeneity among the studies were observed in this meta-analysis ($Q = 678.926$, d.f. = 33, $I^2 = 95.139$, and $P = 0.000$).

Fewer than 5 studies focused on the relationship between abnormal insulin levels and nonpsychotic dementia types other than AD and VD. Hence, we compared only the relationships between abnormal insulin levels and AD or VD because these two subgroups showed high heterogeneity. Thus, we next sought to determine whether there are differences in blood insulin levels between HCs and patients with MCI, mild (or light) nonpsychotic dementia (L, MMSE scores ≥ 16) and moderate or heavy nonpsychotic dementia (MH, MMSE scores < 16).

3.6.3. Associations between Insulin Levels and MCI. Five sets of data were extracted from 5 studies involving a total of 4653 individuals. A random-effects meta-analysis was performed, and the results showed that there were no significant differences in blood insulin levels between the MCI and HC groups (Hedges' $g = 1.557$, 95% CI = −0.253 to 3.367, and $P = 0.092$; Figure 7). A sensitivity analysis was not performed because the number of studies was too small. However, we identified significant heterogeneity among the studies ($Q = 264.128$, $I^2 = 98.486$, and $P < 0.001$).

3.6.4. Associations between Insulin Levels and Patients with Mild (or Light) Nonpsychotic Dementia. Eight sets of data were extracted from 8 studies involving a total of 543 individuals. A random-effects meta-analysis was performed, and the results showed that mild nonpsychotic dementia patients had significantly higher insulin levels than were observed in the HCs (Hedges' $g = 0.520$, 95% CI = 0.284 to 0.757, and $P = 0.000$; Figure 7). A sensitivity analysis indicated that these results were not unduly influenced by any particular study (Additional File 6). Furthermore, low heterogeneity was observed among the studies in this meta-analysis ($Q = 11.531$, d.f. = 7, $I^2 = 39.293$, and $P = 0.117$), demonstrating that the differences among the groups made a negligible contribution to this heterogeneity.

3.6.5. Associations between Insulin Levels and Patients with Moderate or Heavy Nonpsychotic Dementia. Twelve sets of data were extracted from 8 studies involving a total of 610 individuals. A random-effects meta-analysis was performed, and the results showed that the middle and heavy

Meta-analysis

Study name	Subgroup within study	Hedges' g	Standard error	Variance	Lower limit	Upper limit	Z value	P value
		Statistics for each study						
Si-ling Liu, 2011	AD	0.457	0.277	0.077	−0.085	1.000	1.654	0.098
Qin-yun Li, 2015	AD	1.040	0.136	0.018	0.774	1.305	7.670	0.000
Zong-yuan Wang, 2008 a	AD	0.207	0.382	0.146	−0.541	0.956	0.543	0.587
Zong-yuan Wang, 2008 b	AD	0.808	0.441	0.195	−0.057	1.673	1.830	0.067
Angela J .Hanson, 2016	AD	0.359	0.116	0.013	0.132	0.587	3.093	0.002
J.K. Morris, 2016	AD	0.864	0.321	0.103	0.236	1.493	2.696	0.007
G. Stennis Watson, 2009	AD	−0.149	0.332	0.110	−0.800	0.501	−0.450	0.653
Jeffrey M. Burns, 2012	AD	−0.240	0.192	0.037	−0.617	0.137	−1.248	0.212
Auriel A. Willette, 2015 b	AD	−0.271	0.234	0.055	−0.728	0.187	−1.158	0.247
Amber S. Watts, 2013	AD	−0.549	0.167	0.028	−0.876	−0.223	−3.296	0.001
Josh D. oolley, 2014 a	AD	0.808	0.344	0.119	0.133	1.483	2.347	0.019
Xiao-hong Sun, 2010	AD	0.650	0.216	0.047	0.227	1.073	3.013	0.003
Wei-gang Liu, 2009 a	AD	0.463	0.217	0.047	0.038	0.887	2.136	0.033
Wei-gang Liu, 2009 b	AD	0.481	0.237	0.056	0.016	0.946	2.027	0.043
Gui-qing Chen, 2015	AD	0.497	0.153	0.024	0.196	0.797	3.237	0.001
Zhi-juan Wang, 2014 a	AD	−0.204	0.285	0.081	−0.762	0.355	−0.715	0.474
Jun-shi Zhang, 2016	AD	1.047	0.228	0.052	0.600	1.494	4.590	0.000
Jin-geng Li, 2013 a	AD	0.286	0.295	0.087	−0.292	0.863	0.969	0.332
Jin-geng Li, 2013 b	AD	0.198	0.285	0.081	−0.360	0.757	0.697	0.486
Jin-geng Li, 2013 c	AD	0.197	0.299	0.090	−0.390	0.783	0.657	0.511
Zhi-dong Yang, 2007 a	AD	1.089	0.298	0.089	0.504	1.673	3.652	0.000
Zhi-dong Yang, 2007 b	AD	2.186	0.330	0.109	1.540	2.832	6.632	0.000
Hong-mei Yue, 2014 b	AD	1.609	0.183	0.034	1.250	1.968	8.792	0.000
Hong-mei Yue, 2014 c	AD	9.905	0.599	0.358	8.732	11.078	16.549	0.000
Hong-mei Yue, 2014 d	AD	14.217	0.980	0.961	12.296	16.138	14.505	0.000
Liang-mi Li, 2015 a	AD	−0.309	0.164	0.027	−0.630	0.012	−1.886	0.059
Qing-chun Xia, 2015 a	AD	0.616	0.253	0.064	0.119	1.113	2.431	0.015
Qing-chun Xia, 2015 b	AD	0.956	0.279	0.078	0.408	1.503	3.423	0.001
Zhi-juan Wang, 2014 c	AD	−0.090	0.205	0.042	−0.491	0.312	−0.438	0.661
Hong-shan Pan, 2016	AD	−0.358	0.211	0.044	−0.771	0.055	−1.700	0.089
Nan Mu, 2010 a	AD	0.136	0.323	0.105	−0.498	0.770	0.420	0.674
Nan Mu, 2010 b	AD	−0.166	0.333	0.111	−0.818	0.487	−0.497	0.619
Nan Mu, 2010 c	AD	−0.589	0.376	0.141	−1.326	0.147	−1.569	0.117
Hong-li Li, 2013	AD	0.647	0.184	0.034	0.287	1.007	3.523	0.000
		0.852	0.182	0.033	0.494	1.209	4.668	0.000

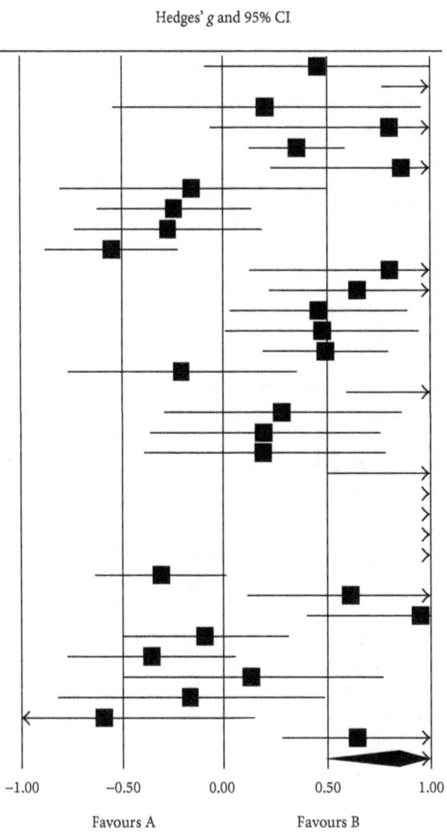

FIGURE 6: Forest plot of the random-effects meta-analysis of differences in blood insulin concentrations between AD patients and HC subjects. In all, 34 sets of data encompassing a total of 8407 individuals were included. The sizes of the squares are proportional to study weight. CI, confidence interval.

nonpsychotic dementia patients had significantly higher insulin levels than were observed in the HCs (Hedges' $g = 2.379$, 95% CI = 1.007 to 3.752, and $P = 0.001$; Figure 7). A sensitivity analysis indicated that the results were not unduly influenced by any particular study (Additional File 7). However, significant heterogeneity was observed among the studies in this meta-analysis ($Q = 531.782$, d.f. = 11, $I^2 = 97.931$, and $P = 0.000$).

The results of the three subgroup analyses demonstrated that the high heterogeneity observed for increased insulin levels in the peripheral blood in patients with nonpsychotic dementia may have been caused by the severity of the dementia as follows: the greater the severity of nonpsychotic dementia, the higher the ESs of peripheral blood insulin levels. Compared with those of the HC group, the insulin levels in the MCI group were not correlated with the MCI.

In a series of metaregression analyses, we assessed whether gender or continuous variables, such as age, could explain the observed between-study differences. Gender was found to have a moderating effect ($P = 0.29$), but age did not significantly contribute to heterogeneity ($P < 0.05$).

Overall, our results indicated that the significant heterogeneity observed in the patients with increased insulin and nonpsychotic dementia could have been caused by a variety of factors, such as gender, sampling differences, and the severity of nonpsychotic dementia.

3.7. Publication Bias. In the abnormal insulin group, no significant publication bias was detected among the studies in a visual inspection of funnel plots (Additional File 8). These results were confirmed in Egger's tests ($t = 0.007$, d.f. = 15, and $P = 0.497$). Moreover, the nonpsychotic dementia group and AD group showed slight publication biases and had the following Egger's test values: for insulin, $t = 3.26$, d.f. = 50, and $P = 0.001$ (Additional File 9); and for AD, $t = 2.399$, d.f. = 32, and $P = 0.011$ (Additional File 10). Because the ESs of small sample studies estimate a large amount of variation, the appearance of extreme ES values is more likely to emerge in small sample studies than in large sample studies. This publication bias was not statistically significant, and we therefore applied Duval and Tweedie's trim and fill method in further analyses.

The classic fail-safe N was used to assess publication bias, and the results revealed that 4805 missing studies would be required for insulin and 1809 missing studies would be required for AD to achieve P values of >0.05. These results support the notion that the observed publication bias was unlikely to have caused the positive results of our meta-analysis.

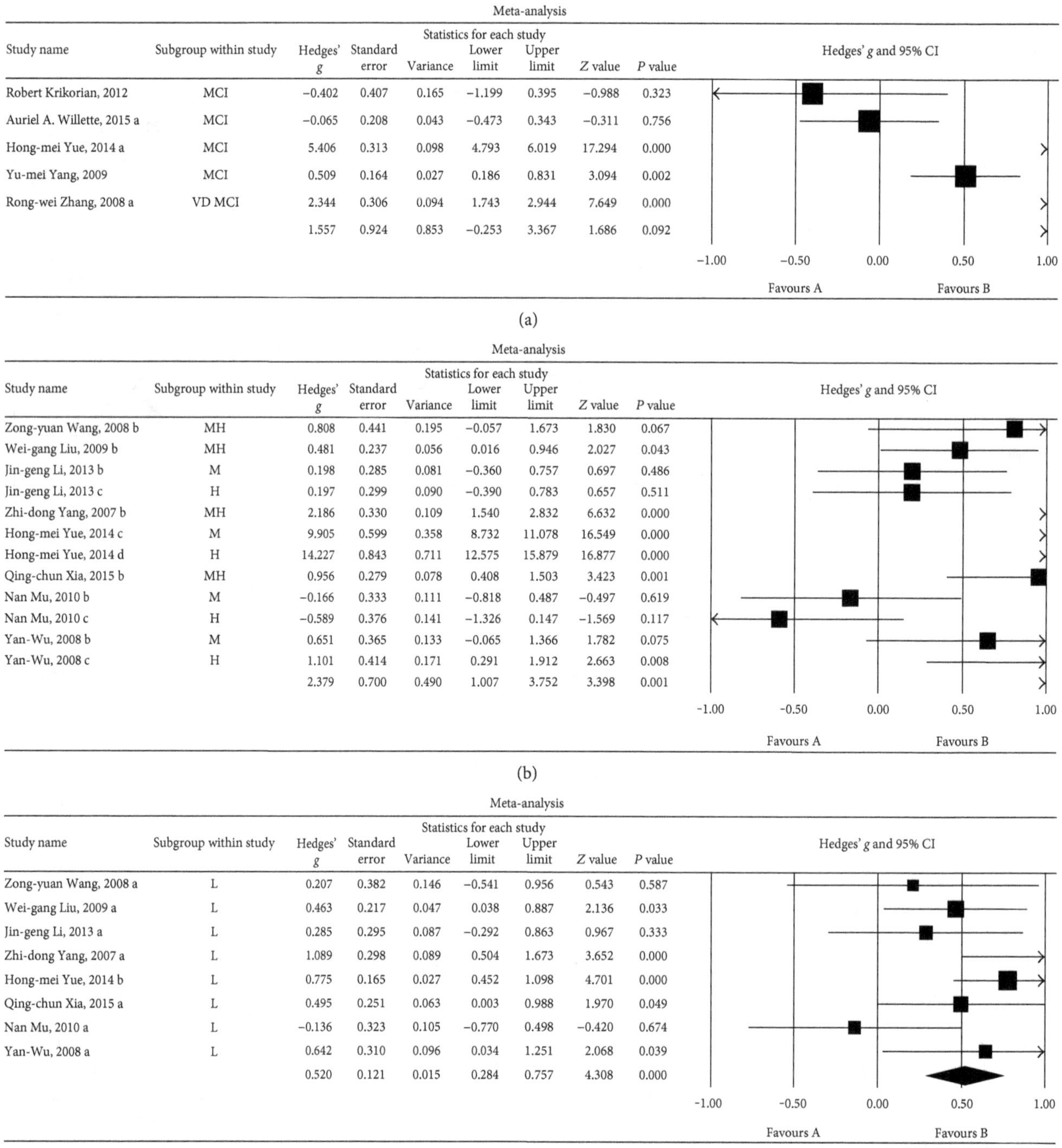

Meta-analysis

Study name	Subgroup within study	Hedges' g	Standard error	Variance	Lower limit	Upper limit	Z value	P value
Robert Krikorian, 2012	MCI	−0.402	0.407	0.165	−1.199	0.395	−0.988	0.323
Auriel A. Willette, 2015 a	MCI	−0.065	0.208	0.043	−0.473	0.343	−0.311	0.756
Hong-mei Yue, 2014 a	MCI	5.406	0.313	0.098	4.793	6.019	17.294	0.000
Yu-mei Yang, 2009	MCI	0.509	0.164	0.027	0.186	0.831	3.094	0.002
Rong-wei Zhang, 2008 a	VD MCI	2.344	0.306	0.094	1.743	2.944	7.649	0.000
		1.557	0.924	0.853	−0.253	3.367	1.686	0.092

(a)

Meta-analysis

Study name	Subgroup within study	Hedges' g	Standard error	Variance	Lower limit	Upper limit	Z value	P value
Zong-yuan Wang, 2008 b	MH	0.808	0.441	0.195	−0.057	1.673	1.830	0.067
Wei-gang Liu, 2009 b	MH	0.481	0.237	0.056	0.016	0.946	2.027	0.043
Jin-geng Li, 2013 b	M	0.198	0.285	0.081	−0.360	0.757	0.697	0.486
Jin-geng Li, 2013 c	H	0.197	0.299	0.090	−0.390	0.783	0.657	0.511
Zhi-dong Yang, 2007 b	MH	2.186	0.330	0.109	1.540	2.832	6.632	0.000
Hong-mei Yue, 2014 c	M	9.905	0.599	0.358	8.732	11.078	16.549	0.000
Hong-mei Yue, 2014 d	H	14.227	0.843	0.711	12.575	15.879	16.877	0.000
Qing-chun Xia, 2015 b	MH	0.956	0.279	0.078	0.408	1.503	3.423	0.001
Nan Mu, 2010 b	M	−0.166	0.333	0.111	−0.818	0.487	−0.497	0.619
Nan Mu, 2010 c	H	−0.589	0.376	0.141	−1.326	0.147	−1.569	0.117
Yan-Wu, 2008 b	M	0.651	0.365	0.133	−0.065	1.366	1.782	0.075
Yan-Wu, 2008 c	H	1.101	0.414	0.171	0.291	1.912	2.663	0.008
		2.379	0.700	0.490	1.007	3.752	3.398	0.001

(b)

Meta-analysis

Study name	Subgroup within study	Hedges' g	Standard error	Variance	Lower limit	Upper limit	Z value	P value
Zong-yuan Wang, 2008 a	L	0.207	0.382	0.146	−0.541	0.956	0.543	0.587
Wei-gang Liu, 2009 a	L	0.463	0.217	0.047	0.038	0.887	2.136	0.033
Jin-geng Li, 2013 a	L	0.285	0.295	0.087	−0.292	0.863	0.967	0.333
Zhi-dong Yang, 2007 a	L	1.089	0.298	0.089	0.504	1.673	3.652	0.000
Hong-mei Yue, 2014 b	L	0.775	0.165	0.027	0.452	1.098	4.701	0.000
Qing-chun Xia, 2015 a	L	0.495	0.251	0.063	0.003	0.988	1.970	0.049
Nan Mu, 2010 a	L	−0.136	0.323	0.105	−0.770	0.498	−0.420	0.674
Yan-Wu, 2008 a	L	0.642	0.310	0.096	0.034	1.251	2.068	0.039
		0.520	0.121	0.015	0.284	0.757	4.308	0.000

(c)

Figure 7: Forest plot of the random-effects meta-analysis of differences in blood insulin concentrations between patients with different severities of dementia and HC subjects. These 3 pictures in (a), (b), and (c) represent a comparison of insulin levels between HC subjects and MCI, mild (L), and moderate to severe (MH) dementia patients, respectively.

4. Discussion

Many studies have focused on the changes that occur in the Pi3k-Akt insulin signaling pathway in nonpsychotic dementia patients. The Pi3k-Akt insulin signaling pathway is an important pathway in insulin metabolism and is also involved in growth and development, metabolism, and vital cognitive activities. Therefore, it is important to determine whether insulin plays a specific role in nonpsychotic dementia. Whether circulating levels of insulin are altered in nonpsychotic dementia patients has been controversial for a long time. Hence, the significance of insulin levels to the etiology of nonpsychotic dementia etiology was not fully known. The results of this study provide strong clinical evidence supporting the notion that nonpsychotic dementia is associated with increased levels of circulating insulin and decreased levels of insulin in the CSF. These results provide new insights into a potential molecular pathway that confers vulnerability to the development of nonpsychotic dementia. A strength of this study is that it is based on a large amount of data and a sufficient number of studies related to nonpsychotic dementia.

We explored the relationship between insulin levels and the occurrence of nonpsychotic dementia from three different perspectives. Our results show that CSF insulin levels are lower in patients with nonpsychotic dementia than in HCs, while insulin levels in the peripheral blood may be higher. Additionally, high insulin levels in the peripheral blood were associated with lower scores in cognitive functions. Because the number of studies that included a CSF group, a VD group, an MCI patient group, an L group, and an MH group was small, our results only reveal that there is a correlation between insulin levels and nonpsychotic dementia in these groups. The results suggest that insulin levels are higher in the peripheral blood in VD, AD, L, and MH patients while CSF insulin levels are lower in nonpsychotic dementia patients. The ES was higher in the VD group than in the AD group and higher in the MH group than in the L group.

Our results show that there was no difference in insulin levels between MCI patients and HCs. Eight sets of data obtained from 4 studies support the finding that there is a relationship between CSF insulin levels and the severity of nonpsychotic dementia. Because the number of enrolled patients was small, the present results show that CSF insulin levels are lower in patients with severe nonpsychotic dementia, and there were no significant differences between MCI patients and HCs. Moreover, when the effects of drugs on insulin metabolism were excluded, a subgroup analysis showed that there was no correlation between nonpsychotic dementia and insulin levels. Therefore, the following two possibilities are considered. First, because MMSE scores were significantly lower in the high insulin subjects than in the HC group, the fact that there was no correlation may be related to the small sample size. Hence, as the study size increased, the trend toward an increase in serum insulin levels in the MCI patients might reach significance, and insulin levels are more likely to vary with the severity of the nonpsychotic dementia. Second, because the severity of nonpsychotic dementia increased with the ages of the affected patients, insulin levels may simply increase with age and may not be a key factor in the pathology of nonpsychotic dementia.

Several studies [44–46] have described insulin levels and MMSE scores in nonpsychotic dementia patients without diabetes, type 2 diabetes patients without dementia, and patients with nonpsychotic dementia and type 2 diabetes, and these studies have reported that there are no significant differences in the ages or genders of these patients. Insulin levels increased in the nonpsychotic dementia patients, and cognitive function scores decreased in subjects with high insulin levels. Further investigations of insulin levels in MCI patients are required to confirm these results.

In this meta-analysis, we found various levels of between-study heterogeneity in the outcomes. Although we attempted to adjust for potential confounders, none of the theoretically relevant categorical or continuous variables that were tested explained the observed heterogeneity. A subgroup analysis showed that serum insulin levels (as opposed to plasma levels) were significantly higher in nonpsychotic dementia patients than in HC subjects and that VD insulin levels (as opposed to AD levels) were significantly higher in nonpsychotic dementia patients than in HC subjects. However, the high level of between-study heterogeneity was not lower in these subgroup analyses. MH insulin levels (but not L levels) were significantly higher in nonpsychotic dementia patients than in HC subjects, and low heterogeneity was found in the L group analysis. The high level of between-study heterogeneity was not reduced in the MH and drug intervention elimination groups. This high level of between-study heterogeneity may have been caused by the differences in the samples (i.e., according to gender, age, or sample type), the type of nonpsychotic dementia, the degree of nonpsychotic dementia, or the drug intervention. In addition, hunger, cold, exogenous diet stimulation, endocrine diseases, and the selection of inspection methods and reagents could potentially have caused an abnormal secretion of insulin. Hence, potential confounders that could contribute to the observed between-study heterogeneity were present in a variety of the analyzed studies and may have been related to patient conditions during sample extraction. Because insulin levels that are determined using blood samples can be affected by handling time and the state of the research subjects, studies that include patients who provide samples while on an empty stomach and who are not affected by other endocrine factors may be required to further investigate whether these factors contributed to the variance observed among the studies in this analysis.

5. Conclusions

Overall, CSF insulin levels were lower in nonpsychotic dementia patients (enrolled sample number < 10, more experimental data are needed to support this finding). The high insulin subjects had significantly lower MMSEs and nonpsychotic dementia events than were observed in the HCs, and blood insulin levels were significantly higher in nonpsychotic dementia patients than in HCs. These results indicate that insulin levels are an important indicator that may be useful in clinical diagnoses of nonpsychotic dementia.

Abbreviations

$A\beta42$:	Beta-amyloid 42
AD:	Alzheimer's disease
APP:	Amyloid precursor protein
CSF:	Cerebrospinal fluid
ESs:	Effect sizes
HC:	Healthy control
HCs:	Healthy control subjects
L:	Light/mild
MH:	Middle and heavy
MCI:	Mild cognitive impairment
MMSE:	Mini-Mental State Examination
NOS:	Newcastle-Ottawa Scale

PRISMA: Reporting Items for Systematic Reviews and Meta-Analysis
s.d.: Standard deviation
VD: Vascular dementia
95% CI: 95% confidence interval.

Additional Points

Availability of Data and Material. The datasets supporting the conclusions of this article are included within the article and its additional files.

Disclosure

The funders had no role in the study design, analysis, decision to publish, or preparation of the manuscript.

Conflicts of Interest

The authors declare that there is no conflict of interest regarding the publication of this article.

Authors' Contributions

Jia-xu Chen and Qiu-xia Pan raised the idea of this study. Qiu-xia Pan and Xiao-juan Li contributed equally as first authors of this manuscript and were the two main reviewers of this study. Fang-fang Wang and Ya-jing Hou contributed to the data collection. You-ming Jiang provided guidance regarding the methodology. Yue-yun Liu took part in the data selection and extraction. Zhi-yi Yan participated in the data extraction. Qiu-xia Pan, Qing-lai Bian, and Wen-qi Qiu cocompleted the primary draft. All authors contributed to the design of this meta-analysis and played a substantial role in the manuscript redaction. All authors approved the final version of this article.

Acknowledgments

The authors thank Yao-wen Zhang for the very helpful and constructive suggestions related to data extraction during this study. This work was funded by the National Natural Science Foundation of China (Grant nos. 81473597 and 81630104), the Beijing Natural Sciences Foundation (Grant no. 7152093), and the 111 Project (no. B07007).

Supplementary Materials

Supplementary 1. Sensitivity analysis of differences in insulin levels in the CSF between nonpsychotic dementia patients and HC subjects.

Supplementary 2. Sensitivity analysis of the random-effects meta-analysis of differences in MMSE scores between patients with abnormal insulin levels and HC subjects.

Supplementary 3. Sensitivity analysis of differences in blood insulin levels between nonpsychotic dementia patients and HC subjects.

Supplementary 4. Sensitivity analysis of differences in blood insulin levels between vascular dementia (VD) patients and HC subjects.

Supplementary 5. Sensitivity analysis of differences in blood insulin levels between AD patients and HC subjects.

Supplementary 6. Sensitivity analysis of differences in insulin levels between L (light/mild) nonpsychotic dementia patients and HC subjects.

Supplementary 7. Sensitivity analysis of differences in insulin levels between MH (moderate to heavy) nonpsychotic dementia patients and HC subjects.

Supplementary 8. Publication bias in MMSE scores between patients with abnormal insulin levels and HC subjects.

Supplementary 9. Publication bias in insulin levels between nonpsychotic dementia patients and HC subjects.

Supplementary 10. Publication bias in insulin levels between AD patients and HC subjects.

Supplementary 11. PRISMA 2009 checklist.

Supplementary 12. PRISMA 2009 flow diagram.

References

[1] C. U. Onyike, "Psychiatric aspects of dementia," *CONTINUUM: Lifelong Learning in Neurology*, vol. 22, no. 2, pp. 600–614, 2016.

[2] H. Umegaki, T. Kawamura, T. Umemura, and N. Kawano, "Factors associated with cognitive decline in older adults with type 2 diabetes mellitus during a 6-year observation," *Geriatrics & Gerontology International*, vol. 15, no. 3, pp. 302–310, 2015.

[3] Z. Chen, Y. Y. Xu, R. Wu et al., "Impaired learning and memory in rats induced by a high-fat diet: involvement with the imbalance of nesfatin-1 abundance and copine 6 expression," *Journal of Neuroendocrinology*, vol. 29, no. 4, 2017.

[4] A. L. Kauffman, J. M. Ashraf, M. R. Corces-Zimmerman, J. N. Landis, and C. T. Murphy, "Insulin signaling and dietary restriction differentially influence the decline of learning and memory with age," *PLoS Biology*, vol. 8, no. 5, article e1000372, 2010.

[5] Q. C. Li, G. I. Wand, B. Y. Li, H. Sun, and N. C. Jiang, "The effect of insulin on the spatial learning and memory abilities of the Alzheimer's disease model rats," *Zhongguo Ying Yong Sheng Li Xue Za Zhi*, vol. 24, no. 4, pp. 494–498, 2008.

[6] J. Q. Wang, J. Yin, Y. F. Song et al., "Brain aging and AD-like pathology in streptozotocin-induced diabetic rats," *Journal of Diabetes Research*, vol. 2014, Article ID 796840, 12 pages, 2014.

[7] A. M. Dorrance, N. Matin, and P. W. Pires, "The effects of obesity on the cerebral vasculature," *Current Vascular Pharmacology*, vol. 12, no. 3, pp. 462–472, 2014.

[8] J. M. Burns, R. A. Honea, E. D. Vidoni, L. J. Hutfles, W. M. Brooks, and R. H. Swerdlow, "Insulin is differentially related to cognitive decline and atrophy in Alzheimer's disease and

aging," *Biochimica et Biophysica Acta (BBA) - Molecular Basis of Disease*, vol. 1822, no. 3, pp. 333–339, 2012.

[9] A. M. Dorrance, N. Matin, and P. W. Pires, "The effects of obesity on the cerebral vasculature," *Current Vascular Pharmacology*, vol. 12, no. 3, pp. 462–472, 2014.

[10] A. M. Dorrance, N. C. Rupp, and E. F. Nogueira, "Mineralocorticoid receptor activation causes cerebral vessel remodeling and exacerbates the damage caused by cerebral ischemia," *Hypertension*, vol. 47, no. 3, pp. 590–595, 2006.

[11] S. Craft, L. D. Baker, T. J. Montine et al., "Intranasal insulin therapy for Alzheimer disease and amnestic mild cognitive impairment: a pilot clinical trial," *Archives of Neurology*, vol. 69, no. 1, pp. 29–38, 2012.

[12] R. O. Roberts, Y. E. Geda, D. S. Knopman et al., "Association of duration and severity of diabetes mellitus with mild cognitive impairment," *Archives of Neurology*, vol. 65, no. 8, pp. 1066–1073, 2008.

[13] J. Y. Jeon, S. R. Kim, H. J. Kim et al., "Risk factors of severe hypoglycemia requiring medical assistance and neurological sequelae in patients with diabetes: a case-control study," *Medicine*, vol. 95, no. 47, article e5365, 2016.

[14] H. Kenna, F. Hoeft, R. Kelley et al., "Fasting plasma insulin and the default mode network in women at risk for Alzheimer's disease," *Neurobiology of Aging*, vol. 34, no. 3, pp. 641–649, 2013.

[15] M. Mwamburi and W. Q. Qiu, "Different associations of premorbid intelligence *vs.* current cognition with BMI, insulin and diabetes in the homebound elderly," *Integrative Molecular Medicine*, vol. 3, no. 3, pp. 547–552, 2016.

[16] A. Liberati, D. G. Altman, J. Tetzlaff et al., "The PRISMA statement for reporting systematic reviews and meta-analyses of studies that evaluate health care interventions: explanation and elaboration," *Journal of Clinical Epidemiology*, vol. 62, no. 10, pp. e1–e34, 2009.

[17] R. L. Ownby, E. Crocco, A. Acevedo, V. John, and D. Loewenstein, "Depression and risk for Alzheimer disease: systematic review, meta-analysis, and metaregression analysis," *Archives of General Psychiatry*, vol. 63, no. 5, pp. 530–538, 2006.

[18] L. Chen, *The Level of Risk Factors for Cognitive Impairment in Insulin Resistance and Diabetes Rat Brain, [M.Sc. Thesis]*, Hebei Medical University, 2009.

[19] Q. H. Fang, *Risk Factors of Mild Cognitive Impairment in Type 2 Diabetes, [M.Sc. Thesis]*, Anhui Medical University, 2014.

[20] D. H. Liu, *Resting-State Functional MRI Study on the Cognitive Impairment in Type 2 Diabetes Mellitus, [M.Sc. Thesis]*, Third Military Medical University, 2015.

[21] J. K. Liu, *The Research of mTOR and Tau Phosphorylated Protein in Hippocampus Tissue of Type 2 Diabetes and Alzheimer's Disease Rats, [M.Sc. Thesis]*, Nanchang University, 2012.

[22] Y. F. Mao, *The Function and Mechanism of Intranasal Insulin on Alzheimer's Disease*, Dr. Dissertation, Zhejiang University, 2016.

[23] W. Shen, *Resting-State Functional Magnetic Resonance Imaging and Neurocognitive Function in Type 2 Diabetes Mellitus, [M.Sc. Thesis]*, Southern Medical University, 2014.

[24] Y. Wang, *Relationship between Cognitive Dysfunction and Vascular Complications in Patients with Type 2 Diabetes Mellitus, [M.Sc. Thesis]*, Shandong University, 2015.

[25] H. Xiong, L. Ding, W. JJ et al., "Effect the impact of insulin on learning and memory of Alzheimer-like mice and its mechanism," *Tianjin Medical Journal*, vol. 41, no. 04, pp. 337–340, 2013.

[26] Y. Y. Xiong, *Prevalence and Risk Factors for Dementia in Diabetics: A Community-Based Case-Control Study [M.Sc. Thesis]*, Fudan University, 2008.

[27] H. Y. Yu, Q. S. Wang, P. Li, and B. X. Yang, "The placebo-controlled study of type 2 diabetes patients with mild cognitive impairment," *Chinese Journal of Gerontology*, vol. 21, pp. 4087–4089, 2011.

[28] T. R. Bomfim, L. Forny-Germano, L. B. Sathler et al., "An anti-diabetes agent protects the mouse brain from defective insulin signaling caused by Alzheimer's disease-associated Aβ oligomers," *The Journal of Clinical Investigation*, vol. 122, no. 4, pp. 1339–1353, 2012.

[29] D. A. Costello, M. Claret, H. Al-Qassab et al., "Brain deletion of insulin receptor substrate 2 disrupts hippocampal synaptic plasticity and metaplasticity," *PLoS One*, vol. 7, no. 2, article e31124, 2012.

[30] M. Hokama, S. Oka, J. Leon et al., "Altered expression of diabetes-related genes in Alzheimer's disease brains: the Hisayama study," *Cerebral Cortex*, vol. 24, no. 9, pp. 2476–2488, 2014.

[31] S. M. Hoscheidt, E. J. Starks, J. M. Oh et al., "Insulin resistance is associated with increased levels of cerebrospinal fluid biomarkers of Alzheimer's disease and reduced memory function in at-risk healthy middle-aged adults," *Journal of Alzheimer's Disease*, vol. 52, no. 4, pp. 1373–1383, 2016.

[32] S. Maimaiti, K. L. Anderson, C. DeMoll et al., "Intranasal insulin improves age-related cognitive deficits and reverses electrophysiological correlates of brain aging," *The Journals of Gerontology Series A: Biological Sciences and Medical Sciences*, vol. 71, no. 1, pp. 30–39, 2016.

[33] T. M. van Himbergen, A. S. Beiser, M. Ai et al., "Biomarkers for insulin resistance and inflammation and the risk for all-cause dementia and Alzheimer disease: results from the Framingham Heart Study," *Archives of Neurology*, vol. 69, no. 5, pp. 594–600, 2012.

[34] W. L. Xu, N. L. Pedersen, L. Keller et al., "*HHEX_23* AA genotype exacerbates effect of diabetes on dementia and Alzheimer disease: a population-based longitudinal study," *PLoS Medicine*, vol. 12, no. 7, article e1001853, 2015.

[35] X. J. Han, P. Yan, L. Wang, L. Cong, and Y. F. Du, "A preliminary study on the changes of insulin signaling pathway in Alzheimer disease," in *National Symposium on Senile Dementia and Related Diseases*, vol. 2013, pp. 74-75, Chinese Pharmacological Society, Nanjing, China, 2013.

[36] Y. Z. Rong, Y. J. Xie, X. M. Chen, and B. R. Zhou, "Analysis of the correlation among insulin resistance ApoE gene polymorphism and mild cognitive impairment," *Hebei Medicine*, vol. 19, no. 11, pp. 1604–1607, 2013.

[37] A. Ernst, A. N. Sharma, K. M. Elased, P. C. Guest, H. Rahmoune, and S. Bahn, "Diabetic *db/db* mice exhibit central nervous system and peripheral molecular alterations as seen in neurological disorders," *Translational Psychiatry*, vol. 3, article e263, 2013.

[38] A. Jayaraman, D. Lent-Schochet, and C. J. Pike, "Diet-induced obesity and low testosterone increase neuroinflammation and impair neural function," *Journal of Neuroinflammation*, vol. 11, p. 162, 2014.

[39] S. D. Ostergaard, S. Mukherjee, S. J. Sharp et al., "Associations between potentially modifiable risk factors and Alzheimer disease: a Mendelian randomization study," *PLoS Medicine*, vol. 12, no. 6, article e1001841, 2015.

[40] J. J. He, Y. Z. Zhang, and X. F. Zhang, "The relationship of cognitive dysfunction in elderly diabetic patients with insulin resistance and care analysis," *China Modern Doctor*, vol. 52, no. 28, pp. 138–140, 2014.

[41] Q. C. Li, G. L. Wang, B. Y. Li, H. Sun, and N. C. Jiang, "Effects of insulin on spatial learning and memory in AD rats," *Chinese Journal of Applied Physiology*, vol. 24, no. 04, pp. 494–498, 2008.

[42] Y. Yang, D. L. Ma, Y. P. Wang, T. Jiang, S. H. Hu, and X. F. Yu, "Intranasal insulin treatment ameliorates Alzheimer disease-like changes in hippocampus in a rat model of type 2 diabetes," *Chinese Journal of Pathophysiology*, vol. 29, no. 01, pp. 56–61, 2013.

[43] T. Kawamura, T. Umemura, and N. Hotta, "Cognitive impairment in diabetic patients: can diabetic control prevent cognitive decline?," *Journal of Diabetes Investigation*, vol. 3, no. 5, pp. 413–423, 2012.

[44] L. J. Cao, "Relationship between cognitive dysfunction and insulin resistance in elderly patients with diabetes mellitus and nursing care," *Nurses Training*, vol. 28, no. 03, pp. 266-267, 2013.

[45] J. Dong, "Relationship between cognitive dysfunction and insulin resistance in elderly patients with diabetes mellitus and nursing care," *World Latest Medicine Information*, vol. 15, no. 105, pp. 303–306, 2015.

[46] M. Li, L. Ma, Y. Fan, Z. Q. Song, and J. Li, "Effect of insulin on patients with type 2 diabetes mellitus complicated with mild cognitive impairment," *Cardiovascular Disease Journal of of integrated Traditional Chinese and Western Medicine*, vol. 14, no. 20, pp. 2417–20, 2016.

[47] N. Mu, S. C. Xu, Q. Chang, D. P. Rao, J. P. Chen, and C. Ma, "Serum lipids, insulin metabolism and 311 gene polymorphism of paraoxonase-2 in patients with different subtypes of Alzheimer's disease," *Chinese Journal of Gerontology*, vol. 34, pp. 5346–5348, 2014.

[48] Z. Shen and Y. Lin, "Significance of fasting serum insulin and C peptide in patients with Alzheimer's disease," *Chinese Journal of Clinical Healthcare*, vol. 15, no. 01, pp. 61-62, 2012.

[49] L. Su, Q. W. Zhang, W. Li et al., "Effect of course on cognitive function and related risk factors in elderly patients with type 2 diabetes mellitus," *Chinese Journal of Geriatric Heart BrainVessel Diseases*, vol. 17, no. 10, pp. 1071–1075, 2015.

[50] L. Y. Tang and W. Tang, "Effect of blood glucose fluctuation on the treatment of senile dementia," *The Word Clinical Medicine*, vol. 9, no. 7, pp. 67-68, 2015.

[51] Q. Tao, "The risk factors of senile patients with type II diabetes," *Modern Hospital*, vol. 15, no. 03, pp. 152-153, 2015.

[52] Q. H. Zhang and Y. F. Du, "Study on the relationship between cognitive impairment and serum levels of TNF-α and IL-6 in middle-aged and elderly patients with type 2 diabetes mellitus," in *National Symposium on Senile Dementia and Related Diseases*, vol. 2013, pp. 67-68, Nanjing: Chinese Pharmacological Society, Nanjing, China, 2013.

[53] M. W. Akhtar, S. Sanz-Blasco, N. Dolatabadi et al., "Elevated glucose and oligomeric β-amyloid disrupt synapses via a common pathway of aberrant protein S-nitrosylation," *Nature Communications*, vol. 7, p. 10242, 2016.

[54] A. M. Barron, E. R. Rosario, R. Elteriefi, and C. J. Pike, "Sex-specific effects of high fat diet on indices of metabolic syndrome in 3xTg-AD mice: implications for Alzheimer's disease," *PLoS One*, vol. 8, no. 10, article e78554, 2013.

[55] L. Devi, M. J. Alldred, S. D. Ginsberg, and M. Ohno, "Mechanisms underlying insulin deficiency-induced acceleration of β-amyloidosis in a mouse model of Alzheimer's disease," *PLoS One*, vol. 7, no. 3, article e32792, 2012.

[56] Y. D. Ke, F. Delerue, A. Gladbach, J. Gotz, and L. M. Ittner, "Experimental diabetes mellitus exacerbates tau pathology in a transgenic mouse model of Alzheimer's disease," *PLoS One*, vol. 4, no. 11, article e7917, 2009.

[57] J. J. Ramos-Rodriguez, S. Molina-Gil, O. Ortiz-Barajas et al., "Central proliferation and neurogenesis is impaired in type 2 diabetes and prediabetes animal models," *PLoS One*, vol. 9, no. 2, article e89229, 2014.

[58] P. Serbedzija, J. E. Madl, and D. N. Ishii, "Insulin and IGF-I prevent brain atrophy and DNA loss in diabetes," *Brain Research*, vol. 1303, pp. 179–194, 2009.

[59] K. Talbot, H. Y. Wang, H. Kazi et al., "Demonstrated brain insulin resistance in Alzheimer's disease patients is associated with IGF-1 resistance, IRS-1 dysregulation, and cognitive decline," *The Journal of Clinical Investigation*, vol. 122, no. 4, pp. 1316–1338, 2012.

[60] H. Y. Mu, "Comparative analysis of insulin resistance in patients with Alzheimer's disease and type 2 diabetes mellitus," in *The 4th National Symposium on Dementia and Cognitive Impairment and Senior Speeches*, vol. 2015, p. 173, Beijing: Chinese Medical Association, Beijing, China, 2015.

[61] C. G. Jolivalt, R. Hurford, C. A. Lee, W. Dumaop, E. Rockenstein, and E. Masliah, "Type 1 diabetes exaggerates features of Alzheimer's disease in APP transgenic mice," *Experimental Neurology*, vol. 223, no. 2, article 19931251, pp. 422–431, 2010.

[62] Y. F. Mao, Z. Guo, T. Zheng et al., "Intranasal insulin alleviates cognitive deficits and amyloid pathology in young adult APPswe/PS1dE9 mice," *Aging Cell*, vol. 15, no. 5, pp. 893–902, 2016.

[63] M. Solas, B. Aisa, M. C. Mugueta, R. J. Del, R. M. Tordera, and M. J. Ramirez, "Interactions between age, stress and insulin on cognition: implications for Alzheimer's disease," *Neuropsychopharmacology*, vol. 35, no. 8, pp. 1664–1673, 2010.

[64] M. Chen, P. Y. Shan, A. F. Liu, L. Ma, and X. L. Yu, "Plasma fasting glucose, fasting insulin and insulin degrading enzyme in Alzheimer's disease," *Journal of Shandong University (Health Sciences)*, vol. 50, no. 03, pp. 75–78, 2012.

[65] R. Y. Huang, J. J. Ren, H. Y. Han, and M. N. Tang, "The correlation between metabolic syndrome and Alzheimer's disease research," *Journal of Psychiatry*, vol. 26, no. 03, pp. 175–177, 2013.

[66] G. X. Wang, "Correlation analysis of insulin resistance and cognitive impairment," *China Practical Medicine*, vol. 6, no. 26, pp. 38-39, 2011.

[67] H. M. Kim, J. M. Seong, and J. Kim, "Risk of hospitalization for hypoglycemia among older Korean people with diabetes mellitus: interactions between treatment modalities and comorbidities," *Medicine*, vol. 95, no. 42, article e5016, 2016.

[68] N. L. Rasgon, H. A. Kenna, T. E. Wroolie et al., "Insulin resistance and hippocampal volume in women at risk for

Alzheimer's disease," *Neurobiology of Aging*, vol. 32, no. 11, pp. 1942–1948, 2011.

[69] E. M. Schrijvers, J. C. Witteman, E. J. Sijbrands, A. Hofman, P. J. Koudstaal, and M. M. Breteler, "Insulin metabolism and the risk of Alzheimer disease: the Rotterdam study," *Neurology*, vol. 75, no. 22, pp. 1982–1987, 2010.

[70] Z. S. Tan, A. S. Beiser, C. S. Fox et al., "Association of metabolic dysregulation with volumetric brain magnetic resonance imaging and cognitive markers of subclinical brain aging in middle-aged adults: the Framingham Offspring Study," *Diabetes Care*, vol. 34, no. 8, pp. 1766–1770, 2011.

[71] M. K. Townsend, O. I. Okereke, W. Xia, T. Yang, D. J. Selkoe, and F. Grodstein, "Relation between insulin, insulin-related factors, and plasma amyloid beta peptide levels at midlife in a population-based study," *Alzheimer Disease and Associated Disorders*, vol. 26, no. 1, pp. 50–54, 2012.

[72] M. van Oijen, O. I. Okereke, J. H. Kang et al., "Fasting insulin levels and cognitive decline in older women without diabetes," *Neuroepidemiology*, vol. 30, no. 3, pp. 174–179, 2008.

[73] A. A. Willette, S. C. Johnson, A. C. Birdsill et al., "Insulin resistance predicts brain amyloid deposition in late middle-aged adults," *Alzheimers Dement*, vol. 11, no. 5, pp. 504–510, 2015.

[74] T. T. Huang, "Effects of insulin resistance on cognitive impairment in patients with Parkinson's disease," *Journal of Bethune Medical Science*, vol. 13, no. 02, pp. 129-130, 2015.

[75] M. Chen, *Relationship of Metabolism Related Factors and Alzheimer's Disease [M.Sc. Thesis]*, Shandong University, 2012.

[76] Z. S. Deng, *Activity of Cholinesterase and Expression of ChAT, Aβof Brain Tissue in Type-2 Diabetic Rat [M.Sc. Thesis]*, Shanxi Medical University, 2008.

[77] W. G. Liu, R. H. Liu, L. Li et al., "Study of CSF levels of glucose, true insulin, $A\beta_{40}$ and $A\beta_{42}$ in patients with Alzheimer's disease," *Journal of Brain and Nervous Diseases*, vol. 17, no. 06, pp. 434–436, 2009.

[78] W. G. Liu, R. Z. Tian, Y. Q. Feng et al., "Level of fasting plasma glucose, true insulin, C-peptide and amyloid Beta-protein in patients with Alzheimer disease," *Chinese Rehabilitation Theory and Practice*, vol. 13, no. 07, pp. 645-646, 2007.

[79] Y. Q. Ma, *Study on the Relationship between PI3K/PKB/mTOR/S6K1 Signaling Pathway and Type 2 Diabetes Mellitus and Alzheimer's Disease*, Dr. Dissertation, Nanchang University, 2013.

[80] L. Zhang, Y. Fang, Y. J. Lian, J. K. Wang, Y. K. Zheng, and Z. Y. Luo, "Study on relationship between the insulin resistant with the concentration of tau protein and β-amyloid protein in cerebrospinal fluid of patients with mild cognitive impairment," *Modern Preventive Medicine*, vol. 38, no. 09, pp. 1774-1775, 2011.

[81] X. H. Zhao, Y. M. Yang, J. Bao, X. Wang, Y. Y. Zhang, and Q. Zhao, "Clinical study on relationship between metabolic syndrome and mild cognitive impairment," *Journal of Kunming Medical University*, vol. 05, pp. 82–86, 2012.

[82] E. Grunblatt, J. Bartl, D. I. Iuhos et al., "Characterization of cognitive deficits in spontaneously hypertensive rats, accompanied by brain insulin receptor dysfunction," *Journal of Molecular Psychiatry*, vol. 3, no. 1, p. 6, 2015.

[83] W. J. Katon, E. H. Lin, L. H. Williams et al., "Comorbid depression is associated with an increased risk of dementia diagnosis in patients with diabetes: a prospective cohort study," *Journal of General Internal Medicine*, vol. 25, no. 5, pp. 423–429, 2010.

[84] L. Ma, M. Feng, Y. Qian et al., "Insulin resistance is an important risk factor for cognitive impairment in elderly patients with primary hypertension," *Yonsei Medical Journal*, vol. 56, no. 1, pp. 89–94, 2015.

[85] M. D. Sullivan, W. J. Katon, L. C. Lovato et al., "Association of depression with accelerated cognitive decline among patients with type 2 diabetes in the ACCORD-MIND trial," *JAMA Psychiatry*, vol. 70, no. 10, pp. 1041–1047, 2013.

[86] B. Y. Ding, *The Incidence and Related Risk Factors of Vascular Cognitive Impairment Not Dementia in Inpatients with Diabetes Mellitus Type 2 and Acute Cerebral Infarction, [M.Sc. Thesis]*, Dalian Medical University, 2015.

[87] J. Hou, *The Study for the Change of CMBs-Related Memory Function and Resting-State Brain Function in T2DM with CMBs, [M.Sc. Thesis]*, Central South University, 2014.

[88] C. H. Shao, K. Li, and X. B. Cao, "Hypertension and related risk factors of vascular dementia," *Chinese Focus Journal*, vol. 27, no. 01, pp. 13–15, 2012.

[89] X. Zhang, *The Control of Glycated Hemoglobin Level and the Use of Insulin Affect the Cognitive Function in Type2 Diabetes, [M.Sc. Thesis]*, Third Military Medical University, 2014.

[90] X. Liu, Y. N. Zhang, L. H. Jiang, and W. Li, "Abnormal expression of insulin receptor and insulin-like growth factor I receptor in hippocampus of Alzheimer's disease," *Chinese Journal of Gerontology*, vol. 07, pp. 1191–1194, 2011.

[91] Y. Ma, D. Wu, W. Zhang, J. Liu, S. Chen, and B. Hua, "Investigation of PI3K/PKB/mTOR/S6K1 signaling pathway in relationship of type 2 diabetes and Alzheimer's disease," *International Journal of Clinical and Experimental Medicine*, vol. 8, no. 10, pp. 18581–18590, 2015.

[92] Z. S. Deng, S. L. Zhang, Y. Zhang, Y. Chen, and X. J. Yang, "The study of expression of β-amyloid of serum and brain tissue in type-2 diabetic rat," *Journal of Practical Medical Techniques*, vol. 15, no. 12, pp. 1503–1505, 2008.

[93] X. Gao, D. Zhao, H. J. Cui, and F. Y. Li, "Study on expression of Aβ in serum and brain tissues in rats with type 2 diabetes mellitus and its relationship with Alzheimer's disease," *Hebei Medical Journal*, vol. 34, no. 22, pp. 3386-3387, 2012.

[94] A. H. Lv, S. K. Zhu, and X. M. Zhang, "Effect of insulin resistance on the expression of Aβ protein in hippocampus of rats and the change of cognitive behavior," *Chinese Journal of Practical Nervous Diseases*, vol. 14, no. 21, pp. 40-41, 2011.

[95] S. H. Yuan, S. Z. Gao, X. P. Liu et al., "The change of cognition function in insulin resistance rats and its brain tissues with Alzheimer-like disease," *Stroke and Neurological Disorders*, vol. 17, no. 03, pp. 139–143, 2010.

[96] X. J. Zhang, S. S. Yang, M. X. Zhang, and Y. Yang, "Common pathogenesis of type 2 diabetes and Alzheimer's disease: a potential mechanism," *Chinese Journal of Pathophysiology*, vol. 26, no. 06, pp. 1107–1114, 2010.

[97] D. Baumeister, R. Akhtar, S. Ciufolini, C. M. Pariante, and V. Mondelli, "Childhood trauma and adulthood inflammation: a meta-analysis of peripheral C-reactive protein, interleukin-6 and tumour necrosis factor-α," *Molecular Psychiatry*, vol. 21, no. 5, pp. 642–649, 2016.

[98] J. Bowden, J. F. Tierney, A. J. Copas, and S. Burdett, "Quantifying, displaying and accounting for heterogeneity in the

meta-analysis of RCTs using standard and generalised Q statistics," *BMC Medical Research Methodology*, vol. 11, p. 41, 2011.

[99] A. Masi, D. S. Quintana, N. Glozier, A. R. Lloyd, I. B. Hickie, and A. J. Guastella, "Cytokine aberrations in autism spectrum disorder: a systematic review and meta-analysis," *Molecular Psychiatry*, vol. 20, no. 4, pp. 440–446, 2015.

[100] P. Langhorne, "Bias in meta-analysis detected by a simple, graphical test. Bias in meta-analysis detected by a simple, graphical test. Prospectively identified trials could be used for comparison with meta-analyses," *BMJ*, vol. 316, no. 7129, article 9492689, p. 471, 1998.

[101] K. L. Soeken and A. Sripusanapan, "Assessing publication bias in meta-analysis," *Nursing Research*, vol. 52, no. 1, pp. 57–60, 2003.

2

Repulsive Environment Attenuation during Adult Mouse Optic Nerve Regeneration

Camila Oliveira Goulart,[1] Henrique Rocha Mendonça,[1,2] Julia Teixeira Oliveira ,[1] Laura Maria Savoldi,[1] Luiza dos Santos Heringer,[1] Alexandre dos Santos Rodrigues,[3] Roberto Paes-de-Carvalho,[3] and Ana Maria Blanco Martinez [1]

[1]*Laboratório de Neurodegeneração e Reparo, Departamento de Patologia, Programa de Pós-graduação em Patologia, Faculdade de Medicina, HUCFF, UFRJ, Rio de Janeiro, RJ, Brazil*
[2]*Pólo Universitário Macaé, Unidade Integrada de Pesquisa em Produtos Bioativos e Biociências, UFRJ, Macaé, RJ, Brazil*
[3]*Departamento de Neurobiologia, Programa de Pós Graduação em Neurociências, UFF, Niterói, RJ, Brazil*

Correspondence should be addressed to Ana Maria Blanco Martinez; anamartinez@hucff.ufrj.br

Academic Editor: Preston E. Garraghty

The regenerative capacity of CNS tracts has ever been a great hurdle to regenerative medicine. Although recent studies have described strategies to stimulate retinal ganglion cells (RGCs) to regenerate axons through the optic nerve, it still remains to be elucidated how these therapies modulate the inhibitory environment of CNS. Thus, the present work investigated the environmental content of the repulsive axon guidance cues, such as Sema3D and its receptors, myelin debris, and astrogliosis, within the regenerating optic nerve of mice submitted to intraocular inflammation + cAMP combined to conditional deletion of PTEN in RGC after optic nerve crush. We show here that treatment was able to promote axonal regeneration through the optic nerve and reach visual targets at twelve weeks after injury. The Regenerating group presented reduced MBP levels, increased microglia/macrophage number, and reduced astrocyte reactivity and CSPG content following optic nerve injury. In addition, Sema3D content and its receptors are reduced in the Regenerating group. Together, our results provide, for the first time, evidence that several regenerative repulsive signals are reduced in regenerating optic nerve fibers following a combined therapy. Therefore, the treatment used made the CNS microenvironment more permissive to regeneration.

1. Introduction

The regenerative capacity of CNS tracts has ever been a great hurdle to regenerative medicine. Only in the last 40 years, CNS regeneration was considered as feasible, with the focus of research on identifying and overcoming the inhibitory nature of CNS to axon growth. From 1980s until early 2000s, it was shown that central axons of the optic nerve were able to regenerate and reinnervate targets when a peripheral nerve bridge was grafted to form a passage where axons could avoid the degenerating central nervous tissue, partially restoring function [1–5]. Additional research by several groups showed that inhibition or degradation of repulsive guidance signals, such as SemaA3 family members, astrocyte-derived chondroitin sulfate proteoglycans (CSPG), and myelin-derived inhibitors such as NOGO-A, oligodendrocyte myelin glycoprotein (OMgp), or myelin-associated glycoprotein (MAG) allow regeneration within CNS paths [6–8]. However, the regeneration achieved by these approaches was not enough to restore function.

During the last 20 years, the research focus has changed to the enhancement of the intrinsic capacity of central neurons to elongate lesioned axons. Approaches that stimulate JAK-STAT and mTOR signaling, such as inflammatory stimuli or genetic deletions of PTEN and/or SOCS3, promoted pronounced regeneration within the optic nerve [9–11], and when these approaches were combined, there was a partial restoration of the visual function [12].

The stimulation of the intrinsic capacity of neurons to regenerate axons can benefit from environmental reduction/inhibition of repulsive guidance cues. Indeed, inflammatory-stimulated retinal ganglion cells regenerate longer distances when NOGO-A is counteracted [13]. Besides, the regenerative capacity of sciatic nerve axons to regenerate is abolished when axons reach an optic nerve graft [14], suggesting that an inhibitory environment prevents the regeneration of intrinsically growth-capable axons. If therapies that target the intrinsic growth capacity of axons also modulates the inhibitory environment of CNS remains to be elucidated.

Thus, the present work investigated the environmental content of the repulsive axon guidance cues, such as Sema3D and its receptors, myelin debris, and astrogliosis, within the regenerating optic nerve of mice submitted to intraocular inflammation + cAMP combined to conditional deletion of PTEN in RGC after optic nerve crush.

2. Methods

2.1. Surgical Procedure. Optic nerve surgery and intraocular injections were performed as previously described [12, 15]. Briefly, to delete pten gene in RGC, pten$^{flx/flx}$ in a C57BL/6 background mice received an intravitreal injection (3 μL) of an adeno-associated virus (AAV2, 10^{12} GC/mL) expressing Cre recombinase (AAV2-Cre under the control of the CMV promoter; Vector Laboratories) (Regenerating group, $n = 5$), as shown to be effective by Kwon et al. [7]. Two weeks after virus injection, the left optic nerve was exposed and crushed with fine forceps (Dumont; WPI) for 5 s. To increase regeneration, zymosan (Sigma; 12.5 μg/μL, sterilized before use) was injected, along with the cAMP analog CPT-cAMP (Sigma; 50 μM, 3 μL), into the posterior chamber of the eye, immediately after surgery. As a control, C57BL/6 mice just had the left optic nerve exposed and crushed for 5 s (Crush-only group, $n = 5$). Before the end of each survival time, animals were injected intraocularly with cholera toxin B fragment (CTB) to trace retinal projections. To all the procedures, mice were anesthetized with either ketamine or xylazine and immobilized in a stereotaxic head holder.

2.2. Tissue Preparation. Two weeks after surgery, mice were perfused transcardially with 4% phosphate-buffered paraformaldehyde (PFA). Optic nerves were carefully dissected, placed in 4% PFA for 1 h, and transferred to 20% sucrose in 0.1 M PBS at 4°C overnight followed by 30% sucrose overnight at 4°C. Optic nerves were then embedded in OCT (Tissue Tek Medium), frozen, and cryostat-sectioned longitudinally at 14 μm thick. Nerve sections were placed on 1% bovine gelatin-coated coverslips and stored at 20°C until used.

In order to analyze central projections, mice were maintained until twelve weeks of survival time and then perfused transcardially with 4% phosphate-buffered paraformaldehyde (PFA). Brains were carefully dissected, placed in 4% PFA for 1 h, and transferred to 20% sucrose in 0.1 M PBS at 4°C overnight followed by 30% sucrose overnight at 4°C. Brains were also embedded in OCT (Tissue Tek Medium), frozen, and sectioned at 40 μm in the coronal plane between the rostral diencephalon and caudal mesencephalon. Sections were maintained in 0.1 M PBS and stored at 4°C until used.

2.3. WFA Histochemistry. Sections were washed three times in 0.1 M PBS (pH 7.4), blocked (PBS containing 0.3% Triton X-100 and 10% normal donkey serum) at room temperature for 1 h, then were incubated in fluorescein Wisteria floribunda lectin (WFA, 1 : 100, Vector) for 2 h at room temperature. Next, the slices were counterstained with DAPI (Molecular Probes) for 5 min and coverslipped with fluoromount (Sigma) for visualization. Staining was analyzed and documented on a laser scanning microscope (LSM 510 META, Zeiss, Germany).

2.4. Immunofluorescence Labeling. Sections were washed three times in 0.1 M PBS (pH 7.4), blocked (PBS containing 0.3% Triton X-100 and 10% normal donkey serum) at room temperature for 1 h, then were incubated overnight in one or more of the following antibodies: rabbit monoclonal anti-CTB (1:500, GenWay), rat polyclonal anti-MBP (myelin basic protein, 1:200, Millipore), mouse monoclonal anti-CC1 (1:200, Abcam), rabbit polyclonal anti-IBA1 (1:250, Wako), rabbit monoclonal anti-TMEM119 (1 : 100, Abcam), and rabbit polyclonal anti-GFAP (glial fibrillary acidic protein, 1 : 100, Sigma). Sections were washed three times in PBS, incubated in the appropriate secondary antibodies (Alexa-fluor 488 Donkey anti-rabbit, Alexa-fluor 594 Donkey anti-rabbit, Alexa-fluor 488 Donkey anti-mouse, and Alexa-fluor 488 Goat anti-rat, 1 :500, Molecular Probes) for 2 h at room temperature, counterstained with DAPI (Molecular Probes) for 5 min, and coverslipped with fluoromount (Sigma) for visualization. Negative control sections were processed identically except that the primary antibodies were omitted. Staining was analyzed and documented on a laser scanning microscope (LSM 510 META, Zeiss, Germany).

Quantification of histochemistry and immunofluorescence data was performed using ImageJ by determining immunostained densities and the number of immunopositive cells [16]. Cell counts were performed identifying DAPI-positive nuclei surrounded by Iba-1 or TMEM119 staining under the microscope. One field at 20x magnification, at a fixed distance of 1.5 mm from the injury site in longitudinal sections of the nerve, was analyzed from five animals per group.

2.5. Electron Microscopy. To observe myelin debris, transmission electron microscopy was performed as described in [17]. Briefly, mice were sacrificed two weeks after injury with an overdose of ketamine/xylazine and perfused transcardially with 4% paraformaldehyde + 2% glutaraldehyde in 0.1 M phosphate buffer pH 7.4. 1 mm long segments of the optic nerve 1.5 mm distal to the lesion site were immersion-fixed in 2.5% glutaraldehyde for 2 h, washed in 0.1 M cacodylate buffer (pH 7.4), and postfixed for 1 h in 1% (wt/vol) osmium tetroxide containing 0.8% potassium ferrocyanide and 5 nM calcium chloride in 0.1 M cacodylate buffer (pH 7.4). Segments were washed in 0.1 M cacodylate buffer (pH 7.4) and distilled water and stained in 1% (wt/vol) uranyl acetate overnight, dehydrated in graded acetone, infiltrated with Poly/Bed 812 resin (Polysciences), and polymerized at 60° for 48 h. Ultrathin cross sections (70 nm) were collected on copper grids and contrasted in uranyl acetate and lead citrate. Microscopy was carried out using a Zeiss 900 transmission electron microscope operated at 80 kV. Several electron micrographs were recorded digitally at ×3000 for each ultrathin nerve section.

2.6. Immunoperoxidase Labeling. Sections were incubated for 10 min with 0.3% H_2O_2 in methanol then washed three times in 0.1 M PBS (pH 7.4). To block nonspecific sites, sections were incubated in PBS containing 0.3% Triton X-100 and 10% normal donkey serum at room temperature for 1 h, then incubated overnight in primary antibodies (goat polyclonal anti-Sema3D, 1:100, Santa Cruz, sc-67943; rabbit polyclonal anti-Plexin, 1:100, Santa Cruz; and mouse polyclonal anti-Neuropilin1, 1:100, Abcan, AB81321). Slides were washed three times in PBS, incubated in the appropriate secondary antibodies (biotinylated horse anti-rabbit; horse anti-goat and goat anti-mouse; 1:500 dilution; Vector Laboratories, Burlingame, CA) for 2 h at room temperature, and then received ABC reagent (1:200 dilution in PBS) treatment (Vectastain Elite ABC kit, Vector, Switzerland). Color reaction used diaminobenzidine (DAB) substrate (Sigma) at room temperature. Slides were coverslipped using fluoromount (Sigma).

Quantification of immunoperoxidase data was performed using ImageJ [18] by determining immunostained densities. Three fields at 20x magnification at 1.5 mm from the injury site in longitudinal sections of the nerve were analyzed, and an average of the optical density was obtained. It used five animals per group.

2.7. Adult Dissociated Retinal Cell Culture. Retinal cultures from mice were prepared as described previously [19]. In brief, retinae were dissected from eyecups and digested in DMEM containing papain (10 U/mL, Worthington) and L-cysteine (0.2 mg/mL, Sigma) at 37°C for 30 minutes. Retinae were then triturated and washed by centrifugation in 50 mL DMEM (7 min at 500 g). Retinal pellets were resuspended in DMEM F12 containing B27-supplement (1:50), 0.25 μg/mL fungizone, 100 μg/mL penicillin/streptomycin, and methylcellulose (1:250). Cells were seeded into 24-well plates coated with poly-D-lysine (0.1 mg/mL, Sigma) and laminin (20 μg/mL, Sigma). After 3 days in culture, cells were fixed in 4% PFA for 1 h. To identify RGCs and search for PlexinA1 receptor, cells were washed in PBS, incubated in blocking solution, and then in the TUJ-1 (1:200; BioLegend) and Plexin A1 primary antibodies (1:100, Santa Cruz). Sections were washed and incubated in appropriate secondary antibody (Alexa-fluor 488 Donkey anti-mouse; Alexa fluor 594 Donkey anti-rabbit). Nuclei were stained with DAPI (Molecular Probes, USA) and mounted with fluoromount (Sigma).

2.8. Retinal Explant Culture. Retinal explant culture was performed as described previously [20]. Briefly, sterile laminules were placed in cell culture plates overnight with 0.3 mL of a 0.25 mg/mL poly-L-lysin (poly-L-lysine hydrobromide, P1274; Sigma, St. Louis, MO) solution in sterile PBS. The wells were rinsed twice with PBS and subsequently coated with 0.3 mL of a 2 μg/mL laminin (Sigma) solution for 2 h and rinsed twice with PBS. Retinal explants were obtained from eye dissection in sterile CMF solution and placed in the wells with the RGC nerve fiber layer contacting the laminule, in 0.5 mL Neurobasal-A medium (Invitrogen), containing 0.4% methylcellulose (Sigma), 1% penicillin/streptomycin, 0.2% fungizone, 0.5% L-glutamine, and 2% B-27 supplement for retina (all from Invitrogen). The explants were cultured at 37°C with 5% CO_2 for 72 h. Daily, 0.25 mL of the explant medium was replaced with fresh medium. Explants were washed in PBS, incubated in blocking solution, and then in the TUJ-1 (1:200; BioLegend) and Plexin A1 primary antibodies (1:100, Santa Cruz). Sections were washed and incubated in appropriate secondary antibody (Alexa-fluor 488 Donkey anti-mouse; Alexa-fluor 594 Donkey anti-rabbit). Nuclei were stained with DAPI (Molecular Probes, USA) and mounted with fluoromount (Sigma).

2.9. Statistical Analysis. Statistical analyses graphs were plotted using GraphPad Prism 5.0 software, and the statistical analysis was performed using unpaired t-test, and differences were considered significant when $^{*}P \leq 0.05$, $^{**}P \leq 0.01$, and $^{***}P \leq 0.001$.

3. Results

3.1. Optic Nerve Regeneration. To confirm that the treatment was able to regenerate axons along the optic nerve, we injected CTB to trace retinal projections. After two weeks, it was already possible to visualize differences between the groups. The untreated group (Crush-only) showed no axons beyond the injury site. Instead, as expected, treated group (Regenerating) exhibited numerous CTB^{+} axons extending the full length of the optic nerve (Figures 1(a)–1(d)). At two weeks after injury and treatment, few axons from the Regenerating group were able to penetrate the chiasm and there were no visible axons crossing this structure.

To search for central projections, animals were left in a longer survival time. Twelve weeks after injury and treatment, animals from the Regenerating group had axons regenerating into appropriate target areas. The contralateral suprachiasmatic nucleus (SCN) exhibited many regenerating axons (Figure 1(e)), and sometimes the projections were bilateral (data not shown). The dorsal lateral geniculate nucleus (dLGN), in the contralateral side to the regenerating nerve, showed a stronger CTB labeling (Figure 1(f)). The contralateral superior colliculus (SC) also exhibited many CTB^{+} fibers (Figure 1(g)). CTB^{+} fibers were never seen in the Crush-only group.

3.2. Myelin Content within the Optic Nerve. To visualize myelin content two weeks after injury, we assessed the major myelin protein, myelin basic protein, in both groups (Figures 2(a)–2(d)). The Regenerating group exhibited

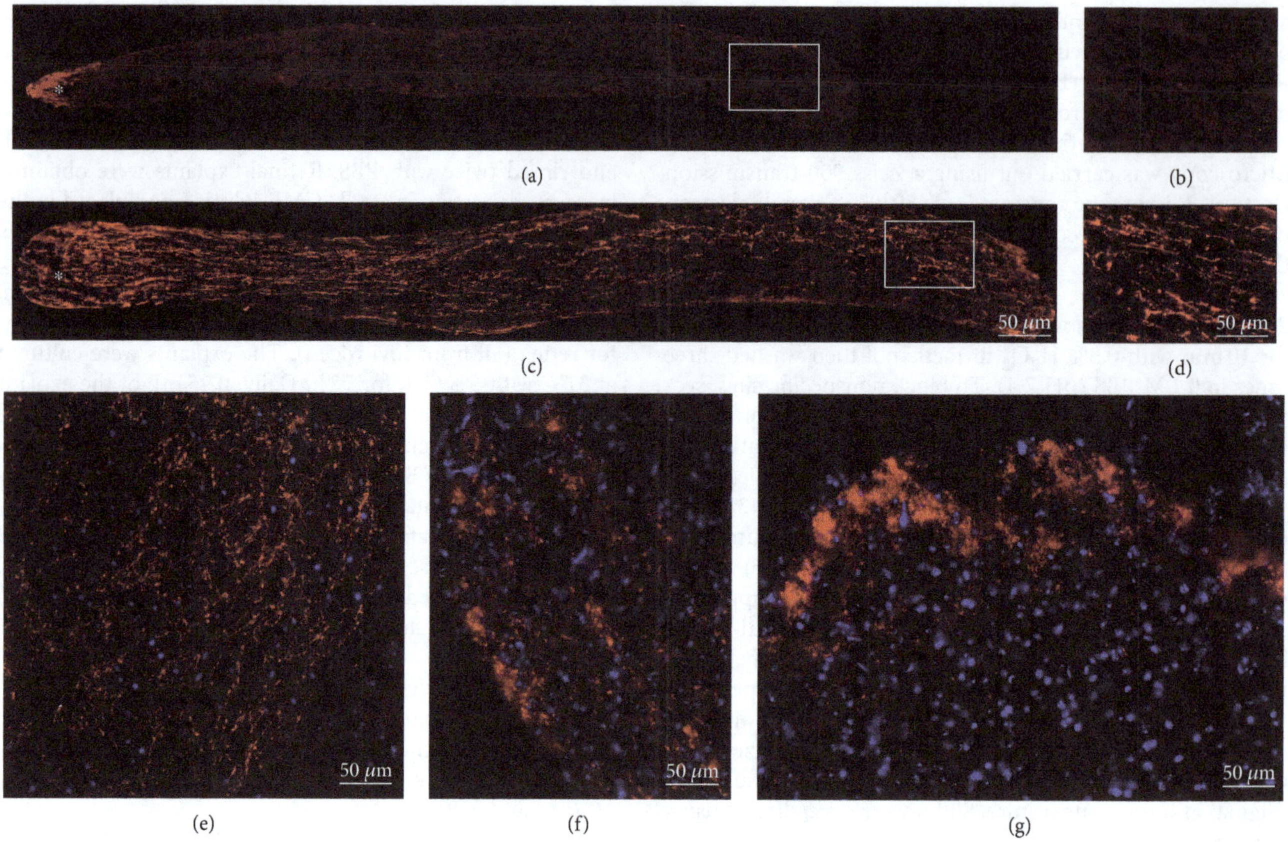

Figure 1: Optic nerve regeneration. (a–d) CTB labeling (red) and nuclear staining (blue) two weeks after optic nerve injury; (a and b) optic nerve from the Crush-only group exhibiting no CTB$^+$ axons (red) beyond injury site; (c and d) optic nerve from the Regenerating group showing full-length axon regeneration; (e–g) CTB (red) and nuclear labeling (blue) showing different levels of reinnervation of the visual nuclei twelve weeks after optic nerve injury. (e) CTB$^+$ axons at the suprachiasmatic nucleus; (f) CTB$^+$ fibers at the lateral geniculate nucleus; (g) CTB$^+$ axons at the superior colliculus. $N = 5$ per group. (a–g) Scale bars: 50 μm.

reduced levels of MBP reactivity compared to the Crush-only group, and our findings were confirmed by the quantification of MBP staining density in the analyzed tissues (Figure 2(e)). Qualitative analysis of electron microscope images also revealed that the Crush-only group showed more myelin debris (arrows) and axons at various stages of degeneration (arrowheads) when compared to the Regenerating group (Figures 2(f)–2(g)).

In order to investigate whether myelin content reduction was due to a reduced oligodendrocyte staining intensity and/or area, we used the oligodendrocyte marker CC1. However, the quantification showed that the CC1 staining was stronger in the Regenerating group compared to the Crush-only group (Figures 2(h)–2(j)), suggesting that the regenerating axons are possibly being myelinated.

3.3. Microglia/Macrophage within the Optic Nerve. Since microglia and macrophages are the cells responsible for the myelin clearance, we decided to investigate the number of these cells in the optic nerves. The Regenerating group exhibited a higher number of Iba-1-positive cells compared to the Crush-only group, and our findings were confirmed by quantification of Iba-1-positive cells in the analyzed tissues (Figures 3(a)–3(c)). In order to visualize only the microglia content, we used a specific microglia marker called TMEM119. The Regenerating group presented an increase in the number of TMEM119-positive cells, when compared to the Crush-only group (Figures 3(d)–3(f)).

3.4. Reactive Astrogliosis within the Optic Nerve. Knowing that one of the inhibitory signs of axonal growth, namely, myelin debris, had been softened after the treatment, we decided to investigate other repulsive signs to axonal regeneration in the central nervous system. Reactive astrogliosis is considered another major inhibitory signal to axonal growth. Following CNS injuries, astrocytes around the injury site are converted into reactive astrocytes and eventually into scar-forming astrocytes that block axon regeneration and neural repair [21]. So, we investigated by means of GFAP immunofluorescence, if the treatment changed the astrocytic reaction after optic nerve injury. Indeed, the Regenerating group presented a decrease in GFAP immunoreactivity (Figures 4(a)–4(c)), when compared to the Crush-only group. As a second step in this process, we examined the expression of CSPG in the optic nerve by staining for *Wisteria floribunda* agglutinin (WFA), a plant lectin reported to selectively bind to N-acetylgalactosamine residues, associated with chondroitin sulfates (CSs) within the extracellular

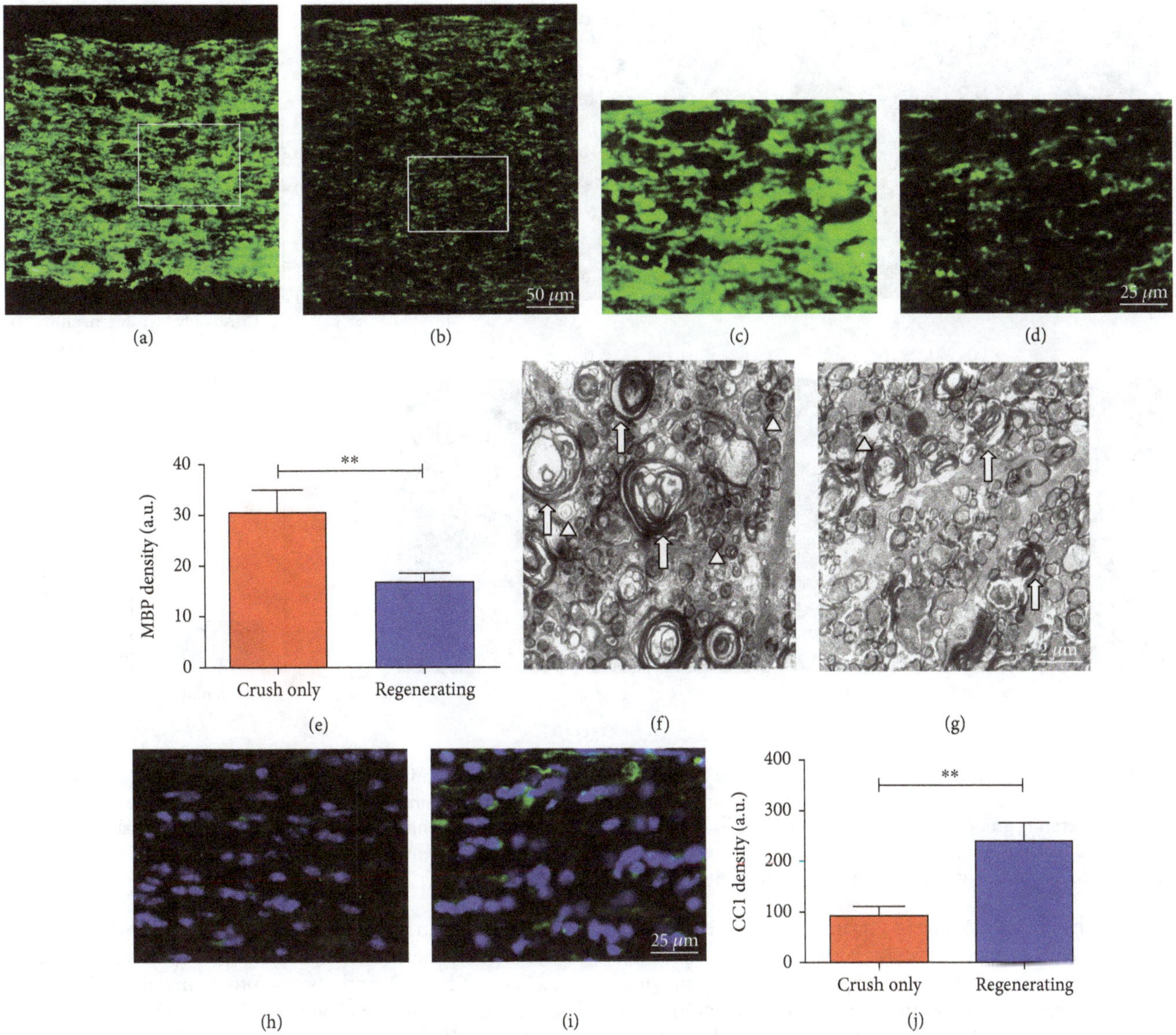

FIGURE 2: Myelin content within the optic nerve. (a–d) MBP labeling (green) two weeks after optic nerve injury. (a and c) Optic nerve from the Crush-only group exhibiting large amount of MBP staining compared to (b and c) optic nerve from the Regenerating group. (e) Quantification of MBP levels. (f, g) EM images showing myelin debris in both groups. Arrows point to myelin debris, whereas arrowheads indicate degenerating nerve fibers; (h–j) CC1 staining (green) two weeks after optic nerve injury; (h) optic nerve from the Crush-only group exhibiting a reduced CC1 staining; (i, j) optic nerve image and quantitative analysis showing a higher density of CC1 staining in the Regenerating group. $N = 5$ per group. Scale bars: (a, b) 50 μm; (c, d) 25 μm; (f, g) 2 μm; (h, i) 25 μm. Error bars in (e) and (j) show SEM. $^{**}P < 0.01$.

matrix. The Regenerating group presented a decrease in WFA staining (Figures 4(d)–4(f)), when compared to the Crush-only group.

3.5. Semaphorin Signaling within the Optic Nerve. Secreted class 3 semaphorins (Sema3s) are also described as repulsive signals which are present after CNS injury [22–24]. We chose to investigate the role of Sema3D and its receptors Plexin A1 and Neuropilin 1. Sema3D is a semaphorin of unknown function during the process of mammal CNS degeneration and regeneration. The immunoreaction for Sema3D showed a diffuse pattern characteristic of secreted molecules. Our results showed a reduction in Sema3D expression on the optic nerves from the Regenerating group compared to the Crush-only group (Figures 5(a)–5(c) and insets). The receptor PlexinA1 also exhibited a smaller density in the Regenerating group compared to the Crush-only group, in a pattern similar to nerve fibers (Figures 5(d)–5(f); black arrows in the insets). However, the Neuropilin 1 receptor showed no difference between groups, presenting a staining pattern that suggest glial cell bodies and its proximal processes (Figures 5(g)–5(i) and red arrows in the insets). Thus, in addition to the reduction in the expression of the inhibitory molecule Sema3D (Figures 5(a)–5(c)), there was also a reduction in the expression of the receptor Plexin A1 (Figures 5(d)–5(f)).

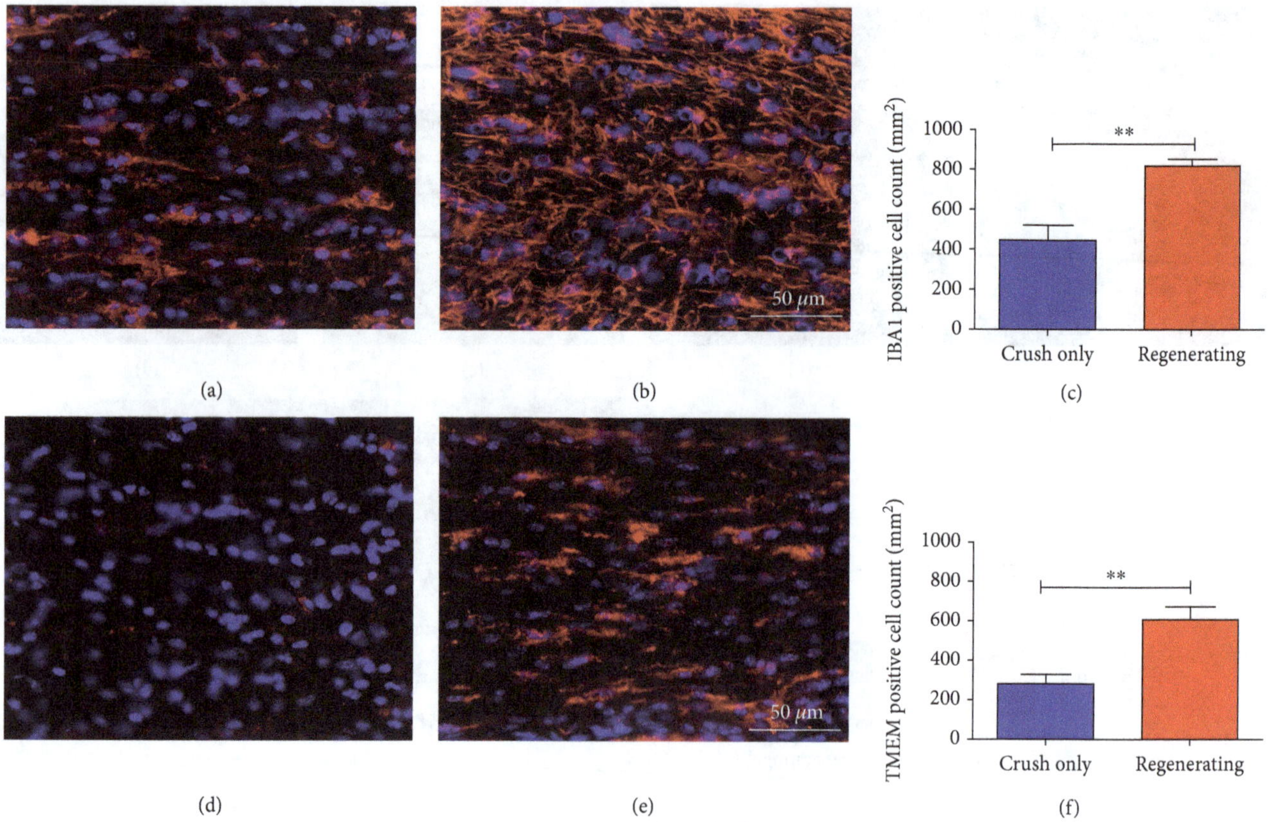

FIGURE 3: Macrophage/microglia within the optic nerve. (a–c) Iba-1 (red) and nuclear staining (blue) two weeks after injury. (a) Optic nerve from the Crush-only group showing a reduced Iba-1 staining; (b and c) optic nerve and quantitative analysis exhibiting intense levels of Iba-1 in the Regenerating group. (d–f) Tmem (red) and nuclear (blue) staining two weeks after injury. (d) Optic nerve from the Crush-only group. (e and f) Optic nerve image and quantitative analysis presenting higher levels of Tmem density in the Regenerating group. $N = 5$ per group. Scale bars: (a, b, d, e) 50 μm. Error bars in (c) and (f) show SEM. $^{**}P < 0.01$.

Since the in vivo staining of Plexin A1 did not lead to certainty that regenerating nerve fibers were Plexin A1-positive within their navigating axons, we used different *in vitro* assays to access it. Analyses of the immunocytochemistry in the retinal dissociated culture and in retinal explants from animals submitted to the same treatment (PTEN gene deletion within retinal ganglion cells, associated to zymosan and cAMP intravitreous injection) indicated that they do express the receptor Plexin A1 in Tuj-1-positive neurites and cell bodies (Figures 6(a)–6(f)).

4. Discussion

Even after stimulation of the intrinsic growth properties of the optic nerve, most regenerating axons are stuck proximal to the glial scar that is formed within the lesion site [25]. Axons that overcome this barrier still undergo U-turns or are incorrectly guided to the wrong axon tract or to the contralateral optic nerve [15, 26, 27]. These findings pointed out the importance of investigating the environmental molecules that drive growth cone guidance during adult CNS regeneration. Even with these barriers, different treatments described full-length optic nerve regeneration, with target reinnervation, synapse formation, and partial function recovery [11, 12, 28]. In the present study, we investigated the effect of the conditional deletion of PTEN in RGC of mice submitted to intraocular inflammation + cAMP during optic nerve regeneration on the content of the repulsive axon guidance cues Sema3D and its receptors, myelin debris, and astrogliosis, within the axon shaft distal to the lesion site.

Our results were able to replicate the data provided by de Lima et al. [12], who found that conditional deletion of PTEN in RGCs followed by intraocular injection of zymosan and cyclic AMP promoted full-length regeneration of optic nerve axons within 2 weeks, reaching SCN, dLGN, and SC, 12 weeks after lesion. On the other hand, Luo et al. [27], using the same stimulatory protocol, argued that they found reinnervation of SCN only. It is possible that the whole-brain 3D imaging employed by Luo et al. [27], although presenting the advantage of allowing the tracing of the path followed by single CTB-traced fascicles, may be less sensitive than the microscopy of thin brain sections employed in the present study and in the study of de Lima et al. [12].

Interestingly, the research that focused in promoting the intrinsic growth capacity of RGC did not investigate if the microenvironment undergoes any modulation in molecules that promotes or inhibits axon regeneration. It is well known that Wallerian degeneration (WD) in the CNS is an inefficient process, since the removal of axon and myelin debris by microglia/macrophages is slow, leaving inhibitory molecules for long period of time, therefore blocking regeneration [29, 30]. In the injured peripheral nervous system (PNS),

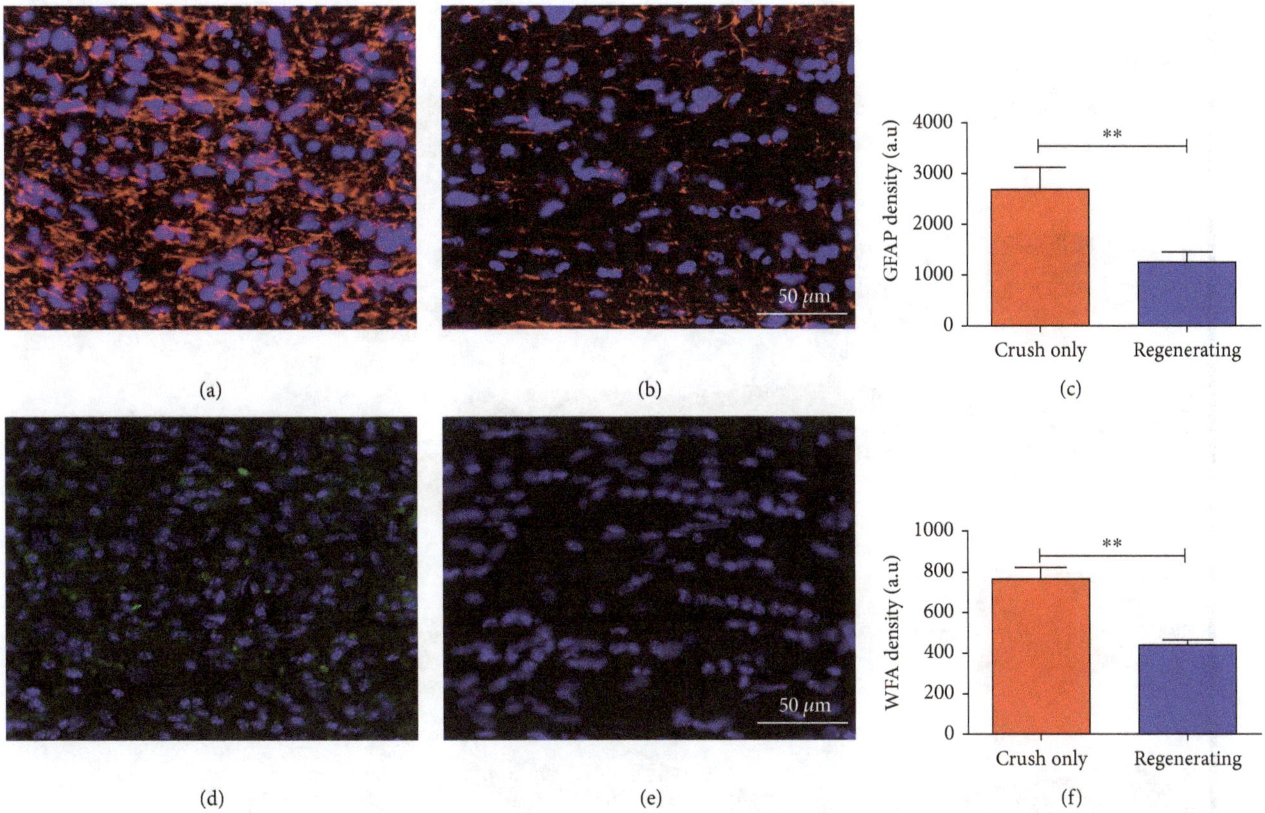

FIGURE 4: Reactive astrogliosis within the optic nerve. (a–c) GFAP (red) and nuclear staining (blue) two weeks after injury. (a) Optic nerve from the Crush-only group showing an intense GFAP staining; (b and c) optic nerve and quantitative analysis exhibiting reduced levels of GFAP in the Regenerating group. (d–f) WFA (green) and nuclear staining (blue) two weeks after injury. (d) Optic nerve from the Crush-only group. (e and f) Optic nerve image and quantitative analysis presenting reduced levels of WFA density in the Regenerating group. $N = 5$ per group. Scale bars: (a, b, d, e) 50 μm. Error bars in (c) and (f) show SEM. $^{**}P < 0.01$.

however, WD takes place in a more effective way resulting in a more efficient nerve regeneration. Accordingly, previous findings of our group [31, 32], in a model of peripheral nerve injury, showed that Galectin-3 knockout mice present earlier sciatic nerve regeneration due to a greater efficiency in the removal of myelin debris by macrophages and Schwann cells favoring an increase in WD speed. Therefore, it is plausible to say that in the present work the reduction in the amount of myelin debris is correlated with the better regeneration found in the treated group. In addition, we analyzed the oligodendrocyte staining and found an increase in CC1 density in the treated group, which corroborates our hypothesis that remyelination is occurring. In fact, this increase in oligodendrocyte staining might be responsible for myelination of regenerating fibers, as suggested by the excitable domain reorganization found after employment of the same protocol by Marin and coworkers [33]. Besides, we observed a higher microglia/macrophage count in the Regenerating group. This increase in phagocytes might be responsible for the better myelin clearance found within this group. Corroborating this idea, Stark and collaborators (2018) recently showed that inflammatory stimulation of ON regeneration promotes an increase in Iba-1 staining, which was correlated to myelin clearance, 7 days after lesion, within the lesion site itself. Considering that all microglia express Iba-1, our results show that most of the IBA-1-positive cells are microglia, suggesting a pivotal role for microglia in myelin clearance outside the lesion site. Contrary to our findings, Hilla and coworkers [34] showed that microglia was irrelevant in promoting optic nerve regeneration after inflammatory stimulus, although microglia depletion delayed the astrocytic repopulation of the crush site. So, further studies are required to fully address the responsible actors of myelin clearance and its role during optic nerve regeneration.

Astrocyte reaction has long been identified as a major event that occurs after CNS lesion that prevents axon passage through the secretion of inhibitory CSPG [35]. Accordingly, we found that the Regenerating group presented less GFAP immunostaining within the optic nerve when compared to the Crush-only group. Besides, *Wisteria floribunda* agglutinin staining revealed less CSPG within the Regenerating group. Corroborating our data, Luo et al. [27] showed that GFAP staining was more prevalent near the lesion site, an area that presented more frequent U-turns of regenerated fascicles after PTEN/SOCS3 conditional deletion in RGC. However, employing only inflammatory stimulation to induce RGC regeneration, Stark and coworkers (2018) found no modulation of GFAP within the lesion site 7 days after lesion. These findings suggest that the reduced astrogliosis observed in our Regenerating group might have allowed the proper regeneration of fibers that otherwise would be trapped into CSPG nets. Additionally, different protocols of

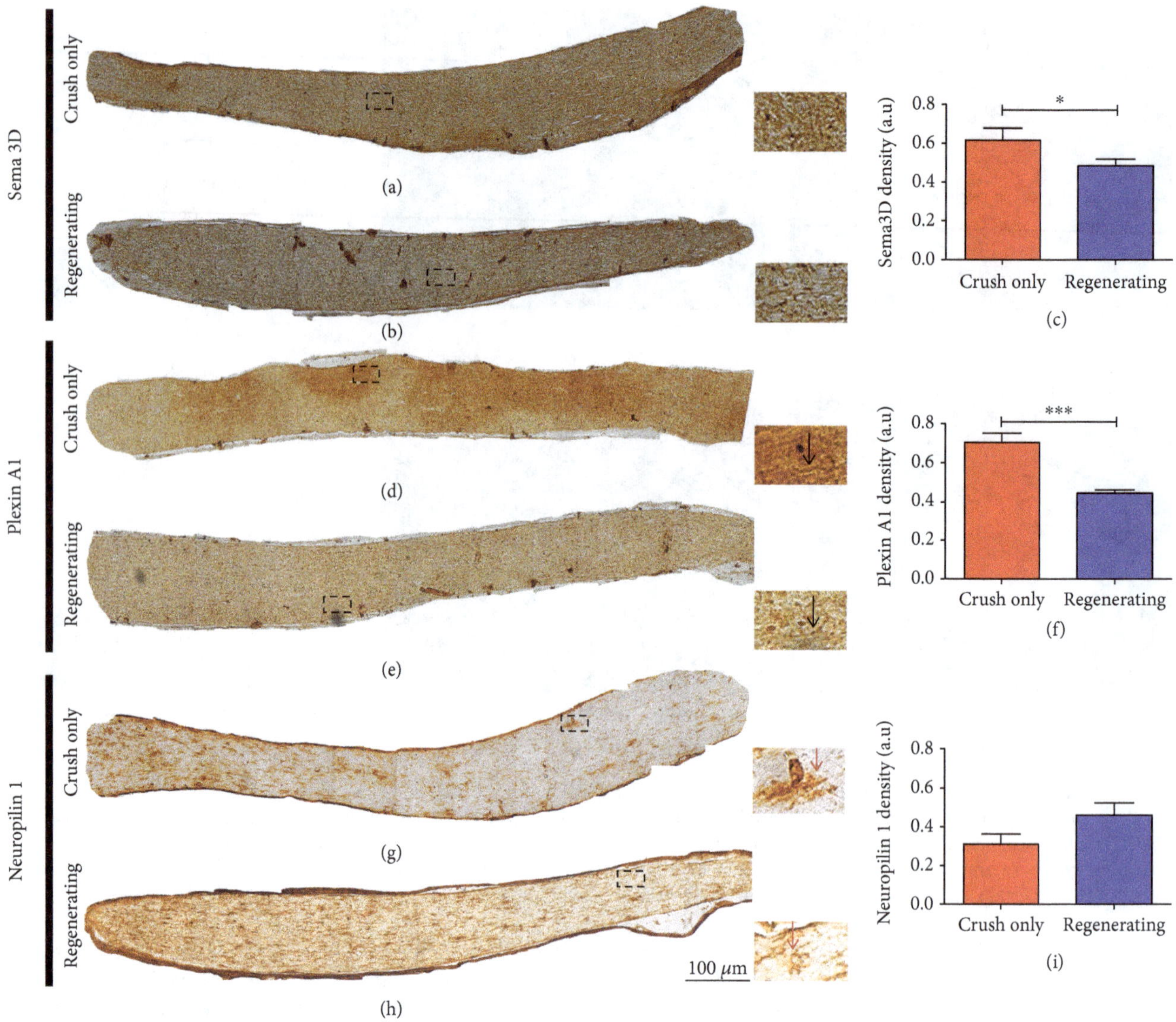

FIGURE 5: Semaphorin signaling within the optic nerve. (a) Optic nerve from the Crush-only group and inset representing the square region; (b) optic nerve from the Regenerating group and inset representing the square region; (c) quantitative analysis of semaphorin staining. (d) Optic nerve from the Crush-only group and inset representing the square region; (e) optic nerve from the Regenerating group and inset representing the square region; (f) quantitative analysis of Plexin A1 staining. (g) Optic nerve from the Crush-only group and inset representing the square region; (h) optic nerve from the Regenerating group and inset representing the square region; (i) quantitative analysis of Neuropilin 1 staining. All analyses were done in the survival time of two weeks after injury. $N = 5$ per group. Scale bars: 100 μm. Error bars in (c, f, i) show SEM $^{*}P < 0.05$ and $^{***}P < 0.001$.

induction of intrinsic growth properties of central axons might elicit different environmental responses.

Since semaphorins are the main molecules known to guide axons within the optic nerve during development, where it builds repulsive walls that confine travelling axons within the optic nerve [36], we investigated their signaling during adult optic nerve regeneration. Family 3 semaphorins correspond to microglia/macrophage, fibroblast, or Schwann cell secreted proteins that bind to the extracellular matrix, where it exerts its repulsive effects onto Plexin and Neuropilin receptors located in growth cones [37]. De Winter et al. [24] showed that several Sema3 family members are upregulated after spinal cord lesion. Nevertheless, SEMA 3D is a secreted member of the SEMA family that was never investigated following mammal SNC lesions. Our results show that Sema3D content is higher in the Crush-only group when compared to the Regenerating group. Besides, Neuropilin 1 receptor was not altered by treatment, while Plexin A1 receptor was also higher in the Crush-only group, where it could signal the collapse of axons [38]. Correspondingly, Plexin A1 staining pattern was putative of nerve fibers, whereas neuropilin 1 staining pattern was similar to soma and proximal processes of putative glial cells. Thus, plexin A1 might be responsible for RGC navigation control during optic nerve regeneration, while Neuropilin1 may not be involved in this process. Since there is no study addressing if adult mice RGCs are able to respond to semaphorins and the immunohistochemistry was not sufficient to prove that

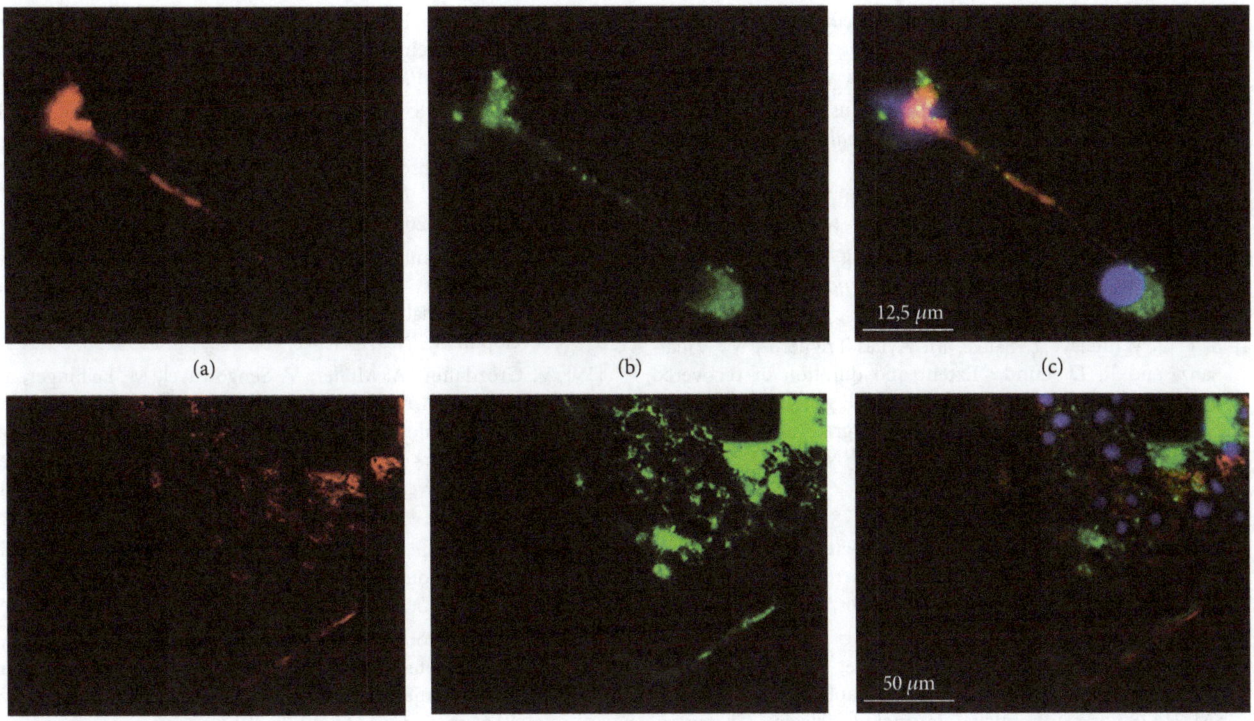

FIGURE 6: *In vitro* expression of Sema3D receptors. (a, b, c) Retinal dissociated culture expressing the receptor Plexin A1 (red) in Tuj-1-positive cells (green) and nuclear staining (DAPI). (d, e, f) Retinal explant cells expressing the receptor Plexina A1 in Tuj-1-positive cells. $N = 3$ per group. Scale bars: (a, b, c) 12.5 μm, (d, e, f) 50 μm.

RGC axons exhibited Sema3 receptors, we employed explant and dissociated retinal cultures that confirmed that adult RGC extending neurites present Plexin A1, therefore being sensitive to Sema3D levels. These results suggest for the first time that Sema3D may be another inhibitory molecule of axonal regeneration in rodent CNS, which could signal through Plexin A1. A repulsive role of Sema3D is consistent with previous works in which RGC growth cones of zebrafish were repelled by Sema3D [39]. Similarly, pharmacological inhibition of Sema3A leads to spinal cord regeneration and protects RGC from axon transection-induced apoptosis [40, 41]. Additionally, chondroitinase ABC treatment reduces Sema3s binding to the extracellular matrix, favoring regeneration (Soleman et al., 2002). Although our and other groups' results suggest that at least a subset of injured adult CNS neurons is inhibited by Sema3D or other Sema3s, future studies employing genetically manipulated mice or other means of blocking semaphorin receptor or intracellular signaling will be required to show without doubt that injured neurons sense and respond to semaphorins following optic nerve injury in vivo.

How PTEN conditional deletion on RGC followed by intravitreal injection of zymosan and cyclic AMP modifies the environment and aids ON regeneration is not currently known. It is possible that zymosan injection might be responsible for the higher proportion of microglia/macrophage number found in our study. Besides, growth cone protrusions, called invadosomes, present metalloproteinases that degrades the extracellular matrix [42] possibly reducing CSPG content and Sema3D content. Corroborating this line of evidence, neuroblastoma-derived growth cones secrete tissue plasminogen activator which activates the serine protease plasminogen, which also degrades extracellular matrix [43].

5. Conclusion

Together, our results provide, for the first time, evidence that several regenerative repulsive signals are reduced in regenerating optic nerve fibers following a combined therapy. Therefore, the treatment used was not only capable to stimulate the intrinsic growth capacity of RGCs but also made the CNS microenvironment more permissive to regeneration.

Conflicts of Interest

The authors declare that they have no conflicts of interest.

Authors' Contributions

Camila Oliveira Goulart and Henrique Rocha Mendonça contributed equally to this work.

References

[1] S. David and A. J. Aguayo, "Axonal regeneration after crush injury of rat central nervous system fibres innervating

peripheral nerve grafts," *Journal of Neurocytology*, vol. 14, no. 1, pp. 1–12, 1985.

[2] M. Vidal-Sanz, G. M. Bray, and A. J. Aguayo, "Regenerated synapses persist in the superior colliculus after the regrowth of retinal ganglion cell axons," *Journal of Neurocytology*, vol. 20, no. 11, pp. 940–952, 1991.

[3] M. Aviles-Trigueros, Y. Sauve, R. D. Lund, and M. Vidal-sanz, "Selective innervation of retinorecipient brainstem nuclei by retinal ganglion cell axons regenerating through peripheral nerve grafts in adult rats," *The Journal of Neuroscience*, vol. 20, no. 1, pp. 361–374, 2000.

[4] S. J. O. Whiteley, Y. Sauvé, M. Avilés-Trigueros, M. Vidal-Sanz, and R. D. Lund, "Extent and duration of recovered pupillary light reflex following retinal ganglion cell axon regeneration through peripheral nerve grafts directed to the pretectum in adult rats," *Experimental Neurology*, vol. 154, no. 2, pp. 560–572, 1998.

[5] M. Vidal-Sanz, M. Aviles-Trigueros, S. J. O. Whiteley, Y. Sauve, and R. D. Lund, "Chapter 33 reinnervation of the pretectum in adult rats by regenerated retinal ganglion cell axons: anatomical and functional studies," *Progress in Brain Research*, vol. 137, pp. 443–452, 2002.

[6] K. Kikuchi, A. Kishino, O. Konishi et al., "*In vitro* and *in vivo* characterization of a novel semaphorin 3A inhibitor, SM-216289 or xanthofulvin," *Journal of Biological Chemistry*, vol. 278, no. 44, pp. 42985–42991, 2003.

[7] B. K. Kwon, E. B. Okon, W. Plunet et al., "A systematic review of directly applied biologic therapies for acute spinal cord injury," *Journal of Neurotrauma*, vol. 28, no. 8, pp. 1589–1610, 2011.

[8] G. Yiu and Z. He, "Glial inhibition of CNS axon regeneration," *Nature Reviews Neuroscience*, vol. 7, no. 8, pp. 617–627, 2006.

[9] S. Leon, Y. Yin, J. Nguyen, N. Irwin, and L. I. Benowitz, "Lens injury stimulates axon regeneration in the mature rat optic nerve," *The Journal of Neuroscience*, vol. 20, no. 12, pp. 4615–4626, 2000.

[10] K. K. Park, K. Liu, Y. Hu et al., "Promoting axon regeneration in the adult CNS by modulation of the PTEN/mTOR pathway," *Science*, vol. 322, no. 5903, pp. 963–966, 2008.

[11] A. Apara and J. L. Goldberg, "Molecular mechanisms of the suppression of axon regeneration by KLF transcription factors," *Neural Regeneration Research*, vol. 9, no. 15, pp. 1418–1421, 2014.

[12] S. de Lima, Y. Koriyama, T. Kurimoto et al., "Full-length axon regeneration in the adult mouse optic nerve and partial recovery of simple visual behaviors," *Proceedings of the National Academy of Sciences of the United States of America*, vol. 109, no. 23, pp. 9149–9154, 2012.

[13] D. Fischer, "Counteracting the Nogo receptor enhances optic nerve regeneration if retinal ganglion cells are in an active growth state," *The Journal of Neuroscience*, vol. 24, no. 7, pp. 1646–1651, 2004.

[14] A. J. Aguayo, R. Dickson, J. Trecarten, M. Attiwell, G. M. Bray, and P. Richardson, "Ensheathment and myelination of regenerating PNS fibres by transplanted optic nerve glia," *Neuroscience Letters*, vol. 9, no. 2-3, pp. 97–104, 1978.

[15] T. Kurimoto, Y. Yin, K. Omura et al., "Long-distance axon regeneration in the mature optic nerve: contributions of oncomodulin, cAMP, and *pten* gene deletion," *The Journal of Neuroscience*, vol. 30, no. 46, pp. 15654–15663, 2010.

[16] S. E. S. Araújo, H. R. Mendonça, N. A. Wheeler et al., "Inflammatory demyelination alters subcortical visual circuits," *Journal of Neuroinflammation*, vol. 14, no. 1, 2017.

[17] C. A. Abreu, S. V. De Lima, H. R. Mendonça, C. de Oliveira Goulart, and A. M. B. Martinez, "Absence of galectin-3 promotes neuroprotection in retinal ganglion cells after optic nerve injury," *Histology and Histopathology*, vol. 32, no. 3, pp. 253–262, 2017.

[18] S. Espírito-Santo, H. R. Mendonça, G. D. Menezes et al., "Intravitreous interleukin-2 treatment and inflammation modulates glial cells activation and uncrossed retinotectal development," *Neuroscience*, vol. 200, pp. 223–236, 2012.

[19] V. Grozdanov, A. Müller, V. Sengottuvel, M. Leibinger, and D. Fischer, "A method for preparing primary retinal cell cultures for evaluating the neuroprotective and neuritogenic effect of factors on axotomized mature CNS neurons," *Current Protocols in Neuroscience*, vol. 53, no. 1, pp. 3.22.1–3.22.10, 2010.

[20] D. Gaublomme, T. Buyens, and L. Moons, "Automated analysis of neurite outgrowth in mouse retinal explants," *Journal of Biomolecular Screening*, vol. 18, no. 5, pp. 534–543, 2013.

[21] D. Sun, S. Moore, and T. C. Jakobs, "Optic nerve astrocyte reactivity protects function in experimental glaucoma and other nerve injuries," *The Journal of Experimental Medicine*, vol. 214, no. 5, pp. 1411–1430, 2017.

[22] R. J. Pasterkamp, F. De Winter, A. J. G. D. Holtmaat, and J. Verhaagen, "Evidence for a role of the chemorepellent semaphorin III and its receptor neuropilin-1 in the regeneration of primary olfactory axons," *The Journal of Neuroscience*, vol. 18, no. 23, pp. 9962–9976, 1998.

[23] R. J. Pasterkamp, R. J. Giger, M. J. Ruitenberg et al., "Expression of the gene encoding the chemorepellent semaphorin III is induced in the fibroblast component of neural scar tissue formed following injuries of adult but not neonatal CNS," *Molecular and Cellular Neurosciences*, vol. 13, no. 2, pp. 143–166, 1999.

[24] F. De Winter, M. Oudega, A. J. Lankhorst et al., "Injury-induced class 3 semaphorin expression in the rat spinal cord," *Experimental Neurology*, vol. 175, no. 1, pp. 61–75, 2002.

[25] E. R. Bray, M. Noga, K. Thakor et al., "3D visualization of individual regenerating retinal ganglion cell axons reveals surprisingly complex growth paths," *Eneuro*, vol. 4, no. 4, 2017.

[26] V. Pernet, S. Joly, D. Dalkara et al., "Long-distance axonal regeneration induced by CNTF gene transfer is impaired by axonal misguidance in the injured adult optic nerve," *Neurobiology of Disease*, vol. 51, pp. 202–213, 2013.

[27] X. Luo, Y. Salgueiro, S. R. Beckerman, V. P. Lemmon, P. Tsoulfas, and K. K. Park, "Three-dimensional evaluation of retinal ganglion cell axon regeneration and pathfinding in whole mouse tissue after injury," *Experimental Neurology*, vol. 247, pp. 653–662, 2013.

[28] F. Bei, H. H. C. Lee, X. Liu et al., "Restoration of visual function by enhancing conduction in regenerated axons," *Cell*, vol. 164, no. 1-2, pp. 219–232, 2016.

[29] J. W. Fawcett and R. A. Asher, "The glial scar and central nervous system repair," *Brain Research Bulletin*, vol. 49, no. 6, pp. 377–391, 1999.

[30] S. Rotshenker, "Wallerian degeneration: the innate-immune response to traumatic nerve injury," *Journal of Neuroinflammation*, vol. 8, no. 1, p. 109, 2011.

[31] M. S. Narciso, B. S. Mietto, S. A. Marques et al., "Sciatic nerve regeneration is accelerated in galectin-3 knockout mice," *Experimental Neurology*, vol. 217, no. 1, pp. 7–15, 2009.

[32] B. S. Mietto, S. Jurgensen, L. Alves et al., "Lack of galectin-3 speeds Wallerian degeneration by altering TLR and pro-inflammatory cytokine expressions in injured sciatic nerve," *The European Journal of Neuroscience*, vol. 37, no. 10, pp. 1682–1690, 2013.

[33] M. A. Marin, S. de Lima, H.-Y. Gilbert, R. J. Giger, L. Benowitz, and M. N. Rasband, "Reassembly of excitable domains after CNS axon regeneration," *The Journal of Neuroscience*, vol. 36, no. 35, pp. 9148–9160, 2016.

[34] A. M. Hilla, H. Diekmann, and D. Fischer, "Microglia are irrelevant for neuronal degeneration and axon regeneration after acute injury," *The Journal of Neuroscience*, vol. 37, no. 25, pp. 6113–6124, 2017.

[35] S. Soleman, P. K. Yip, D. A. Duricki, and L. D. F. Moon, "Delayed treatment with chondroitinase ABC promotes sensorimotor recovery and plasticity after stroke in aged rats," *Brain*, vol. 135, no. 4, pp. 1210–1223, 2012.

[36] S. F. Oster, "Invariant Sema5A inhibition serves an ensheathing function during optic nerve development," *Development*, vol. 130, no. 4, pp. 775–784, 2003.

[37] V. Mecollari, B. Nieuwenhuis, and J. Verhaagen, "A perspective on the role of class III semaphorin signaling in central nervous system trauma," *Frontiers in Cellular Neuroscience*, vol. 8, 2014.

[38] K. Venkova, A. Christov, Z. Kamaluddin, P. Kobalka, S. Siddiqui, and K. Hensley, "Semaphorin 3A signaling through neuropilin-1 is an early trigger for distal axonopathy in the SOD1^{G93A} mouse model of amyotrophic lateral sclerosis," *Journal of Neuropathology & Experimental Neurology*, vol. 73, no. 7, pp. 702–713, 2014.

[39] Y. Liu, "Semaphorin3D guides retinal axons along the dorsoventral axis of the tectum," *The Journal of Neuroscience*, vol. 24, no. 2, pp. 310–318, 2004.

[40] S. Kaneko, A. Iwanami, M. Nakamura et al., "A selective Sema3A inhibitor enhances regenerative responses and functional recovery of the injured spinal cord," *Nature Medicine*, vol. 12, no. 12, pp. 1380–1389, 2006.

[41] A. Shirvan, M. Kimron, V. Holdengreber et al., "Anti-semaphorin 3A antibodies rescue retinal ganglion cells from cell death following optic nerve axotomy," *The Journal of Biological Chemistry*, vol. 277, no. 51, pp. 49799–49807, 2002.

[42] M. Santiago-Medina, K. A. Gregus, R. H. Nichol, S. M. O'Toole, and T. M. Gomez, "Regulation of ECM degradation and axon guidance by growth cone invadosomes," *Development*, vol. 142, no. 3, pp. 486–496, 2015.

[43] A. Krystosek and N. W. Seeds, "Plasminogen activator release at the neuronal growth cone," *Science*, vol. 213, no. 4515, pp. 1532–1534, 1981.

3

Oscillatory Corticospinal Activity during Static Contraction of Ankle Muscles is Reduced in Healthy Old versus Young Adults

Meaghan Elizabeth Spedden,[1] **Jens Bo Nielsen,**[2,3] **and Svend Sparre Geertsen**[1,2]

[1]*Department of Nutrition, Exercise and Sports, University of Copenhagen, Copenhagen, Denmark*
[2]*Department of Neuroscience, University of Copenhagen, Copenhagen, Denmark*
[3]*Elsass Institute, Charlottenlund, Denmark*

Correspondence should be addressed to Svend Sparre Geertsen; ssgeertsen@nexs.ku.dk

Academic Editor: Claudio A. Mastronardi

Aging is accompanied by impaired motor function, but age-related changes in neural networks responsible for generating movement are not well understood. We aimed to investigate the functional oscillatory coupling between activity in the sensorimotor cortex and ankle muscles during static contraction. Fifteen young (20–26 yr) and fifteen older (65–73 yr) subjects were instructed to match a target force by performing static ankle dorsi- or plantar flexion, while electroencephalographic (EEG) activity was recorded from the cortex and electromyographic (EMG) activity was recorded from dorsi- (proximal and distal anterior tibia) and plantar (soleus and medial gastrocnemius) flexor muscles. EEG-EMG and EMG-EMG beta band (15–35 Hz) coherence was analyzed as an index of corticospinal activity. Our results demonstrated that beta cortico-, intra-, and intermuscular coherence was reduced in old versus young subjects during static contractions. Old subjects demonstrated significantly greater error than young subjects while matching target forces, but force precision was not related to beta coherence. We interpret this as an age-related decrease in effective oscillatory corticospinal activity during steady-state motor output. Additionally, our data indicate a potential effect of alpha coherence and tremor on performance. These results may be instrumental in developing new interventions to strengthen sensorimotor control in elderly subjects.

1. Introduction

Aging is accompanied by increased incidence of gait and balance problems, greater movement variability, reduced force steadiness, and worsened coordination [1–3], but age-related changes in neural control of motor function have yet to be fully elucidated. Previous studies have primarily focused on characterizing structural mechanisms, whereas knowledge regarding functional changes in the neural networks involved in generating movements is limited. A better understanding of how activity patterns in descending tracts controlling motor function are modified with age is of particular importance, as these tracts directly mediate motor signals from the brain to the spinal cord.

The corticospinal tract is a major descending pathway governing voluntary movement in humans and appears to be vulnerable to age-related deterioration. Diffusion tensor imaging has revealed declining fractional anisotropy (FA) in the posterior limb of the internal capsule, indicating degeneration in white matter microstructure [4, 5]. The functional significance of these declines is supported by associations between internal capsule FA and motor performance [6]. Input-output characteristics of the corticospinal system also appear to be modulated with age. Studies using transcranial magnetic stimulation indicate that the amplitude of motor-evoked responses is lower in old than in young adults [7–9], which suggests that aging may entail reduced excitability in the corticospinal pathway.

Another functional marker of corticospinal integrity is corticomuscular coherence, which quantifies the degree of task-related oscillatory coupling between the sensorimotor cortex and contralateral muscle. In healthy young adults, coherent oscillations are present between the cortex and muscle at beta frequencies (15–35 Hz) during isometric contractions and are mediated by the corticospinal tract [10–16]. Coherent beta oscillations may also be seen between different pools of motor neurons in synergists and within the same muscle [15, 17–19]. This intra- and intermuscular coherence shares several similarities with corticomuscular coherence and is generally assumed to be generated by similar mechanisms, and both inter- and intramuscular coherence are therefore often used as an indirect measure of the corticospinal activity [18, 19]. Coherent oscillations are also present in the alpha band (5–15 Hz) between pairs of motor units [17] but are only rarely seen between the cortex and the muscles [20, 21]. The origin of alpha coherence is debated, but some evidence suggests a central origin [21] and a relation to physiological tremor [22].

Previous investigations of age-related changes in beta band coherence have produced equivocal results. Studies have demonstrated reduced [23], increased [24], and unchanged [25] amplitudes of corticomuscular coherence in old versus young adults, whereas studies examining inter- or intramuscular coherence have shown both unchanged [26, 27] and increased [27, 28] magnitudes. However, the use of different motor tasks and muscle groups may render direct comparisons across studies inappropriate or, in the least, less straightforward. Studies exploring age-related changes in coherence have primarily focused on hand and arm muscles [23–25, 28]. Less is known about the cortical control of ankle muscles, which is of interest due to their important role in postural control and gait. For example, during gait, ankle dorsiflexors lift the toes in order to clear the ground in the swing phase, and plantar flexors play a crucial role in forward propulsion during the late stance phase [29]. To date, age-related changes in intermuscular coherence in ankle muscles during a simple phasic task [26] and during uni- and bipedal stance [27] have been explored, but investigation of the direct corticomuscular coupling is lacking.

We aimed to investigate cortico-, intra-, and intermuscular coherence in ankle muscles during static dorsi- and plantar flexion in old versus young adults. It was hypothesized that older adults would display less beta coherence than young adults, indicative of reduced oscillatory corticospinal activity. Additionally, we wanted to explore if beta coherence estimates were positively associated with task performance.

2. Methods

2.1. Subjects. Fifteen young (mean: 22.1 ± 1.7, range 20–26 yr; 7 men) and fifteen older (mean: 68.3 ± 2.7, range 65–73 yr; 7 men) participants were recruited (see Table 1). The sample size was chosen based on previous studies comparing coherence between groups [24, 25]. Subjects were free from neurological disorders and afflictions impairing leg motor function. No subjects were taking medication expected to affect neuromuscular function. There was no indication of cognitive impairment in any subjects as determined by the Mini-Mental State Examination (MMSE; all scores ≥ 26 out of 30) [30]. According to the Waterloo Footedness Questionnaire [31], 21 subjects were right-footed, 2 were left-footed, and 7 were equally right- and left-footed.

Table 1: Subject characteristics.

Group	Young ($n = 15$)	Old ($n = 15$)
Age (years)	22.1 ± 1.7	68.3 ± 2.7
Gender (M/F)	7/8	7/8
Body mass (kg)	72.95 ± 15.89	81.45 ± 14.12
Height (m)	1.76 ± 0.08	1.73 ± 0.11
BMI	23.43 ± 4.29	27.31 ± 4.14*
MMSE (score out of 30)	29.0 ± 1.1	28.9 ± 1.0
Footedness (R/L/B)	11/1/3	10/1/4

Values are presented at mean ± standard deviation where applicable. Significant differences between young and old groups are indicated by $^*p < 0.05$. MMSE: Mini-Mental State Examination. Footedness indicates foot preference. R: right; L: left; B: both.

Prior to participation in the study, subjects provided written, informed consent. All procedures were approved by the ethics committee for the Capital Region of Denmark (approval number H-16021214), and experiments were conducted in accordance with the Helsinki declaration.

2.2. Protocol. Subjects were seated in a rigid chair with the left foot firmly fastened to a force pedal containing a strain gauge that measured force exerted on the pedal. The leg was positioned with ~90° flexion at the hip joint, ~115° flexion at the knee joint, and ~120° dorsiflexion at the ankle joint.

First, subjects performed three maximal isometric dorsiflexion contractions (MVC), separated by 30 s rest, as a measure of maximal voluntary dorsiflexion strength. Online visual feedback of force production was projected onto the wall in front of subjects as a moving yellow trace on a black background. The projector (TDP-T 255; Toshiba) was attached to the ceiling 148 cm from the wall, resulting in a screen size of 125 cm by 167 cm. During MVC, verbal encouragement was provided to ensure maximal efforts. MVC was determined as peak force production across the three trials.

Subsequently, subjects performed a static contraction, where they were asked to maintain a force level of 10% MVC during isometric dorsiflexion for two minutes. The target force level was displayed on the wall as a horizontal line, and subjects were instructed to follow this line as precisely as possible with the moving yellow trace depicting real-time force production (Figure 1).

Following a short rest, subjects repeated the MVC procedure and static contraction for plantar flexion. During periods where data was recorded, subjects were asked to relax face and neck muscles to minimize artifacts in electroencephalographic (EEG) signals.

2.3. Electrophysiological Recordings. EEG and electromyographic (EMG) activity were recorded using active surface electrodes (BioSemi, The Netherlands) and ActiView acquisition software (version 6.05). EEG was measured using 64 pin electrodes plugged into a headcap (BioSemi) that ensured positioning in accordance with the 10/20 layout system. EMG was recorded from four pairs of electrodes placed on left lower leg muscles (interelectrode distance ~ 1.5 cm) after

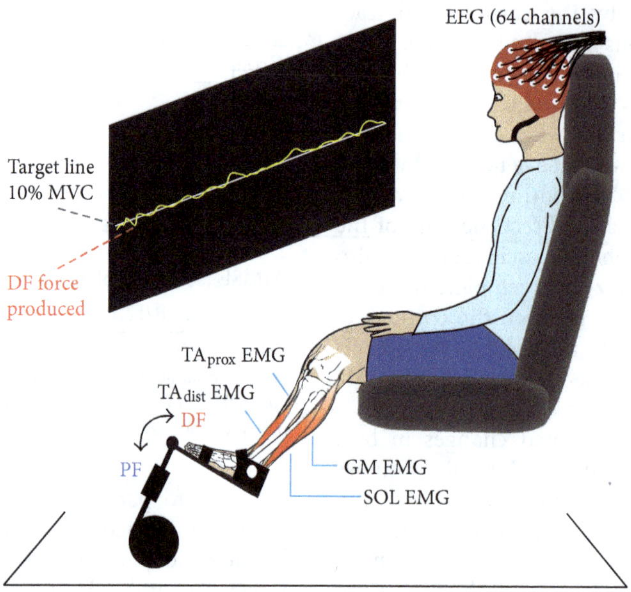

FIGURE 1: Experimental setup and static contractions. Subjects sat in a chair with their left foot fastened to a force pedal and maintained a force level of 10% of their maximal voluntary contraction (MVC) for 2 min, first for dorsiflexion (DF) and subsequently for plantar flexion (PF). The target force level was projected onto the wall as a horizontal line that subjects were asked to follow as precisely as possible with a yellow force trace showing online force production. During contractions, electroencephalographic (EEG) and electromyographic (EMG) signals from the proximal and distal ends of the anterior tibial muscle (TA_{prox} and TA_{dist}), soleus (SOL), and medial gastrocnemius (GM) were recorded.

preparation of the skin with shaving, abrasion, and cleaning with alcohol. Pairs of EMG electrodes were positioned over the proximal (TA_{prox}) and distal (TA_{dist}) ends of the anterior tibial muscle (mean distance between electrode pairs ~ 12 cm) and over the center of the medial gastrocnemius (MG) and soleus (SOL) muscles. As per the BioSemi system design, signals were recorded in reference to a common mode sense active electrode, while a driven right leg electrode was used to cancel signals measured at the common mode sense electrode. Analog signals were sampled at 2048 Hz, and offset was contained to $\pm 25\,\mu V$.

2.4. Data Analysis and Statistics. All data analysis was performed in MATLAB (Version R2016b, MathWorks, MA, USA). Electrophysiological data was preprocessed using the EEGLAB toolbox (v14.0.0). Initially, EEG and EMG signals were downsampled to 256 Hz. EEG signals were then rereferenced to an average reference excluding noisy and high impedance channels and band pass filtered between 0.5 to 120 Hz. Independent component analysis was performed in EEGLAB [32] and was used to remove EEG signal components displaying unequivocal spatial and temporal characteristics of eye blinks and/or face and neck muscle activity [33]. EMG signals were band pass filtered between 5 and 120 Hz then full-wave rectified to emphasize information about timing of motor unit action potentials in the signals [34] and to improve coherence detection [35].

In order to examine the coupling between EEG-EMG and EMG-EMG signals in the frequency domain, coherence estimates were constructed [36]. Coherence describes the linear association between two signals at each frequency of interest and is a measure of phase consistency between signals. Coherence estimates are defined over the range [0, 1] where 0 indicates no association between signals and 1 indicates a strong association. To calculate coherence, auto- and cross-spectra were constructed by dividing signals into nonoverlapping segments, after which discrete Fourier transforms were performed on each segment and averaged. Coherence was then determined as the squared modulus of the cross-spectrum for the two signals $f_{xy}(\lambda)$ normalized by the product of the two autospectra, $f_{xx}(\lambda)$ and $f_{yy}(\lambda)$:

$$|Rxy(\lambda)|^2 = \frac{\left|f_{xy}(\lambda)\right|^2}{f_{xx}(\lambda) f_{yy}(\lambda)}. \tag{1}$$

EEG-EMG coherence thus quantifies the strength and frequency range of the coupling between cortical and muscular activity, whereas EMG-EMG coherence quantifies common rhythmic drive to two muscles or motor neuron pools. The statistical significance of individual coherence estimates was assessed according to an upper 95% confidence limit determined as

$$1 - 0.05^{\frac{1}{(L-1)}}, \tag{2}$$

where L indicates the number of data segments used for the analysis [36].

For data obtained during static dorsiflexion, coherence was calculated between EEG and TA_{prox}; EEG and TA_{dist}; and between TA_{prox} and TA_{dist}. For static plantar flexion, coherence analysis was likewise performed for EEG and SOL; EEG and MG; and between SOL and MG. For all analyses, 120 seconds of data and a frequency resolution of 1 Hz were utilized.

Initially, EEG-EMG coherence was calculated for all EEG electrodes. Scalp plots indicated that beta band (15–35 Hz) coherence was localized at the vertex (Cz), assumedly corresponding to the sensorimotor cortex (Figure 2). Accordingly, further analysis was performed using coherence at the Cz electrode (see example in Figure 3).

All EMG-EMG coherence data was visually inspected for signs of crosstalk, that is, high coherence across a wide range of frequencies and close to zero lag synchronization in the time domain as evidenced in cumulant density plots [37]. No data was observed displaying these characteristics, so all data was included in pooled analyses.

To undertake a population analysis, coherence for each age group was pooled, resulting in single group estimates at each frequency of interest. Group differences were investigated using the χ^2 extended difference of coherence test [38], a nonparametric test that provides the amount of pooled coherence difference between groups at each frequency in relation to an upper 95% confidence interval limit.

Coherence was also quantified as the sum (i.e., area) of alpha (5–15 Hz), total beta (15–35), low (15–25 Hz), and high (25–35 Hz) beta coherence. These values were transformed logarithmically to symmetrize distributions for statistical analyses. Additionally, we registered the frequency at which peak beta coherence occurred as well as the sum of EMG power in alpha and beta bands.

Performance during static contractions was quantified as the root mean square (RMS) error, that is, the RMS deviation of the raw force signal from the target force level.

One-way ANOVA was used to evaluate effects of age group on dependent variables, that is, logarithmic coherence area estimates, frequency for peak beta coherence, summed EMG power, RMS error, and subject characteristics (MMSE score, height, weight, and body mass index (BMI)). Model assumptions were checked by visual inspection of residual and normal probability plots. ANOVA was also utilized to explore if gender and/or laterality (footedness) affected the area of beta coherence.

Associations between task performance and coherence estimates, as well as performance and power were assessed by means of Pearson correlations. The significance level used to reject the null hypothesis was $\alpha = 0.05$, but tendencies were also noted for $p < 0.1$. Values are presented as mean ± standard deviation where applicable.

3. Results

Subject characteristics are summarized in Table 1. Young and old subjects were comparable in height ($p = 0.349$), body mass ($p = 0.133$), and MMSE score ($p = 0.726$), whereas older subjects had significantly greater BMI ($p = 0.018$).

EEG, EMG, autospectra, and coherence results from a single young subject during static dorsiflexion are shown in Figure 3. For this subject, sizeable coherence peaks were observed in the beta band (~20 Hz) for both cortico- and intramuscular coherence.

3.1. EMG Power. Figure 4 shows summed EMG power for young and older subjects. Alpha EMG power was greater in old subjects for TA_{dist} ($p = 0.011$) and SOL ($p = 0.023$), whereas group differences were not significant for TA_{prox} ($p = 0.312$) or GM ($p = 0.218$). In the beta band, old subjects had significantly greater power for TA_{prox} ($p = 0.005$), but no other differences were detected (TA_{dist}, $p = 0.413$; SOL, $p = 0.666$; GM, $p = 0.363$).

3.2. Coherence during Static Dorsiflexion. Pooled coherence for young and old groups during the dorsiflexion task is presented in Figure 5. For both groups, pooled beta coherence estimates exceeded significance levels for cortico- and intramuscular coherence measures and indicated greater coherence in young than in old subjects (Figures 5(a), 5(c), and 5(e)). The χ^2 extended difference of coherence test confirmed that group means differed significantly at beta frequencies for both cortico- and intramuscular coherence (Figures 5(b), 5(d), and 5(f)). The χ^2 test also revealed significant group differences in intramuscular coherence in the alpha band (~10 Hz), where young subjects had greater coherence than old subjects.

Estimates for coherence area in alpha, beta, and high and low beta bands are presented in Figure 6. Differences between young and old subjects were most consistent in the high beta band, where coherence area was greater for young than old subjects for all three coherence measures, though group differences in total and low beta area were also significant for TA_{prox}-TA_{dist} coherence and tended towards significance for the total beta band in Cz-TA_{prox}. Using this approach, no differences between young and old subjects were present in the area of alpha coherence.

Visual inspection of pooled group plots suggested that coherence in old adults appeared to be slightly shifted toward earlier frequencies, but review of single-subject plots indicated that this trend was driven by three older subjects showing pronounced coherence at alpha to early beta frequencies. In addition, the frequency at which peak beta coherence occurred did not differ significantly between groups for corticomuscular coherence (Cz-TA_{prox}, $p = 0.420$, Cz-TA_{dist}, $p = 0.742$), although it tended to be lower in old subjects for intramuscular coherence (TA_{prox}-TA_{dist}, $p = 0.088$).

No significant effects of gender (all $p > 0.2$) or footedness (all $p > 0.3$) on beta band coherence area during dorsiflexion were present.

3.3. Coherence during Static Plantar Flexion. Pooled coherence data from the plantar flexion task demonstrated trends similar to those observed for the dorsiflexion task, though amplitudes were lower in both age groups (Figures 7(a), 7(c), and 7(e)). Group estimates indicated statistically significant beta coherence in both young and old subjects for all three measures. Pooled plots suggested that the magnitude of beta coherence was consistently larger for young subjects, which was corroborated by the χ^2 extended difference of coherence test (Figures 7(b), 7(d), and 7(f)). For intermuscular coherence, pooled estimates indicated the presence of alpha coherence in both age groups, but group differences at these frequencies did not reach the significance level. Thus,

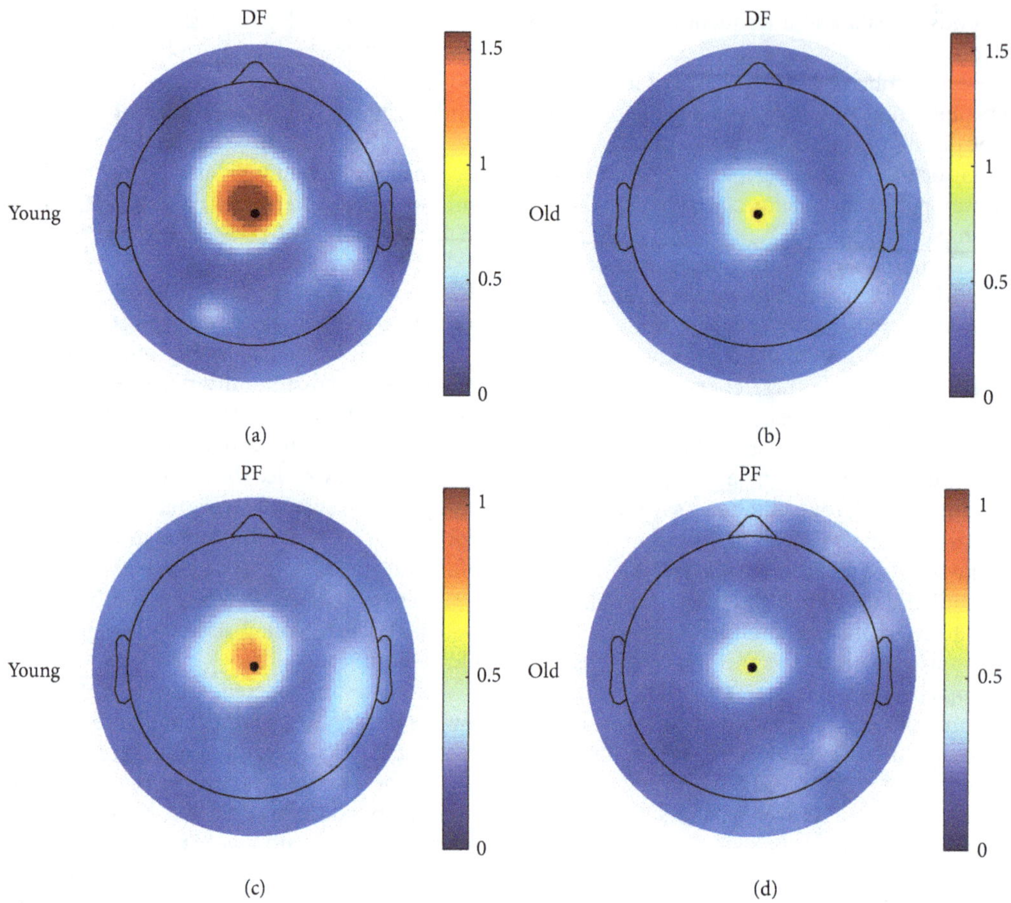

FIGURE 2: Coherence head plots. Spatial localization of summed beta band (15–35 Hz) corticomuscular coherence for single young (a, c) and old (b, d) subjects during static dorsiflexion (a, b; EEG-TA_{prox} coherence) and plantar flexion (c, d; EEG-SOL coherence).

the χ^2 test indicated that group differences were confined to the beta band.

The area of beta coherence differed between groups in a more widespread manner than for dorsiflexion (Figure 6); Cz-SOL coherence only tended to be greater in young subjects for the high beta band, whereas for Cz-GM and SOL-GM, significant differences in total, low, and high beta bands were observed. In the alpha band, a significant group difference was observed for Cz-GM, where coherence area was greater in old subjects.

Similar to what was observed in dorsiflexion, pooled coherence data suggested that coherence in old subjects was present at slightly lower frequencies than in young subjects. Upon inspection of individual coherence estimates, it was again apparent that the same three old subjects were responsible for this trend. Correspondingly, the frequency at which peak beta coherence occurred did not differ in young and old adults for Cz-GM ($p = 0.754$) or SOL-GM ($p = 0.673$), but a tendency towards lower frequency beta coherence in older adults was present for Cz-SOL ($p = 0.081$).

As for dorsiflexion, beta band coherence during plantar flexion was neither affected by gender (all $p > 0.4$) nor footedness (all $p > 0.3$).

3.4. Task Performance and Associations with Power and Coherence. Figure 8 shows group differences in force precision during static dorsi- and plantar flexion contractions. RMS error during dorsiflexion was greater for old (14.5 ± 8.2 mV) than for young (9.5 ± 3.1 mV) adults ($p = 0.035$). During plantar flexion, RMS error for old adults (16.8 ± 6.3 mV) was likewise greater than for young adults (11.1 ± 3.1 mV; $p = 0.004$).

To examine if low-frequency rhythmicity in EMG bursts was related to task performance, associations between EMG alpha power and RMS error were explored. EMG alpha power in TA_{prox} was positively associated with RMS error ($r = 0.47$, $p = 0.008$), and a tendency towards a positive correlation between TA_{dist} and RMS error was also present ($r = 0.36$, $p = 0.054$), while alpha power in SOL and GM was not related to RMS error during plantar flexion (SOL, $p = 0.323$, GM, $p = 0.776$).

Furthermore, we investigated possible associations between coherence estimates and performance. Surprisingly, neither cortico- nor intramuscular beta coherence area was correlated with RMS error during the dorsiflexion task (Cz-TA_{prox}, $p = 0.783$; Cz-TA_{dist}, $p = 0.745$; TA_{prox}-TA_{dist}, $p = 0.306$), suggesting that the amount of beta coherence was not related to task performance. For the plantar flexion task, RMS error was also unrelated to beta coherence area (Cz-SOL, $p = 0.327$; Cz-GM, $p = 0.870$; SOL-GM, $p = 0.946$). Correlations between RMS error and low and high beta coherence were similarly nonsignificant for

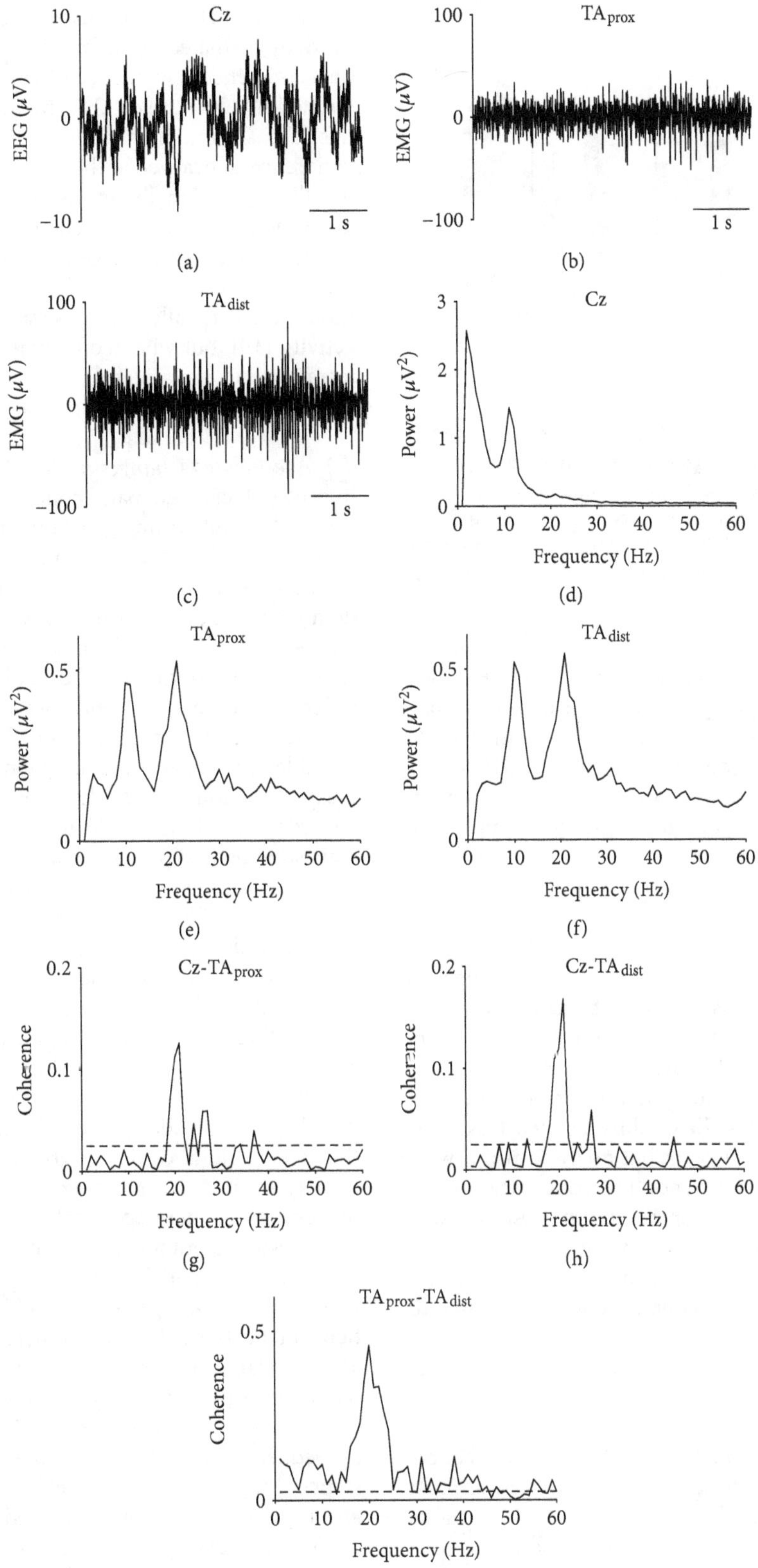

FIGURE 3: Raw EEG and EMG traces, autospectra, and coherence results from a single young subject. EEG from Cz (a), EMG from proximal (b), and distal (c) ends of the anterior tibial muscle (TA_{prox} and TA_{dist}, resp.); autospectra for Cz (d), TA_{prox} (e), TA_{dist} (f); and coherence for Cz-TA_{prox} (g), Cz-TA_{dist} (h), and TA_{prox}-TA_{dist} (i) during static dorsiflexion. Dashed lines on coherence plots indicate upper 95% confidence interval limits.

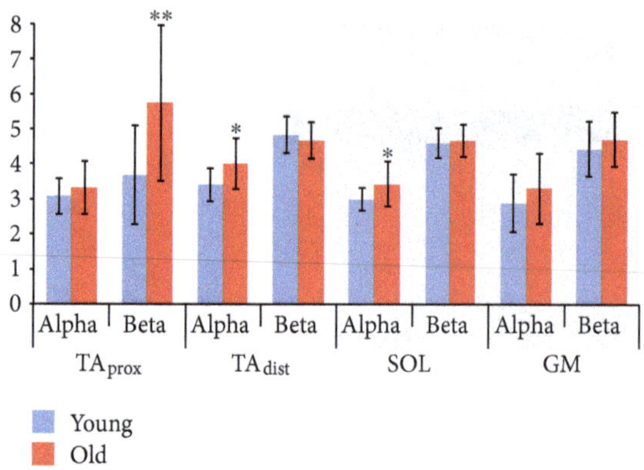

FIGURE 4: EMG power. Summed EMG power in alpha (5–15 Hz) and beta (15–35 Hz) bands for young and old subjects during dorsiflexion (white background) and plantar flexion (grey background). Significant differences between young and old groups are indicated by $^*p < 0.05$; $^{**}p < 0.01$. TA_{prox}: proximal end of anterior tibial; TA_{dist}: distal end of anterior tibial; SOL: soleus; GM: medial gastrocnemius.

both dorsi- and plantar flexion tasks (range for p values: 0.175–0.971). Interestingly, alpha coherence area was positively correlated with RMS error for both tasks in five out of six coherence measures (range for p values: 0.010–0.062, range for r: 0.34–0.46), demonstrating that greater coherence in the alpha band was accompanied by less precision in force production across groups.

4. Discussion

The aim of this study was to examine age-related changes in cortico-, intra-, and intermuscular beta band coherence in lower leg muscles during static dorsi- and plantar flexion. We found that beta band coherence estimates were significantly lower in old versus young adults for all coherence measures during both tasks. Error during force tasks was greater for old than young subjects, but no associations were observed between task performance and coherence area in the beta band. Collectively, our results suggest an age-related reduction in oscillatory corticospinal activity in the beta band during a simple task requiring steady state motor output, but the amount of beta coherence was not related to precision in force production. Interestingly, our data indicate a potential effect of alpha coherence and EMG alpha power on task performance.

4.1. Beta Band Coherence. For subjects with significant coherence, cortico-, intra-, and intermuscular coherence was most prominent in the beta band, which agrees with previous results demonstrating beta coherence during isometric contractions [10, 11, 13–17, 20]. That this oscillatory coupling in the beta band specifically reflects task-related corticospinal activity is confirmed by multiple lines of evidence. In the monkey, it has been demonstrated that local field potentials in the primary motor cortex are coherent with EMG in the beta band during static contractions, and that these local field potentials were phase-locked with pyramidal cell firing, indicating that corticomuscular coherence is, in the least, partially mediated by the corticospinal tract [39]. Moreover, beta coherence is weakened or absent in patients with central stroke [40]. The use of EEG, MRI, and TMS in combination has also shown, in healthy humans, that corticomuscular coherence is localized at the same site as the muscle's hotspot for TMS [41]. Finally, it has been shown that subthreshold TMS increases corticomuscular coherence, suggesting a role for cortical cells in the generation of beta band coherence [42]. Cortico-, intra-, and intermuscular coherence are thought to generally reflect the same oscillatory corticospinal activity [19], but when considering the indirect measures of intra and intermuscular coherence, contributions from other common neural drives cannot be excluded.

4.2. Age-Related Changes in Beta Band Coherence. Our findings of reduced beta band coherence in older subjects are in line with results from a previous study suggesting weakened corticomuscular coherence in older adults during static contractions of arm muscles [23], although other studies have demonstrated unchanged or greater beta coherence in older adults [24–28]. These inconsistencies are not easily reconciled, but considering that beta coherence is task-dependent, differences in task details across studies are likely of utmost importance. One study examined intermuscular coherence in ankle muscles during a simple motor task across the adult lifespan and found no evidence of age-related changes in beta coherence amplitude [26]. However, this study utilized a task consisting of brief phasic dorsiflexions, where visual feedback of EMG traces was provided, but where contraction strength was not controlled, which may contribute to explaining the seemingly divergent results. What is more, this study only examined the corticomuscular coupling indirectly, that is, via intermuscular coherence.

Another recent study investigated intermuscular coherence in triceps surae muscles during stance and found greater beta band coherence in older versus young adults during the uni- but not bipedal posture [27]. These findings indicate that older adults deployed greater oscillatory corticospinal activity during a demanding task, possibly as a strategy to manage their increased postural sway. Interestingly, beta coherence was not greater in older adults during the simpler task, that is, bipedal stance, suggesting that task difficulty may modulate the age-related mobilization of oscillatory corticospinal activity. Our task differed considerably from uni- and bipedal stance, making direct comparisons difficult, but one interesting factor may be differences in the costs of failure in task performance; for static dorsiflexion, there is no consequence to poor performance, whereas during unipedal stance, there is likely a perceived risk of falling that could affect the neural strategy employed.

The age-related reduction we observed in beta coherence, indicative of decreased oscillatory corticospinal activity, is plausibly related to both structural and functional declines in the nervous system. There does not appear to be an age-related loss of neurons in the primary motor cortex [43], but the deterioration in white matter microstructure that occurs with aging likely affects corticospinal connectivity [4, 5]. Decreases in synaptic density [44] and dendritic

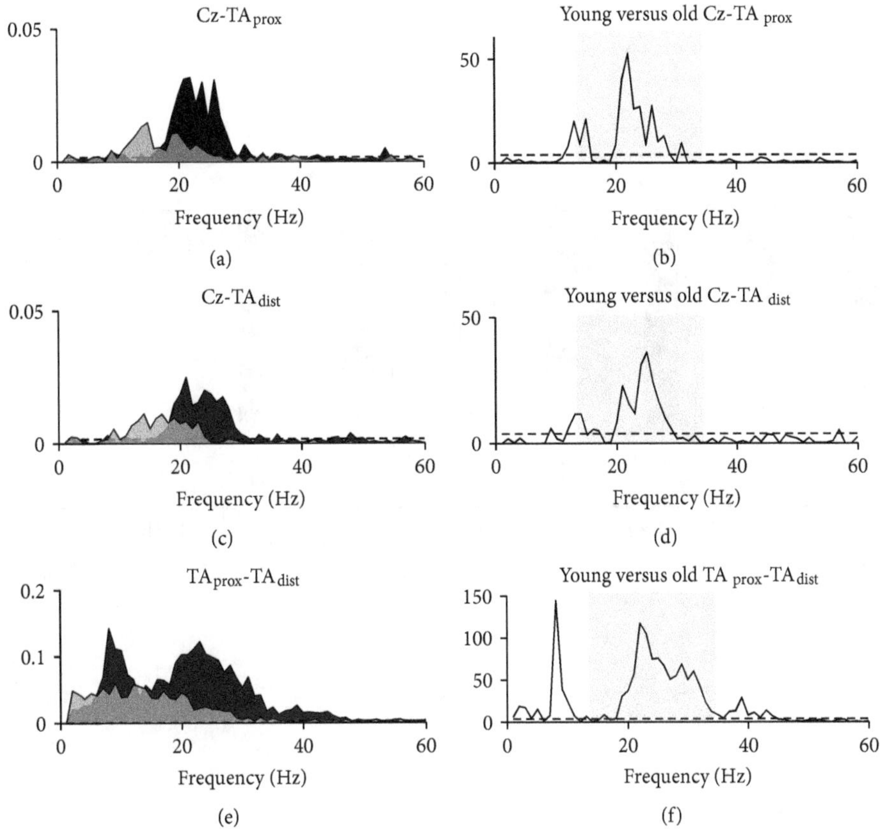

FIGURE 5: Pooled coherence during dorsiflexion. Pooled coherence estimates for young (black areas) and old (light grey areas) groups during static dorsiflexion (a, c, e) and χ^2 test statistics as a function of frequency (b, d, f) illustrating frequencies at which group means differed. Shaded boxes in b, d, and f mark the beta band (15–35 Hz). Dashed lines indicate upper 95% confidence interval limits. TA_{prox}: proximal end of anterior tibial muscle; TA_{dist}: distal end of anterior tibial muscle.

arborization [45] may likewise contribute to reduced corticomuscular coherence in older adults.

Age-related changes in the functional organization of sensorimotor networks have also been demonstrated. Functional MRI studies suggest that aging entails greater and more widespread cortical activation including regions involved in sensory processing and cognitive control, even during simple motor tasks [46–48]. The reduction we observed in functional corticospinal involvement is not necessarily inconsistent with these findings but may rather be a consequence of age-related de-differentiation of networks, that is, more defocalized and nonspecific activation patterns may entail a less focused and effective corticospinal coupling. Alternatively, decreased corticospinal involvement may represent a fundamental decline in the sensorimotor system compelling compensatory activation in, for example, cognitive or sensory processing regions. Synchronous activity has been theorized as a particularly efficient mode of corticospinal interaction in tasks with relatively low computational demands [39, 49]; accordingly, decreased coherence in older adults may indicate decreased efficiency in the corticospinal system necessitating compensatory strategies in order to perform a given task. The relationship between age-related reductions in beta coherence and modifications of sensorimotor networks should be explored in future studies.

When we examined group estimates for pooled coherence, we noticed that the area of significant coherence was shifted towards lower frequencies (late alpha-early beta) in older subjects. However, this shift appeared to be primarily driven by three older subjects and was not statistically evident when comparing the frequency for peak beta coherence in old versus young groups. We only investigated this apparent shift within the confines of the beta band, as the origin of this activity is well-established, but it is possible that the frequency band reflecting oscillatory corticospinal activity shifts slightly with aging and is thus present at somewhat lower frequencies (~10–25 Hz). This would be in line with previous results indicating that cortical activity and corticomuscular coherence slow with aging [24]; thus, this potential shift towards lower frequencies should be explored in further projects.

It should be noted that we found higher BMI in the older subjects, but we do not believe that this could explain the observed differences in coherence. Although more subcutaneous fat could affect the EMG amplitude, it would not be expected to affect the frequency of the signals, which is what is used for coherence analyses.

4.3. Mechanisms Contributing to Decreased Performance in Older Subjects. The functional significance of the observed decline in beta band coherence is unclear. We expected that

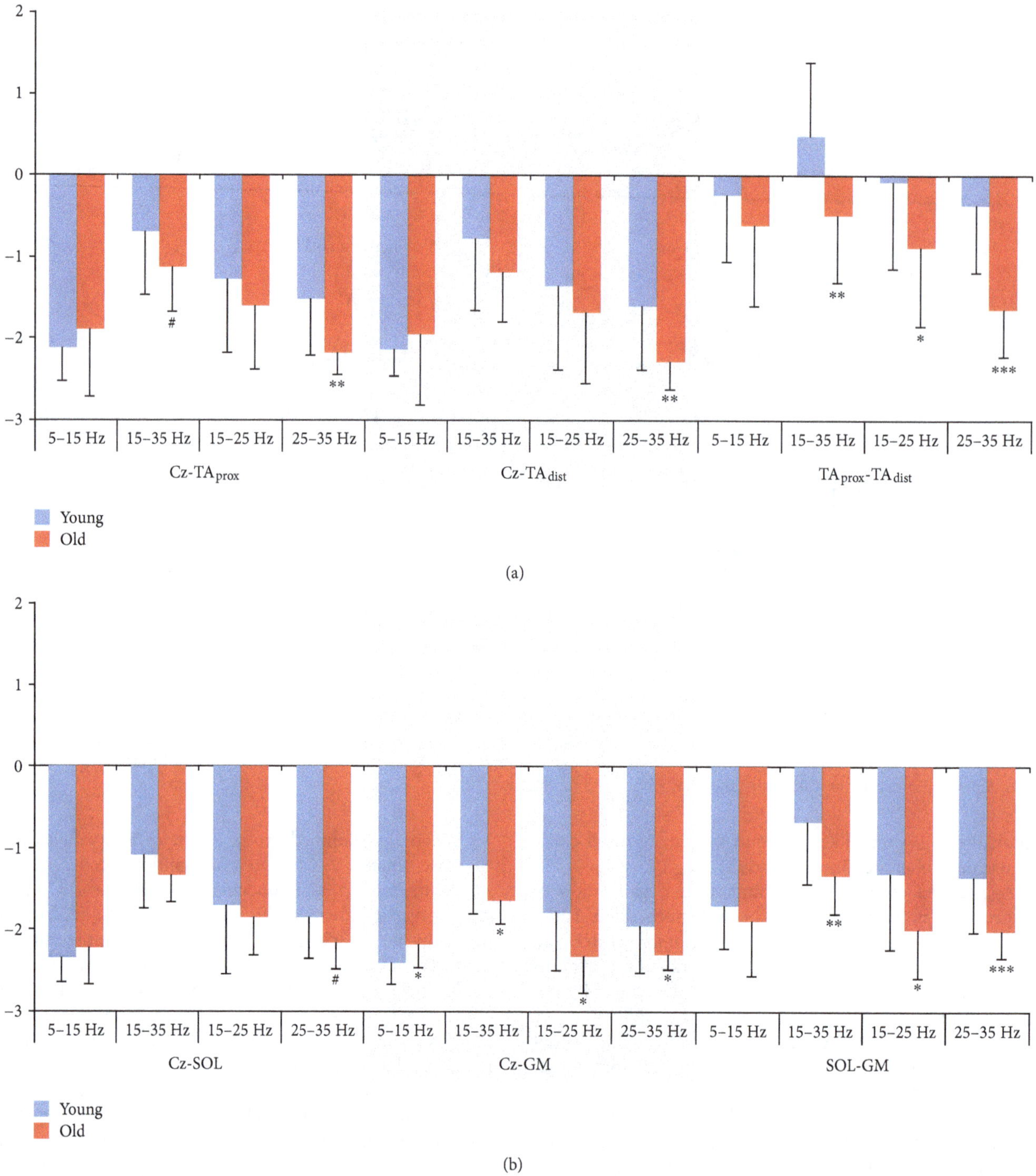

FIGURE 6: Coherence area estimates. Logarithmic coherence area in alpha (5–15 Hz), beta (15–35 Hz), low (15–25 Hz), and high (25–35 Hz) beta during static dorsiflexion (a) and plantar flexion (b) for young and old subjects. Significant differences between young and old groups are indicated by $^{*}p < 0.05$; $^{**}p < 0.01$; $^{***}p < 0.001$; $^{\#}p < 0.1$. TA_{prox}: proximal end of anterior tibial; TA_{dist}: distal end of anterior tibial; SOL: soleus; GM: medial gastrocnemius.

greater oscillatory corticospinal activity would be positively related to precision in force production, as suggested by a previous study [49], but our results indicated no association between beta coherence and force precision; older adults demonstrated greater error and less beta coherence, but the two parameters were not related. As a more challenging visuomotor task was used by Kristeva and colleagues [49], requiring subjects to respond precisely to an applied force of 4% MVC, this divergence may reflect that our task was not sufficiently demanding to detect a positive effect of beta coherence on performance. On the other hand, other studies have found that greater beta coherence was associated with

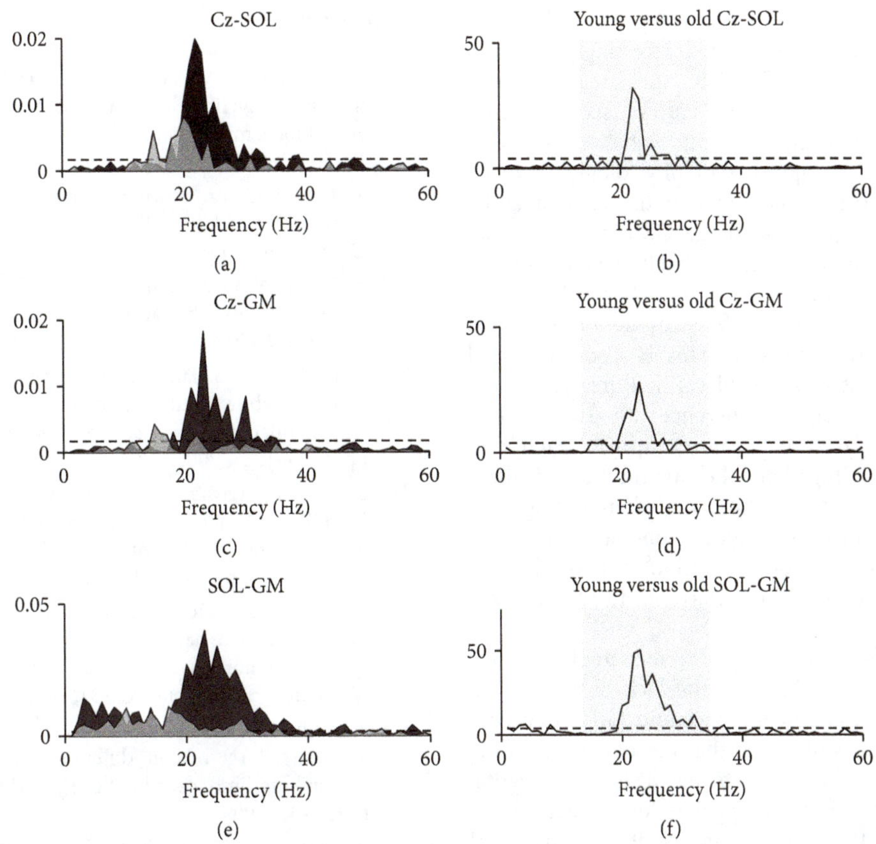

FIGURE 7: Pooled coherence during plantar flexion. Pooled coherence estimates for young (black areas) and old (light grey areas) groups during static plantar flexion (a, c, e) and χ^2 test statistics as a function of frequency (b, d, f) illustrating frequencies at which group means differed. Shaded boxes in b, d, and f mark the beta band (15–35 Hz). Dashed lines indicate upper 95% confidence interval limits. SOL: soleus; GM: medial gastrocnemius.

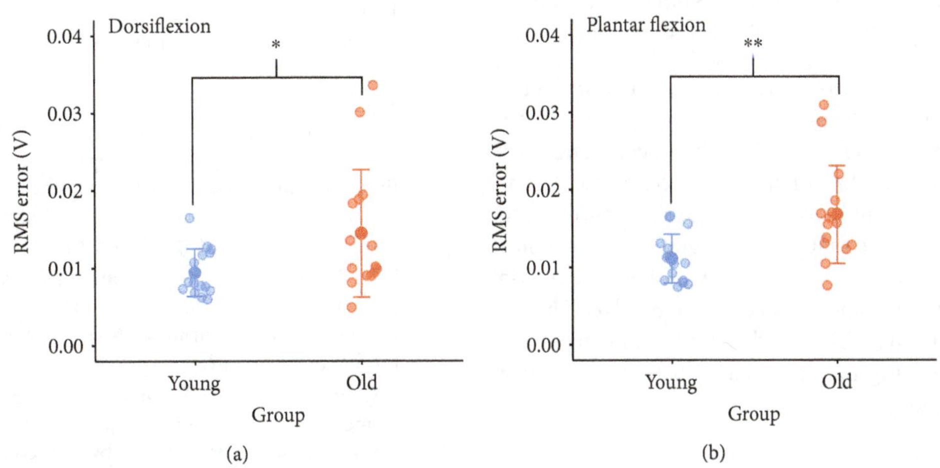

FIGURE 8: Performance during static contractions. Group differences in force precision during submaximal dorsiflexion (a) and plantar flexion (b). Significant differences between young and old groups are indicated by $^*p < 0.05$, $^{**}p < 0.01$. RMS: root mean square.

worsened precision [14, 25], which emphasizes that the functional significance of beta coherence probably also differs according to task demands.

We also investigated the presence of age-related physiological (or essential) tremor as a possible explanation for decreased force precision in older adults [50]. EMG power in the alpha band was greater in TA_{dist} and SOL for old versus young subjects, indicating greater tremor in older subjects in these muscles, as would be expected. Alpha power was also positively associated with RMS error across groups for TA_{prox} and tended strongly to be associated with error for TA_{dist}, which suggests that the degree of rhythmic bursting in EMG had a negative effect on the ability to precisely maintain the target force. Interestingly, we also found positive correlations between the area of alpha coherence and RMS error for five out of six coherence measures. It has been suggested that alpha coherence is related to the central component of physiological tremor [22, 51]; however, group differences in the area of alpha coherence were only significant for Cz-GM, indicating that the area of alpha coherence is not a likely explanation for worsened force precision in older subjects but rather a factor contributing to individual differences in the ability to maintain a target force precisely. This is also supported by the observation that young subjects had greater magnitude of intramuscular alpha coherence at ~10 Hz when coherence was compared between groups at each frequency of interest. Altogether, the significance of these correlations is ambiguous, particularly when taking into account the low magnitudes of alpha coherence area estimates, but the consistency of correlations across different muscles and coherence measures warrants further investigation in future studies.

Nonetheless, greater physiological tremor in older adults may by some means be related to the lack of association observed between beta band coherence and force precision. Though speculative, it is plausible that mechanisms leading to increased tremor in older subjects may have a detrimental effect on the ability to effectively regulate force precision via beta oscillations and thus obscure any positive influence of beta coherence on performance.

5. Conclusion

We have shown that the amount of beta band cortico-, intra-, and intermuscular coherence in ankle muscles is reduced in old versus young adults during static contraction, suggesting an age-related decrease in the strength of oscillatory corticospinal activity during steady-state motor output. Our data also indicate a potential effect of alpha band coherence and tremor on precision control of muscle force. These results may be instrumental in developing new preventive and therapeutic interventions that may strengthen sensorimotor control in elderly subjects. Future projects should focus on delineating the relationship between beta band coherence and specific motor deficits in older adults and exploring mechanisms underlying the observed reduction in effective corticospinal coupling.

Conflicts of Interest

The authors declare that there is no conflict of interest regarding the publication of this article.

Funding

This work was supported by grants from the Danish Medical Research Council (FSS) and the Elsass Fonden.

References

[1] R. D. Seidler, J. A. Bernard, T. B. Burutolu et al., "Motor control and aging: links to age-related brain structural, functional, and biochemical effects," *Neuroscience & Biobehavioral Reviews*, vol. 34, no. 5, pp. 721–733, 2010.

[2] M. Cruz-Jimenez, "Normal changes in gait and mobility problems in the elderly," *Physical Medicine and Rehabilitation Clinics of North America*, vol. 28, no. 4, pp. 713–725, 2017.

[3] N. M. C. W. Oomen and J. H. van Dieën, "Effects of age on force steadiness: s literature review and *meta*-analysis," *Ageing Research Reviews*, vol. 35, pp. 312–321, 2017.

[4] D. H. Salat, D. S. Tuch, D. N. Greve et al., "Age-related alterations in white matter microstructure measured by diffusion tensor imaging," *Neurobiology of Aging*, vol. 26, no. 8, pp. 1215–1227, 2005.

[5] S. Sala, F. Agosta, E. Pagani, M. Copetti, G. Comi, and M. Filippi, "Microstructural changes and atrophy in brain white matter tracts with aging," *Neurobiology of Aging*, vol. 33, no. 3, pp. 488–498.e2, 2012.

[6] E. V. Sullivan, T. Rohlfing, and A. Pfefferbaum, "Quantitative fiber tracking of lateral and interhemispheric white matter systems in normal aging: relations to timed performance," *Neurobiology of Aging*, vol. 31, no. 3, pp. 464–481, 2010.

[7] H. Fujiyama, M. I. Garry, O. Levin, S. P. Swinnen, and J. J. Summers, "Age-related differences in inhibitory processes during interlimb coordination," *Brain Research*, vol. 1262, pp. 38–47, 2009.

[8] A. Oliviero, P. Profice, P. A. Tonali et al., "Effects of aging on motor cortex excitability," *Neuroscience Research*, vol. 55, no. 1, pp. 74–77, 2006.

[9] J. B. Pitcher, K. M. Ogston, and T. S. Miles, "Age and sex differences in human motor cortex input–output characteristics," *The Journal of Physiology*, vol. 546, no. 2, pp. 605–613, 2003.

[10] B. A. Conway, D. M. Halliday, S. F. Farmer et al., "Synchronization between motor cortex and spinal motoneuronal pool during the performance of a maintained motor task in man," *The Journal of Physiology*, vol. 489, no. 3, pp. 917–924, 1995.

[11] D. M. Halliday, B. A. Conway, S. F. Farmer, and J. R. Rosenberg, "Using electroencephalography to study functional coupling between cortical activity and electromyograms during voluntary contractions in humans," *Neuroscience Letters*, vol. 241, no. 1, pp. 5–8, 1998.

[12] S. N. Baker, "Synchronization in monkey motor cortex during a precision grip task. II. Effect of oscillatory activity on corticospinal output," *Journal of Neurophysiology*, vol. 89, no. 4, pp. 1941–1953, 2002.

[13] S. Chen, J. Entakli, M. Bonnard, E. Berton, and J. B. De Graaf, "Functional corticospinal projections from human supplementary motor area revealed by corticomuscular coherence during precise grip force control," *PLoS One*, vol. 8, no. 3, article e60291, 2013.

[14] J. Ushiyama, J. Yamada, M. Liu, and J. Ushiba, "Individual difference in β-band corticomuscular coherence and its relation to force steadiness during isometric voluntary ankle dorsiflexion in healthy humans," *Clinical Neurophysiology*, vol. 128, no. 2, pp. 303–311, 2017.

[15] A. Reyes, C. M. Laine, J. J. Kutch, and F. J. Valero-Cuevas, "Beta band corticomuscular drive reflects muscle coordination strategies," *Frontiers in Computational Neuroscience*, vol. 11, p. 17, 2017.

[16] R. Matsuya, J. Ushiyama, and J. Ushiba, "Inhibitory interneuron circuits at cortical and spinal levels are associated with individual differences in corticomuscular coherence during isometric voluntary contraction," *Scientific Reports*, vol. 7, article 44417, 2017.

[17] S. F. Farmer, F. D. Bremner, D. M. Halliday, J. R. Rosenberg, and J. A. Stephens, "The frequency content of common synaptic inputs to motoneurones studied during voluntary isometric contraction in man," *Physiology*, vol. 470, no. 1, pp. 127–155, 1993.

[18] P. Grosse, M. J. Cassidy, and P. Brown, "EEG–EMG, MEG–EMG and EMG–EMG frequency analysis: physiological principles and clinical applications," *Clinical Neurophysiology*, vol. 113, no. 10, pp. 1523–1531, 2002.

[19] J. M. Kilner, S. N. Baker, S. Salenius, V. Jousmäki, R. Hari, and R. N. Lemon, "Task-dependent modulation of 15-30 Hz coherence between rectified EMGs from human hand and forearm muscles," *The Journal of Physiology*, vol. 516, no. 2, pp. 559–570, 1999.

[20] S. Salenius, K. Portin, M. Kajola, R. Salmelin, and R. Hari, "Cortical control of human motoneuron firing during isometric contraction," *Journal of Neurophysiology*, vol. 77, no. 6, pp. 3401–3405, 1997.

[21] S. Hansen, N. L. Hansen, L. O. D. Christensen, N. T. Petersen, and J. B. Nielsen, "Coupling of antagonistic ankle muscles during co-contraction in humans," *Experimental Brain Research*, vol. 146, no. 3, pp. 282–292, 2002.

[22] J. Raethjen, M. Lindemann, M. Dümpelmann et al., "Corticomuscular coherence in the 6–15 Hz band: is the cortex involved in the generation of physiologic tremor?," *Experimental Brain Research*, vol. 142, no. 1, pp. 32–40, 2002.

[23] M. B. Bayram, V. Siemionow, and G. H. Yue, "Weakening of corticomuscular signal coupling during voluntary motor action in aging," *The Journals of Gerontology: Series A*, vol. 70, no. 8, pp. 1037–1043, 2015.

[24] D. Kamp, V. Krause, M. Butz, A. Schnitzler, and B. Pollok, "Changes of cortico-muscular coherence: an early marker of healthy aging?," *Age*, vol. 35, no. 1, pp. 49–58, 2013.

[25] S. Graziadio, A. Basu, L. Tomasevic, F. Zappasodi, F. Tecchio, and J. A. Eyre, "Developmental tuning and decay in senescence of oscillations linking the corticospinal system," *The Journal of Neuroscience*, vol. 30, no. 10, pp. 3663–3674, 2010.

[26] S. R. Jaiser, M. R. Baker, and S. N. Baker, "Intermuscular coherence in normal adults: variability and changes with age," *PLoS One*, vol. 11, no. 2, article e0149029, 2016.

[27] T. Watanabe, K. Saito, K. Ishida, S. Tanabe, and I. Nojima, "Coordination of plantar flexor muscles during bipedal and unipedal stances in young and elderly adults," *Experimental Brain Research*, pp. 1–11, 2018.

[28] J. G. Semmler, "Motor-unit coherence during isometric contractions is greater in a hand muscle of older adults," *Journal of Neurophysiology*, vol. 90, no. 2, pp. 1346–1349, 2003.

[29] J. B. Nielsen, "How we walk: central control of muscle activity during human walking," *The Neuroscientist*, vol. 9, no. 3, pp. 195–204, 2003.

[30] M. F. Folstein, S. E. Folstein, and P. R. McHugh, "'Mini-mental state'. A practical method for grading the cognitive state of patients for the clinician," *Journal of Psychiatric Research*, vol. 12, no. 3, pp. 189–198, 1975.

[31] L. J. Elias and M. P. Bryden, "Footedness is a better predictor of language lateralisation than handedness," *Laterality: Asymmetries of Body, Brain and Cognition*, vol. 3, no. 1, pp. 41–52, 1998.

[32] A. Delorme and S. Makeig, "EEGLAB: an open source toolbox for analysis of single-trial EEG dynamics including independent component analysis," *Journal of Neuroscience Methods*, vol. 134, no. 1, pp. 9–21, 2004.

[33] M. Chaumon, D. V. M. Bishop, and N. A. Busch, "A practical guide to the selection of independent components of the electroencephalogram for artifact correction," *Journal of Neuroscience Methods*, vol. 250, pp. 47–63, 2015.

[34] D. M. Halliday and S. F. Farmer, "On the need for rectification of surface EMG," *Journal of Neurophysiology*, vol. 103, no. 6, article 3547, 2010.

[35] N. J. Ward, S. F. Farmer, L. Berthouze, and D. M. Halliday, "Rectification of EMG in low force contractions improves detection of motor unit coherence in the beta-frequency band," *Journal of Neurophysiology*, vol. 110, no. 8, pp. 1744–1750, 2013.

[36] D. M. Halliday, J. R. Rosenberg, A. M. Amjad, P. Breeze, B. A. Conway, and S. F. Farmer, "A framework for the analysis of mixed time series/point process data—theory and application to the study of physiological tremor, single motor unit discharges and electromyograms," *Progress in Biophysics and Molecular Biology*, vol. 64, no. 2-3, pp. 237–278, 1995.

[37] S. F. Farmer, J. Gibbs, D. M. Halliday et al., "Changes in EMG coherence between long and short thumb abductor muscles during human development," *The Journal of Physiology*, vol. 579, no. 2, pp. 389–402, 2007.

[38] A. M. Amjad, D. M. Halliday, J. R. Rosenberg, and B. A. Conway, "An extended difference of coherence test for comparing and combining several independent coherence estimates: theory and application to the study of motor units and physiological tremor," *Journal of Neuroscience Methods*, vol. 73, no. 1, pp. 69–79, 1997.

[39] S. N. Baker, J. M. Kilner, E. M. Pinches, and R. N. Lemon, "The role of synchrony and oscillations in the motor output," *Experimental Brain Research*, vol. 128, no. 1-2, pp. 109–117, 1999.

[40] S. F. Farmer, M. Swash, D. A. Ingram, and J. A. Stephens, "Changes in motor unit synchronization following central nervous lesions in man," *The Journal of Physiology*, vol. 463, no. 1, pp. 83–105, 1993.

[41] T. Mima, C. Gerloff, J. Steger, and M. Hallett, "Frequency-coding of motor control system—coherence and phase estimation between cortical rhythm and motoneuronal firing in humans," *Society for Neuroscience - Abstracts*, vol. 24, article 1768, 1998.

[42] N. L. Hansen and J. B. Nielsen, "The effect of transcranial magnetic stimulation and peripheral nerve stimulation on corticomuscular coherence in humans," *The Journal of Physiology*, vol. 561, no. 1, pp. 295–306, 2004.

[43] H. Haug and R. Eggers, "Morphometry of the human cortex cerebri and corpus striatum during aging," *Neurobiology of Aging*, vol. 12, no. 4, pp. 336–338, 1991.

[44] P. R. Huttenlocher, "Synaptic density in human frontal cortex — developmental changes and effects of aging," *Brain Research*, vol. 163, no. 2, pp. 195–205, 1979.

[45] B. Anderson and V. Rutledge, "Age and hemisphere effects on dendritic structure," *Brain*, vol. 119, no. 6, pp. 1983–1990, 1996.

[46] V. S. Mattay, F. Fera, A. Tessitore et al., "Neurophysiological correlates of age-related changes in human motor function," *Neurology*, vol. 58, no. 4, pp. 630–635, 2002.

[47] S. Heuninckx, N. Wenderoth, F. Debaere, R. Peeters, and S. P. Swinnen, "Neural basis of aging: the penetration of cognition into action control," *The Journal of Neuroscience*, vol. 25, no. 29, pp. 6787–6796, 2005.

[48] S. Heuninckx, N. Wenderoth, and S. P. Swinnen, "Systems neuroplasticity in the aging brain: recruiting additional neural resources for successful motor performance in elderly persons," *The Journal of Neuroscience*, vol. 28, no. 1, pp. 91–99, 2008.

[49] R. Kristeva, L. Patino, and W. Omlor, "Beta-range cortical motor spectral power and corticomuscular coherence as a mechanism for effective corticospinal interaction during steady-state motor output," *NeuroImage*, vol. 36, no. 3, pp. 785–792, 2007.

[50] F. Gövert, J. S. Becktepe, and G. Deuschl, "Current concepts of essential tremor," *Revue Neurologique*, vol. 172, no. 8-9, pp. 416–422, 2016.

[51] J. F. Marsden, P. Brown, and S. Salenius, "Involvement of the sensorimotor cortex in physiological force and action tremor," *Neuroreport*, vol. 12, no. 9, pp. 1937–1941, 2001.

4

Brain-Specific SNAP-25 Deletion Leads to Elevated Extracellular Glutamate Level and Schizophrenia-Like Behavior in Mice

Hua Yang,[1] Mengjie Zhang,[1] Jiahao Shi,[1] Yunhe Zhou,[1] Zhipeng Wan,[1] Yicheng Wang,[2] Yinghan Wan,[2] Jun Li,[2] Zhugang Wang,[2] and Jian Fei[1,2]

[1]*School of Life Science and Technology, Tongji University, Shanghai 200092, China*
[2]*Shanghai Engineering Research Center of Model Organisms (SRCMO/SMOC), Shanghai 201203, China*

Correspondence should be addressed to Jian Fei; jfei@tongji.edu.cn

Academic Editor: Depei Li

Several studies have associated reduced expression of synaptosomal-associated protein of 25 kDa (SNAP-25) with schizophrenia, yet little is known about its role in the illness. In this paper, a forebrain glutamatergic neuron-specific SNAP-25 knockout mouse model was constructed and studied to explore the possible pathogenetic role of SNAP-25 in schizophrenia. We showed that SNAP-25 conditional knockout (cKO) mice exhibited typical schizophrenia-like phenotype. A significantly elevated extracellular glutamate level was detected in the cerebral cortex of the mouse model. Compared with Ctrls, SNAP-25 was dramatically reduced by about 60% both in cytoplasm and in membrane fractions of cerebral cortex of cKOs, while the other two core members of SNARE complex: Syntaxin-1 (increased ~80%) and Vamp2 (increased ~96%) were significantly increased in cell membrane part. Riluzole, a glutamate release inhibitor, significantly attenuated the locomotor hyperactivity deficits in cKO mice. Our findings provide *in vivo* functional evidence showing a critical role of SNAP-25 dysfunction on synaptic transmission, which contributes to the developmental of schizophrenia. It is suggested that a SNAP-25 cKO mouse, a valuable model for schizophrenia, could address questions regarding presynaptic alterations that contribute to the etiopathophysiology of SZ and help to consummate the pre- and postsynaptic glutamatergic pathogenesis of the illness.

1. Introduction

Schizophrenia (SZ), a complicated psychiatric disorder, affects almost 1 percent of the general population in the world [1, 2]. While the etiology and pathophysiology of SZ remain elusive, genetic risk factors are recognized as an important contributing factor to the pathogenesis of this neuropsychiatric disorder [3]. It has been documented that the synaptosomal-associated protein of 25 kDa (SNAP-25) is a candidate risk gene for SZ, as supported by the following lines of evidence: (1) Genetic association and linkage studies have revealed that chromosome region 20p12.2 which SNAP-25 locates in has significant linkage with SZ [4, 5]. (2) Large-scale genome-associated case-control studies have revealed that several single nucleotide polymorphisms (SNPs) of SNAP-25 are significantly associated with SZ [6]. (3) Various postmortem analyses have found that the expression of SNAP-25 is reduced in prefrontal cortex (PFC) and hippocampus in brain of patients with SZ [7–9]. However, how the reduction of SNAP-25 level is involved in the pathological phenotype remains unknown.

In the brain, SNAP-25 proteins are abundantly expressed in glutamatergic terminals, while relatively lower amounts of the protein are detectable in GABAergic terminals [10]. The primary role of SNAP-25 is a fundamental component of soluble N-ethylmaleimide-sensitive factor attachment protein receptor (SNARE). Together with cell membrane protein syntaxin and vesicle-associated membrane protein (VAMP), SNAP-25 mediates presynaptic vesicle docking and exocytosis [11]. In addition to regulation of synaptic transmission, SNAP-25 is also believed to regulate intracellular calcium dynamics through negative modulation of voltage-gated calcium channels. It also plays a role in other neuronal processes, including spine morphogenesis, postsynaptic receptor trafficking, and neuronal plasticity [12]. But the underlying cellular mechanisms still need to be explored.

Over the past few decades, several mouse models have been constructed to elucidate the physiological role of SNAP-25 *in vivo*. Complete knockout of SNAP-25 in mice leads to no evoked exocytosis and death of the animal at birth. However, heterozygous mice are able to survive and exhibit locomotor hyperactivity and learning deficiencies. SNAP-25 knock-in mice, which have a single amino acid substitution of Ala for Ser187, have been shown to display epilepsy and anxiety-related behavior. The blind-drunk (Bdr) mouse expresses a dominant point mutant SNAP-25b protein, resulting in impaired sensorimotor gating and ataxia, while SNAP-25b-deficient model has developmental defects, seizures, and impaired synaptic plasticity. Conclusively, SNAP-25 mouse mutants occupied a series of psychophenotypes. However, the results derived from different models were inconsistent or conflicting, and no convincing evidence has supported an association between SNAP-25 and SZ. Therefore, additional investigations are necessary to demonstrate the possible role of SNAP-25 in SZ.

Taking into account that the cerebral cortex and hippocampus are the critical brain areas associated with SZ, brain-specific SNAP-25 knockout mice are most suitable to explore the relationship between SNAP-25 and SZ. Furthermore, SNAP-25 has been highly expressed both in neuron and endocrine cells, so brain-targeted SNAP-25 modification is capable of excluding interference signals from the surrounding system. In this study, we designed a brain-specific SNAP-25 knockout mouse, through behavioral phenotyping, molecular detection, and drug treatment within this model, to explore the possible pathogenetic role of SNAP-25 in SZ.

2. Materials and Methods

2.1. Animals. Mice were maintained in a specific pathogen-free (SPF) facility under a 12 h light/dark cycles. All animal protocols were approved by the Institutional Animal Care and Use Committee at Shanghai Research Center for Model Organisms (number 2015-0005). Mice were sacrificed with carbon dioxide when experiments were completed.

2.2. Generation of SNAP-25 cKO Mice. Genomic DNA of SCR012 ES cells isolated from 129S6/SvEv mouse strain was utilized to amplify SNAP-25 homologous fragments. The targeting strategy is flanking exon 4 of the mouse SNAP-25 gene with two loxP cassettes. Chimera mice were constructed by injecting recombination-positive ES cells into blastocyst and backcrossed to C57BL/6J mice. SNAP-$25^{L2/L2}$: CaMKIIα-$Cre^{+/wt}$ mice were obtained by regular breeding procedure between SNAP-$25^{L2/L2}$ mice and CaMKIIα-Cre strain (The Jackson Laboratory, stock number 005359) in which Cre-recombinase is extensively expressed in forebrain excitatory neurons by p20 [13, 14]. PCR genotyping was performed with genomic DNA isolated from mouse tail tissue. The primers used for genotyping were designed for identifying loxP (forward: 5′-CACTGCAGAGATTGCA GTATCACTA-3′, reverse: 5′- CAATGCACAGTTATTG TATTGAAGG-3′), and Cre sequences (forward: 5′- AGCG ATGGATTTCCGTCTCTGG-3′, reverse: 5′- AGCTTGCAT GATCTCCGGTATTGAA -3′).

2.3. Western Blot Analysis. Cell cytosolic or membrane protein lysates of mouse brain tissues were prepared using Mem-PER Plus Membrane Protein Extraction Kit (Thermo Scientific, 89842). Then, the lysates were separated by SDS–PAGE and probed with specific antibodies: SNAP-25 (Abcam, ab66066), SNAP-23 (Abcam, ab3340), syntaxin (Santa Cruz, sc-12736), Vamp2 (Abcam, ab6276), Munc-18 (SYSY, 116002), Phospho-Synaptotagmin (R&D Systems, PPS085), β-ACTIN (Abcam, ab6276), TUBULIN (Abcam, ab15246), and Na/K ATPase (Millipore, 05-369). For quantification, the densitometry measurement of each band was first normalized to that of β-ACTIN, TUBULIN, or Na/K ATPase (used as loading control) and then averaged from at least three independent samples.

2.4. Immunofluorescence Staining. Sagittal brain sections (15 μm in thickness) were prepared from a fixed brain with 4% paraformaldehyde, and immunostaining was performed as described [15]. Antibodies used for the immunostaining were SNAP-25 (Abcam, ab66066) and VGLUT1 (SYSY, 135304). Fluorescence was analyzed on a Nikon A1R confocal microscope (Nikon Instruments, Shanghai, CN).

2.5. Behavioral Testing. Behavioral phenotyping was performed on age-paired adult male mice (8 to 12 weeks for both cKO and Ctrl littermates). Prior to testing, mice were habituated to the testing room for 2 h.

2.5.1. Open-Field Test. The open field is a square arena ($40 \times 42 \times 30$ cm). 8 cm width elongated area along the wall is defined as the "peripheral zone," approximately 66% of the total area. We place the mouse in the center of the box and enable it to move freely for 15 mins, and an infrared tracking system (Kinder Scientific, Julian, USA) was borrowed to record the movement.

2.5.2. Prepulse Inhibition of the Startle Response. The Acoustic Startle Reflex Starter Package and Startle Reflex 5 software system (Med Associates Inc., St. Albans, VT) was used to assess prepulse inhibition (PPI). The test began with placing the mouse in the chamber's cylinder to acclimate for 5 mins. The remainder of the test consisted of two blocks of trials. A 65 dB background sound was presented throughout the session. The first block consisted of twenty trials of 20 ms and 105 dB sound served as startle stimuli and presented with different intertrial intervals (10–30 s). The second block consisted of 50 trials, with five varying trial types: startle only, or a 10 ms prepulse sound at 70, 75, 80, and 85 dB appeared 50 ms before the startle stimulus. The trial types were presented in random order with intertrial interval range from 10 to 30 s. Percent PPI of the startle response was calculated as the following formula: [1 – (startle response to prepulse + startle/startle response to startle only)] × 100.

2.5.3. Social Approach-Avoidance. The test was carried out as previously described [16]. Approach-avoidance behaviors toward an unfamiliar social partner were recorded by an infrared tracking system. The arena was a plastic open field (42 × 42 cm) containing an empty wire mesh cage (10 × 8 cm) located at one side of the field. During the first session ("no target"), the experimental mouse was introduced into the field and its trajectory was tracked for 5 mins. During the second session ("target 1"), the conditions were identical except that a social target animal (an unfamiliar C57BL/6J male mouse) had been introduced into the cage, and for the third session ("target 2"), the social target mouse was an unfamiliar C57BL/6J female. The tracking data from both the "no target" and "target" conditions were used to determine the time spent by the experimental mouse in the "interaction zone" (an 8 cm wide corridor surrounding the cage) and in the "corners" of the open field opposite to the location of the cage.

2.5.4. Hole-Board Test. The apparatus was a white wooden board (25 × 25 cm) with 16 evenly spaced holes. The number of head-dips was recorded by KS motor infrared monitor system over a 30-minute period.

2.5.5. Nest Building Assay. The nest building test was performed as previously described [17]. Briefly, one square piece of material made of cotton fibre (5 × 5 cm) was put in a cage with an individual mouse. Pictures of the nests were taken 16 h later. The quality of the nest was assessed using the following score: 1, nest not noticeably touched; 2, nest partially torn up; 3, mostly shredded but not identifiable nest site; 4, an identifiable but flat nest; 5, a well-defined nest with walls.

2.5.6. Passive Avoidance Task. The apparatus employed in the passive avoidance task is composed of compartment shuttle chambers, one dark with shock generator and other illuminated compartments. In acquisition trials (2 days), the mouse was allowed to explore the apparatus freely for 5 mins. It would encounter an electric shock (0.5 mA, 2 s duration) once it was inside of the dark chamber with all four paws. On the third day of the trial, the mouse was positioned in the illuminated compartment. Its latency to enter the dark compartment (step-through latency) was recorded automatically.

2.6. In Vivo Brain Microdialysis. In vivo brain microdialysis was carried out to measure glutamate content in the extracellular fluid in the cerebral cortex as previously described [18]. After mice had been anesthetized with inhaled isofluorane (3%), the cerebral cortex was surgically exposed and a microdialysis probe (MAB6.14.2) was inserted into the following coordinates relative to the bregma in mm: −2 to the anterior/posterior axis, ±2.0 to the lateral/medial axis, and −2.5 to the dorsal/ventral axis. Microdialysis was performed by perfusing of the probe with artificial cerebrospinal fluid at a flow rate of 2 μL/min via a microinfusing pump. The total volume of each dialysate sample (20 mins) was 40 μL. Samples were stored at −80°C until use.

2.7. Preparation of Tissue Samples for HPLC. Cerebral cortex and hippocampus tissues were isolated from the brains of *SNAP-25* cKO mice and their age- and sex-paired control littermates. After weighing, the samples were homogenized in ice-cold 0.4 M $HClO_4$ and centrifuged at 10,000*g* for 15 mins at 4°C. Then, 1 μL of supernatant was mixed with 750 μL of 2 M $KHCO_3$ and centrifuged at 3,000*g* for 5 mins. Supernatant was gathered and stored at −80°C until use.

2.8. High-Performance Liquid Chromatography (HPLC). HPLC analyses were performed in the State Key Laboratory of Medical Neurobiology of Fudan University as previously described [19]. The Agilent 1260 series neurotransmitter analyzer (Agilent Technologies, Santa Clara, CA) was utilized to detect the concentrations of amino acid neurotransmitters. Peaks and relative concentrations were identified by comparison to known external standards (Sigma-Aldrich).

2.9. Drug Treatments. Clozapine and LY354740 were purchased from Sigma-Aldrich (St. Louis, MO, USA), and lamotrigine was the product of Glaxosmithkline (Brentford, Middlesex, UK). For stock solutions, clozapine was dissolved in 0.1 M HCl and buffered with NaOH to achieve a final pH of 6.5–7.5. Riluzole was suspended in 10 *w*/*v*% cyclodextrin/saline, and LY354740 or lamotrigine was dissolved in saline. Vehicle was developed in an identical manner without the addition of drug, respectively. Concentrated aliquots of both drugs and vehicles were stored at −20°C. On the day of dosing, aliquots were thawed and diluted to their final concentration in sterile saline. Vehicles or clozapine (2.5 mg/kg), riluzole (10 mg/kg), and LY354740 (15 mg/kg) were injected intraperitoneally into age-matched male mice (8–12 weeks old), respectively, and submitted to the open-field test 30 mins later. Lamotrigine was administered to mice by gavage at a dose of 60 mg/kg per day for 2 weeks, followed by behavior testing.

The dose of drug was selected according to previously used doses in mouse behavioral studies [20–23] and our preliminary tests.

2.10. Statistical Analysis. Results are shown as the mean ± SEM. Student's *t*-test was utilized to compare two means and two-way ANOVA followed by Bonferroni test to compare multiple means. The nest building scores were treated as nonparametric data, and statistical analysis was performed using Kruskal-Wallis one-way analysis on ranks followed by multiple comparison using Dunn's method. All statistical analyses were performed using Excel 2010 (Microsoft) or GraphPad Prism 5.0. $P < 0.05$ was examined statistically significant.

3. Results

3.1. Generation of SNAP-25 Forebrain-Specific KO Mice. We generated the SNAP-25-floxed mouse strain SNAP-$25^{L2/L2}$ through inserting of loxP cassettes in the flank sequence of exon4 loci, which caused a frame shifting by Cre-loxP recombinant mechanism (Figure 1(a)). The mouse strain was crossed with CaMKIIα-Cre transgenic mice to generate forebrain-specific SNAP-25 cKO (SNAP-$25^{L2/L2}$:

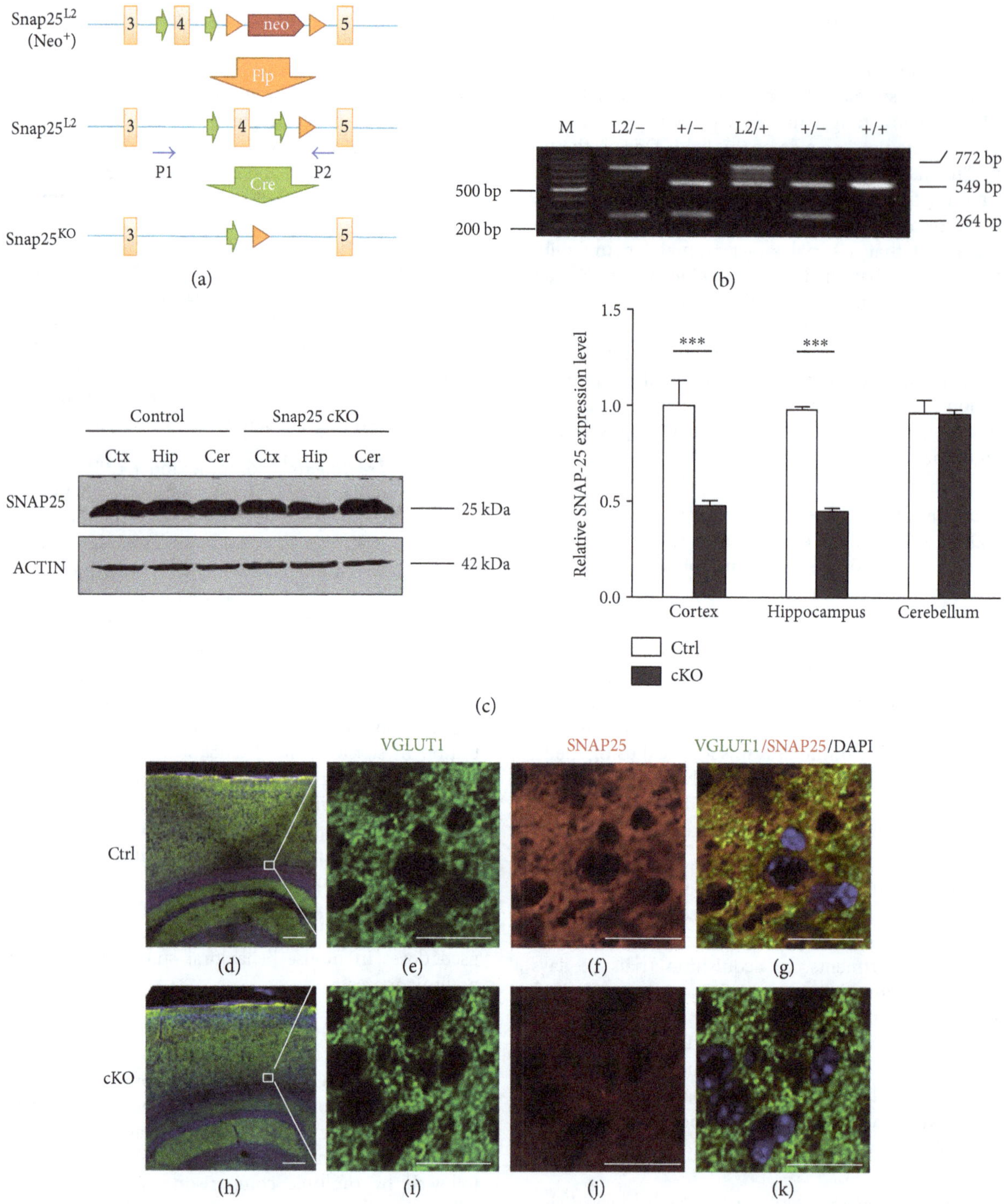

FIGURE 1: Generation of SNAP-25 forebrain-specific KO mice. (a) Targeting strategy used for the deletion of the SNAP-25 exon 4. P1-2 referred to PCR primers for genotyping, which is located on intron flank exon 4 separately. (b) PCR genotyping of recombinant SNAP-25 locus. (c) Western blot analysis of brain extracts of Ctrl and mutant mice. Right panel: quantitative analysis of western blot images. $n = 3$ per group. $^{***}P < 0.001$ compared with control littermates. (d–k) Immunostaining with anti-SNAP-25 (red) and anti-VGLUT1 (green) of cortex of sagittal sections from adult mice brains. Scale bars are 20 μm in (d) and 200 μm in (e).

CaMKIIα-Cre$^{+/wt}$) model. As we expected, the PCR product of wild-type SNAP-25 allele was 549 bp, whereas the floxed SNAP-25 allele (L2) was 772 bp and the knockout one (L-) was 264 bp. The accuracy of fragments was verified by sequencing (Figure 1(b)). SNAP-25 deletion in different brain areas was confirmed at protein levels. Dramatic reduction of SNAP-25 expression was observed in the cortex and hippocampus but no obvious change in the cerebellum of cKO mice (Figure 1(c)). Furthermore, we executed immunofluorescence examination with anti-SNAP-25 and anti-VGLUT1 (glutamatergic neuron marker) staining. It was found that abundant SNAP-25-positive glutamatergic

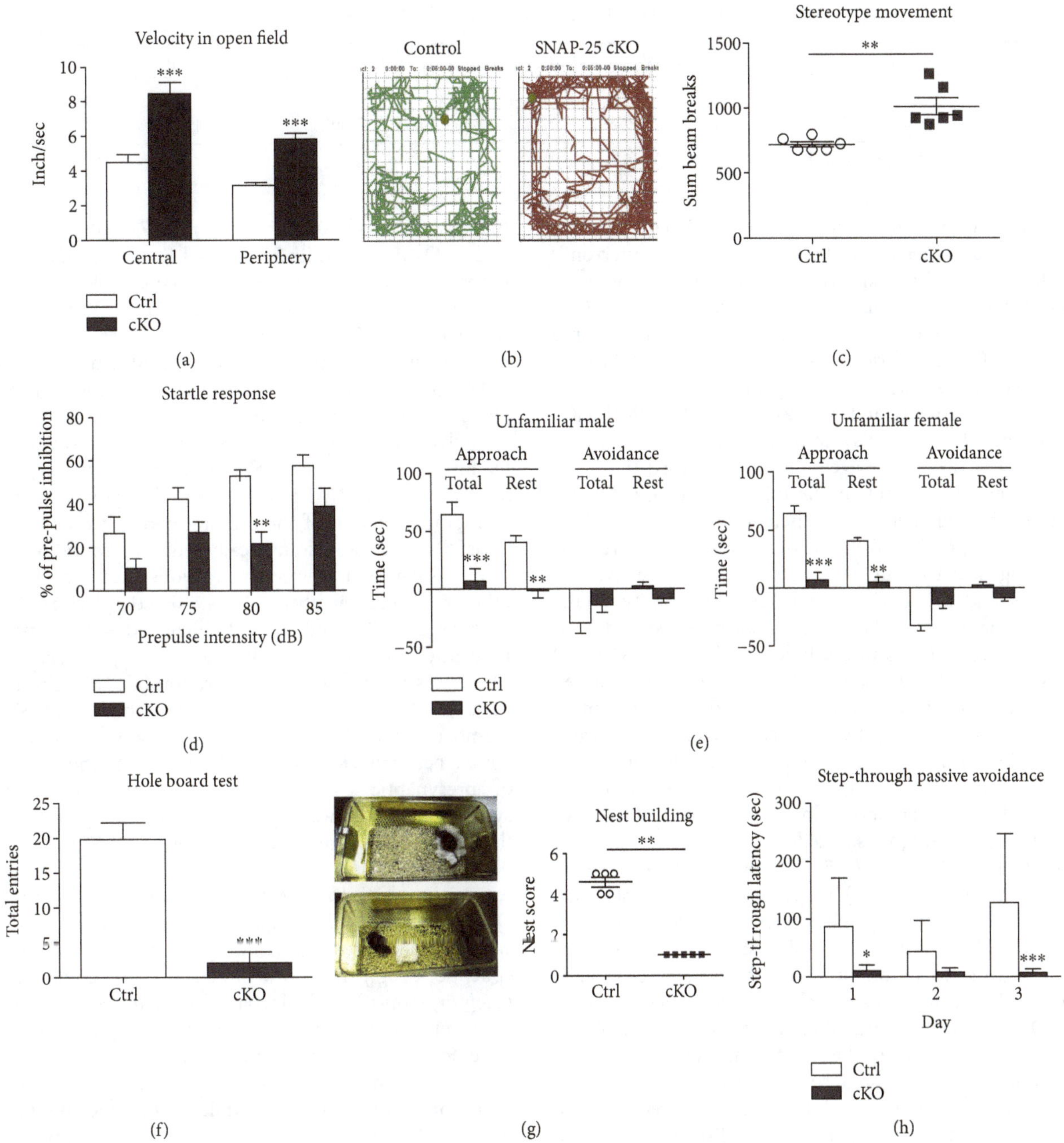

FIGURE 2: SNAP-25 cKO mice exhibit schizophrenia-like phenotype. (a–d) Summary plots of velocity, movement trajectory, stereotype movement in the open-field test ($n = 6$), and reduced prepulse inhibition ($n = 5$). (e) cKOs display deficient social skills as shown by social approach-avoidance test ($n = 10$). (f) cKOs occupy an impaired tendency to explore novel environment in hole-board test ($n = 6$). (g) Nest building. Left panel: pictures show the results of nesting of different genotypic mice. Right panel: statistical results of nesting scores ($n = 5$). (h) cKOs display impaired learning and memory in the step-through passive avoidance task ($n = 10$). $^{*}P < 0.05$, $^{**}P < 0.01$, and $^{***}P < 0.001$ compared with control littermates.

neurons were detected in the cerebral cortex of Ctrl mice, whereas little staining was found in those of cKOs, confirming that SNAP-25 was inactivated in forebrain glutamatergic neurons (Figures 1(d), 1(e), 1(f), 1(g), 1(h), 1(i), 1(j), and 1(k)).

3.2. SNAP-25 cKO Mice Exhibit SZ-Like Phenotype. To determine whether SNAP-25 cKO mice occupy behavioral impairments, we subjected these animals to a battery of behavioral tests. First, in the open-field test, cKO mice showed a significant increased locomotion (3.326 ± 0.160 versus 5.879 ± 0.334 inch/sec, $P < 0.0001$, $n = 6$) and remarkably enhanced stereotype movements (718.50 ± 20.74 versus 1012.00 ± 64.42 breaks, $P < 0.05$, $n = 6$) compared with their control littermates (SNAP-25$^{L2/L2}$, Ctrl, hereafter), demonstrating the abnormal hyperactivity and stereotypical behavior of cKOs (Figures 2(a), 2(b), and 2(c)). Acoustic startle test revealed that prepulse inhibition (PPI) was

Table 1: Mating and nursing test of SNAP-25 cKO females (crossed with C57BL/6 J male).

Genotype	Total pairs	Pregnant females	Born pups	Mean ± SEM	Survival pups	Mean ± SEM
Ctrl	10	9	57	5.70 ± 0.76	57	5.70 ± 0.76
cKO	10	4	25	2.50 ± 1.05*	13	1.30 ± 0.87**

*$P < 0.05$ and **$P < 0.01$ compared with Ctrl.

significantly decreased in the group of cKOs compared to Ctrls [F (1, 8) = 24.37, $P < 0.0001$, $n = 5$], and Bonferroni's post hoc comparison showed a significant disruption of PPI at the prepulse level of 80 dB ($P < 0.01$) (Figure 2(d)). There was no significant difference in the startle response between cKOs and Ctrls, suggesting no apparent hearing deficit (data not shown). Thus, hyperactivity, enhanced stereotypical movements and reduced PPI of SNAP-25 cKO mice fit into the positive symptoms of SZ.

For social behavior judgement, first, we used the social approach-avoidance test to probe animals for their voluntary initiation of social interaction. When presented with an unfamiliar partner, Ctrls had the tendency to spend more time interacting socially, but cKOs displayed intense aversive responses and spent less time in close proximity to the stranger (Figure 2(e)). Also, the significantly reduced head dipping times of cKOs in the hole-board test (19.83 ± 2.39 versus 1.67 ± 1.31 entries, $P < 0.0001$, $n = 6$) also reflected an impaired tendency to explore a novel environment (Figure 2(f)). By mating two genotypic females with wild-type C57BL/6J males, paired for a 4-month period, we observed that both the pregnancy rate and survival pups of cKO females were significantly lower than Ctrls, but the litter size per pregnant mother showed no difference between two groups (6.33 ± 0.47 versus 6.25 ± 0.63 pups/mother, $P = 0.92$, Ctrls $n = 9$, and cKOs $n = 4$), which indicates that both mating and maternal nursing behaviors were defective in cKOs (Table 1). While Ctrls could build clean and typical nests after 16 h with the nesting material, the nests of cKO mice were poorly formed. Substantially decreased nesting score of cKO mice demonstrated their impaired self-care ability (Figure 2(g)). Collectively, the results of the above behavioral tests showed that impaired social skills, exploratory tendency, self-care, and nursing abilities have occurred in cKOs. The cKO mice thus fit the criteria established for negative symptoms of SZ.

To determine whether cKOs have deficits in hippocampus-dependent learning and memory processes, we subjected mice to the step-through passive avoidance task. During the 3-day experiment, cKOs stepped faster into the darker-shock chamber than Ctrls. After subjected to electric shock, the step-through latencies of cKOs were more statistically pronounced compared with Ctrls, which indicated impaired learning and memory of cKOs (Figure 2(h)).

3.3. Elevated Glutamate Level in the Cortex of SNAP-25 cKO Mice. We measured the content of glutamate in cerebral cortex and hippocampus of two mice groups by combining *in vivo* microdialysis and HPLC. As indicated in Figure 3(a), a significant increase in glutamate concentration was detected in the microdialysis fluid of the cerebral cortex (0.27 ± 0.02 versus 0.72 ± 0.14 μg/mL, $P < 0.05$, Ctrls $n = 5$, and cKOs $n = 6$), while unchanged level were inspected in hippocampus area (0.48 ± 0.12 versus 0.58 ± 0.17 μg/mL, $P = 0.63$, Ctrls $n = 5$, and cKOs $n = 6$) in cKOs compared with Ctrl mice. However, there was no observable alteration between the concentration of amino acid neurotransmitters of homogenates freshly prepared from the same brain subregions of the cKO and Ctrl mice (Figure 3(b)).

Subsequently, by using TUBULIN and Na/K ATPase as loading controls, respectively, we examined the expression level of all three SNARE members in the cytoplasm and cell membrane fraction of the cerebral cortex. Compared with Ctrls, SNAP-25 was dramatically reduced around 60% both in cytoplasm and membrane fractions of cKOs, while the other two core members of SNARE complex: Syntaxin-1 (increased ~80%) and Vamp2 (increased ~96%) were significantly increased in cell membrane part (Figure 4). There was no difference in expression of SNAP-25 homologous molecule—SNAP-23 or another important SNARE member—Munc-18 in the cell membrane of the cerebral cortex between cKOs and Ctrls. However, the expression of presynaptic calcium sensor protein—phosphorylated synaptotagmin-1—was significantly elevated about 93% in the cell membrane of the cerebral cortex of cKOs.

3.4. Antipsychotic Drugs Attenuated Locomotor Hyperactivity Deficits in cKO Mice. Antipsychotic drugs, clozapine (atypical schizophrenic drug), lamotrigine (broad-spectrum antiepileptic drug), LY354740 (metabotropic glutamate 2/3 receptor agonist), and riluzole (glutamate release inhibitor) were selected to examine their effects on the locomotor hyperactivities and stereotype behavior of cKO mice. Compared with controls, LY354740 treatment has no detectable effects on all four test index, while lamotrigine could reduce the stereotype movement of cKOs. Administration of either clozapine or riluzole was able to significantly attenuate the hyperactivity and stereotype movements of the SNAP-25 cKO mice (Figure 5).

4. Discussion

SNAP-25 is a key molecule involved in synaptic vesicle docking and neurotransmitter release. In line with its central role in neuronal function, it is thought that SNAP-25 is related to human neurological syndromes, especially SZ. In this study, we specifically deleted SNAP-25 gene in forebrain glutamatergic neurons with utilization of the Cre/LoxP strategy. The phenotypes observed in this model fit into SZ-like behaviors, which include positive symptoms (such as hyperlocomotion and reduced PPI), negative symptoms (decreased motivation and impaired social skills), and

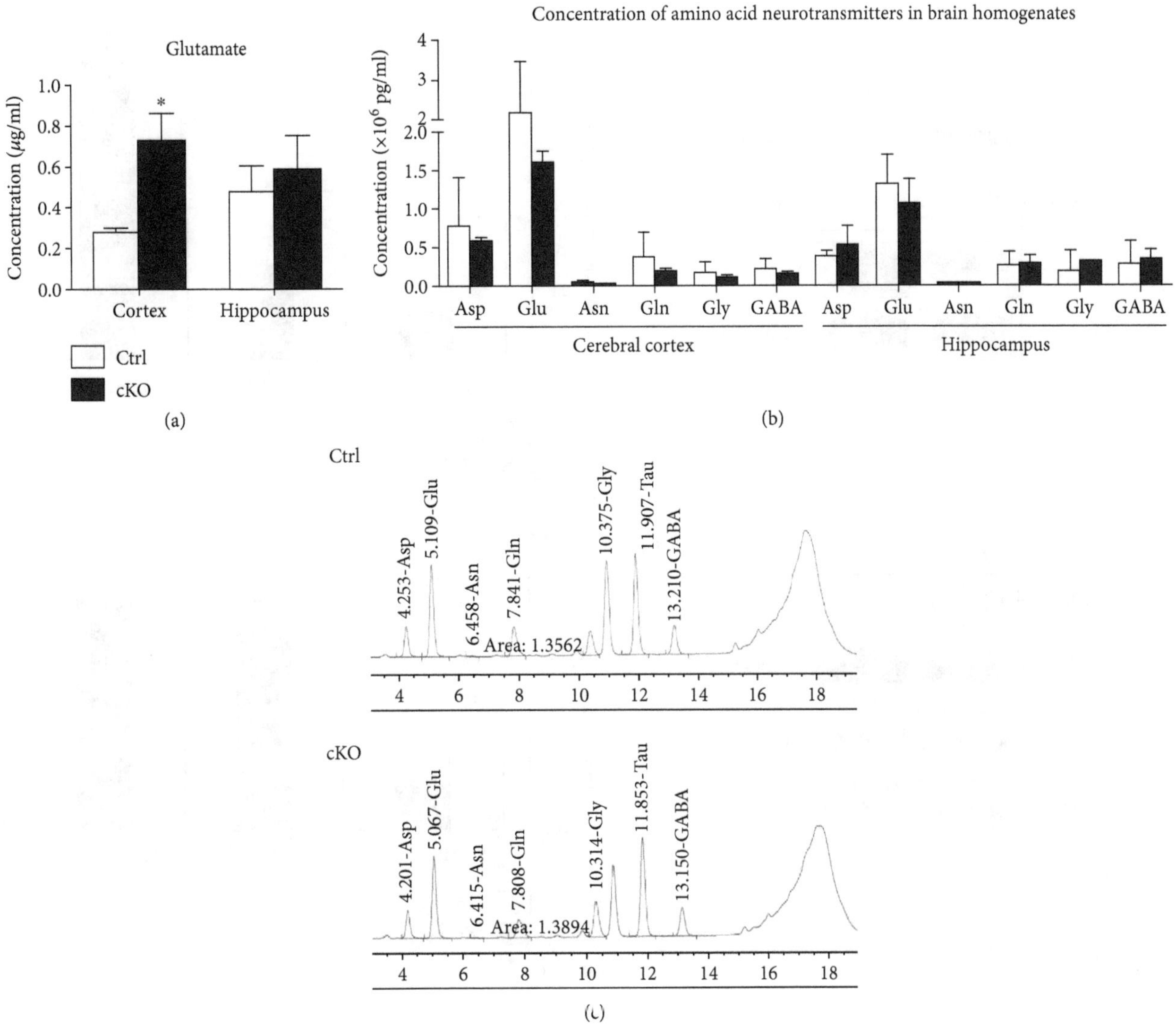

FIGURE 3: Elevated cortex glutamate level of SNAP-25 cKO mice. (a) The concentration of glutamate (μg/mL) in the microdialysis fluid (Ctrls, $n = 5$; cKOs, $n = 6$). (b) The concentration of amino acid neurotransmitters ($\times 10^6$ pg/mL) in brain homogenates ($n = 5$ per group). (c) The original representative HPLC figures of different genotypic mice. $^*P < 0.05$ compared with control littermates. Asp: aspartate; Glu: glutamate; Asn: asparaginate; Gln: glutamine; Gly: glycine; GABA: γ-aminobutyric acid.

memory deficit. Our results provided *in vivo* functional evidence to support that altered SNAP-25 expression in the forebrain glutamatergic neurons lead to a greater effect of the illness, confirming the strong association between SNAP-25 and SZ.

It is well known that SNAP-25 plays a key role in medicating neurotransmitter release. Previous studies provided evidence that botulinum neurotoxin type A (BoNT/A) could block synaptic vesicle neuroexocytosis by proteolytic cleavage of SNAP-25, indicating that SNAP-25-deficiency could inhibit neurotransmitter release [24]. However, by *in vivo* brain microdialysis, we found the remarkable elevation of extracellular glutamate levels in cerebral cortex of SNAP-25 cKO mice. No noticeable difference in the total content of amino acid neurotransmitters in the same brain subregions was found between the two groups. Subsequent western blot test revealed the elevated gathering of the SNARE proteins on the cell membrane, which indicated the possibility of increased synaptic vesicle assembly and release. SNAP-25 inactivation seemed not only to fail to block synaptic transmission but also to enhance glutamatergic neurotransmitter in the cortex of cKOs. Previously, Antonucci et al. reported that reduced SNAP-25 levels lead to enhanced evoked glutamatergic transmission in hippocampal cultures and identified that this consequence was not due to changes in a releasable pool of synaptic vesicles [25]. However, we did not detect a statistical difference in hippocampus microdialysis, and we do not know the exact reason yet. We noticed that there were several differences between our and their works: (1) the developmental state of animals (adult mice and E18 mice embryos); (2) the experimental condition (intact animal under physiological condition and *in vitro* cultured cell model); and (3) the detective method (*in vivo* brain microdialysis and whole-cell patch-clamp recording). All

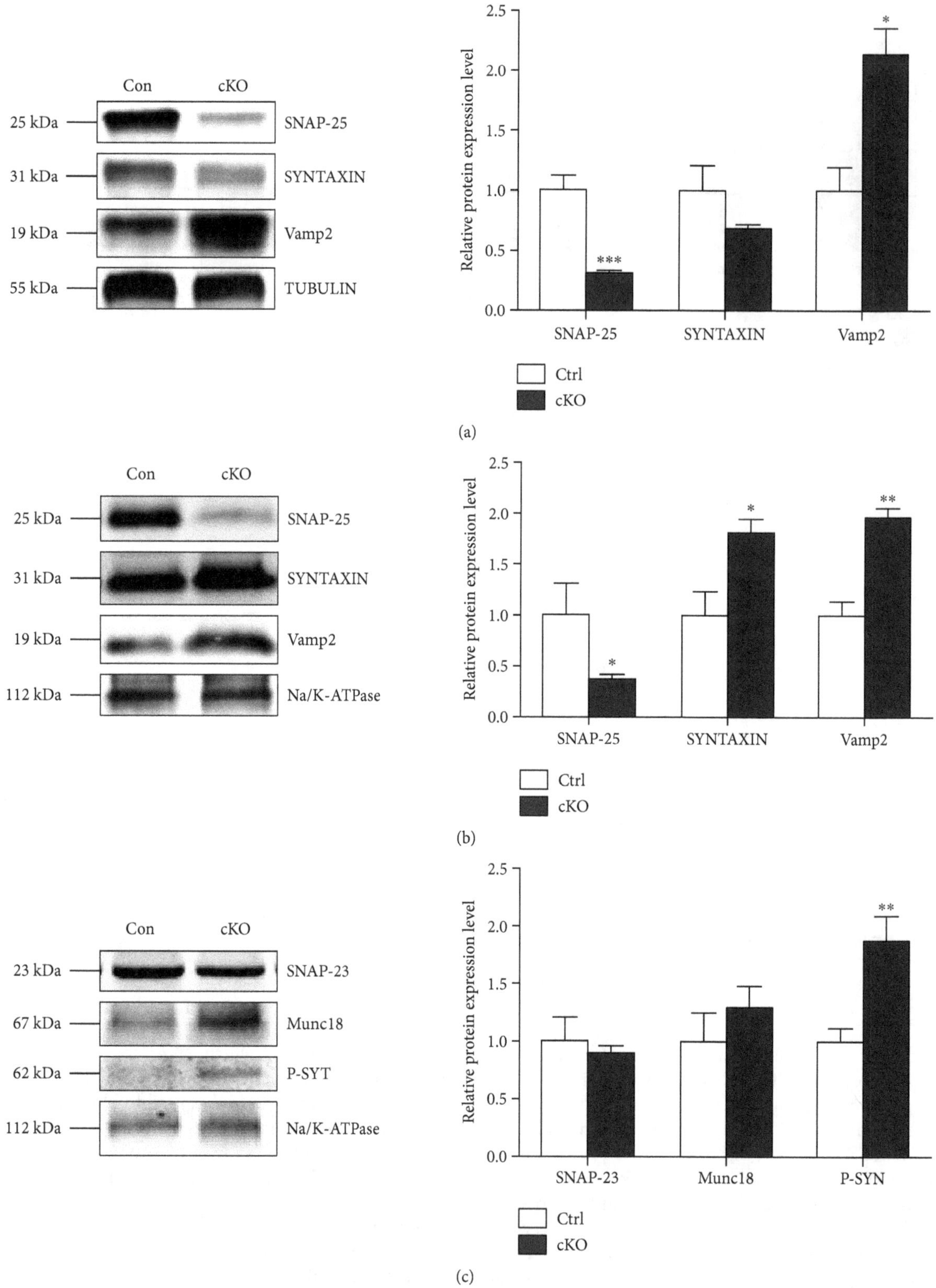

FIGURE 4: Alteration of expression pattern of SNARE-related proteins. Representative western blot (left) and densitometric analysis (right) of proteins in the cytosolic (a) and membrane (b and c) fractions prepared from mouse cerebral cortex ($n = 3$ per group). $^{*}P < 0.05$, $^{**}P < 0.01$, and $^{***}P < 0.001$ compared with control littermates. P-SYT: phosphorylated synaptotagmin-1.

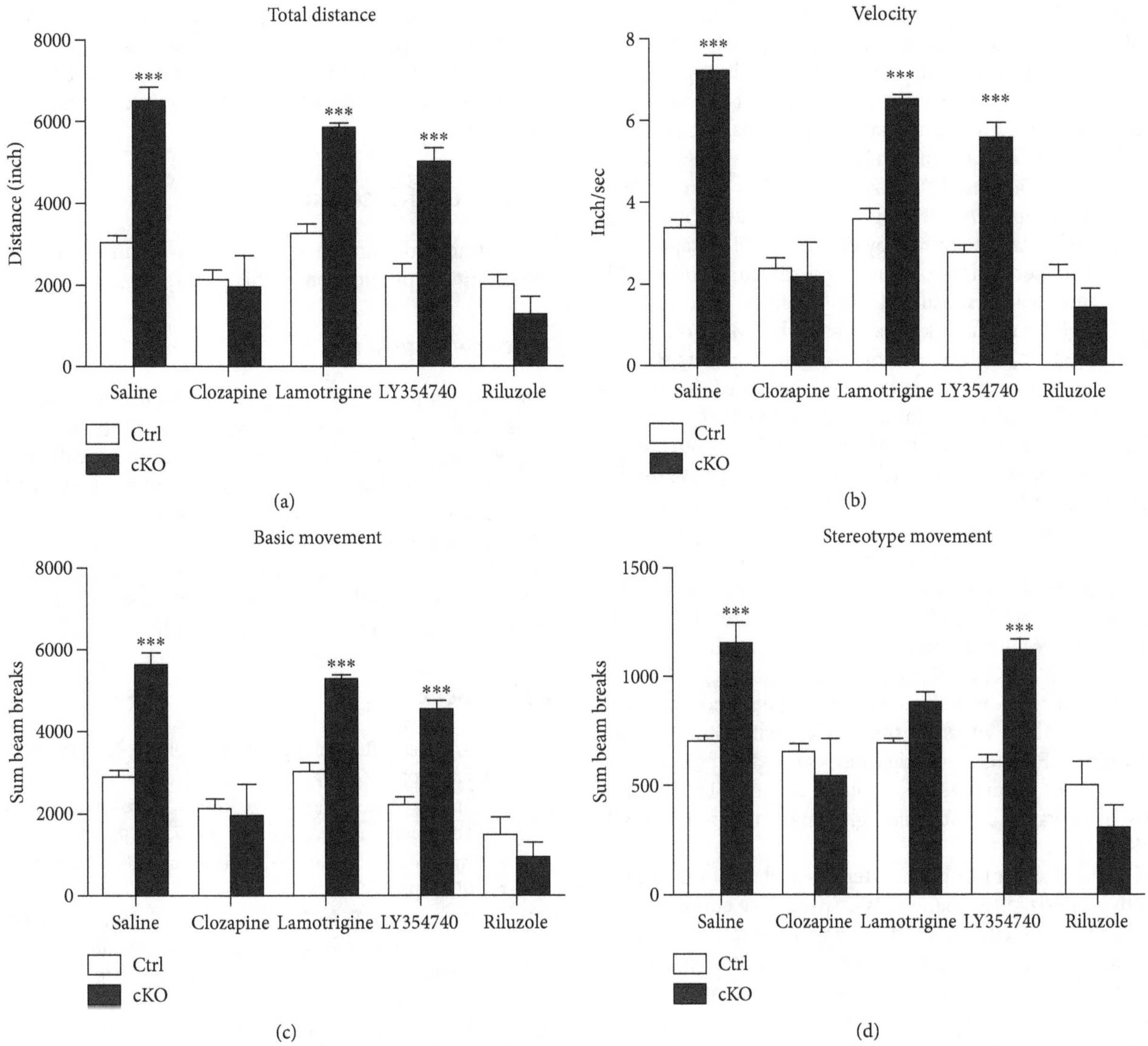

FIGURE 5: Antipsychotic drugs could attenuate the locomotor hyperactivity deficits in cKO mice. Summary plots of total distance (a), activity velocity (b), basic (c), and stereotype (d) movement in the open-field test. $^{***}P < 0.001$ compared with control littermates. Ctrls: $n = 5$; cKOs: $n = 8$.

above factors may contribute to the inconsistent results we have made.

Thus, the emerging question is how synaptic exocytosis could be enhanced without SNAP-25. To investigate the intrinsic mechanism of this phenomenon, we detected the expression level of three molecules, which are functionally related to SNAP-25 closely. These were (1) SNAP-23, the closest homolog of SNAP-25, which may be the substitution for SNAP-25 to mediate synaptic vesicle fusion [26]; (2) mammalian uncoordinated-18 (Munc-18), which has been found to have dual binding ability to syntaxin-1 and Vamp2, classified as the fourth crucial member of SNARE-pin assembly and may be another alternative for mediating neurotransmitter release [27, 28]; and (3) as the synaptic vesicle Ca^{2+} sensor, synaptotagmin-1 could be phosphorylated with calcium influx and trigger the synaptic release subsequently. Endogenous SNAP-25 negatively modulates neuronal voltage-gated calcium channels (VGCCs) [11, 29]. Therefore, SNAP-25 deficiency may release VGCC activity from SNAP-25-mediated inhibition, thus resulting in exaggerated calcium influx and triggering exocytic release of glutamate. Accordingly, our molecular detection results showed the phosphorylated synaptotagmin-1 was obviously elevated, which indicated the active of VGCCs and enhanced calcium influx that may lead to greater synaptic release at the presynaptic terminal.

Moreover, we assessed the effects of commonly used antipsychotic drugs on the locomotor hyperactivities and stereotype behavior of cKO mice. The atypical antipsychotic clozapine can bind to receptors of serotonin, dopaminergic, and glutamatergic system. Multitarget actions make clozapine one of the most efficacious antipsychotics. It is therefore considered the "gold standard" for the treatment of SZ [30]. In regard to the cortical hyperglutamatergic state within our model, we chose three drugs that aim to inhibit presynaptic glutamate release through different pathways. These were (1) LY354740, a presynaptic metabotropic glutamate receptor 2/3 (mGlu2/3) receptor agonist, which helps suppress the release of neurotransmitters, including glutamate and GABA [31]; (2) lamotrigine, which acts primarily through inhibition of glutamate release via blockade of voltage-sensitive sodium channels and stabilization of neuronal membrane [32]; and (3) riluzole, which has diverse effects on multiple components of the glutamatergic system, such as inhibition of glutamate release by depression of voltage-gated ion channels (sodium, potassium, and calcium) and inhibition of autoreceptors. Riluzole also affects glial cells by increasing glutamate uptake, trafficks with AMPA receptors, and so on [33, 34]. Subsequent open-field test results showed that (1) clozapine could attenuate heightened locomotor activity of cKO mice. Its validity illustrated that SNAP-25 cKO mice could respond effectively to antipsychotics drug, which is the qualifying standard for an animal disease model; (2) glutamate release inhibitors occupied different efficacies on our mice and administration of riluzole has significantly corrected the hyperactivity of the SNAP-25 cKOs, whereas lamotrigine could only alleviate the stereotype movements of the mouse model, and LY354740 did not alter the activity at all. These results suggested that the hyperglutamatergic phenotype of our model may be associated closely with enhanced calcium influx rather than impaired mGlu2/3 receptor function, which corresponded with our previous observation. Further investigations are still required to provide more evidences to explore the detailed mechanisms of elevated extracellular glutamate tones in SNAP-25 cKO mice.

The involvement of glutamatergic mechanism in SZ has been hypothesized for many years. SZ-relative abnormalities have been well documented in mice with mutations in postsynaptic components of glutamatergic transmission, such as NMDAR [35, 36], glycine transporter [37], and metabotropic glutamate receptor [38]. The hypofunction of postsynaptic NMDAR on inhibitory neurons that leads to disinhibition of glutamate transmission and glutamate excitotoxicity has formed the bedrock of the glutamate hypothesis of SZ. However, influence of presynaptic glutamatergic deficits is less well understood. Being a key component of glutamatergic neurotransmission at presynaptic locus, SNAP-25 deficiency induced typical SZ-like behavior demonstrated the strong association between presynaptic dysfunction and the outbreak of SZ. SNAP-25 cKO mice would be a useful novel tool for investigating presynaptic alterations that contribute to the etiopathophysiology of SZ. This research helps to consummate the pre- and postsynaptic glutamatergic pathogenesis of SZ.

5. Conclusion

This study showed that the forebrain glutamatergic neuron-specific SNAP-25 cKO lead to a typical SZ-like phenotype. The deficiency of SNAP-25 may lead to enhanced calcium influx and exaggerated glutamatergic release and may result in the elevated extracellular glutamate level. Riluzole attenuates the locomotor hyperactivity deficits in cKO mice. Our results provided new insight that SNAP-25 dysfunction has direct consequences on synaptic transmission and contributes to developmental of SZ. SNAP-25 cKO mouse could be a valuable new model for SZ and could be used to address questions regarding pathophysiology and etiology of the illness.

Conflicts of Interest

The authors declare that there is no conflict of interests regarding the publication of this paper.

Acknowledgments

The authors gratefully acknowledge Professor Fang Huang (The State Key Laboratory of Medical Neurobiology, Fudan University) for the technical assistance and critically reading the manuscript. This work was supported by the grant from the National Natural Science Foundation of China (no. 81271483), the Funds of Science and Technology Commission of Shanghai Municipality (nos. 14140904300 and 16DZ2280800), and the Fundamental Research Funds for the Central Universities (no. 2000219140).

References

[1] T. R. Insel, "Rethinking schizophrenia," *Nature*, vol. 468, no. 7321, pp. 187–193, 2010.

[2] J. Van Os, G. Kenis, and B. P. Rutten, "The environment and schizophrenia," *Nature*, vol. 468, no. 7321, pp. 203–212, 2010.

[3] J. Van Os and S. Kapur, "Schizophrenia," *Lancet*, vol. 374, no. 9690, pp. 635–645, 2009.

[4] C. M. Lewis, D. F. Levinson, L. H. Wise et al., "Genome scan meta-analysis of schizophrenia and bipolar disorder, part II: schizophrenia," *American Journal of Human Genetics*, vol. 73, no. 1, pp. 34–48, 2003.

[5] A. H. Fanous, M. C. Neale, B. T. Webb et al., "Novel linkage to chromosome 20p using latent classes of psychotic illness in 270 Irish high-density families," *Biological Psychiatry*, vol. 64, no. 2, pp. 121–127, 2008.

[6] Q. Wang, Y. Wang, W. Ji et al., "SNAP25 is associated with schizophrenia and major depressive disorder in the Han Chinese population," *The Journal of Clinical Psychiatry*, vol. 76, no. 1, pp. e76–e82, 2015.

[7] V. E. Barakauskas, A. Moradian, A. M. Barr et al., "Quantitative mass spectrometry reveals changes in SNAP-25 isoforms in schizophrenia," *Schizophrenia Research*, vol. 177, no. 1-3, pp. 44–51, 2016.

[8] C. N. Karson, R. E. Mrak, K. O. Schluterman, W. Q. Sturner, J. G. Sheng, and W. S. T. Griffin, "Alterations in synaptic proteins and their encoding mRNAs in prefrontal cortex in schizophrenia: a possible neurochemical basis for 'hypofrontality'," *Molecular Psychiatry*, vol. 4, no. 1, pp. 39–45, 1999.

[9] S. H. Fatemi, J. A. Earle, J. M. Stary, S. Lee, and J. Sedgewick, "Altered levels of the synaptosomal associated protein SNAP-25 in hippocampus of subjects with mood disorders and schizophrenia," *Neuroreport*, vol. 12, no. 15, pp. 3257–3262, 2001.

[10] M. Matteoli, D. Pozzi, C. Grumelli et al., "The synaptic split of SNAP-25: different roles in glutamatergic and GABAergic neurons?," *Neuroscience*, vol. 158, no. 1, pp. 223–230, 2009.

[11] S. B. Condliffe, I. Corradini, D. Pozzi, C. Verderio, and M. Matteoli, "Endogenous SNAP-25 regulates native voltage-gated calcium channels in glutamatergic neurons," *The Journal of Biological Chemistry*, vol. 285, no. 32, pp. 24968–24976, 2010.

[12] F. Antonucci, I. Corradini, G. Fossati, R. Tomasoni, E. Menna, and M. Matteoli, "SNAP-25, a known presynaptic protein with emerging postsynaptic functions," *Frontiers in Synaptic Neuroscience*, vol. 8, p. 7, 2016.

[13] J. Z. Tsien, D. F. Chen, D. Gerber et al., "Subregion- and cell type-restricted gene knockout in mouse brain," *Cell*, vol. 87, no. 7, pp. 1317–1326, 1996.

[14] M. He, Y. Liu, X. Wang, M. Q. Zhang, G. J. Hannon, and Z. J. Huang, "Cell-type-based analysis of microRNA profiles in the mouse brain," *Neuron*, vol. 73, no. 1, pp. 35–48, 2012.

[15] I. H. Kim, S. K. Park, S. T. Hong et al., "Inositol 1,4,5-trisphosphate 3-kinase a functions as a scaffold for synaptic Rac signaling," *The Journal of Neuroscience*, vol. 29, no. 44, pp. 14039–14049, 2009.

[16] O. Berton, C. A. Mcclung, R. J. Dileone et al., "Essential role of BDNF in the mesolimbic dopamine pathway in social defeat stress," *Science*, vol. 311, no. 5762, pp. 864–868, 2006.

[17] H. Zhang, E. Kang, Y. Wang et al., "Brain-specific Crmp2 deletion leads to neuronal development deficits and behavioural impairments in mice," *Nature Communications*, vol. 7, 2016.

[18] Y. K. Wang, D. Shen, Q. Hao et al., "Overexpression of angiotensin-converting enzyme 2 attenuates tonically active glutamatergic input to the rostral ventrolateral medulla in hypertensive rats," *American Journal of Physiology. Heart and Circulatory Physiology*, vol. 307, no. 2, pp. H182–H190, 2014.

[19] M. Han, X. Xiao, Y. Yang et al., "SIP30 is required for neuropathic pain-evoked aversion in rats," *The Journal of Neuroscience*, vol. 34, no. 2, pp. 346–355, 2014.

[20] C. L. Schmid, J. M. Streicher, H. Y. Meltzer, and L. M. Bohn, "Clozapine acts as an agonist at serotonin 2A receptors to counter MK-801-induced behaviors through a *β*arrestin2-independent activation of Akt," *Neuropsychopharmacology*, vol. 39, no. 8, pp. 1902–1913, 2014.

[21] C. Procaccini, M. Maksimovic, T. Aitta-Aho, E. R. Korpi, and A. M. Linden, "Reversal of novelty-induced hyperlocomotion and hippocampal c-Fos expression in GluA1 knockout male mice by the mGluR2/3 agonist LY354740," *Neuroscience*, vol. 250, pp. 189–200, 2013.

[22] M. Y. Zhang, C. Y. Zheng, M. M. Zou et al., "Lamotrigine attenuates deficits in synaptic plasticity and accumulation of amyloid plaques in APP/PS1 transgenic mice," *Neurobiology of Aging*, vol. 35, no. 12, pp. 2713–2725, 2014.

[23] N. Egashira, R. Okuno, S. Harada et al., "Effects of glutamate-related drugs on marble-burying behavior in mice: implications for obsessive-compulsive disorder," *European Journal of Pharmacology*, vol. 586, no. 1-3, pp. 164–170, 2008.

[24] I. Matak and Z. Lackovic, "Botulinum neurotoxin type a: actions beyond SNAP-25?," *Toxicology*, vol. 335, pp. 79–84, 2015.

[25] F. Antonucci, I. Corradini, R. Morini et al., "Reduced SNAP-25 alters short-term plasticity at developing glutamatergic synapses," *EMBO Reports*, vol. 14, no. 7, pp. 645–651, 2013.

[26] S. Arora, I. Saarloos, R. Kooistra, R. van de Bospoort, M. Verhage, and R. F. Toonen, "SNAP-25 gene family members differentially support secretory vesicle fusion," *Journal of Cell Science*, vol. 130, no. 11, pp. 1877–1889, 2017.

[27] A. Pertsinidis, K. Mukherjee, M. Sharma et al., "Ultrahigh-resolution imaging reveals formation of neuronal SNARE/Munc18 complexes in situ," *Proceedings of the National Academy of Sciences of the United States of America*, vol. 110, no. 30, pp. E2812–E2820, 2013.

[28] D. Parisotto, J. Malsam, A. Scheutzow, J. M. Krause, and T. H. Sollner, "SNAREpin assembly by Munc18-1 requires previous vesicle docking by synaptotagmin 1," *The Journal of Biological Chemistry*, vol. 287, no. 37, pp. 31041–31049, 2012.

[29] S. B. Condliffe and M. Matteoli, "Inactivation kinetics of voltage-gated calcium channels in glutamatergic neurons are influenced by SNAP-25," *Channels*, vol. 5, no. 4, pp. 304–307, 2011.

[30] H. Y. Meltzer, "Update on typical and atypical antipsychotic drugs," *Annual Review of Medicine*, vol. 64, no. 1, pp. 393–406, 2013.

[31] R. Farazifard and S. H. Wu, "Metabotropic glutamate receptors modulate glutamatergic and GABAergic synaptic transmission in the central nucleus of the inferior colliculus," *Brain Research*, vol. 1325, pp. 28–40, 2010.

[32] A. L. Meehan, X. Yang, B. D. McAdams, L. Yuan, and S. M. Rothman, "A new mechanism for antiepileptic drug action: vesicular entry may mediate the effects of levetiracetam," *Journal of Neurophysiology*, vol. 106, no. 3, pp. 1227–1239, 2011.

[33] N. Lamanauskas and A. Nistri, "Riluzole blocks persistent Na^+ and $Ca2^+$ currents and modulates release of glutamate via presynaptic NMDA receptors on neonatal rat hypoglossal motoneurons *in vitro*," *The European Journal of Neuroscience*, vol. 27, no. 10, pp. 2501–2514, 2008.

[34] R. Machado-Vieira, G. Salvadore, L. A. Ibrahim, N. Diaz-Granados, and C. A. Zarate Jr, "Targeting glutamatergic signaling for the development of novel therapeutics for mood disorders," *Current Pharmaceutical Design*, vol. 15, no. 14, pp. 1595–1611, 2009.

[35] K. Nakazawa, V. Jeevakumar, and K. Nakao, "Spatial and temporal boundaries of NMDA receptor hypofunction leading to schizophrenia," *NPJ Schizophrenia*, vol. 3, no. 1, p. 7, 2017.

[36] D. Timucin, O. Ozdemir, and M. Parlak, "The role of NMDAR antibody in the etiopathogenesis of schizophrenia," *Neuropsychiatric Disease and Treatment*, vol. 12, pp. 2327–2332, 2016.

[37] E. Dunayevich, R. W. Buchanan, C. Y. Chen et al., "Efficacy and safety of the glycine transporter type-1 inhibitor AMG 747 for the treatment of negative symptoms associated with schizophrenia," *Schizophrenia Research*, vol. 182, pp. 90–97, 2017.

[38] J. Maksymetz, S. P. Moran, and P. J. Conn, "Targeting metabotropic glutamate receptors for novel treatments of schizophrenia," *Molecular Brain*, vol. 10, no. 1, p. 15, 2017.

5

Repetitive Transcranial Electrical Stimulation Induces Quantified Changes in Resting Cerebral Perfusion Measured from Arterial Spin Labeling

Matthew S. Sherwood,[1,2] **Aaron T. Madaris**,[1,2] **Casserly R. Mullenger**,[1] **and R. Andy McKinley**[3]

[1]*Infoscitex, a DCS company, 4027 Colonel Glenn Hwy, Beavercreek, OH 45431, USA*
[2]*Department of Biomedical, Industrial & Human Factors Engineering, Wright State University, 3640 Colonel Glenn Hwy, Dayton, OH 45435, USA*
[3]*Air Force Research Laboratory, U.S. Air Force, 2510 Fifth Street, Bldg 840, Wright-Patterson AFB, OH 45433-7951, USA*

Correspondence should be addressed to Matthew S. Sherwood; matt.sherwood@wright.edu

Academic Editor: Junichi Ushiba

The use of transcranial electrical stimulation (TES) as a method to augment neural activity has increased in popularity in the last decade and a half. The specific application of TES to the left prefrontal cortex has been shown to produce broad cognitive effects; however, the neural mechanisms underlying these effects remain unknown. In this work, we evaluated the effect of repetitive TES on cerebral perfusion. Stimulation was applied to the left prefrontal cortex on three consecutive days, and resting cerebral perfusion was quantified before and after stimulation using arterial spin labeling. Perfusion was found to decrease significantly more in a matched sham stimulation group than in a group receiving active stimulation across many areas of the brain. These changes were found to originate in the locus coeruleus and were broadly distributed in the neocortex. The changes in the neocortex may be a direct result of the stimulation or an indirect result via the changes in the noradrenergic system produced from the altered activity of the locus coeruleus. These findings indicate that anodal left prefrontal stimulation alters the activity of the locus coeruleus, and this altered activity may excite the noradrenergic system producing the broad behavioral effects that have been reported.

1. Introduction (AM)

Transcranial electrical stimulation (TES) has experienced increased interest over the last 15 years [1]. The application of TES using a weak, constant current delivered to the scalp is referred to as transcranial direct current stimulation (tDCS) [2]. This method has been presented by many groups as a feasible process for stimulation of the brain to augment neural activity [3–7]. The specific application of tDCS with the anode placed over the left prefrontal cortex has been routinely applied in the literature with demonstrable behavioral effects in combating performance decrements associated with vigilance [8], decreasing the effect of fatigue on cognitive performance [9, 10], accelerating learning processes [2, 3, 11, 12], enhancing multitasking performance [13], and improving procedural memory [14].

Clark et al. [11] implemented 2 mA anodal left prefrontal tDCS while performing a task involving the identification of threat-related objects in a naturalistic environment. Using dynamic Bayesian network analysis, they indicated that the right frontal and parietal cortices were involved in the learning processes of their identification task. Furthermore, they reported that the group receiving full-current (2 mA) tDCS performed significantly better than the one that received low-current (0.1 mA) stimulation. McKinley et al. [12] provided support for the findings of Clark and colleagues using a realistic visual search task implanted with synthetic aperture radar images. They stated that participants who received anodal left prefrontal tDCS attained enhanced visual search accuracies compared to those supplied with sham or no stimulation. Effects of anodal left prefrontal tDCS have also been observed in decreasing the effects of fatigue on cognitive performance. Using a cohort of 30 participants (10 placebo gum, 10 caffeine gum with sham tDCS, and 10 2 mA anodal left prefrontal tDCS with placebo gum), McIntire et al. [9] performed psychomotor vigilance tasks, delayed matching-to-sample working memory tasks, and the Mackworth clock test throughout 30 hours of continuous wakefulness. They reported improved latencies in working memory tasks and faster reaction times in psychomotor tasks in the groups receiving active tDCS and caffeine gum compared to placebo throughout the sleep deprivation period. Altogether, these findings provide evidence for the central role of the prefrontal cortex in vigilance, accelerated learning, fatigue, and multitasking performance but indicate that tDCS may be utilized to maintain performance levels in environments requiring little to no rest or settings required sustained attentional focus.

Despite the broad applications of tDCS and those specific to anodal left prefrontal stimulation, the neural mechanisms underlying tDCS are not well understood. It has been suggested that anodal tDCS increases excitability in the neocortex [6] by altering neuronal membrane potentials [15]. This theory is supported by findings of enhanced glutamatergic activity following the application of anodal tDCS [2]. Neuroplasticity, the ability of the brain to form and restructure synaptic connections [16], is thought to coincide with increased glutamatergic activity [2] as evidenced in the lasting behavioral effects from tDCS (e.g., [9, 10]) and the acceleration of learning processes [3, 11, 12]. However, recent evidence suggests that the neuroplastic effects of tDCS have some dependence on synaptic activity during stimulation [7].

A growing method for studying neural processes is through the measurement of cerebral perfusion. The *in vivo* quantification of cerebral perfusion (referred to as cerebral blood flow (CBF) mL/100 mg/min) can be performed noninvasively using magnetic resonance imaging (MRI) through an arterial spin labeling (ASL) pulse sequence [17, 18]. ASL is a clinical method that has been used to identify early pathophysiological changes in Alzheimer's disease and other disorders such as dementia [18, 19]. In comparison to signals based on blood oxygen, CBF has better reliability and intersubject variability [20]. Furthermore, CBF is directly responsible for the delivery of glucose and oxygen. Both oxygen and glucose are necessary to maintain adenosine triphosphate (ATP) production and need to be replenished to support continued neural activity. Although CBF is not a direct measure of neural activity, it is a tightly coupled correlate: CBF changes with neural activity such as that which occurs during task activation or with changing metabolism [21]. Evidence published just this year indicates that this coupling is electrical: extracellular K^+ activates capillary endothelial cells which then signal upstream arteriolar dilation [22]. The extracellular concentration of K^+ increases during neural activity, thereby signaling enhanced vasodilation and increased blood flow to the supporting capillary bed.

The study of resting CBF in anodal left prefrontal tDCS may provide critical insights as increased glutamatergic activity associated with anodal tDCS would manifest as enhanced cerebral perfusion. Few previous studies have utilized ASL to assess the neural effects of tDCS. In some studies, anodal tDCS led increased regional CBF in the brain tissue underneath the stimulation site, with reliable and reproducible results within and between subjects. Furthermore, transfer effects were observed in brain regions functionally connected to the stimulation site [7]. Importantly, immediate and lasting changes in CBF have been associated with anodal left prefrontal tDCS [23]. The goal of this study is to enhance our understanding of the underlying neural mechanisms associated with repetitive anodal tDCS to the left prefrontal cortex through the study of resting cerebral perfusion. The study consisted of anodal left prefrontal tDCS applied on three consecutive days with the same procedures performed on each day to assess the additive effects of tDCS. In this work, we present preliminary findings of a larger, ongoing study.

2. Materials and Methods

2.1. Participants. A total of 28 healthy, active duty, Air Force military members recruited from Wright-Patterson Air Force Base volunteered to participate in this study. Participants were excluded from participation if they had any neurological or psychological diagnoses; vision, hearing, or motor control impairments; or recent trauma or hospitalization. Participants were also excluded if they currently took any medication which may affect cognitive function or if they were dependent on alcohol, caffeine, or nicotine. Written informed consent was obtained from each participant prior to any experimental procedures which were approved by the Air Force Research Laboratory Institutional Review Board at Wright-Patterson Air Force Base under Protocol number FWR20130126H. Participants eligible for compensation (i.e., if participation occurred in an off-duty status) received equal remuneration. Of the 28 participants recruited, eight were excluded due to medical disqualification ($n = 2$), incomplete data or corrupted data ($n = 2$), or failure to complete all three sessions in three consecutive days ($n = 4$).

Participants were randomly assigned to one of two groups. Both groups received the same instructions and performed the same tasks with the exception of the stimulation that was received. In the experimental group (ACT, $n = 11$, mean age = 24.5 ± 2.6), 2 mA stimulation was provided for 30 minutes while in the control group (CON, $n = 9$, mean age = 25.9 ± 3.2) sham stimulation consisting of 2 mA stimulation for 30 s. Participants in each group were blinded to the validity of the simulation (i.e., not aware of the stimulation condition) and naïve to TES (i.e., first time receiving TES).

All participants completed three experimental sessions on three consecutive days. Each session was separated by 24 hours. The sessions were conducted in the evening so as to not conflict with the working day but also due to the MRI availability. Participants completed the experimental sessions in groups of two with staggered start times (see Table 1). Start

Table 1: Starting times for the experimental procedures. Participants completed the three sessions in groups of two with staggered start times.

Procedure	Participant 1 Local start time	Participant 1 ASL scan time	Participant 1 Local end time	Participant 2 Local start time	Participant 2 ASL scan time	Participant 2 Local end time
Prestimulation MRI	5:00 pm	6:10 pm	6:15 pm	6:15 pm	7:25 pm	7:30 pm
Transcranial DC stimulation	6:30 pm	n/a	7:00 pm	7:55 pm	n/a	8:25 pm
Poststimulation MRI	7:30 pm	8:40 pm	8:45 pm	8:45 pm	9:55 pm	10:00 pm

times were held consistent across the three sessions and were counterbalanced across groups.

2.2. Transcranial DC Stimulation. On each of the three sessions, anodal stimulation was applied to the left prefrontal cortex (approximately F3) with the cathode placed on the contralateral bicep. During stimulation, participants completed a 30 min laboratory vigilance task [24]. The electric stimulation (MagStim DC Stimulator, Magstim Company Limited, Whitland, UK) delivered a constant 2 mA through a ring of five custom Na/NaCl electrodes. The electrodes were arranged in a 1.6 cm radius circle and separated by 0.1 cm (outer edge to outer edge). The same ring configuration was used at the cathode location. The 2 mA stimulation was distributed evenly among the five electrodes. The stimulator is battery-powered and utilizes multistage current monitoring to ensure constant current levels are delivered to the anode. Each electrode was placed in a small "cup" and secured to the participant using medical bandages. The electrode cups were filled with highly conductive gel (SignaGel, Parker Laboratories, Fairfield, NJ) to ensure current transfer to the scalp.

2.3. MRI Acquisition. At each session, MRI data was acquired prior to and approximately 0.5 hours following the application of tDCS. The MRI acquisition consisted of the following sequences: a 12 min resting-state functional MRI (fMRI), three 10 min task fMRIs, T1-weighted MRI, diffusion tensor imaging (DTI), magnetic resonance spectroscopy (MRS), and resting ASL. As this work is part of a larger, ongoing study, we will only be presenting the resting ASL data in this work. However, it is important to discuss the three task fMRIs where participants completed a dual (verbal and spatial) n-back task. This task was conducted in a boxcar design with 48 s control and task blocks, each with 16–3 s trials. During each trial, a letter was displayed on a 3×3 grid for 500 ms. Participants were asked to provide one response if the current letter was the same as the nth previous letter that was presented and another response if the current letter was in the same position on a 3×3 grid as the nth previous letter. For control blocks, the letter was replaced with a dot and participants were instructed to provide one response if the dot was on the right side of the grid and another for the left. For the first run, n was set to 2. n for the second run was determined from the performance of the first run (if performance was 90 or above, n incremented; if less than 70, n decremented; otherwise, n remained the same) and the third run from the second.

Structural (T1-weighted) images were acquired using a 3D brain volume imaging (BRAVO) pulse sequence which uses an inversion recovery prepared fast spoiled gradient echo (FSPGR). The structural images were acquired using a 256×256 element matrix, 172 slices oriented to the anterior commissure- (AC-) posterior commissure (PC) plane, 1 mm^3 isotropic voxels, 0.8 phase field of view factor, inversion time (TI) = 450 ms, TE = 3.224 ms, a flip angle of 13°, and an autocalibrated reconstruction for Cartesian sampling with a phase acceleration factor of 1.0 for the first session and 2.0 for all remaining sessions. All MRI procedures were conducted on a 3 Tesla (T) MRI (Discovery 750w, GE Healthcare, Madison, WI) using a 24-channel head coil.

Images of cerebral perfusion were acquired approximately 20 minutes prior to the application of tDCS and approximately 1.5 hours after the conclusion of stimulation using a pseudocontinuous arterial spin labeling (pcASL) technique [25] with inversion (tagging) pulses administered immediately inferior to the imaging volume. All images were acquired true axial (oriented perpendicular to the scanner bore) using a postlabel delay time (PLD) of 2025 ms. Five background suppression pulses were applied to reduce the signal of stationary tissues [26–28] and improve signal-to-noise ratio (SNR) of arterial blood. A 3D fast spin echo (3D FSE) sequence was used for acquisition of the imaging volume. To reduce motion sensitivity, improve acquisition time, and minimize susceptibility artifacts, a stack-of-spirals readout gradient starting at the center of the k-space was used [29]. A total of 8 spiral arms were used for k-space sampling. Echoes were rebinned to Cartesian space in a 128×128 matrix, with TR = 4640 ms, TE = 10.7 ms, voxel size = 1.875×1.875 mm, slice thickness = 4 mm, and flip angle = 111°. The sequence acquired a total of 3 tag/control pairs. The total acquisition time was 4 min 46 s. During the scan, participants were instructed to remain awake and focus on a fixation dot presented on the display. This condition has demonstrated significantly greater reliability in resting-state functional MRI across all within-network connections, as well as within default-mode, attention, and auditory networks when compared to eyes open (no specified fixation) and closed methods [30].

2.4. Data Processing and Analysis. Cerebral perfusion was quantified from ASL. CBF maps were computed from the automated functions in the GE reconstruction software. First, the 3 tagged and 3 control volumes were averaged in place (without motion correction). Then, difference images were calculated for all participants by subtracting the average tagged volume from the average control volume. Finally, quantitative CBF maps were generated from the difference images, the associated proton

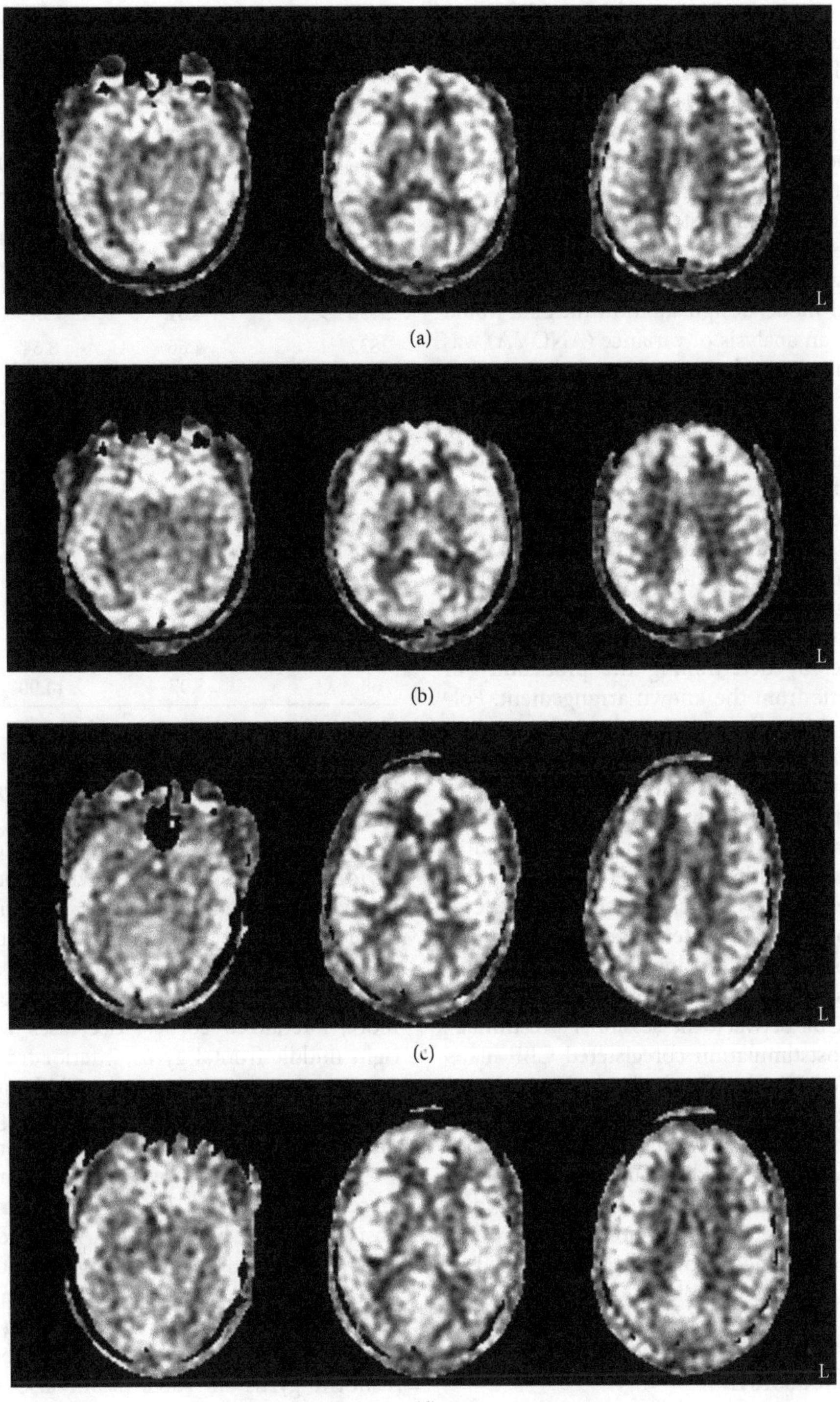

Figure 1: Raw CBF maps for (a) day 1 prestimulation and (b) day 3 poststimulation from a single CON participant and (c) day 1 prestimulation and (d) day 3 poststimulation from a single ACT participant.

density- (PD-) weighted volumes, and a standard single compartment model [31–33].

The CBF maps from each day and session were exported from the MRI scanner and processed using the FMRIB Software Library (FSL) [34, 35] on a 74-core Rocks Cluster Distribution (http://www.rocksclusters.org) high-performance computing system capable of running 120 threads in parallel (see Figure 1, e.g., CBF maps). First, the PD-weighted images acquired were registered to the individual's high-resolution structural image by estimating motion from a boundary-based registration method which includes a fieldmap-based distortion correction [36]. Then, the individual's high-resolution structural image was registered to the MNI-152 T1-weighted 2 mm template provided in FSL [37, 38] using a 12-parameter model [39, 40]. In order to coregister all volumes, the CBF maps were converted to standard space using the transforms responsible for morphing the PD-weighted image of each data set to the structural image and the structural image to the template.

Next, group nonparametric statistical analyses were performed on the session 1 prestimulation and session 3 poststimulation coregistered CBF maps in a voxelwise fashion. Due to our mixed-model design and how the data would need to be permuted, an analysis of variance (ANOVA) was not possible using this approach. Instead, two separate analyses were performed. In the first, analyses were conducted separately for each group to evaluate the effect of the session. This analysis determined the statistical significance of differences in CBF (evaluated as increased perfusion from session 1 prestimulation to session 3 poststimulation) using permutation testing implemented in FSL's randomise [41, 42]. Null t distributions for contrasts representative of the main effect of the session were derived by performing 500,000 random permutations of the data [43]. A final t statistic was computed for each voxel by determining the probability of exceeding the t statistic from the known arrangement. Following this analysis, we implemented a clustering method to account for false positives due to the multiple comparisons [44]. This method considered adjacent voxels with a t statistic of 1.96 or greater to be a cluster. The significance of each cluster was estimated and compared to a threshold of $p < 0.05$ using Gaussian random field theory. The significance of voxels that either did not pass the significance level threshold or do not belong to a cluster was set to zero.

The second analysis assessed the interaction of the group and session using a single unpaired approach. Prior to this analysis, changes in CBF between the session 1 prestimulation and session 3 poststimulation coregistered CBF maps were calculated at the individual level. Then, the statistical significance of the variation in CBF between sessions and groups was determined using permutation testing implemented in FSL's randomise. Null t distributions for contrasts representative of the interaction of the session and group were derived by performing 500,000 random permutations. The clustering method outlined above was implemented to account for false positives due to multiple comparisons.

3. Results and Discussion

Paired permutation testing revealed a few small clusters with significant increases in resting CBF resulting from repetitive 2 mA stimulation of the left prefrontal cortex (Table 2, Figure 2). Localized increases in CBF were observed in several regions of the brainstem and cerebellum including the substantia nigra (SN). Cortically, bilateral changes in CBF were observed in the middle frontal, superior frontal, and inferior frontal gyri. Lateralized cortical changes were observed in the right rectal gyrus and precuneus and in the left supramarginal gyrus, paracentral lobule, parahippocampal gyrus, thalamus, caudate, and posterior cingulate cortex (PCC). However, the majority of the cortical effects appeared in white matter.

Table 2: The largest 15 clusters identified with an average increase in perfusion between prestimulation at session 1 and poststimulation at session 3 (ΔCBF) for the ACT group.

Volume (mm^3)	Max t-statistic	Max ΔCBF (mL/100 mg/min)	Max ΔCBF location (mm) X	Y	Z
8000	7.23	13.45	−4	16	64
3824	5.28	15.00	16	−52	34
3320	3.76	10.27	−36	−60	52
3136	4.61	15.73	50	14	28
2832	4.66	8.64	−8	−12	10
2632	5.39	9.09	6	−12	12
2312	4.21	9.45	29	−40	38
2280	3.68	17.82	0	−28	44
1984	4.87	11.73	42	12	34
1800	5.00	13.09	−34	−26	−22
1528	6.58	10.09	40	32	4
1048	3.57	12.00	40	−72	−52
1032	3.79	9.18	−22	−36	10
864	6.59	13.73	0	−44	28
768	3.07	14.00	−6	−48	−52

In contrast to the ACT group, paired permutation testing performed on the group receiving repetitive sham stimulation identified significant decreases in resting CBF (Table 3, Figure 3). This included a large cluster encompassing multiple subcortical brain regions. This also comprised of a bilateral decrease in the superior frontal gyrus. Furthermore, lateralized cortical decreases were observed in the right middle frontal gyrus, inferior frontal gyrus, precentral gyrus, superior temporal gyrus, thalamus, and putamen and in the left cuneus, precuneus, cingulate gyrus, fusiform gyrus, middle temporal gyrus, and medial frontal gyrus.

The unpaired permutation testing analyzed the difference in resting CBF from session 1 prestimulation to session 3 poststimulation between the ACT and CON groups. This analysis revealed an overall significantly larger decrease in resting CBF for the CON group (Tables 4 and 5). This included a large cluster encompassing multiple subcortical and cortical brain regions. This cluster is identified as the fusiform gyrus in Table 4 but also included projections beginning in the locus coeruleus (LC) and projecting through the SN and PCC. This also comprised of localized clusters across several cortical regions. CBF in the bilateral superior frontal gyrus was found to increase in the ACT group but decrease in the CON group. This effect also appeared in right-lateralized regions: inferior frontal and middle frontal gyri. Left-lateralized clusters in the medial frontal gyrus and fusiform and right-lateralized clusters in the precentral gyrus, thalamus, and putamen showed a significant decrease in perfusion in the CON group, but no significant changes were observed in the ACT group. The opposite was observed for the left inferior parietal lobule.

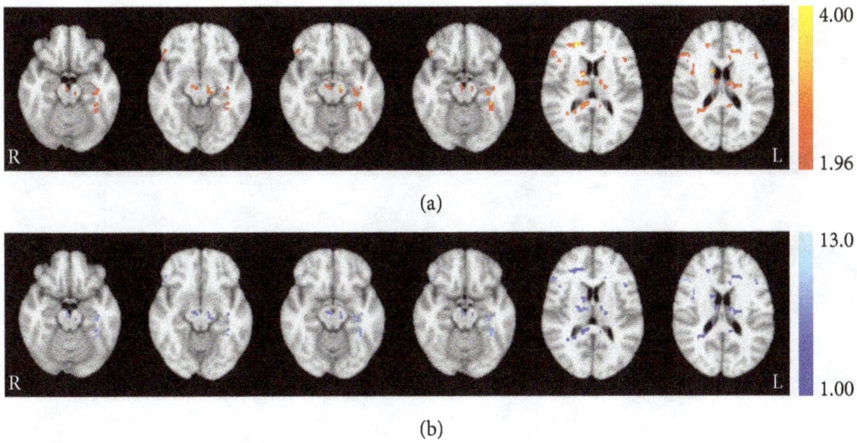

FIGURE 2: Session effect revealed from permutation testing for the ACT group. (a) Statistically significant (t-statistic) regions with altered CBF from baseline to session 3 poststimulation and (b) corresponding increases in quantified perfusion (mL/100 mg/min). Axial images taken at MNI coordinates $x = -18, -12, -14, -16, 12,$ and 18 mm.

TABLE 3: The largest 15 clusters identified with an average decrease in perfusion between prestimulation at session 1 and poststimulation at session 3 (ΔCBF) for the CON group.

Volume (mm^3)	Max t-statistic	Max ΔCBF (mL/100 mg/min)	Max ΔCBF location (mm) X	Y	Z
204,208	11.3	−23.00	−4	76	64
4016	7.41	−12.78	16	−20	34
3528	4.83	−24.56	−36	−60	52
2912	5.37	−12.67	50	14	28
2560	3.91	−13.11	−8	−12	10
1976	8.95	−13.89	6	−12	12
1344	4.34	−12.22	32	−40	38
1336	5.01	−9.44	0	−28	44
1296	5.84	−9.56	42	12	34
1112	4.75	−15.33	−34	−26	−22
944	5.48	−13.00	40	32	4
840	5.35	−20.44	40	−72	−52
832	4.62	−9.89	−22	−36	10
824	7.72	−22.11	0	−44	28
816	4.38	−9.89	−16	−42	30

Systematic group variations in thickness or atrophy in gray matter and/or different gyrification patterns are plausible and may have resulted in some or all of the effects observed. To evaluate the possibility of anatomical variations between groups, we performed voxel-based morphometry (VBM) to investigate voxelwise differences in local gray matter volume and/or topography. This analysis utilized brain-extracted structural images to first produce a template. In order to not bias the template towards one group, 2 random subjects from the ACT group were not included in this step to ensure an equal number of samples represent each group. The brain-extracted images were segmented automatically into gray matter, affine-registered to the gray matter International Consortium for Brain Mapping (ICBM) 152 template [38], concatenated, and averaged. The average image was flipped along the x-axis, and the mirror images were reaveraged. The gray matter images were reregistered to the average template using nonlinear registration, concatenated, averaged, and flipped along the x-axis. A final symmetric gray matter template was created by averaging the mirror images from the nonlinear registration. Next, gray matter templates for all subjects were created and nonlinearly registered to the custom gray matter template. A compensation for gray matter variations due to the nonlinear transformation was introduced using the Jacobian of the warp field [45]. All the registered gray matter volumes were spatially smoothed using a Gaussian kernel (sigma = 4 mm). Finally, an unpaired t-test was performed to compare the gray matter volumes across groups using a permutation (number of permutations = 500,000) approach performed in FSL randomise. A threshold-free cluster enhancement method was utilized to correct for multiple comparisons. No significant findings were observed in this analysis indicating neither the thickness or atrophy in gray matter nor different gyrification patterns existed between groups. Furthermore, this suggests that these anatomical variations could not have caused the observed variations in perfusion.

The unpaired permutation analysis represents the interaction between the session and group and, thus, reveals the effects on cerebral perfusion attributable to the application of anodal left prefrontal tDCS. Cerebral perfusion measured from ASL is a correlate of metabolic processes [21]. In general, small, focal increases in perfusion were found in the group receiving 2 mA anodal left prefrontal tDCS across 3 consecutive days while a widespread decrease was observed in the group receiving sham stimulation. This implies metabolism was consistent in recurrent tDCS, and decreased metabolism is associated with sham stimulation.

Our study population was limited to active duty military members, and the study was executed in the evening after typical work days, although we did not measure or control

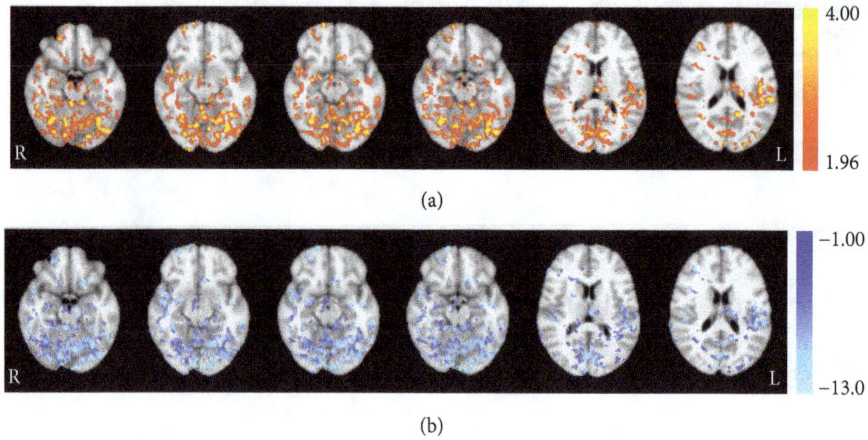

Figure 3: Session effect revealed from permutation testing for the CON group. (a) Statistically significant (t-statistic) regions with altered CBF from baseline to session 3 poststimulation and (b) corresponding decreases in quantified perfusion (mL/100 mg/min). Axial images taken at MNI coordinates $x = -18, -12, -14, -16, 12$, and 18 mm.

Table 4: Clusters identified with a significantly larger increase in perfusion from prestimulation at session 1 to session 3 poststimulation for the ACT group than for the CON group.

Hemisphere	Lobe	Gyrus	Volume (mm^3)	Max t-statistic	Max t-statistic location (mm)		
					X	Y	Z
Left	Temporal	Fusiform gyrus	15,784	5.14	−44	−56	−12
Right	Frontal	Inferior frontal gyrus	1445	5.66	60	20	4
Left	Parietal	Inferior parietal lobule	981	4.09	−32	−28	38
Left	Frontal	Superior frontal gyrus	715	4.09	−16	50	−20
Right	Parietal	Inferior parietal lobule	454	4.13	38	12	26
Left	Parietal	Superior parietal lobule	412	3.96	−44	−58	58
Left	Frontal	Precentral gyrus	293	4.43	−36	2	24
Right	Temporal	Fusiform gyrus	252	3.87	50	−32	−28
Right	Temporal	Middle temporal gyrus	210	3.93	42	0	−26
Right	Temporal	Inferior temporal gyrus	208	5.34	68	−30	−18
Right	Limbic	Cingulate	206	4.82	20	−4	42
Right	Parietal	Postcentral gyrus	177	3.24	62	−12	24
Right	Frontal	Precentral gyrus	176	3.08	50	2	48
Right	Limbic	Anterior cingulate cortex	166	3.67	12	22	−12
Left	Frontal	Medial frontal gyrus	148	3.42	−12	2	60
Left	Frontal	Superior frontal gyrus	131	3.93	−6	32	62
Right	Frontal	Superior frontal gyrus	101	3.78	18	70	−6
Right		Thalamus	95	3.64	8	−10	18
Right	Frontal	Middle frontal gyrus	87	3.37	22	20	64
Right	Parietal	Postcentral gyrus	86	3.54	44	−20	46
Left	Limbic	Anterior cingulate cortex	82	3.35	−14	30	22
Right	Limbic	Cingulate	80	3.53	24	−18	44
Left	Frontal	Medial frontal	80	3.28	−8	30	40
Left	Frontal	Superior frontal gyrus	77	2.91	−2	68	18
Left	Temporal	Fusiform gyrus	73	4.27	−46	−12	−28
Left	Frontal	Precentral gyrus	73	3.35	−38	−6	46
Right	Occipital	Lingual gyrus	71	3.45	26	−102	−6
Right		Putamen	71	3.09	−32	−8	−2

Table 5: Average CBF (±SEM) for each session/group from the clusters identified with a significantly larger increase in perfusion from prestimulation at session 1 to session 3 poststimulation for the ACT group than for the CON group.

Cluster	ACT		CON	
	Day 1 prestimulation CBF (mg/100 mL/min)	Day 3 poststimulation CBF (mg/100 mL/min)	Day 1 prestimulation CBF (mg/100 mL/min)	Day 3 poststimulation CBF (mg/100 mL/min)
L. fusiform gyr.	46.05 ± 1.67	49.12 ± 2.72	54.32 ± 2.95	44.92 ± 3.11
R. inf. front. gyr.	45.66 ± 1.74	51.35 ± 2.66	55.39 ± 2.14	48.77 ± 1.80
L. inf. par. lob.	41.91 ± 2.33	46.66 ± 2.85	53.84 ± 2.97	48.20 ± 2.31
L. sup. front. gyr.	43.85 ± 1.66	49.38 ± 2.28	54.18 ± 3.77	45.59 ± 2.08
R. inf. par. lob.	54.02 ± 2.71	60.72 ± 3.61	62.01 ± 2.61	56.53 ± 2.17
L. sup. par. lob.	46.36 ± 2.06	51.62 ± 2.46	57.50 ± 3.72	51.70 ± 2.37
L. precentral gyr.	47.67 ± 2.56	54.85 ± 3.32	60.10 ± 3.59	53.57 ± 2.24
R. fusiform gyr.	45.13 ± 1.75	49.94 ± 2.78	54.71 ± 2.83	47.77 ± 2.10
R. mid. temp. gyr.	35.97 ± 1.72	38.91 ± 2.66	44.12 ± 3.19	36.85 ± 2.29
R. inf. temp. gyr.	54.20 ± 2.66	60.18 ± 3.50	67.23 ± 3.00	59.48 ± 3.20
R. cingulate	26.44 ± 1.62	29.40 ± 1.67	31.46 ± 1.57	26.75 ± 1.24
R. postcentral gyr.	55.16 ± 2.92	58.52 ± 3.74	66.35 ± 2.57	58.83 ± 3.34
R. precentral gyr.	50.97 ± 2.50	55.60 ± 3.57	59.40 ± 2.75	52.78 ± 2.22
R. ant. cing. cort.	43.86 ± 2.98	47.93 ± 3.31	50.55 ± 1.89	43.44 ± 2.40
L. med. front. gyr.	38.35 ± 2.21	44.37 ± 2.64	50.01 ± 2.87	44.60 ± 1.31
L. sup. front. gyr.	45.39 ± 2.39	51.99 ± 1.73	58.87 ± 3.47	52.62 ± 2.46
R. sup. front. gyr.	55.52 ± 1.68	61.90 ± 3.42	70.82 ± 5.29	59.93 ± 2.77
R. thalamus	37.73 ± 2.26	43.27 ± 2.47	42.38 ± 1.91	39.36 ± 2.03
R. mid. front. gyr.	47.86 ± 3.26	54.08 ± 3.30	60.84 ± 2.89	52.83 ± 2.26
R. postcentral gyr.	44.32 ± 1.83	49.13 ± 2.65	51.83 ± 3.68	45.45 ± 3.21
L. ant. cing. cort.	26.56 ± 1.71	31.58 ± 1.28	38.40 ± 4.57	31.94 ± 1.78
R. cingulate	45.18 ± 3.25	49.41 ± 3.54	54.01 ± 2.76	46.79 ± 1.87
L. med. front. gyr.	21.89 ± 1.24	26.22 ± 1.71	27.54 ± 1.55	24.80 ± 1.47
L. sup. front. gyr.	48.97 ± 1.86	54.11 ± 4.37	60.99 ± 5.80	51.25 ± 3.37
L. fusiform gyr.	43.57 ± 2.65	49.91 ± 3.64	58.01 ± 2.42	52.00 ± 2.71
L. precentral gyr.	37.09 ± 1.91	40.43 ± 2.50	47.73 ± 3.50	39.29 ± 2.63
R. lingual gyr.	39.00 ± 1.94	41.87 ± 1.60	46.74 ± 3.45	40.15 ± 2.49
R. putamen	47.96 ± 3.36	48.57 ± 2.53	56.82 ± 4.07	46.27 ± 3.81

sleep/wake times. After three consecutive days of study participation as outlined in Table 1, it is only reasonable that the participants would be experiencing symptoms of fatigue. Hypoperfusion measured from ASL has been observed and detailed in patients with chronic fatigue syndrome [46–48] and associated with cognitive fatigue in healthy individuals [49]. Furthermore, hypometabolism has been observed in patients with chronic fatigue syndrome [50] and multiple sclerosis with fatigue [51]. The results from our CON group are consistent with this postulation and these previous findings; however, the findings from our ACT group are not. We theorize that left prefrontal tDCS provides some neural mechanism that counteracts this neural effect of fatigue. Behaviorally, left prefrontal tDCS has been shown to reduce the cognitive decline associated with fatigue in a similar group of active duty military members in an extended wakefulness study [9]. Anodal tDCS applied to the motor cortex has also been shown to have behavioral effects from fatigue in patients with multiple sclerosis [52]. However, there are no studies to date that have evaluated the neural effects of tDCS on fatigue.

The altered perfusion observed in this work can be traced to the LC. The LC is well known as the largest noradrenergic nucleus in the brain. The noradrenergic system is responsible for the synthesis, storage, and release of norepinephrine. Although the LC is relatively small, it is the primary source of norepinephrine for the neocortex. Projections from the LC are diverse, innervating most of the central nervous system [53]. Norepinephrine is a neurotransmitter associated with increased arousal and alertness [46–48], enhances long-term and working memory processes [54], and promotes vigilance and sensory processing [55]. The evidence presented in this work suggests that repetitive 2 mA tDCS applied to the left prefrontal cortex sustains the metabolic activity of the LC (Figure 4) which may result in an increased production of norepinephrine and a decreased effect of fatigue. In this work, measurements of resting perfusion were collected approximately

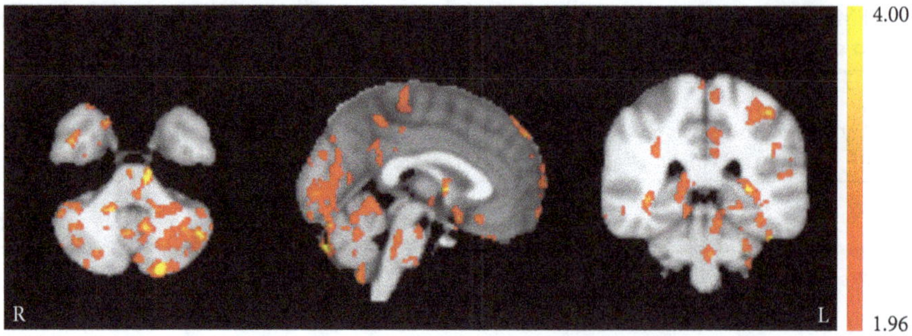

FIGURE 4: Session/group interaction effects (t-statistic) in the locus coeruleus revealed from permutation testing. The ACT group had significantly larger perfusion increases in the locus coeruleus from baseline to session 3 poststimulation compared to the CON group. The axial (left), sagittal (middle), and coronal (right) images were taken from MNI coordinates $z = -40$ mm, $y = -36$ mm, and $x = 0$ mm, respectively.

1.5 hrs following the conclusion of stimulation. Therefore, this effect remains following stimulation; however, it is not known how long this effect persists. Previous sleep deprivation studies utilizing anodal left prefrontal tDCS observed single-session behavioral effects that persisted for many hours [9, 10]. Effects such as this and the current findings could be derived from activation of the noradrenergic system.

Attention involves both top-down and bottom-up modulation. In bottom-up modulation, salient stimuli capture attention involuntarily while top-down modulation can direct attention as well as inhibit bottom-up processes. The ability to voluntarily direct attention (i.e., attentional control) varies significantly and substantially across individuals [56]. Top-down modulation of attention involves a variety of brain regions including the middle frontal gyrus, ACC, and superior parietal lobule. Each of these regions were found to have enhanced perfusion following repetitive 2 mA anodal tDCS to the left prefrontal cortex (Figure 5), suggestive of increased attentional control.

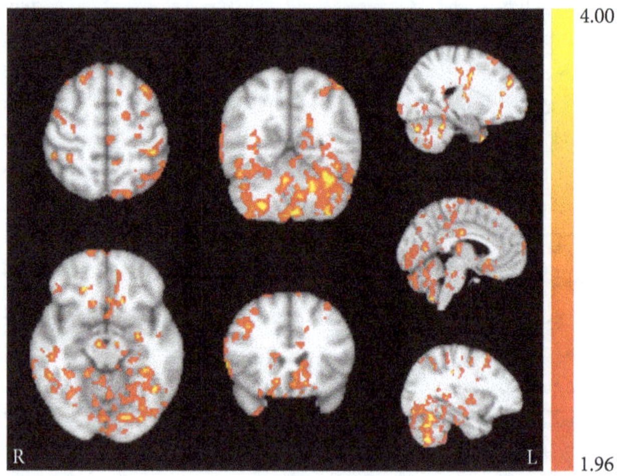

FIGURE 5: Session/group interaction effects (t-statistic) in the top-down attentional control network revealed from permutation testing. The ACT group had significantly larger perfusion increases in the right middle frontal gyrus, bilateral ACC, and left superior lobule from baseline to session 3 poststimulation compared to the CON group. The axial (left) images were taken from MNI coordinates $z = -14$ (top) and 56 (bottom) mm, sagittal (middle) images were taken from $y = -58$ (top) and 22 (bottom) mm, and coronal (right) images were taken from $x = 35$ (top), 47 (center), and 61 (bottom) mm.

Objects can be classified based upon the observation of physical properties such as shape, color, and texture. Semantic memory, general knowledge that has accumulated through life, can aid the classification process. The fusiform gyrus is theorized to largely contribute to processes involving semantic memory [57]. The large increase in perfusion in the occipital cortex, including the fusiform gyrus (Figure 6), is suggestive of enhanced utilization of semantic processes, increased semantic memory, and/or a heightened ability to recognize objects.

4. Conclusions

This study examined the effect of repetitive tDCS on cerebral perfusion. Anodal left prefrontal tDCS was used to apply 2 mA to the scalp for 30 minutes on three consecutive days. Measures of resting cerebral perfusion were acquired before and after stimulation on each day using ASL. Widespread increases in perfusion, indicative of increased metabolism, were observed; however, general decreases were observed in a matched group receiving sham tDCS. Furthermore, perfusion increased significantly more in the active stimulation group across many areas of the brain. These increases originated in the LC and spread extensively to regions in the neocortex supporting functions such as object recognition and top-down attentional modulation. The changes in the neocortex may be a direct result of the stimulation or an indirect result via the changes in the noradrenergic system produced from the altered LC activity. These findings help understand the broad behavioral effects that have been demonstrated using anodal left prefrontal tDCS. Future work is necessary to identify if the observed changes in perfusion correlate with altered metabolism but should also address the transiency of these effects.

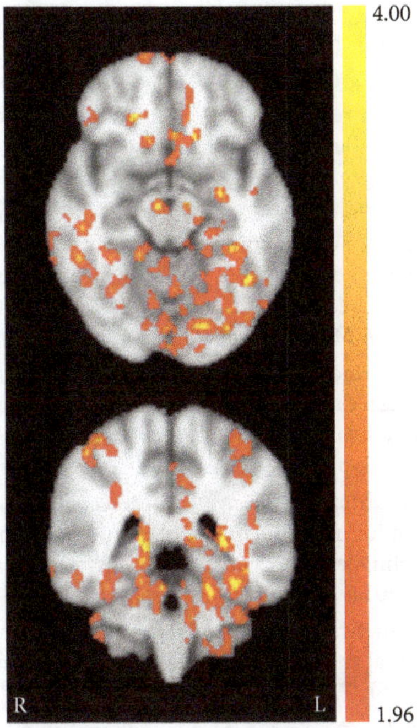

FIGURE 6: Session/group interaction effects (t-statistic) in the fusiform gyrus revealed from permutation testing. The ACT group had significantly larger perfusion increases in the right middle frontal gyrus, bilateral ACC, and left superior lobule from baseline to session 3 poststimulation compared to the CON group. The axial (top) and coronal (bottom) images were taken from MNI coordinates $z = -14$ mm and $y = -40$ mm, respectively.

Disclosure

The opinions expressed herein belong solely to the authors. They do not represent and should not be interpreted as being those of or endorsed by the Department of Defense or any other branch of the federal government. The U.S. Government is authorized to reproduce and distribute reprints for governmental purposes notwithstanding any copyright notation thereon. The voluntary, fully informed consent of the subjects used in this research was obtained as required by 32 CFR 210 and DODI 3216.02_AFI 40-402.

Conflicts of Interest

Matthew Sherwood received compensation for this work as a consultant through DCS Corporation and is also employed by Wright State University. Dr. Sherwood serves an unpaid role as a member of Aaron Madaris' Dissertation Committee at Wright State University. Aaron Madaris received compensation for this work as an intern through DCS Corporation and is also a student at Wright State University. All other authors declare no conflicts of interest.

Acknowledgments

This work was supported by the Air Force Research Laboratory (AFRL) under the Human Interface and Research Technology program (Contract FA8650-14-D-6500).

References

[1] F. Fregni, M. A. Nitsche, C. K. Loo et al., "Regulatory considerations for the clinical and research use of transcranial direct current stimulation (tDCS): review and recommendations from an expert panel," *Clinical Research and Regulatory Affairs*, vol. 32, no. 1, pp. 22–35, 2015.

[2] B. A. Coffman, M. C. Trumbo, R. A. Flores et al., "Impact of tDCS on performance and learning of target detection: interaction with stimulus characteristics and experimental design," *Neuropsychologia*, vol. 50, no. 7, pp. 1594–1602, 2012.

[3] L. M. Bullard, E. S. Browning, V. P. Clark et al., "Transcranial direct current stimulation's effect on novice versus experienced learning," *Experimental Brain Research*, vol. 213, no. 1, pp. 9–14, 2011.

[4] V. P. Clark, B. A. Coffman, M. C. Trumbo, and C. Gasparovic, "Transcranial direct current stimulation (tDCS) produces localized and specific alterations in neurochemistry: a 1H magnetic resonance spectroscopy study," *Neuroscience Letters*, vol. 500, no. 1, pp. 67–71, 2011.

[5] N. Lang, H. R. Siebner, N. S. Ward et al., "How does transcranial DC stimulation of the primary motor cortex alter regional neuronal activity in the human brain?," *The European Journal of Neuroscience*, vol. 22, no. 2, pp. 495–504, 2005.

[6] D. Liebetanz, "Pharmacological approach to the mechanisms of transcranial DC-stimulation-induced after-effects of human motor cortex excitability," *Brain*, vol. 125, no. 10, pp. 2238–2247, 2002.

[7] X. Zheng, D. C. Alsop, and G. Schlaug, "Effects of transcranial direct current stimulation (tDCS) on human regional cerebral blood flow," *NeuroImage*, vol. 58, no. 1, pp. 26–33, 2011.

[8] J. T. Nelson, R. A. McKinley, E. J. Golob, J. S. Warm, and R. Parasuraman, "Enhancing vigilance in operators with prefrontal cortex transcranial direct current stimulation (tDCS)," *NeuroImage*, vol. 85, pp. 909–917, 2014.

[9] L. K. McIntire, R. A. McKinley, C. Goodyear, and J. Nelson, "A comparison of the effects of transcranial direct current stimulation and caffeine on vigilance and cognitive performance during extended wakefulness," *Brain Stimulation*, vol. 7, no. 4, pp. 499–507, 2014.

[10] L. McIntire, R. Andy McKinley, J. Nelson, and C. Goodyear, "Transcranial direct current stimulation (tDCS) versus caffeine to sustain wakefulness at night when dosing at start-of-shift," in *Advances in Neuroergonomics and Cognitive Engineering*, K. Hale and K. Stanney, Eds., vol. 488 of Advances in Intelligent Systems and Computing, pp. 157–172, Springer International Publishing, Cham, 2017.

[11] V. P. Clark, B. A. Coffman, A. R. Mayer et al., "TDCS guided using fMRI significantly accelerates learning to identify concealed objects," *NeuroImage*, vol. 59, no. 1, pp. 117–128, 2012.

[12] R. A. McKinley, L. McIntire, N. Bridges, C. Goodyear, and M. P. Weisend, "Acceleration of image analyst training with transcranial direct current stimulation," *Behavioral Neuroscience*, vol. 127, no. 6, pp. 936–946, 2013.

[13] J. Nelson, R. A. McKinley, C. Phillips et al., "The effects of transcranial direct current stimulation (tDCS) on multitasking throughput capacity," *Frontiers in Human Neuroscience*, vol. 10, p. 589, 2016.

[14] R. Andy McKinley, L. McIntire, J. Nelson, J. Nelson, and C. Goodyear, "The effects of transcranial direct current stimulation (tDCS) on training during a complex procedural task," in *Advances in Neuroergonomics and Cognitive Engineering*,

K. Hale and K. Stanney, Eds., vol. 488 of Advances in Intelligent Systems and Computing, Springer, Cham, 2017.

[15] L. J. Bindman, O. C. J. Lippold, and J. W. T. Redfearn, "Long-lasting changes in the level of the electrical activity of the cerebral cortex produced by polarizing currents," *Nature*, vol. 196, no. 4854, pp. 584-585, 1962.

[16] C. Pittenger and R. S. Duman, "Stress, depression, and neuroplasticity: a convergence of mechanisms," *Neuropsychopharmacology*, vol. 33, no. 1, pp. 88–109, 2008.

[17] D. S. Williams, D. J. Grandis, W. Zhang, and A. P. Koretsky, "Magnetic resonance imaging of perfusion in the isolated rat heart using spin inversion of arterial water," *Magnetic Resonance in Medicine*, vol. 30, no. 3, pp. 361–365, 1993.

[18] G. Xu, H. A. Rowley, G. Wu et al., "Reliability and precision of pseudo-continuous arterial spin labeling perfusion MRI on 3.0 T and comparison with ^{15}O-water PET in elderly subjects at risk for Alzheimer's disease," *NMR in Biomedicine*, vol. 23, no. 3, pp. n/a–293, 2010.

[19] M. Grade, J. A. Hernandez Tamames, F. B. Pizzini, E. Achten, X. Golay, and M. Smits, "A neuroradiologist's guide to arterial spin labeling MRI in clinical practice," *Neuroradiology*, vol. 57, no. 12, pp. 1181–1202, 2015.

[20] M. J. Weber, J. A. Detre, S. L. Thompson-Schill, and B. B. Avants, "Reproducibility of functional network metrics and network structure: a comparison of task-related BOLD, resting ASL with BOLD contrast, and resting cerebral blood flow," *Cognitive, Affective, & Behavioral Neuroscience*, vol. 13, no. 3, pp. 627–640, 2013.

[21] A. Borogovac and I. Asllani, "Arterial spin labeling (ASL) fMRI: advantages, theoretical constrains and experimental challenges in neurosciences," *International Journal of Biomedical Imaging*, vol. 2012, Article ID 818456, 13 pages, 2012.

[22] T. A. Longden, F. Dabertrand, M. Koide et al., "Capillary K +-sensing initiates retrograde hyperpolarization to increase local cerebral blood flow," *Nature Neuroscience*, vol. 20, no. 5, pp. 717–726, 2017.

[23] C. J. Stagg, R. L. Lin, M. Mezue et al., "Widespread modulation of cerebral perfusion induced during and after transcranial direct current stimulation applied to the left dorsolateral prefrontal cortex," *The Journal of Neuroscience*, vol. 33, no. 28, pp. 11425–11431, 2013.

[24] N. H. Mackworth, "The breakdown of vigilance during prolonged visual search," *Quarterly Journal of Experimental Psychology*, vol. 1, no. 1, pp. 6–21, 1948.

[25] A. C. Silva and S.-G. Kim, "Pseudo-continuous arterial spin labeling technique for measuring CBF dynamics with high temporal resolution," *Magnetic Resonance in Medicine*, vol. 42, no. 3, pp. 425–429, 1999.

[26] W. T. Dixon, M. Sardashti, M. Castillo, and G. P. Stomp, "Multiple inversion recovery reduces static tissue signal in angiograms," *Magnetic Resonance in Medicine*, vol. 18, no. 2, pp. 257–268, 1991.

[27] S. Mani, J. Pauly, S. Conolly, C. Meyer, and D. Nishimura, "Background suppression with multiple inversion recovery nulling: applications to projective angiography," *Magnetic Resonance in Medicine*, vol. 37, no. 6, pp. 898–905, 1997.

[28] F. Q. Ye, J. A. Frank, D. R. Weinberger, and A. C. McLaughlin, "Noise reduction in 3D perfusion imaging by attenuating the static signal in arterial spin tagging (ASSIST)," *Magnetic Resonance in Medicine*, vol. 44, no. 1, pp. 92–100, 2000.

[29] G. H. Glover, "Spiral imaging in fMRI," *NeuroImage*, vol. 62, no. 2, pp. 706–712, 2012.

[30] R. Patriat, E. K. Molloy, T. B. Meier et al., "The effect of resting condition on resting-state fMRI reliability and consistency: a comparison between resting with eyes open, closed, and fixated," *NeuroImage*, vol. 78, pp. 463–473, 2013.

[31] D. C. Alsop, J. A. Detre, X. Golay et al., "Recommended implementation of arterial spin-labeled perfusion MRI for clinical applications: a consensus of the ISMRM perfusion study group and the European consortium for ASL in dementia," *Magnetic Resonance in Medicine*, vol. 73, no. 1, pp. 102–116, 2015.

[32] D. C. Alsop and J. A. Detre, "Reduced transit-time sensitivity in noninvasive magnetic resonance imaging of human cerebral blood flow," *Journal of Cerebral Blood Flow & Metabolism*, vol. 16, no. 6, pp. 1236–1249, 1996.

[33] H. J. M. M. Mutsaerts, R. M. E. Steketee, D. F. R. Heijtel et al., "Inter-vendor reproducibility of pseudo-continuous arterial spin labeling at 3 Tesla," *PLoS One*, vol. 9, no. 8, article e104108, 2014.

[34] S. M. Smith, M. Jenkinson, M. W. Woolrich et al., "Advances in functional and structural MR image analysis and implementation as FSL," *NeuroImage*, vol. 23, Supplement 1, pp. S208–S219, 2004.

[35] M. W. Woolrich, S. Jbabdi, B. Patenaude et al., "Bayesian analysis of neuroimaging data in FSL," *NeuroImage*, vol. 45, no. 1, Supplement 1, pp. S173–S186, 2009.

[36] D. N. Greve and B. Fischl, "Accurate and robust brain image alignment using boundary-based registration," *NeuroImage*, vol. 48, no. 1, pp. 63–72, 2009.

[37] D. L. Collins, C. J. Holmes, T. M. Peters, and A. C. Evans, "Automatic 3-D model-based neuroanatomical segmentation," *Human Brain Mapping*, vol. 3, no. 3, pp. 190–208, 1995.

[38] J. Mazziotta, A. Toga, A. Evans et al., "A probabilistic atlas and reference system for the human brain: international consortium for brain mapping (ICBM)," *Philosophical Transactions of the Royal Society B: Biological Sciences*, vol. 356, no. 1412, pp. 1293–1322, 2001.

[39] M. Jenkinson and S. Smith, "A global optimisation method for robust affine registration of brain images," *Medical Image Analysis*, vol. 5, no. 2, pp. 143–156, 2001.

[40] M. Jenkinson, P. Bannister, M. Brady, and S. Smith, "Improved optimization for the robust and accurate linear registration and motion correction of brain images," *NeuroImage*, vol. 17, no. 2, pp. 825–841, 2002.

[41] M. J. Anderson and J. Robinson, "Permutation tests for linear models," *Australian & New Zealand Journal of Statistics*, vol. 43, no. 1, pp. 75–88, 2001.

[42] A. M. Winkler, G. R. Ridgway, M. A. Webster, S. M. Smith, and T. E. Nichols, "Permutation inference for the general linear model," *NeuroImage*, vol. 92, pp. 381–397, 2014.

[43] T. Nichols and A. Holmes, "Nonparametric permutation tests for functional neuroimaging," in *Human Brain Function: Second Edition*, pp. 887–910, Academic Press, 2004.

[44] K. J. Worsley, "Statistical analysis of activation images," in *Functional MRI: An Introduction to Methods*, P. M. Matthews, P. Jezzard, and S. M. Smith, Eds., pp. 251–270, Oxford UP, London, 2001.

[45] C. D. Good, I. S. Johnsrude, J. Ashburner, R. N. A. Henson, K. J. Friston, and R. S. J. Frackowiak, "A voxel-based morphometric study of ageing in 465 normal adult human brains," *Neuroimage*, vol. 14, no. 1, pp. 21–36, 2001.

[46] B. Biswal, P. Kunwar, and B. H. Natelson, "Cerebral blood flow is reduced in chronic fatigue syndrome as assessed by arterial spin labeling," *Journal of the Neurological Sciences*, vol. 301, no. 1-2, pp. 9–11, 2011.

[47] S. M. MacHale, S. M. Lawrie, J. T. O. Cavanagh et al., "Cerebral perfusion in chronic fatigue syndrome and depression," *The British Journal of Psychiatry*, vol. 176, no. 6, pp. 550–556, 2000.

[48] D. C. Costa, C. Tannock, and J. Brostoff, "Brainstem perfusion is impaired in chronic fatigue syndrome," *QJM*, vol. 88, no. 11, pp. 767–773, 1995.

[49] J. Lim, W.-C. Wu, J. Wang, J. A. Detre, D. F. Dinges, and H. Rao, "Imaging brain fatigue from sustained mental workload: an ASL perfusion study of the time-on-task effect," *NeuroImage*, vol. 49, no. 4, pp. 3426–3435, 2010.

[50] U. Tirelli, F. Chierichetti, M. Tavio et al., "Brain positron emission tomography (PET) in chronic fatigue syndrome: preliminary data," *The American Journal of Medicine*, vol. 105, no. 3, pp. 54S–58S, 1998.

[51] U. Roelcke, L. Kappos, J. Lechner-Scott et al., "Reduced glucose metabolism in the frontal cortex and basal ganglia of multiple sclerosis patients with fatigue: a 18F-fluorodeoxyglucose positron emission tomography study," *Neurology*, vol. 48, no. 6, pp. 1566–1571, 1997.

[52] R. Ferrucci, M. Vergari, F. Cogiamanian et al., "Transcranial direct current stimulation (tDCS) for fatigue in multiple sclerosis," *NeuroRehabilitation*, vol. 34, no. 1, pp. 121–127, 2014.

[53] D. J. Chandler, "Evidence for a specialized role of the locus coeruleus noradrenergic system in cortical circuitries and behavioral operations," *Brain Research*, vol. 1641, Part B, pp. 197–206, 2016.

[54] V. Sterpenich, A. D'Argembeau, M. Desseilles et al., "The locus ceruleus is involved in the successful retrieval of emotional memories in humans," *The Journal of Neuroscience*, vol. 26, no. 28, pp. 7416–7423, 2006.

[55] C. W. Berridge, B. E. Schmeichel, and R. A. España, "Noradrenergic modulation of wakefulness/arousal," *Sleep Medicine Reviews*, vol. 16, no. 2, pp. 187–197, 2012.

[56] K. Fukuda and E. K. Vogel, "Human variation in overriding attentional capture," *The Journal of Neuroscience*, vol. 29, no. 27, pp. 8726–8733, 2009.

[57] M. Mion, K. Patterson, J. Acosta-Cabronero et al., "What the left and right anterior fusiform gyri tell us about semantic memory," *Brain*, vol. 133, no. 11, pp. 3256–3268, 2010.

6

Neurorehabilitation in Parkinson's Disease: A Critical Review of Cognitive Rehabilitation Effects on Cognition and Brain

María Díez-Cirarda, Naroa Ibarretxe-Bilbao, Javier Peña, and Natalia Ojeda

Department of Methods and Experimental Psychology, Faculty of Psychology and Education, University of Deusto, Bilbao, Spain

Correspondence should be addressed to Naroa Ibarretxe-Bilbao; naroa.ibarretxe@deusto.es

Academic Editor: Toshiyuki Fujiwara

Background. Parkinson's disease (PD) patients experience cognitive impairment which has been related to reduced quality of life and functional disability. These symptoms usually progress until dementia occurs. Some studies have been published assessing the efficacy of cognitive treatments on improving cognition, functional outcome, and producing changes in brain activity. *Objective.* A critical review was performed to present up-to-date neurorehabilitation effects of cognitive rehabilitation in PD, with special emphasis on the efficacy on cognition, quality of life aspects, brain changes, and the longitudinal maintenance of these changes. *Results.* After exclusions, 13 studies were reviewed, including 6 randomized controlled trials for the efficacy on cognition, 2 randomized controlled trials regarding the brain changes after cognitive training, and 5 studies which evaluated the long-term effects of cognitive treatments. *Conclusions.* Cognitive rehabilitation programs have demonstrated to be effective on improving cognitive functions, but more research is needed focusing on the efficacy on improving behavioral aspects and producing brain changes in patients with PD. Moreover, there is a need of randomized controlled trials with long-term follow-up periods.

1. Introduction

Parkinson's disease (PD) is a common neurodegenerative disease, being most of the cases diagnosed at around 60 years [1]. Traditionally, PD has been considered a motor disorder, and the core motor symptoms are rigidity, tremor, bradykinesia (akinesia), and postural instability. In addition, freezing of gait (difficulty to initiate or continue walking) and flexed posture have been included in the cardinal motor symptoms of the disease [2]. Nowadays, it is known that this neurodegenerative process produces a wide range of motor and nonmotor symptoms in PD patients; hence, PD is considered a multiple system neurodegenerative disorder [3]. Among these nonmotor symptoms, cognitive impairment is an important nonmotor symptom due to its prevalence among PD patients (20–50%) [4, 5]. In addition, PD patients might develop cognitive impairment from the early stages of the disease [4, 5]. These cognitive deficits may deteriorate with the progression of the disease until dementia occurs [6, 7]. The analysis of cognitive impairment and dementia in PD patients is relevant because both have shown relationship with reduced quality of life and functional disability in PD patients [8, 9].

These cognitive impairments in PD have been related to grey matter (GM) atrophy, white matter (WM) alterations, brain functional connectivity (FC), and brain activation alterations. PD patients with Mild Cognitive Impairment (MCI) diagnosis have shown GM volume reduction in the frontal, temporal, and parietal lobes, but also in the hippocampus, amygdala, and putamen [10, 11]. Additionally, PD patients with MCI have shown widespread cerebral WM deterioration [11–13]. Interestingly, WM alterations have been found to appear before GM volume reduction in PD patients, which highlights the importance to explore the relationship between WM indexes and cognitive impairment [14]. In addition, cognitive deficits have also been related to functional brain alterations, showing altered FC and brain activation values both during resting state and during cognitive tasks inside the scanner [15, 16].

With the progression of the disease, cognitive deficits usually deteriorate until dementia occurs after 10 to 20 years [6, 17]. A study followed newly diagnosed PD patients over time and found that after 20 years, dementia was present in up to 80% of PD patients [6]. In addition, recent studies showed that the presence of MCI diagnosis in PD patients contributes to the development of dementia [7], and results support that MCI could be considered as a prodromal stage for dementia in PD [18]. Cognitive deterioration is accompanied by GM volume loss [19], WM alterations [20], and functional brain changes [21, 22]. When dementia occurs in PD patients, cortical degeneration has been extended to frontal, temporal, parietal, and occipital areas [23].

Due to the relevance of cognitive deficits, therapeutic strategies are needed to treat cognitive decline. A common cognitive rehabilitation program could be described as a behavioral treatment for cognitive impairment which focused on cognitive abilities and daily living activities, which is based on the restoration, compensation, and optimization of the cognitive functions [24, 25]. Cognitive rehabilitation programs have demonstrated their efficacy on improving cognition in different studies in PD. Several reviews [26–28] and meta-analyses [29, 30] have been published in the field. The efficacy of cognitive rehabilitation on improving cognition has been shown, but these reviews and meta-analyses highlight the importance of continuing with research focused on the efficacy of the cognitive rehabilitation approach in PD.

The main objective of the present study is to perform a critical review to present up-to-date neurorehabilitation effects of cognitive rehabilitation in PD. The first objective was to examine the efficacy of cognitive rehabilitation programs on cognition and behavioral aspects. The second objective was to review the evidence of the brain changes found after cognitive treatments. Finally, the present study analyzed the long-term effects of cognitive rehabilitation in PD.

2. Methods

2.1. Review Strategy. Studies were included from inception to December 2017. Focusing on the first objective of this critical review, which was to analyze those randomized controlled trials focused on the efficacy of cognitive rehabilitation programs on cognition, we selected only those studies that fulfilled the following criteria: (1) randomized controlled trials; (2) PD patients underwent a cognitive rehabilitation program; (3) the main objective was to investigate the change in cognition; and (4) studies including a PD control group. Among the studies that fulfilled these specific criteria, we also reported (if included in the studies) the results of the efficacy on behavioral or mood aspects, such as depression, apathy, functional disability, and quality of life aspects.

Regarding the second objective of the present review, the efficacy of cognitive rehabilitation programs in producing brain changes in PD was determined based on the following criteria: (1) randomized controlled trials; (2) PD patients underwent a cognitive rehabilitation program; (3) studies including a PD control group; and (4) brain changes were evaluated.

Finally, focusing on the last objective of the present study, the review about the long-term effects of cognitive rehabilitation programs was based on the following criteria: (1) PD patients underwent a cognitive rehabilitation program; (2) a longitudinal follow-up evaluation was performed; and (3) the main objective was to investigate the change in cognition at follow-up. In this specific section, we included both randomized controlled trials and nonrandomized trials, due to the scarce number of published studies and to have a wider perspective.

Databases included were PubMed, Medline, and Google Scholar. The search terms were specified to be found in the title of the studies. The terms were (1) Parkinson's disease/Parkinson disease; (2) cognitive rehabilitation/cognitive training/cognitive remediation; (3) attention rehabilitation/attention training/attention remediation; (4) executive training/executive rehabilitation/executive remediation; (5) memory training/memory rehabilitation/memory remediation; (6) randomized controlled trial/randomized controlled trial; and (7) cognition. The search term combinations in the databases were (1) + (2); (1) + (3); (1) + (4); (1) + (5); and (1) + (6) + (7).

A summary of study selection is shown in Figure 1. The results of the selected studies were divided into 3 different sections. First, the studies evaluating the cognitive and behavioral changes are shown in Table 1. Then, Table 2 shows the studies that assessed the brain changes after cognitive rehabilitation in PD. In addition, the longitudinal effects of cognitive rehabilitation programs are shown in Table 3. In Tables 1 and 3, different characteristics of the studies are shown, such as the sample size, characteristics of the cognitive rehabilitation program used, cognitive domains analyzed, significant results found, and limitations of each study. In Table 2, MRI acquisition, preprocessing, and analysis specifications are included for each study, along with the brain significant results and the study limitations.

3. Results

3.1. Efficacy on Improving Cognition and Behavioral Aspects. A summary of the included cognitive rehabilitation studies in PD is shown in Table 1. Studies were included if they followed guidelines for randomized controlled trials, the intervention was a cognitive rehabilitation program, and the main objective of the study was to improve cognition. As previously reported in other reviews and meta-analyses, cognitive rehabilitation improves cognition in PD [27, 29, 30]. However, there is a need for studies with larger samples and double-blind randomized controlled trials to reach generalized conclusions in PD.

A less studied aspect of cognitive rehabilitation is its efficacy on improving mood symptoms or functional disability related to the disease. Following the review-specific criteria, among the randomized controlled trials in PD, only five studies have evaluated the change in functionality and mood aspects [31–35] and two of them found positive effects [31, 32] (Table 1). Petrelli et al. compared a structured and a nonstructured cognitive training program in PD patients and found that the symptoms of depression were reduced only in those PD patients that attended the nonstructured cognitive program [32]. Peña et al. found that functional disability scores were reduced in the experimental group (3 months of cognitive training) compared to the

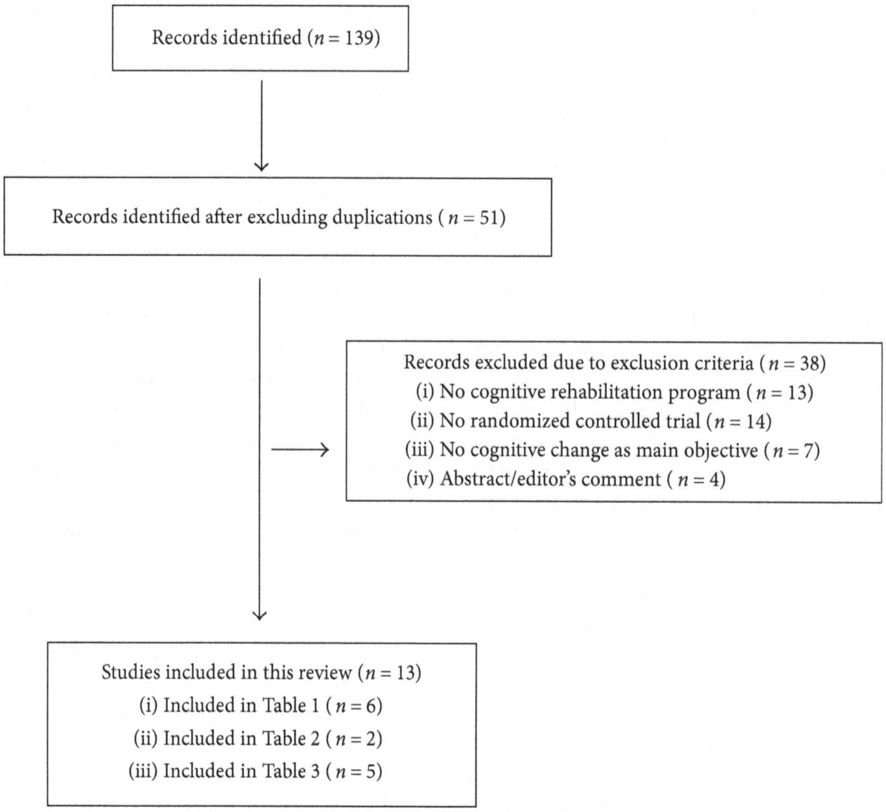

FIGURE 1: Summary of studies identified and included in the review.

active control group [31]. On the contrary, París et al. evaluated the change in quality of life, depressive symptoms, and activities of daily life after attending a cognitive rehabilitation program [35]. No significant changes were found in any scale, and authors related the absence of significant changes in quality of life to the short time of training (12 sessions in 1 month). In the same line, PD patients in the study of Cerasa et al. also attended a cognitive training program during 12 sessions and showed no significant changes in mood status [33]. However, in the study of Edwards et al., PD patients attended a cognitive training program during a longer period of time (3 months), but patients showed no changes in behavioral measures [34]. Among clinical symptoms of the disease, the change in depressive symptoms has been usually assessed in cognitive training studies in PD, but despite some significant changes, the overall results point to the absence of efficacy in reducing depression symptomatology after treatment [30]. However, these studies excluded patients with depression diagnosis or with severe symptoms of depression prior to participation. Therefore, this criterion could have influenced the absence of significant changes. With all, the mechanisms that make possible the improvement in quality of life aspects after a cognitive rehabilitation program are not clear. The duration of treatment and degree of structuration of the sessions could be two relevant variables to take into account when assessing transfer effects to clinical variables, but other variables seem to influence this process. Interestingly, in schizophrenia studies, the presence of a therapist during the training sessions and the group format of the training program have been suggested to influence the results on mood symptoms [36]. The cognitive sessions carried in a group format enhance social interactions between participants, and the presence of a therapist may increase the motivation and give positive feedback to the patients, which could have an impact in the affective state of patients. In fact, the two PD studies that found transfer effects to functional aspects or depressive symptoms performed a group-based cognitive training, and the training was guided by a qualified therapist [31, 32].

Moreover, detecting variables that predict the efficacy of cognitive treatments is an important aspect to take into account in order to understand the cognitive rehabilitation process, which could guide researchers to develop more effective programs and clinicians to personalize treatments for patients (Table 1). Despite the large amount of studies assessing the efficacy of cognitive rehabilitation in PD, few studies have investigated the predictors of the efficacy of cognitive treatments in PD. These PD studies found that lower age at diagnosis and longer disease duration were predictors of higher degree of cognitive improvements after rehabilitation [34], but higher scores in working memory and flexibility at baseline were related with lower degree of improvements after rehabilitation [37].

3.2. Changes in Brain Activity after Cognitive Rehabilitation. Little is known about the neurobiological effects of cognitive rehabilitation programs in PD. To date, literature is scarce about the presence of cerebral changes associated with cognitive rehabilitation programs assessed with structural and functional MRI techniques in PD. Table 2 summarized the main findings of the two randomized controlled trials in

Table 1: Summary of the randomized controlled trials in assessing the efficacy of cognitive rehabilitation programs in PD.

Authors	Sample	H&Y	Cognitive rehabilitation program Duration	Paper-pencil—P Computerized—C	Cogn. domains trained	Format	Tests[1]	Predictors of greater improvement	MRI (Table 2)	Results	Long-term follow-up (Table 3)	Limitations/ risk of bias
París et al. [35]	**28 PD** 16 CR 12 ACG	1–3	**12 sessions** 4 weeks 3 times/ week 45 min/ session	CR—"SmartBrain tool" (P + C) ACG— speech therapy	(i) Attention (ii) WM (iii) Memory (iv) Psychomotor speed (v) EF (vi) Visuospatial ability (vii) Language (viii) Calculation skills (ix) Culture	Group + home	(i) Attention (ii) WM (iii) EF (iv) Processing speed (v) Verbal memory (vi) Visual memory (vii) Visuoconstruction (viii) Visuospatial ability (ix) Verbal fluency (x) *Depression* (xi) *Quality of life* (xii) *Daily living activities*	—	—	**Improvements** (i) Attention/WM (ii) Information processing speed (iii) Visual memory (iv) Visuospatial ability (v) Visuoconstructive ability (vi) Semantic fluency (vii) EF	—	Small sample size
Edwards et al. [34]	**74 PD** 32 CR 42 CG	1–3	**36 sessions** 3 months 3 times/ week 1 h/session	CR—"InSight version of SOPT" (C)	(i) Information processing speed	Home	(i) Speed of processing (self-reported) (ii) Perception of cognitive and everyday functioning (self-reported) (iii) *Depression*	<Age at PD diagnosis >Disease duration	—	**Improvements** (i) Speed of processing	—	No ACG Only 1 domain trained Self-reported test for cognition and functionality
Cerasa et al. [33]	**15 PD** 8 CR 7 ACG	1–3	**12 sessions** 6 weeks 2 times/ week 1 h/session	CR—"RehaCom" (C) ACG—visuomotor coordination tapping task. In-house software (C)	(i) Attention (ii) Information processing	Group	(i) Attention/ processing speed (ii) EF (iii) WM (iv) Spatial memory (v) Verbal memory (vi) Visuospatial orientation (vii) Verbal fluency (viii) *Depression* (ix) *Anxiety* (x) *Quality of life*	—	Yes	**Improvements** (i) Attention/ processing speed (ii) WM	—	Small sample size
Zimmermann et al. [37]	**39 PD** 19 CR 20 ACG	2[a]	**12 sessions** 4 weeks 3 times/ week	CR—"CogniPlus" (C) ACG—"Nintendo Wii" (C)	(i) Attention (ii) Working memory (iii) EF	Group	(i) Attention (ii) WM (iii) EF (iv) Episodic memory (v) Visuoconstruction	(i) WM score (ii) Flexibility score	—	(i) ACG improved attention compared to CR	—	Small sample size No change in functionality evaluated

Table 1: Continued.

Authors	Sample	H&Y	Duration	Cognitive rehabilitation program: Paper-pencil—P Computerized—C	Cognitive rehabilitation program: Cogn. domains trained	Format	Tests[1]	Predictors of greater improvement	MRI (Table 2)	Results	Long-term follow-up (Table 3)	Limitations/ risk of bias
Petrelli et al. [32]	**65 PD** 22 CR-NV 22 CR-MT 21 CG	1–3	12 sessions 6 weeks 2 times/ week 90 min/ session	P "NEUROvitalis"—NV P "mentally fit"—MF	**NV** (i) Attention (ii) Memory (iii) EF **MF** (i) Attention (ii) Memory (iii) Creativity	Group + individual	(i) Attention (ii) Memory (iii) EF (iv) Visuoconstruction (v) *Depression* (vi) *Quality of life*	—	—	**Improvements NV versus CG** (i) Working memory (ii) Short-term memory **Improvements MF versus CG** (i) *Depression* **Improvements NV versus MT** (i) Working memory	12 months	Small sample size No ACG
Peña et al. [31]	**42 PD** 20 PD-CR 22 PD-ACG	1–3	39 sessions 13 weeks 3 times/ week 1 h/session	CR—"REHACOP" (P) ACG—occupational activities (P)	(i) Attention (ii) Memory (iii) Language (iv) EF (v) Social cognition (vi) PS	Group	(i) Processing speed (ii) Memory (iii) Executive functions (iv) Social cognition (v) *Functional disability* (vi) *Apathy* (vii) *Depression*	—	Yes	**Improvements PD-CR versus PD-ACG** (i) Processing speed (ii) Visual memory (iii) Social cognition (iv) *Functional disability*	18 months	Small sample size

ACG = active control group; CG = control group; CR = cognitive rehabilitation; EF = executive functions; HC = healthy controls; H&Y = Hoehn and Yahr; MRI = magnetic resonance image; PD = Parkinson's disease; WM = working memory. [1]Tests assessing mood, clinical, and functionality aspects are shown in *italics*. [a]Median.

Table 2: Summary of randomized controlled trials in assessing brain changes related to cognitive rehabilitation programs in PD.

Authors	MRI sample	H&Y	Cognitive rehabilitation program	MRI acquisition/ preprocessing/analysis	MRI statistical analysis	MRI results	Correlation with cognitive measures	Limitations/risk of bias
Cerasa et al. [33]	**15 PD** 8 CR 7 ACG	1–3	RehaCom computer program Training: (i) Attention (ii) Information processing	Resting-state fMRI/ICA in FSL/FC analysis	ANOVA (group × time) Region of interests Dorsolateral PFC Ventrolateral PFC ACC Sup + inf parietal left Caudate Cerebellum	Increased functional activity: (i) Left dorsolateral PFC (executive network) (ii) Superior parietal left (attention network)	—	Small sample size Only one type of MRI acquisition
Díez-Cirarda et al. [38] (cognitive results in [31])	**30 PD** 15 CR 15 ACG	1–3	"REHACOP" program Training: (i) Attention (ii) Memory (iii) Language (iv) EF (v) Social cognition	Resting-state fMRI/ROI-to-ROI approach in CONN toolbox Memory fMRI paradigm/ model-based approach in SPM Diffusion weighted/TBSS in FSL T1 weighted/VBM in FSL	ANOVA (group × time) Paired t-test Whole brain	Increased FC between BA9L-BA20L and BA9R-BA20L Increased brain activation Learning task: left frontal inferior lobe Increased brain activation Memory task: left middle temporal lobe — —	Yes	Small sample size and reduced at long-term follow-up Memory fMRI paradigm results at FWE uncorrected

ACC = anterior cingulate cortex; ACG = active control group; BA = Brodmann area; CR = cognitive rehabilitation; EF = executive functions; FC = functional connectivity; fMRI = functional magnetic resonance imaging; FSL = FMRIB Software Library; H&Y = Hoehn and Yahr; ICA = independent component analysis; MRI = magnetic resonance image; PD = Parkinson's disease; PFC = prefrontal cortex; TBSS = tract-based spatial statistics; VBM = voxel-based morphometry.

Table 3: Summary of cognitive rehabilitation studies in PD with longitudinal follow-up evaluation.

Authors	Sample	H&Y	Duration	Cognitive rehabilitation program: Paper-pencil—P Computerized—C	Cognitive rehabilitation program: Cogn. domains trained	Format	Tests[1]	MRI (Table 2)	Results (pre- and posttreatment)	Long-term follow-up (T0/T1/T2)	Limitations/risk of bias
Nonrandomized/noncontrolled trials											
Sinforiani et al. [39]	**20 PD**	1.5 ±0.6	**12 sessions** 6 weeks + 12 h MT	C "TNP"	(i) Attention (ii) Abstract reasoning (iii) Visuospatial	Group	(i) MMSE (ii) Digit span (iii) Corsi's test (iv) Babcock's story (v) FAS phonetic (vi) Raven matrix (vii) WCST (viii) Stroop test	—	**Improvements:** (i) Babcock (recall) (ii) FAS phonetic (iii) Raven matrix	**6 months without training: maintenance (no statistical data)** (i) Babcock (recall) (ii) FAS phonetic (iii) Raven matrix	No CG No differentiation of the efficacy of motor or cognitive training No statistical data at follow-up
Reuter et al. [40]	**222 PD** Gr A—CR = 71 Gr B—CR-TT = 75 Gr C—CR-TT-MT = 76 (plus psychoeducation with caregivers)	2–4	**14 sessions** 4 weeks 4 times/week 60 min/session	P + C Group A: cognitive training Group B: cognitive + transfer training Group C: cognitive + transfer + motor training	(i) Attention (ii) Concentration (iii) EF (iv) WM (v) Memory (vi) Processing speed	Individual	(i) ADAS-Cog (ii) SCOPA-Cog (iii) EF-BADS (iv) PS-PASAT (v) *Depression* (vi) *Anxiety* (vii) *PDQ-39*	—	**Improvements in all groups:** (i) ADAS-Cog (ii) BADS (iii) PASAT **Greater improvements in group C:** (i) ADAS-Cog (ii) SCOPA-Cog (iii) BADS (iv) PASAT	**6 months with home training: group C performed more training sessions (T2 > T0)** (i) ADAS-Cog (ii) SCOPA-Cog (iii) BADS (iv) PASAT	No ACG No PDQ-39 scores at baseline Different number of sessions between posttreatment and long-term evaluation
Adamski et al. [45]	**6 PD-CR 12 HC-CR 7 HC-CG**	—	**16 sessions** 4 weeks 4 times/week 45 min/session	C "BrainStim"	(i) WM (ii) Encoding (iii) Recall (iv) EF (v) Visuospatial ability	Group	(i) Attention (ii) WM (iii) Short-term memory (iv) Long-term memory (v) PS (vi) EF (vii) *Depression* (viii) *Fatigue*	—	**Improvements in PD group:** (i) Short-term memory (ii) Long-term memory **Improvements in HC groups:** (iii) Diverse cognitive domains	**3 months without training: PD group increased (T2 > T0)** (i) Short-term memory	Small sample size No PD-ACG Baseline differences between groups

Table 3: Continued.

Authors	Sample	H&Y	Duration	Cognitive rehabilitation program Paper-pencil—P Computerized—C	Cogn. domains trained	Format	Tests[1]	MRI (Table 2)	Results (pre- and posttreatment)	Long-term follow-up (T0/T1/T2)	Limitations/risk of bias
Randomized controlled trials											
Petrelli et al. [42]	**65 PD** 22 CR-NV 22 CR-MF 21 CG	1–3	**12 sessions** 6 weeks 2 times/week 90 min/session	P "NEUROvitalis"—NV P "mentally fit"—MF	**NV** (i) Attention (ii) Memory (iii) EF **MF** (i) Attention (ii) Memory (iii) Creativity	Group + individual	(i) Attention (ii) Memory (iii) EF (iv) Visuoconstruction (v) *Depression* (vi) *Quality of life*	—	**Improvements in NV versus CG:** (i) Working memory (ii) Short-term memory **Improvements in MF versus CG:** (i) *Depression* **Improvements in NV versus MT:** (i) Working memory	**12 months without training: NV group maintenance (T2 = T0)** (i) MMSE (ii) DemTect	Small sample size No ACG Long-term evaluation with screening tests
Díez-Cirarda et al. [41]	**42 PD** 20 PD-CR 22 PD-ACG	1–3	**39 sessions** 13 weeks 3 times/week 60 min/session	CR—"REHACOP" (P) ACG—occupational activities (P)	(i) Attention (ii) Memory (iii) Language (iv) EF (v) Social cognition (vi) PS	Group	(i) PS (ii) Memory (iii) Executive functions (iv) Social cognition (v) *Functional disability* (vi) *Apathy* (vii) *Depression*	Yes	**Improvements in PD-CR versus PD-ACG:** (i) PS (ii) Visual memory (iii) Social cognition (iv) *Functional disability* (v) Brain functional changes	**18 months without training: PD-CR increased (T2 > T0):** (i) Verbal memory (ii) Visual memory (iii) EF (iv) ToM (v) *Functional disability* (vi) Brain functional activity	Small sample size Absence of CG at follow-up

ACG = active control group; CG = control group; CR = cognitive rehabilitation; EF = executive functions; FAS = phonetic fluency test; HC = healthy controls; H&Y = Hoehn and Yahr; MMSE = minimental state examination; MRI = magnetic resonance image; MT = motor training; TT = transfer training; PD = Parkinson's disease; PS = processing speed; WCST = Wisconsin card sorting task; WM = working memory.
[1]Tests assessing mood, clinical, and functionality aspects are shown in *italics*.

evaluating brain changes after a cognitive rehabilitation program in PD.

One study evaluated the effects of group-based attention rehabilitation on brain functional activity in PD patients [33]. PD patients were included in the trial if they had attention impairment but no other cognitive domain impaired. At pre- and post-treatment assessments, patients underwent an extensive neuropsychological assessment and resting-state fMRI were acquired. PD patients were randomly divided into experimental group and active control group. The experimental group received attention rehabilitation using "RehaCom" computer program, while the control group attended in-house software which focused on visuomotor coordination. The attention rehabilitation consisted in computer-assisted tasks which trained attention and information processing during 6 weeks. Specifically, attention rehabilitation tasks were focused on concentration and attention tasks and vigilance program and divided attention from the RehaCom software. After rehabilitation, PD patients showed improvements in attention and processing speed tasks and increased brain activation in the left dorsolateral prefrontal cortex (part of the executive resting-state network) and the left superior parietal cortex (part of the attentional resting-state network) [33] (Table 2).

A later study in PD patients evaluated the changes in brain activity after a 3-month integrative cognitive rehabilitation program [38]. PD patients underwent an extensive neuropsychological assessment at pre- and post-treatment. Regarding MRI acquisition, GM and WM changes were analyzed as well as brain activity changes during resting-state and during a memory paradigm. The cognitive rehabilitation program used was the REHACOP, a paper/pencil rehabilitation program, which trained attention, processing speed, memory, language, executive functions, and social cognition during 3 months. PD patients after cognitive rehabilitation showed increased brain FC between frontal and temporal lobes and increased brain activation during the memory paradigm in frontal and temporal areas (see Table 2). No brain structural changes were found after rehabilitation. These brain FC and activation values at post-treatment showed correlations with post-treatment cognitive performance in PD patients from the experimental group. Specifically, during resting state, FC values between frontal and temporal lobes at post-treatment correlated with executive function performance at post-treatment. Additionally, during the learning fMRI task, the brain activation values after treatment correlated with the visual memory performance at post-treatment [38].

These studies suggest that brain activity changes are possible after a cognitive rehabilitation program in PD. Further studies are needed to replicate and complement these findings.

3.3. Long-Term Effects of Cognitive Rehabilitation. Furthermore, the ultimate goal of cognitive treatments is to ensure that benefits are maintained over long periods of time, but little is known about the maintenance of cognitive improvements over time in PD patients, and a few studies have evaluated it [39–42, 45]. A summary of these studies is shown in Table 3.

The first study to evaluate the long-term effects of cognitive rehabilitation was published in 2004 by Sinforiani et al. and showed that PD patients attending a cognitive training program combined with motor training during one month showed maintenance of the cognitive benefits after 6 months [39]. However, the study did not include statistical analyses for the follow-up period. Moreover, this study did not include a control group; therefore, we cannot conclude that these possible benefits were related to the cognitive or motor training or the combination of treatments.

Another study in PD compared three training groups: "group A" which attended cognitive training, "group B" which attended cognitive training and transfer training, and "group C" which attended cognitive, transfer, and motor training [40] (Table 3). The authors found that the three groups benefited from training, but those PD patients that attended cognitive training combined with transfer training and physical activity benefited significantly more in the short term. Moreover, over the next 6 months, patients from "group C" were more motivated to spend more time training at home compared to the other groups and showed greater maintenance of cognitive improvements after 6 months [40]. However, because patients from group C spent more hours in training at home over the next 6 months compared to the other groups, these results may be influenced by the difference of hours spent in training. Finally, this study also included an intervention therapy with caregivers focusing on psychoeducation, which helped the patients to continue the training tasks at home [40] (Table 3).

A later study in PD assessed the long-term effects of cognitive rehabilitation for a longer period of time (12 months) [42]. At baseline, these PD patients were randomized to a structured cognitive rehabilitation program (NEUROvitalis), to a nonstructured cognitive rehabilitation program (mentally fit), or to a control group. After 12 months from post-treatment, PD patients that attended NEUROvitalis training program showed reduced cognitive performance compared to post-treatment, but scores were similar compared to baseline. Moreover, the risk of conversion to MCI was found higher in the control group than in any of the cognitive training groups. Regarding depression, the "mentally fit" group was the only group that showed significant reduction in depressive symptoms after training, but these changes were not maintained at follow-up (Table 3). With all, the authors concluded that a structured cognitive treatment could prevent cognitive decline [42].

Regarding the maintenance of neuroimaging changes, to date, only one study has been published assessing the longitudinal effects of cognitive rehabilitation [41]. PD patients attended a 3-month cognitive rehabilitation program and showed increased brain connectivity and activation in the frontal and temporal lobes after treatment. These patients underwent a neuropsychological and neuroimaging assessment after 18 months from post-treatment. The results showed that not only improvements in cognitive performance and functionality were maintained after 18 months but also increased FC was found at follow-up [41]. In addition, PD patients also showed maintenance of the increased brain activation during the memory paradigm at long-term compared to baseline, but the level of activation at long-term was reduced compared to post-treatment. This study showed promising findings regarding the maintenance of brain changes in a neurodegenerative disease; however, the sample size was small, and the control group was not evaluated in the long term. The results need to be replicated.

These few studies suggest the maintenance of cognitive improvements after attending a cognitive rehabilitation program in PD patients (Table 3). However, literature is scarce in this pathology and more research needs to be done, especially including neuroimaging assessment at follow-up.

4. Discussion

The studies on the efficacy of cognitive rehabilitation programs in PD suggest that cognitive rehabilitation programs are effective in improving cognition but further research is needed in this field to clarify its efficacy on functional disability and brain activity changes. Also, very little is known about the long-term maintenance of cognitive changes after rehabilitation. There are few cognitive rehabilitation studies in PD which followed the Consolidated Standards of Reporting Trials (CONSORT) guidelines for randomized controlled trials. These make more difficult to find conclusive findings. Future studies should implement these guidelines in order to improve the research quality and validity of findings.

All randomized controlled trials in PD for cognitive rehabilitation programs point to the efficacy in improving cognition. However, most of them highlighted the small sample size as a limitation, which makes it difficult to generalize the findings. Additionally, all of them used different types of cognitive training programs, with different duration and type of exercises. One of the future steps to be taken towards understanding the efficacy of cognitive rehabilitation is identifying the characteristics that make an integrative cognitive rehabilitation program effective against cognitive impairment. A review of cognitive rehabilitation concluded that better results may be obtained in a group-based format compared to an individual format [28]. However, while most of the rehabilitation studies in PD are group-based, this question has not been directly addressed. In addition, a recent meta-analysis compared the efficacy of standardized with tailored (individualized) cognitive interventions, but found that there were insufficient studies for a statistical comparison [29]. Furthermore, other variables are also to be defined, such as the most appropriate number of sessions, their frequency, and the duration of the treatment. Also, the number of cognitive domains trained may also influence the results. Moreover, predictors of the efficacy of cognitive treatments are useful in the disease to adequate cognitive treatment to the patient. Very few studies have evaluated this aspect, and research is needed in the field.

Regarding patients' characteristics, most of the randomized controlled trials in PD have been performed with PD patients at the early Hoehn and Yahr stages of the disease. Future studies should also include PD patients at more advanced stages to evaluate whether cognitive treatments could also benefit these patients. Interestingly, a study protocol was recently published addressing the efficacy of a cognitive rehabilitation in PD patients with dementia, but results are pending [43].

Moreover, transfer effects to clinical aspects have been found in some cognitive rehabilitation studies in PD; however, other studies found no significant changes. The mechanisms that make possible to transfer benefits to clinical variables are unknown. There is an urgent need of studies analyzing this subject. The last goal of cognitive rehabilitation programs is to improve quality of life of patients. Future studies should also include clinical and functionality scales in pre- and post-treatment neuropsychological assessments.

On the other hand, promising findings have been found regarding brain changes after treatment in PD, which support the efficacy of cognitive rehabilitation programs in the disease. Results showing brain connectivity and activation increments after a cognitive treatment of less than 3 months in patients with a neurodegenerative disease are relevant in the field of neurorehabilitation. Future studies should include the MRI acquisition as part of the protocol assessment to evaluate brain changes after treatment and replicate the findings.

All these changes have been analyzed at follow-up, and some studies found maintenance of these improvements. Future randomized controlled trials should include follow-up periods in order to replicate previous findings and assess whether the improvements after training could be maintained over time. It would be also interesting to examine the maintenance of these changes in PD patients with and without booster sessions.

Another aspect to be taken into account during the rehabilitation process of the patient is the role of the caregiver. Some cognitive rehabilitation studies have included an intervention which focused on psychoeducation with the caregivers of the PD patients [40, 44]. The psychoeducation usually addresses aspects of the disease, patients' care management, information about help aids, and the importance of the self-care [40, 44]. These studies found that the caregivers gain self-confidence and felt more confident to take care of the person with the disease.

In conclusion, cognitive rehabilitation programs have demonstrated to be effective in improving cognitive functions and may also improve functional disability and produce brain changes in patients with PD. In addition, to provide a complete or integrative treatment, the combination of cognitive training with other types of trainings or the intervention with the caregivers should be further analyzed. More research should be performed in the field, with a view to reaching generalized conclusions and including cognitive rehabilitation in the standard of care of PD patients.

Disclosure

This article is a contribution to the special issue entitled Neurorehabilitation: Neural Plasticity and Functional Recovery 2018.

Conflicts of Interest

Natalia Ojeda and Javier Peña are coauthors and copyright holders of the REHACOP cognitive rehabilitation program, published by Parima Digital, S.L. (Bilbao, Spain). María Díez-Cirarda and Naroa Ibarretxe-Bilbao have no conflicts of interest to report.

Acknowledgments

The authors thank ASPARBI (Parkinson's Disease Association in Biscay) and all the patients involved in the study. This study was supported by the Department of Health of the Basque Government (2011111117), the Ministerio de Economía y Competitividad (PSI2012-32441), and the Department of Education and Science of the Basque Government (Equipo A) (IT946-16).

References

[1] L. Hirsch, N. Jette, A. Frolkis, T. Steeves, and T. Pringsheim, "The incidence of Parkinson's disease: a systematic review and meta-analysis," *Neuroepidemiology*, vol. 46, no. 4, pp. 292–300, 2016.

[2] R. Xia and Z.-H. Mao, "Progression of motor symptoms in Parkinson's disease," *Neuroscience Bulletin*, vol. 28, no. 1, pp. 39–48, 2012.

[3] E. Tolosa, C. Gaig, J. Santamaria, and Y. Compta, "Diagnosis and the premotor phase of Parkinson disease," *Neurology*, vol. 72, no. 7, Supplement 2, pp. S12–S20, 2009.

[4] D. Muslimovic, B. Post, J. D. Speelman, and B. Schmand, "Cognitive profile of patients with newly diagnosed Parkinson disease," *Neurology*, vol. 65, no. 8, pp. 1239–1245, 2005.

[5] A. J. Yarnall, D. P. Breen, G. W. Duncan et al., "Characterizing mild cognitive impairment in incident Parkinson disease: the ICICLE-PD study," *Neurology*, vol. 82, no. 4, pp. 308–316, 2014.

[6] M. A. Hely, W. G. J. Reid, M. A. Adena, G. M. Halliday, and J. G. L. Morris, "The Sydney multicenter study of Parkinson's disease: the inevitability of dementia at 20 years," *Movement Disorders*, vol. 23, no. 6, pp. 837–844, 2008.

[7] J. Hoogland, J. A. Boel, R. M. A. de Bie et al., "Mild cognitive impairment as a risk factor for Parkinson's disease dementia," *Movement Disorders*, vol. 32, no. 7, pp. 1056–1065, 2017.

[8] I. Leroi, K. McDonald, H. Pantula, and V. Harbishettar, "Cognitive impairment in Parkinson disease: impact on quality of life, disability, and caregiver burden," *Journal of Geriatric Psychiatry and Neurology*, vol. 25, no. 4, pp. 208–214, 2012.

[9] E. Rosenthal, L. Brennan, S. Xie et al., "Association between cognition and function in patients with Parkinson disease with and without dementia," *Movement Disorders*, vol. 25, no. 9, pp. 1170–1176, 2010.

[10] T. R. Melzer, R. Watts, M. R. MacAskill et al., "Grey matter atrophy in cognitively impaired Parkinson's disease," *Journal of Neurology, Neurosurgery, & Psychiatry*, vol. 83, no. 2, pp. 188–194, 2012.

[11] G. W. Duncan, M. J. Firbank, A. J. Yarnall et al., "Gray and white matter imaging: a biomarker for cognitive impairment in early Parkinson's disease?," *Movement Disorders*, vol. 31, no. 1, pp. 103–110, 2016.

[12] Z. Zheng, S. Shemmassian, C. Wijekoon, W. Kim, S. Y. Bookheimer, and N. Pouratian, "DTI correlates of distinct cognitive impairments in Parkinson's disease," *Human Brain Mapping*, vol. 35, no. 4, pp. 1325–1333, 2014.

[13] H. Matsui, K. Nishinaka, M. Oda, H. Niikawa, T. Kubori, and F. Udaka, "Dementia in Parkinson's disease: diffusion tensor imaging," *Acta Neurologica Scandinavica*, vol. 116, no. 3, pp. 177–181, 2007.

[14] I. Rektor, A. Svátková, L. Vojtíšek et al., "White matter alterations in Parkinson's disease with normal cognition precede grey matter atrophy," *PLoS One*, vol. 13, no. 1, article e0187939, 2018.

[15] R. Cabeza and L. Nyberg, "Imaging cognition II: an empirical review of 275 PET and fMRI studies," *Journal of Cognitive Neuroscience*, vol. 12, no. 1, pp. 1–47, 2000.

[16] L. Christopher and A. P. Strafella, "Neuroimaging of brain changes associated with cognitive impairment in Parkinson's disease," *Journal of Neuropsychology*, vol. 7, no. 2, pp. 225–240, 2013.

[17] C. H. Williams-Gray, S. L. Mason, J. R. Evans et al., "The CamPaIGN study of Parkinson's disease: 10-year outlook in an incident population-based cohort," *Journal of Neurology, Neurosurgery, & Psychiatry*, vol. 84, no. 11, pp. 1258–1264, 2013.

[18] D. K. Johnson, Z. Langford, M. Garnier-Villarreal, J. C. Morris, and J. E. Galvin, "Onset of mild cognitive impairment in Parkinson disease," *Alzheimer Disease & Associated Disorders*, vol. 30, no. 2, pp. 127–133, 2016.

[19] B. Ramírez-Ruiz, M. J. Martí, E. Tolosa et al., "Longitudinal evaluation of cerebral morphological changes in Parkinson's disease with and without dementia," *Journal of Neurology*, vol. 252, no. 11, pp. 1345–1352, 2005.

[20] Y. Zhang, I. W. Wu, D. Tosun, E. Foster, N. Schuff, and the Parkinson's Progression Markers Initiative, "Progression of regional microstructural degeneration in Parkinson's disease: a multicenter diffusion tensor imaging study," *PLoS One*, vol. 11, no. 10, article e0165540, 2016.

[21] C. Huang, C. Tang, A. Feigin et al., "Changes in network activity with the progression of Parkinson's disease," *Brain*, vol. 130, no. 7, pp. 1834–1846, 2007.

[22] B. Segura, N. Ibarretxe-Bilbao, R. Sala-Llonch et al., "Progressive changes in a recognition memory network in Parkinson's disease," *Journal of Neurology, Neurosurgery, & Psychiatry*, vol. 84, no. 4, pp. 370–378, 2013.

[23] E. Mak, L. Su, G. B. Williams, and J. T. O'Brien, "Neuroimaging correlates of cognitive impairment and dementia in Parkinson's disease," *Parkinsonism & Related Disorders*, vol. 21, no. 8, pp. 862–870, 2015.

[24] A. Bahar-Fuchs, L. Clare, and B. Woods, "Cognitive training and cognitive rehabilitation for persons with mild to moderate dementia of the Alzheimer's or vascular type: a review," *Alzheimer's Research & Therapy*, vol. 5, no. 4, p. 35, 2013.

[25] T. Wykes and W. D. Spaulding, "Thinking about the future cognitive remediation therapy—what works and could we do better?," *Schizophrenia Bulletin*, vol. 37, Supplement 2, pp. S80–S90, 2011.

[26] J. V. Hindle, A. Petrelli, L. Clare, and E. Kalbe, "Nonpharmacological enhancement of cognitive function in Parkinson's disease: a systematic review," *Movement Disorders*, vol. 28, no. 8, pp. 1034–1049, 2013.

[27] R. Biundo, L. Weis, E. Fiorenzato, and A. Antonini, "Cognitive rehabilitation in Parkinson's disease: is it feasible?," *Archives of Clinical Neuropsychology*, vol. 32, no. 7, pp. 840–860, 2017.

[28] C. C. Walton, S. L. Naismith, A. Lampit, L. Mowszowski, and S. J. G. Lewis, "Cognitive training in Parkinson's disease: a

theoretical perspective," *Neurorehabilitation and Neural Repair*, vol. 31, no. 3, pp. 207–216, 2017.

[29] B. J. Lawrence, N. Gasson, R. S. Bucks, L. Troeung, and A. M. Loftus, "Cognitive training and noninvasive brain stimulation for cognition in Parkinson's disease: a meta-analysis," *Neurorehabilitation and Neural Repair*, vol. 31, no. 7, pp. 597–608, 2017.

[30] I. H. Leung, "Cognitive training in Parkinson disease," *Neurology*, vol. 85, pp. 1–9, 2015.

[31] J. Peña, N. Ibarretxe-Bilbao, I. García-Gorostiaga, M. A. Gomez-Beldarrain, M. Díez-Cirarda, and N. Ojeda, "Improving functional disability and cognition in Parkinson disease: randomized controlled trial," *Neurology*, vol. 83, no. 23, pp. 2167–2174, 2014.

[32] A. Petrelli, S. Kaesberg, M. T. Barbe et al., "Effects of cognitive training in Parkinson's disease: a randomized controlled trial," *Parkinsonism & Related Disorders*, vol. 20, no. 11, pp. 1196–1202, 2014.

[33] A. Cerasa, M. C. Gioia, M. Salsone et al., "Neurofunctional correlates of attention rehabilitation in Parkinson's disease: an explorative study," *Neurological Sciences*, vol. 35, no. 8, pp. 1173–1180, 2014.

[34] J. D. Edwards, R. A. Hauser, M. L. O'Connor, E. G. Valdés, T. A. Zesiewicz, and E. Y. Uc, "Randomized trial of cognitive speed of processing training in Parkinson disease," *Neurology*, vol. 81, no. 15, pp. 1284–1290, 2013.

[35] A. P. París, H. G. Saleta, M. de la Cruz Crespo Maraver et al., "Blind randomized controlled study of the efficacy of cognitive training in Parkinson's disease," *Movement Disorders*, vol. 26, no. 7, pp. 1251–1258, 2011.

[36] M. Cella, A. Preti, C. Edwards, T. Dow, and T. Wykes, "Cognitive remediation for negative symptoms of schizophrenia: a network meta-analysis," *Clinical Psychology Review*, vol. 52, pp. 43–51, 2017.

[37] R. Zimmermann, U. Gschwandtner, N. Benz et al., "Cognitive training in Parkinson disease: cognition-specific vs nonspecific computer training," *Neurology*, vol. 82, no. 14, pp. 1219–1226, 2014.

[38] M. Díez-Cirarda, N. Ojeda, J. Peña et al., "Increased brain connectivity and activation after cognitive rehabilitation in Parkinson's disease: a randomized controlled trial," *Brain Imaging and Behavior*, vol. 11, no. 6, pp. 1640–1651, 2017.

[39] E. Sinforiani, L. Banchieri, C. Zucchella, C. Pacchetti, and G. Sandrini, "Cognitive rehabilitation in Parkinson's disease," *Archives of Gerontology and Geriatrics*, vol. 38, pp. 387–391, 2004.

[40] I. Reuter, S. Mehnert, G. Sammer, M. Oechsner, and M. Engelhardt, "Efficacy of a multimodal cognitive rehabilitation including psychomotor and endurance training in Parkinson's disease," *Journal of Aging Research*, vol. 2012, Article ID 235765, 15 pages, 2012.

[41] M. Díez-Cirarda, N. Ojeda, J. Peña et al., "Long-term effects of cognitive rehabilitation on brain, functional outcome and cognition in Parkinson's disease," *European Journal of Neurology*, vol. 25, no. 1, pp. 5–12, 2018.

[42] A. Petrelli, S. Kaesberg, M. T. Barbe et al., "Cognitive training in Parkinson's disease reduces cognitive decline in the long term," *European Journal of Neurology*, vol. 22, no. 4, pp. 640–647, 2015.

[43] J. V. Hindle, T. J. Watermeyer, J. Roberts et al., "Cognitive rehabilitation for Parkinson's disease dementia: a study protocol for a pilot randomised controlled trial," *Trials*, vol. 17, no. 1, p. 152, 2016.

[44] L. E. I. A'Campo, N. G. A. Spliethoff-Kamminga, M. Macht, R. A. C. Roos, and The EduPark Consortium, "Caregiver education in Parkinson's disease: formative evaluation of a standardized program in seven European countries," *Quality of Life Research*, vol. 19, no. 1, pp. 55–64, 2010.

[45] N. Adamski, M. Adler, K. Opwis, and I. K. Penner, "A pilot study on the benefit of cognitive rehabilitation in Parkinson's disease," *Therapeutic Advances in Neurological Disorders*, vol. 9, no. 3, pp. 153–164, 2016.

7

Function of Connexins in the Interaction between Glial and Vascular Cells in the Central Nervous System and Related Neurological Diseases

Yinan Zhao,[1] Yanguo Xin,[2] Zhiyi He ,[1] and Wenyu Hu [3]

[1]*Department of Neurology, The First Affiliated Hospital of China Medical University, Shenyang, Liaoning 110001, China*
[2]*Department of Cardiology, West China Hospital of Sichuan University, Chengdu, Sichuan 610041, China*
[3]*Department of Cardiology, The First Affiliated Hospital of China Medical University, Shenyang, Liaoning 110001, China*

Correspondence should be addressed to Zhiyi He; hezhiyi0320@yahoo.co.jp and Wenyu Hu; huwen0320@sohu.com

Academic Editor: Jean-Pierre Mothet

Neuronal signaling together with synapse activity in the central nervous system requires a precisely regulated microenvironment. Recently, the blood-brain barrier is considered as a "neuro-glia-vascular unit," a structural and functional compound composed of capillary endothelial cells, glial cells, pericytes, and neurons, which plays a pivotal role in maintaining the balance of the microenvironment in and out of the brain. Tight junctions and adherens junctions, which function as barriers of the blood-brain barrier, are two well-known kinds in the endothelial cell junctions. In this review, we focus on the less-concerned contribution of gap junction proteins, connexins in blood-brain barrier integrity under physio-/pathology conditions. In the neuro-glia-vascular unit, connexins are expressed in the capillary endothelial cells and prominent in astrocyte endfeet around and associated with maturation and function of the blood-brain barrier through a unique signaling pathway and an interaction with tight junction proteins. Connexin hemichannels and connexin gap junction channels contribute to the physiological or pathological progress of the blood-brain barrier; in addition, the interaction with other cell-cell-adhesive proteins is also associated with the maintenance of the blood-brain barrier. Lastly, we explore the connexins and connexin channels involved in the blood-brain barrier in neurological diseases and any programme for drug discovery or delivery to target or avoid the blood-brain barrier.

1. Introduction

In the 1900s, the term "blood-brain barrier (BBB)" was firstly proposed to explain the reason that certain medicines failed to treat brain conditions [1]. The previous concept of BBB is a pure endothelial barrier of the brain, a physical barrier comprised of tight junctions (TJs) and adherens junctions (AJs) that limit paracellular diffusion of solutes between the blood and the brain [2, 3]. Currently, BBB is more likely to be considered as "a neuro-glia-vascular unit" [4, 5], a functional unit composed of capillar endothelial cells (ECs), glial cells, pericytes, and neurons and which interacts with local segments of blood vessels. Functionally, in healthy conditions, BBB serves as a higher selective barrier, protecting and separating the central nervous system (CNS) from toxic and damaging blood-borne compounds and peripheral neurotransmitter pools, protecting the synaptic and axonal signaling from ionic fluctuations, permitting the entry of required chemical molecules, and clearing larger molecules and brain metabolites, maintaining the balance of the brain microenvironment [6, 7]. In pathological conditions, brain-targeted diseases may be the origins, followed by vasculopathy, change of blood flow, and altered secretion of matrix molecules. Microglia activated and recruited by signals from astrocytes and neurons secrete more inflammatory cytokines, ultimately causing neuronal injury and synaptic dysfunction [5, 8–10].

According to previous studies, it is well known that the two kinds of vascular endothelial cell-cell junction, TJs and AJs, play key roles in the barrier function of BBB [2, 11];

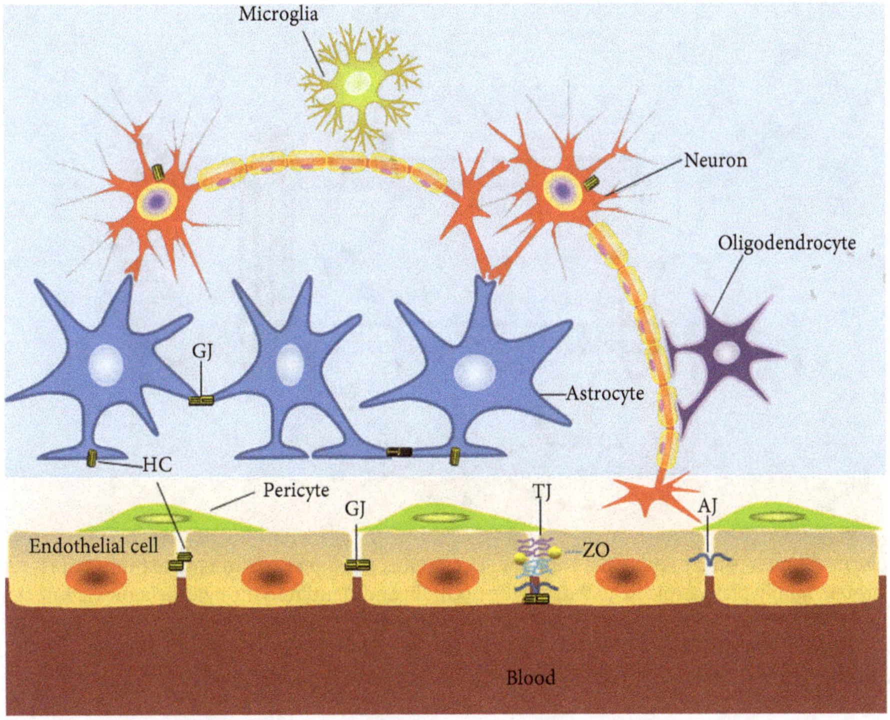

FIGURE 1: Connexin-based channels in BBB. A functional unit composed of capillary endothelial cells (ECs), glial cells, pericytes, neurons, and interaction with local segments of blood vessels.

nevertheless, very recently, researchers discovered a third category, gap junction (GC) channels, and the cross work with other cell-cell junctions in maintaining the barrier function [12]. Gap junction intercellular communication (GJIC) is formed by two hemichannels (HCs) located on the opposing cell membranes; each one is composed of six transmembrane proteins termed as connexins (Cxs) [13, 14]. Cx channels contribute to the intercellular communication between different cellular compartments. In addition, crapping around the capillary endothelial cells in CNS, dysfunction of vascular barriers caused by deficiency of Cxs on the membrane of astrocytes has been observed [15], indicating that Cx channels on astrocyte endfeet also play a pivotal role in the maintenance of function in BBB. However, it is still unclear how Cx channels work on astrocyte endfeet and contribute to the regulation of BBB. In addition, some believe that Cxs on the membrane of ECs rather than astrocytes are involved in the permeability status of BBB [16]. Accordingly, there are still debates about where and how Cxs regulate the barrier function and interact with other junctional proteins in CNS, hence the problem. This review focuses on the pivotal roles of Cxs and Cx channels in regulating the permeability of CNS/PNS barriers and related diseases caused by dysfunction of the "neuro-glia-vascular unit."

2. BBB Structure

BBB is considered as a functional unit, and glial cell is one of the important constituent structures, which forms a continuous membranous network around the vessels, where molecular signaling through pericytes and ECs is organized (Figure 1). This "highly selective permeability barrier" maintains brain homeostasis through permitting the entry of required nutrients and excluding potentially harmful compounds into the CNS [17, 18]. Thus, BBB plays a pivotal role in protecting the specific neuron function from biochemical attack in the systemic circulation.

Capillary ECs, another constituent structure of BBB, supply a junctional complex comprising of AJs and TJs and control paracellular diffusion of solute between the blood and the brain [2, 4, 11, 19] (Figure 2). TJs contain a complex of proteins spanning the intercellular cleft (occludin and claudin) and junctional adhesion molecules [2, 20]. The zona occludin protein family (ZO-1, ZO-2, and ZO-3) plays a key role in anchoring the occludin and claudin to the cytoskeleton via interaction with actin [21]. The AJ protein, cadherin (α, β, and γ), spans the intercellular cleft and provides structural support [2]. Recently, more focus is on the significant role of Cx proteins in the junctional complex [22, 23]. Unlike TJ and AJ proteins, Cx proteins do not form a tight seal between the connecting cytoplasm and adjacent cells, despite adhesive properties indispensable for the adjacent cells.

3. Cxs in Glial Cells and Neurons

GJs constitute connected exchange channels between adjacent cells for the interchange of cytoplasm components, small molecules, ions, and so on, and maintain metabolic cooperation [24–26], completeness of intercellular signaling pathways, liquid buffer, and electric coupling [27, 28]. GJs

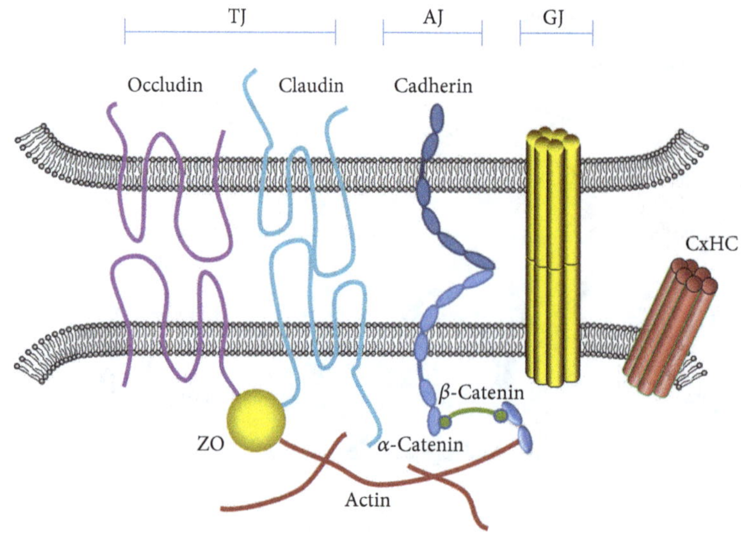

FIGURE 2: Cx channels form the intercellular junctional complex. TJ contains a complex of proteins spanning the intercellular cleft (occludin and claudin). The ZO protein family plays a role in anchoring the occludin and claudin to the cytoskeleton via interaction with actin. The AJ protein, cadherin, spans the intercellular cleft and provides structural support. Transmembrane Cx proteins constitute a third partner in the intercellular junctional complex. GJ is formed by two HCs located on the opposing cell membranes, which are composed of six transmembrane Cx proteins.

are formed by two HCs located on the opposing cell membranes (Figure 2), which are composed of six transmembrane proteins termed as Cxs. The Cx superfamily is comprised of 21 isoforms in humans and 20 isoforms in mice in a tissue-specific expression pattern and named according to their molecular weight (Figure 3) [29, 30].

Eleven kinds of Cxs have been detected in the rodent brain [31]; Cx30 and Cx43 are two major categories expressed in astrocytes. The expression of astrocytic Cxs varies by brain region and stage of development [31]. For instance, the time pattern of the postnatal expression of Cx30 (from P12) and Cx43 (from P2) in astrocyte endfeet correlates with the maturation of the BBB [15, 32]. White matter astrocytes express minimal or no Cx30 [33]. In contrast, expression of Cx30 is higher compared with that in white matter, even more than Cx43, in the thalamus [34]. Lack of Cx43 leads to the reduction of coupling and absence of both Cx43 and Cx30 abolishment of interastrocyte coupling [35–37], indicating that Cx43 and Cx30 are the major components of a direct intercellular communication between astrocytes. Cx36, together with a site-specific expression of Cx45 and Cx57, is the principal connexin expressed in neurons. Cx36 was firstly reported to be expressed specifically in mammalian neurons [38]. The expression of Cx36 is sharply reduced during the course of postnatal maturation and is sparsely expressed in the neocortex; however, it remains enriched in subsets of interneurons in the hippocampus, olfactory bulb, and thalamus [38–40]. There was evidence indicating the absence of GJs between neurons and glial cells in the mammalian CNS [31, 41, 42]; however, both electrical and dye coupling between Bergmann glial cells and Purkinje neurons has been observed in adult rats [43].

4. Cxs in Different Regions of Vascular Tree (Arteries, Arterioles/Venous System, and Lymphatic System)

The expression regions of Cx40, Cx37, and Cx43 are mainly restricted on the cytomembrane of vascular ECs [44]. Cx37 and Cx40 are widely expressed in arteries and arterioles, while Cx43 in the regions is consistent with turbulent blood flow [45–47]. Cx37 expression is prominent in the straight portion of carotid arteries, but reduced from the carotid bifurcation [48]. Cx43 is robustly expressed at branching vessels; turbulent shear stress caused by disturbed blood flow makes the endothelium of these small vessels prone to developing atherosclerotic lesions [46, 49].

Very limited studies focused on the expression pattern of Cxs in the venous/lymphatic system. Cxs expression (Cx37, Cx40, and Cx43) in the venous system also exhibited the same manner as in the arterial systems, which is a regional variation [50].

Kanady et al. observed Cx37, Cx43, and Cx47, especially the first two which exhibited a regional and dynamic variation of expression manner in mice. Interestingly, coexpression of Cx47 and Cx43 was observed in the region upstream of the adult valve. A knockout mouse model showed that Cx37 and Cx43 but not Cx47 affected lymphatic morphology [51–53].

Microvasculature is the region where the exchange of nutrients and materials between tissue and blood takes place. As mentioned above, the expression of Cx43 is higher in microvasculature compared with that in macrovasculature [54], indicating that Cx43 is a major regulator of vascular permeability. Upregulation of Cx43 in ECs, associated with the vascular hyperpermeability, has been verified to be consistent with the above conclusion [54–57].

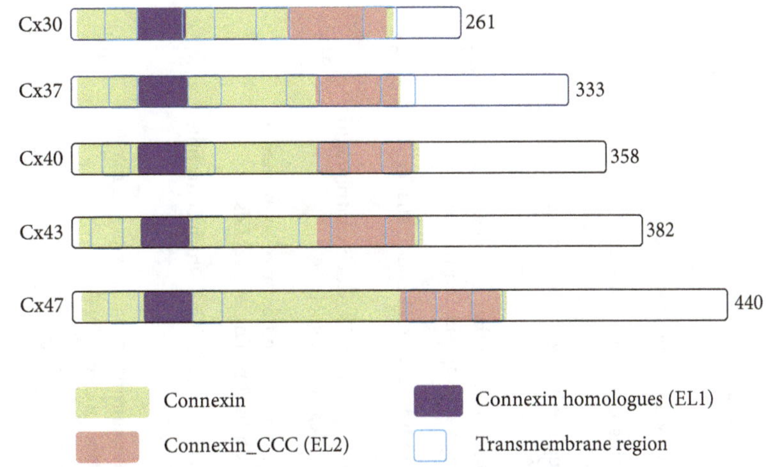

FIGURE 3: Schematic representation of connexins. Each Cx is a four-pass transmembrane (red frame) protein comprising two extracellular loops (EL1, purple region; EL2, green region) and a C-terminal cytoplasmic tail. The domains and motifs of connexins are depicted according to the size.

5. Function of Endothelial Cxs in BBB

Endothelial cells individually or jointly express Cx37, Cx40, and Cx43, in a vessel type-dependent manner as mentioned above. Several evidences point to the possible contribution of endothelial Cxs in maintaining the permeability status of the BBB. Cx40 and Cx43 are associated with TJ proteins (occludin and claudin-5) in porcine brain ECs through cytoplasmic scaffold proteins, such as ZO-1. GJ blocker 18 β-glycyrrhetinic acid and oleamide did weaken the barrier function of TJs, but did not influence the expression or distribution of Cxs or TJ proteins in porcine BBB ECs [12] (Table 1). Damaged BBB permeability was considered to be caused by loss of function of GJIC and TJs without morphological change; however, the mechanism needs further research. In contrast with pathological conditions, the expression of Cx43 in the endothelial wall of healthy blood vessels appears low and increases after inflammation occurred, especially in the endothelial cells of smaller blood vessels including those of the BBB [55, 58]. Cx43 antisense treatment further reduces vascular permeability and invasion of neutrophils in spinal cord injury (SCI) [55] (Table 2). Very recently, increased expression of Cx43 and permeability of BBB were observed in familial cerebral cavernous malformation type III (FCCM3) lesions of mouse model brains [59], partly consistent with the observation in *ccm3* knockdown brain microvascular ECs, which was accompanied by dislocation of ZO-1, limitation to formation, and transinteraction of TJs *in vitro*. Gap27, a Cx43 GJ inhibitor, rescued CCM3KD hyperpermeability through inhibiting Cx43 GJs, restoring ZO-1 to TJ structures, and reducing plaque accumulation in Cx43 GJs, indicating that Cx43 GJs are increased in Fccm3 and regulate barrier permeability in a TJ-dependent manner [59] (Table 1). It is unclear by what mechanism CCM3 regulates Cx43 and whether Cx43 is exclusive to participate in the formation of TJs.

6. Involvement of Glial and Neuronal Connexins and BBB Function

In the nervous system, astrocytic Cx is unique and contributes pivotally to brain metabolism and processing [60]. Cx30 and Cx43 are two major Cx proteins expressed by astrocytes and that form Cx-based channels to mediate intercellular signaling, especially that involving Ca^{2+} and maintaining the BBB integrity [15, 32]. A knockout model was induced to clarify the role of astroglial Cxs in the morphology and function of BBB. The combination of global *Cx30* and astrocyte-specific *Cx43* deletion (conditional knockout from glial fibrillary acidic protein-expressing cells) downregulates aquaporin 4 (AQP4), which is located in astrocytes throughout the CNS in the brain, spinal cord, and optic nerve and is particularly concentrated in foot processes adjacent to microvessels at BBB [61] (Table 2). In contrast, TJ proteins, occludin, and ZO-1 show no difference in expression or morphology, compared with the WT mice [15]. Consequently, double knockout of astrocytic *Cx43* and *Cx30* leads to systemic astrocyte endfeet swell and increased BBB permeability with the increase in vascular and shear stress [15]. However, absence of Cx30 did not affect organization or permeability of BBB according to a further analysis of the separate role of Cx30 [62] (Table 2). Absence of astroglial Cx43 compromises the ability of the brain to maintain immune quiescence [63]; recruitment of T cells, B cells, macrophages, and neutrophils; enhanced antigen presentation; and autoimmune reaction [64–66] (Table 2). Immune cell recruitment is not the consequence of BBB breakdown in *Cx43-KO* mouse brain, despite progressively weakened BBB permeability under shear and pressure [64]. Loss of immune-quiescent, immune-competent cells abnormally crossing the BBB and developing autoimmune mechanisms could be harmful as suggested in pathological conditions linked to a decreased expression of Cx43 in multiple sclerosis (MS) and neuromyelitis optica (NMO) patients [67, 68]. Deficiency of Cx43

Table 1: Connexin inhibitors link to the BBB permeability *in vitro*.

Cell type	Stimulus	Treatment	Main outcome	Reference
Porcine BBB ECs		18β-Glycyrrhetinic acid and oleamide	Inhibits the barrier function of TJs and GJIC without morphological change	[12]
Mouse brain CCM3KD ECs		Gap27	Inhibits BBB hyperpermeability through blocking Cx43 GJs, restoring ZO-1 to TJ structures	[59]
Rat brain RBE4 cells	Bradykinin	Gap27, *Cx37*-siRNA, and *Cx43*-siRNA	Inhibits endothelial hyperpermeability through reducing intracellular calcium oscillations	[57]
Rat brain RBE4 cells	A reduction in extracellular Ca^{2+} concentration	Gap27	Inhibits endothelial hyperpermeability through blocking the intercellular Ca^{2+} waves and repressing PKC, CaMKII, and actomyosin contraction	[77]
Rat brain (RBE4, GP8 cells)	TNF-α	Gap26	No effect on the elevated baseline ATP release from rat brain endothelial cells treated by TNF-α	[82]
Rat brain GP8 cells		Gap26 and Gap27	Inhibits intracellular ATP release through blocking Cx43-HCs which contribute to the intercellular propagation of calcium signals	[81]
Organotypic hippocampal slices from 7-day-old Wistar rats	Albumin	Carbenoxolone, Gap27, and SLS peptide	In developing hippocampal networks, the generation and initiation of spontaneous recurrent seizure-like activity depend on the opening of glial GJs	[119]
Astrocytes from the cortex and spinal cord of the SCI mouse model	TNF-α	Gap26, Gap27, and *Cx43*-siRNA	TNF-α activated Cx43-HCs, rather than GJIC, to release CXCL1 which contribute to neuropathic pain	[94]
Astrocytes from cortex of Sprague-Dawley rat	Aβ-peptide	Octanol (an uncoupler of gap junctions)	Functional GJs are not required for calcium-wave propagation; they play a role in the enhancement of calcium waves induced by Aβ.	[110]

ECs: endothelial cells; SCI: spinal cord injury; TJs: tight junctions; GJs: gap junctions; ZO: zona occludin; PKC: protein kinase C; CaMKII: Ca^{2+}/calmodulin-dependent kinase II; HCs: hemichannels; GJIC: gap junction intercellular communication; Aβ: amyloid β.

Table 2: Connexin inhibitors link to the BBB permeability *in vivo*.

	Disease model	Interference	Main outcome	Reference
Spinal cord	SCI	Cx43-asODN	Reduce vascular permeability and invasion of neutrophils in spinal cord injury	[55]
BBB	Neuroinflammation	Gap27	Gap27 coadministered together with bradykinin reduced leakage of reporter dye from the vascular lumen into the tissue	[57]
BBB		Global *Cx30* and astrocytic-specific *Cx43* deletion	Systemic astrocyte endfeet swell and increased BBB permeability with the increase in vascular and shear stress	[61]
BBB		Global *Cx30* deletion	Not affecting organization or permeability of BBB	[62]
BBB		Astrocytic-specific *Cx43* deletion	Compromises the ability of the brain to maintain immune quiescence and recruitment of immune cells without BBB breakdown	[63–66]
Embryo		*Cx43* deletion	Migration impairment of neurons through adhesive interaction with radial fibers	[69, 70]
Brain	AD	INI-1602 (microglia HC blocker)	Improve memory deficits	[114]

SCI: spinal cord injury; HCs: hemichannels; BBB: brain-blood barrier.

nonchannel function is associated with migration impairment of neurons through adhesive interaction with radial fibers during embryogenesis [69, 70] (Table 2). However, the mechanism by which knockdown of Cx43 leads to the migration of immune-competent cells abnormally crossing the BBB and the Cx-channel-dependent or nondependent function important to mediate the migration process needs to be clarified further.

In an ultrasound-induced BBB opening Wistar rat model [71], reorganization of neuronal Cx36-containing GJs with an increase in gap-junctional plaque size was found, similar to the results in another study [72]; neuronal Cx36 interacts with a ZO-1 PDZ domain, the same as in astrocytic Cx43, thus indicating that ultrasound-induced disruption of ZO-1 might lead to an increase in Cx36 plaque size. However, in the same BBB opening model [71], changes in Cx36 plaque size were not as striking as in astrocytic Cx43 plaques, suggesting the key role of astrocytes for the maintenance of homeostasis of BBB.

7. The Roles of Cx Channels in BBB Function

Several factors, such as inflammatory cytokines and growth factors, contribute to the regulation of Cx-HC and GJ channels in physiological or pathological progress and modulatory mechanism of BBB. Accumulating evidence indicated that Ca^{2+} transients in astrocyte endfeet may induce dilation and constrictions in the adjacent arterioles and may further precede changes in blood flow and disturbance of the healthy brain function [73, 74]. One research showed an increased BBB and bovine brain capillary EC permeability through triggering calcium oscillations involved in Cx-HC opening, indicating that HCs may play a vital role in the process of calcium signaling and propagation of ICW [57]. Divergent functional properties of Cx43 channels have been set forth in inflammatory conditions. Retamal et al. found that the proinflammatory cytokines IL-1β and TNF-α reduced the intercellular communication via Cx43 GJIC, whereas it increased the cellular exchange with the extracellular milieu via Cx43 HCs [75]. Inhibition of GJIC that is observed under the condition of inflammation indicates that the increased membrane permeability may be attributable to active HCs [75, 76]. On the other hand, the effect of proinflammatory cytokines enhanced the uptake and reduced the intercellular diffusion of glucose, which might explain the change of metabolic status in astrocytes under inflammatory conditions. Accordingly, such opposite regulation effects of Cx channels may impact glucose trafficking and modify the metabolic status of astrocytes involved in brain inflammation [75]. Connexin channels provide a target to manipulate brain endothelial calcium dynamics and BBB permeability [57]. Bradykinin, a typical inflammatory messenger, increases BBB and rat brain endothelial (RBE4) cell permeability through triggering calcium oscillations involved in Cx-HC opening. Gap27, a GJ mimetic peptide identical to part of the second extracellular loop of Cx37 and Cx43 structurally, reduced intracellular oscillations in RBE4 cells in response to bradykinin, in accordance with the Cx37/Cx43-targeted siRNA [57] (Table 1). Another group indicated that intercellular Ca^{2+} waves (ICWs) increased the endothelial permeability by lowering the extracellular Ca^{2+}. The endothelial permeability increase was furthermore inhibited by Gap27, which also blocked the ICWs, and with inhibition of protein kinase, Ca^{2+}/calmodulin-dependent kinase II, and actomyosin contraction. In conclusion, ICWs significantly increase endothelial permeability and the Cxs underlying Ca^{2+} wave propagation form a target to limit BBB alteration [77] (Table 1).

GJs mimetic peptides, Gap26 and Gap27, which specifically target Cx channels, are widely used to close the HCs and, in certain conditions, gap junction communication [78]. ATP is the best known signaling factor linked to Cx-HC activity and released from astrocytes directly through Cx43-HCs [79]. Gap26 binds to the first extracellular loop

Table 3: Cxs/Cx-channels in BBB in CNS pathology.

CNS pathology	Cxs/Cx channel remodeling	BBB dysfunction	Reference
MOG-induced EAE mouse model	Deletion of both *Cx30* and *Cx43*	None	[126]
Carrageenan-induced inflammatory pain rat model	Not mentioned	Increased expression of ZO-1 in TJs and permeability of the BBB	[92]
MCAO mouse model	*Cx43* $^{+/-}$, GJIC reduction	Weakened barrier function of BBB and exacerbated ischemic injury	[98]
Age-related neurodegenerative disease mouse model	Increased expression and relocalization of Cx43 in ECs	An increase in the permeability of the BBB without change of ZO-1	[108]
4-AP-induced epilepsy rat model	Gradually elevated expression of Cx43 and GJIC remodeling	Not mentioned	[118]
HIV-infected neuroAIDS macaque model	HIV amplified by GJs	Compromised BBB integrity	[123]

Cx: connexin; TJs: tight junctions; GJs: gap junctions; ZO: Zona occludin; GJIC: gap junction intercellular communication; BBB: brain-blood barrier; 4-AP: 4-aminopyridine.

of Cx43 and blocks Cx43-HCs in ECs, demonstrating that intracellular ATP is released through Cx-HCs in a Cx-dependent manner, which contributes to the intercellular propagation of calcium signals, thereby affecting the postulated spatial spread of BBB opening [80, 81] (Table 1). Nevertheless, one *in vitro* study showed that Gap26 has no effect on the elevated baseline ATP from rat brain ECs treated by TNF-α, suggesting that ATP release is non-Cx-dependent under proinflammatory cytokine-stimulated conditions [82] (Table 1). Gap27 targets the second extracellular loop of Cx37 and Cx43, and exposure to Gap27 upon short time (minutes) inhibits Cx-HC-mediated ATP release and dye uptake [32, 81, 83], while longer exposure duration (hours) blocks junctional coupling, as well [81, 84]. Gap27 limits BBB permeability induced by bradykinin *in vivo* through reducing intracellular calcium oscillations without modifications of TJs and cytoskeletal proteins such as occludin or ZO-1 [57] (Table 2). Some problems remain to be solved. First, some GJ mimetic peptides are widely used to inhibit the HC and GJ channels; however, what role GJ channels and HCs play in glial endfeet and how they contribute to regulation of BBB permeability need to be explained in detail. Secondly, Wnt, together with the Sonic hedgehog (Shh) signaling pathway, regulates the maturation of the BBB during development [85–87]; however, which signaling molecules that passed through Cx channels contribute to astrocyte endfeet structure adhesion and affect the integrity of BBB also needs to be clarified.

8. Cxs and Cx Channels in Nervous System Diseases

8.1. Multiple Sclerosis. Downregulation of oligodendrocytic Cx32, Cx47, and astrocytic Cx43 had been identified in the active lesions of CNS in MS patients and EAE mice [88–90]. Lutz et al. reported that deletion of both *Cx30* and *Cx43* in the EAE model did not aggravate clinical signs or pathological progress; moreover, no difference was observed in BBB permeability [91], indicating that absence of astrocytic Cx43 and Cx30 does not contribute to the pathology progress of the nerve tissue or further weaken BBB intensity under inflammatory condition (Table 3).

8.2. Neuropathic Pain. Inflammatory-mediated pain alters in TJs; ZO-1 expression was significantly increased, increasing the permeability of the BBB of the carrageenan-induced inflammatory pain rat model [92] (Table 3). An in vivo evidence suggests that carrageenan-induced spinal IL-1β inhibits astrocyte activation during the early phase of inflammation through the suppression of Cx43 expression [93]. Cx43 has been reported to induce chemokine CXCL1 (keratinocyte-derived cytokine) release to contribute to neuropathic pain. TNF-α activated Cx43-HCs, rather than GJIC, to release CXCL1 [94], which could be blocked by Gap26, Gap27, and *Cx43*-siRNA in cultured astrocytes from the cortex and spinal cord of the SCI mouse model, a mouse model for chronic neuropathic pain (Table 1). Cx43 is increased in cervical level 6 to 8 dorsal root ganglia, and specific peptide inhibitors of Cx43 ameliorated established tactile allodynia after severe SCI. Notably, SCI-induced mechanical allodynia was prevented in *Cx43/Cx30* double-knockout mice, highlighting the importance of glial intercommunication in chronic neuropathic pain [95, 96].

8.3. Stroke. *Cx43* deficiency not only creates intercellular communication reduction and weakened barrier function of BBB but also exacerbates ischemic injury [15, 97, 98] (Table 3). After ischemia-reperfusion, endothelial Cx expression is upregulated and Cx-HCs open [57, 99, 100], leading to glutamate excitotoxicity and inflammatory mediator release including nitric oxide [101] and further leading to EC edema and rupture [56, 102], astrocyte activity, T cell and monocyte migration, and increased inflammatory reaction, ultimately inducing tissue damage [103–105]. Inhibition of astrocytic GJs by octanol, for instance, could restrict the flow of neurotoxins, which exacerbate neuronal damage of cerebral ischemia [106]. In addition, Cx43 mimetic peptide, a Cx43 inhibitor, exhibited protective effects after cerebral and retinal ischemia [58, 107], which proves the point in reverse.

8.4. Alzheimer's Disease (AD). An age-related decline in BBB integrity correlates with the loss of sex steroids and increase in gonadotropins with menopause [108]. Ovarietomy of young female mice induces an increased expression and dislocation of Cx43 in ECs accompanied by a rise in the permeability of the BBB without change of TJ protein, ZO-1 [108] (Table 3). It implicates Cx43 in regulating changes in BBB permeability and serum gonadotropins in the cerebral pathophysiology of neurodegenerative diseases, such as AD. One study reported that amyloid β (Aβ) peptide, a self-aggregating 40–42-amino-acid protein that is crucially involved in AD as the main component of the amyloid plaques, did harm to neurons resulting in their dysfunction and death [109], contributing to AD pathology through dramatically enhancing GJC/HC-mediated Ca^{2+} wave propagation in astrocytes [110] (Table 1). Recently, several studies [111–113] indicated that expression of astroglial Cxs is increased at amyloid plaques and that there is an increase in HC activity in reactive astrocytes that should certainly have an impact on gliovascular interaction. Until recently, INI-0602, a putative HC blocker, was verified to inhibit LPS-induced glutamate release from microglia *in vivo* and improve memory deficits in double transgenic mice expressing human amyloid precursor protein with K595N and M596L mutations and presenilin 1 with A264E mutation as an AD mouse model [114] (Table 2). An important next step underlying *Cx32* conditional knockout in microglia will be needed to demonstrate the unique regulation of microglial HCs in the progress of AD.

8.5. Epilepsy. TGF-β signaling is a key trigger of albumin-induced epileptogenesis, following BBB breakdown, which can be inhibited by the TGF-β pathway blocker and can manifest the TGF-β pathway as a novel therapeutic target for preventing injury-related epileptogenesis [115, 116]. Downregulation of GJ proteins Cx43 and Cx30, inwardly rectifying K^+ channels (Kir4.1), the glial excitatory amino acid transporters (EAAT1 and EAAT2), and dislocation of aquaporins (AQP4), represents astrocyte activation induced by BBB disruption, as well as by focal application of albumin or TGF-β. These data indicate that activation of astrocytes is a critical step in epileptogenesis preceding alteration in neuronal function [115, 117]. Although many of those signaling cascades are altered in activated astrocytes, very little is known about neurovascular coupling in epilepsy. In the immature rat brain, GJIC is involved in rhythm genesis and synchronization of cortical activity and may enhance the epileptogenicity of the 4-aminopyridine- (4-AP-) induced epilepsy model [118]. In addition, repeated seizures can induce changes in different Cx gene (Cx26, 32, and 43) expression during the postnatal development, especially gradually elevated expression of Cx43 and GJIC remodeling [118] (Table 3). Assuming a selective inhibition of a Cx43-dependent process by the mimetic peptides and preferential localization of this Cx isoform in astrocytes suggests that in developing hippocampal networks, the generation and initiation of spontaneous recurrent seizure-like activity may depend in large part upon the opening of glial GJs [119] (Table 1).

8.6. NeuroAIDS. The main cells infected with HIV within the CNS are macrophages, microglia, and a small fraction of astrocytes [120–122]. Both *in vitro* and *in vivo* evidence uncovered a novel mechanism of bystander BBB toxicity mediated by low numbers of HIV-infected astrocytes and amplified by GJs [123] (Table 3). Few HIV-infected astrocytes compromise BBB integrity through blocking GJ channels, indicating that HIV affects the CNS by a GJ-dependent manner [123].

9. Discussion

Homeostasis of metabolites and ions is strictly regulated by the barrier between blood and nerve tissue. The BBB shields the direct contact between systemic circulation and the brain, as well as the spinal cord and peripheral nerve. TJs and AJs, two pivotal junctional complexes physically located in the ECs, are considered as the main structural components of the barriers. In this review, we introduce a third junctional component, Cx proteins, as an important player in the interactions with other junctional complexes that occur at the neuro-glia-vascular interface. In a cerebral microenvironment, Cx-forming channels of both astrocytes and ECs are critical in the control of BBB function. Interestingly, GJ channels and HC channels of BBB appear to play opposite roles in the regulation of BBB permeability. GJIC contributes to maintaining BBB integrity, while HCs are associated with ATP signaling release and necessary to generate the Ca^{2+} oscillations linked to BBB disruption induced by proinflammatory signals. A cluster of papers have provided strong evidence in favor of a Cx channel-dependent manner contributing to the regulation of BBB function; however, few researchers focus on a Cx channel-independent manner, adhesive contact, and gene expression, for instance [16, 124, 125]. It remains to be demonstrated how nonchannel Cxs interact with other cell-cell-adhesive proteins to maintain the barrier. Cxs have been considered as novel therapy targets for neurologic diseases in connection with BBB dysfunctions. Astrocytic and endothelial Cx channels are vital to BBB permeability change caused by neurologic pathology, especially inflammation. Microglial cells also play an important role in activating immune cells; however, the role of Cxs in the intercellular cross talk between BBB endothelial cells and microglia, and microglia in the BBB development in physiological or pathologic conditions, remains unclear. More studies should be focused on the mechanism of microglia-endothelial Cx channels in BBB permeability regulation.

Conflicts of Interest

The authors declare no competing interests.

Acknowledgments

The authors gratefully acknowledge financial support from the China Scholarship Council.

References

[1] S. A. Liddelow, "Fluids and barriers of the CNS: a historical viewpoint," *Fluids and Barriers of the CNS*, vol. 8, no. 1, p. 2, 2011.

[2] H. Wolburg and A. Lippoldt, "Tight junctions of the blood-brain barrier: Development, composition and regulation," *Vascular Pharmacology*, vol. 38, no. 6, pp. 323–337, 2002.

[3] M. M. Tenreiro, R. Ferreira, L. Bernardino, and M. A. Brito, "Cellular response of the blood-brain barrier to injury: potential biomarkers and therapeutic targets for brain regeneration," *Neurobiology of Disease*, vol. 91, pp. 262–273, 2016.

[4] N. J. Abbott, A. A. K. Patabendige, D. E. M. Dolman, S. R. Yusof, and D. J. Begley, "Structure and function of the blood-brain barrier," *Neurobiology of Disease*, vol. 37, no. 1, pp. 13–25, 2010.

[5] J. Lok, P. Gupta, S. Guo et al., "Cell-cell signaling in the neurovascular unit," *Neurochemical Research*, vol. 32, no. 12, pp. 2032–2045, 2007.

[6] B. V. Zlokovic, "The blood-brain barrier in health and chronic neurodegenerative disorders," *Neuron*, vol. 57, no. 2, pp. 178–201, 2008.

[7] N. J. Abbott, L. Ronnback, and E. Hansson, "Astrocyte-endothelial interactions at the blood-brain barrier," *Nature Reviews Neuroscience*, vol. 7, no. 1, pp. 41–53, 2006.

[8] S. Boillee, C. Vande Velde, and D. W. Cleveland, "ALS: a disease of motor neurons and their nonneuronal neighbors," *Neuron*, vol. 52, no. 1, pp. 39–59, 2006.

[9] B. V. Zlokovic, "Neurovascular mechanisms of Alzheimer's neurodegeneration," *Trends in Neurosciences*, vol. 28, no. 4, pp. 202–208, 2005.

[10] C. Iadecola, "Neurovascular regulation in the normal brain and in Alzheimer's disease," *Nature Reviews. Neuroscience*, vol. 5, no. 5, pp. 347–360, 2004.

[11] I. Bechmann, I. Galea, and V. H. Perry, "What is the blood-brain barrier (not)?," *Trends in Immunology*, vol. 28, no. 1, pp. 5–11, 2007.

[12] K. Nagasawa, H. Chiba, H. Fujita et al., "Possible involvement of gap junctions in the barrier function of tight junctions of brain and lung endothelial cells," *Journal of Cellular Physiology*, vol. 208, no. 1, pp. 123–132, 2006.

[13] R. Bruzzone, T. W. White, and D. L. Paul, "Connections with connexins: the molecular basis of direct intercellular signaling," *European Journal of Biochemistry*, vol. 238, no. 1, pp. 1–27, 1996.

[14] D. W. Laird, "Life cycle of connexins in health and disease," *Biochemical Journal*, vol. 394, no. 3, pp. 527–543, 2006.

[15] P. Ezan, P. André, S. Cisternino et al., "Deletion of astroglial connexins weakens the blood-brain barrier," *Journal of Cerebral Blood Flow & Metabolism*, vol. 32, no. 8, pp. 1457–1467, 2012.

[16] N. Prochnow and R. Dermietzel, "Connexons and cell adhesion: a romantic phase," *Histochemistry and Cell Biology*, vol. 130, no. 1, pp. 71–77, 2008.

[17] L. L. Rubin and J. M. Staddon, "The cell biology of the blood-brain barrier," *Annual Review of Neuroscience*, vol. 22, no. 1, pp. 11–28, 1999.

[18] R. Daneman and A. Prat, "The blood-brain barrier," *Cold Spring Harbor Perspectives in Biology*, vol. 7, no. 1, article a020412, 2015.

[19] S. Ge, L. Song, and J. S. Pachter, "Where is the blood-brain barrier ... really?," *Journal of Neuroscience Research*, vol. 79, no. 4, pp. 421–427, 2005.

[20] H. Wolburg, S. Noell, A. Mack, K. Wolburg-Buchholz, and P. Fallier-Becker, "Brain endothelial cells and the glio-vascular complex," *Cell and Tissue Research*, vol. 335, no. 1, pp. 75–96, 2009.

[21] E. Dejana, "Endothelial cell-cell junctions: happy together," *Nature Reviews Molecular Cell Biology*, vol. 5, no. 4, pp. 261–270, 2004.

[22] M. Derangeon, D. C. Spray, N. Bourmeyster, D. Sarrouilhe, and J. C. Herve, "Reciprocal influence of connexins and apical junction proteins on their expressions and functions," *Biochimica et Biophysica Acta (BBA) - Biomembranes*, vol. 1788, no. 4, pp. 768–778, 2009.

[23] R. A. Meyer, D. W. Laird, J. P. Revel, and R. G. Johnson, "Inhibition of gap junction and adherens junction assembly by connexin and A-CAM antibodies," *The Journal of Cell Biology*, vol. 119, no. 1, pp. 179–189, 1992.

[24] G. S. Goldberg, P. D. Lampe, and B. J. Nicholson, "Selective transfer of endogenous metabolites through gap junctions composed of different connexins," *Nature Cell Biology*, vol. 1, no. 7, pp. 457–459, 1999.

[25] G. S. Goldberg, A. P. Moreno, and P. D. Lampe, "Gap junctions between cells expressing connexin 43 or 32 show inverse permselectivity to adenosine and ATP," *The Journal of Biological Chemistry*, vol. 277, no. 39, pp. 36725–36730, 2002.

[26] Y. Qu and G. Dahl, "Function of the voltage gate of gap junction channels: selective exclusion of molecules," *Proceedings of the National Academy of Sciences of the United States of America*, vol. 99, no. 2, pp. 697–702, 2002.

[27] S. M. Lee and M. G. Clemens, "Subacinar distribution of hepatocyte membrane potential response to stimulation of gluconeogenesis," *The American Journal of Physiology-Gastrointestinal and Liver Physiology*, vol. 263, no. 3, pp. G319–G326, 1992.

[28] S. Rohr, "Role of gap junctions in the propagation of the cardiac action potential," *Cardiovascular Research*, vol. 62, no. 2, pp. 309–322, 2004.

[29] R. Dobrowolski and K. Willecke, "Connexin-caused genetic diseases and corresponding mouse models," *Antioxidants & Redox Signaling*, vol. 11, no. 2, pp. 283–296, 2009.

[30] A. Pfenniger, A. Wohlwend, and B. R. Kwak, "Mutations in connexin genes and disease," *European Journal of Clinical Investigation*, vol. 41, no. 1, pp. 103–116, 2011.

[31] J. I. Nagy, F. E. Dudek, and J. E. Rash, "Update on connexins and gap junctions in neurons and glia in the mammalian nervous system," *Brain Research Reviews*, vol. 47, no. 1-3, pp. 191–215, 2004.

[32] W. H. Evans, E. De Vuyst, and L. Leybaert, "The gap junction cellular internet: connexin hemichannels enter the signalling limelight," *Biochemical Journal*, vol. 397, no. 1, pp. 1–14, 2006.

[33] J. I. Nagy, D. Patel, P. A. Y. Ochalski, and G. L. Stelmack, "Connexin30 in rodent, cat and human brain: selective expression in gray matter astrocytes, co-localization with connexin43 at gap junctions and late developmental appearance," *Neuroscience*, vol. 88, no. 2, pp. 447–468, 1999.

[34] S. Griemsmann, S. P. Höft, P. Bedner et al., "Characterization of panglial gap junction networks in the thalamus, neocortex,

and hippocampus reveals a unique population of glial cells," *Cerebral Cortex*, vol. 25, no. 10, pp. 3420–3433, 2015.

[35] N. Rouach, A. Koulakoff, V. Abudara, K. Willecke, and C. Giaume, "Astroglial metabolic networks sustain hippocampal synaptic transmission," *Science*, vol. 322, no. 5907, pp. 1551–1555, 2008.

[36] L. Roux, K. Benchenane, J. D. Rothstein, G. Bonvento, and C. Giaume, "Plasticity of astroglial networks in olfactory glomeruli," *Proceedings of the National Academy of Sciences of the United States of America*, vol. 108, no. 45, pp. 18442–18446, 2011.

[37] A. Wallraff, R. Köhling, U. Heinemann, M. Theis, K. Willecke, and C. Steinhäuser, "The impact of astrocytic gap junctional coupling on potassium buffering in the hippocampus," *The Journal of Neuroscience*, vol. 26, no. 20, pp. 5438–5447, 2006.

[38] D. F. Condorelli, R. Parenti, F. Spinella et al., "Cloning of a new gap junction gene (Cx36) highly expressed in mammalian brain neurons," *European Journal of Neuroscience*, vol. 10, no. 3, pp. 1202–1208, 1998.

[39] D. F. Condorelli, A. Trovato-Salinaro, G. Mudo, M. B. Mirone, and N. Belluardo, "Cellular expression of connexins in the rat brain: neuronal localization, effects of kainate-induced seizures and expression in apoptotic neuronal cells," *European Journal of Neuroscience*, vol. 18, no. 7, pp. 1807–1827, 2003.

[40] M. R. Deans, J. R. Gibson, C. Sellitto, B. W. Connors, and D. L. Paul, "Synchronous activity of inhibitory networks in neocortex requires electrical synapses containing connexin36," *Neuron*, vol. 31, no. 3, pp. 477–485, 2001.

[41] J. E. Rash, T. Yasumura, F. E. Dudek, and J. I. Nagy, "Cell-specific expression of connexins and evidence of restricted gap junctional coupling between glial cells and between neurons," *Journal of Neuroscience*, vol. 21, no. 6, pp. 1983–2000, 2001.

[42] J. E. Rash, T. Yasumura, K. G. V. Davidson, C. S. Furman, F. E. Dudek, and J. I. Nagy, "Identification of cells expressing Cx43, Cx30, Cx26, Cx32 and Cx36 in gap junctions of rat brain and spinal cord," *Cell Communication & Adhesion*, vol. 8, no. 4–6, pp. 315–320, 2001.

[43] P. Pakhotin and A. Verkhratsky, "Electrical synapses between Bergmann glial cells and Purkinje neurones in rat cerebellar slices," *Molecular and Cellular Neurosciences*, vol. 28, no. 1, pp. 79–84, 2005.

[44] S. Johnstone, B. Isakson, and D. Locke, "Chapter 2 biological and biophysical properties of vascular connexin channels," *International Review of Cell and Molecular Biology*, vol. 278, pp. 69–118, 2009.

[45] R. Bruzzone, J. A. Haefliger, R. L. Gimlich, and D. L. Paul, "Connexin40, a component of gap junctions in vascular endothelium, is restricted in its ability to interact with other connexins," *Molecular Biology of the Cell*, vol. 4, no. 1, pp. 7–20, 1993.

[46] J. E. Gabriels and D. L. Paul, "Connexin43 is highly localized to sites of disturbed flow in rat aortic endothelium but Connexin37 and Connexin40 are more uniformly distributed," *Circulation Research*, vol. 83, no. 6, pp. 636–643, 1998.

[47] J. A. Haefliger, P. Nicod, and P. Meda, "Contribution of connexins to the function of the vascular wall," *Cardiovascular Research*, vol. 62, no. 2, pp. 345–356, 2004.

[48] A. Pfenniger, C. Wong, E. Sutter et al., "Shear stress modulates the expression of the atheroprotective protein Cx37 in endothelial cells," *Journal of Molecular and Cellular Cardiology*, vol. 53, no. 2, pp. 299–309, 2012.

[49] B. R. Kwak, P. Silacci, N. Stergiopulos, D. Hayoz, and P. Meda, "Shear stress and cyclic circumferential stretch, but not pressure, alter connexin43 expression in endothelial cells," *Cell Communication & Adhesion*, vol. 12, no. 5-6, pp. 261–270, 2005.

[50] T. Inai and Y. Shibata, "Heterogeneous expression of endothelial connexin (Cx) 37, Cx40, and Cx43 in rat large veins," *Anatomical Science International*, vol. 84, no. 3, pp. 237–245, 2009.

[51] J. D. Kanady, M. T. Dellinger, S. J. Munger, M. H. Witte, and A. M. Simon, "Connexin37 and Connexin43 deficiencies in mice disrupt lymphatic valve development and result in lymphatic disorders including lymphedema and chylothorax," *Developmental Biology*, vol. 354, no. 2, pp. 253–266, 2011.

[52] A. Sabine, Y. Agalarov, H. Maby-el Hajjami et al., "Mechanotransduction, PROX1, and FOXC2 cooperate to control connexin37 and calcineurin during lymphatic-valve formation," *Developmental Cell*, vol. 22, no. 2, pp. 430–445, 2012.

[53] M. J. Meens, I. Kutkut, V. Rochemont et al., "Cx47 fine-tunes the handling of serum lipids but is dispensable for lymphatic vascular function," *PLoS One*, vol. 12, no. 7, article e0181476, 2017.

[54] H. H. Wang, C. H. Su, Y. J. Wu et al., "Reduction of connexin43 in human endothelial progenitor cells impairs the angiogenic potential," *Angiogenesis*, vol. 16, no. 3, pp. 553–560, 2013.

[55] M. Cronin, P. N. Anderson, J. E. Cook, C. R. Green, and D. L. Becker, "Blocking connexin43 expression reduces inflammation and improves functional recovery after spinal cord injury," *Molecular and Cellular Neuroscience*, vol. 39, no. 2, pp. 152–160, 2008.

[56] H. V. Danesh-Meyer, R. Huang, L. F. B. Nicholson, and C. R. Green, "Connexin43 antisense oligodeoxynucleotide treatment down-regulates the inflammatory response in an *in vitro* interphase organotypic culture model of optic nerve ischaemia," *Journal of Clinical Neuroscience*, vol. 15, no. 11, pp. 1253–1263, 2008.

[57] M. De Bock, M. Culot, N. Wang et al., "Connexin channels provide a target to manipulate brain endothelial calcium dynamics and blood-brain barrier permeability," *Journal of Cerebral Blood Flow & Metabolism*, vol. 31, no. 9, pp. 1942–1957, 2011.

[58] H. V. Danesh-Meyer, N. M. Kerr, J. Zhang et al., "Connexin43 mimetic peptide reduces vascular leak and retinal ganglion cell death following retinal ischaemia," *Brain*, vol. 135, no. 2, pp. 506–520, 2012.

[59] A. M. Johnson, J. P. Roach, A. Hu et al., "Connexin 43 gap junctions contribute to brain endothelial barrier hyperpermeability in familial cerebral cavernous malformations type III by modulating tight junction structure," *The FASEB Journal*, vol. 32, no. 5, pp. 2615–2629, 2018.

[60] C. Giaume, A. Koulakoff, L. Roux, D. Holcman, and N. Rouach, "Astroglial networks: a step further in neuroglial and gliovascular interactions," *Nature Reviews Neuroscience*, vol. 11, no. 2, pp. 87–99, 2010.

[61] S. Nielsen, E. Arnulf Nagelhus, M. Amiry-Moghaddam, C. Bourque, P. Agre, and O. Petter Ottersen, "Specialized membrane domains for water transport in glial cells: high-

resolution immunogold cytochemistry of aquaporin-4 in rat brain," *Journal of Neuroscience*, vol. 17, no. 1, pp. 171–180, 1997.

[62] A.-C. Boulay, B. Saubaméa, S. Cisternino et al., "The Sarcoglycan complex is expressed in the cerebrovascular system and is specifically regulated by astroglial Cx30 channels," *Frontiers in Cellular Neuroscience*, vol. 9, 2015.

[63] A. Lampron, A. Elali, and S. Rivest, "Innate immunity in the CNS: redefining the relationship between the CNS and its environment," *Neuron*, vol. 78, no. 2, pp. 214–232, 2013.

[64] A. C. Boulay, A. Mazeraud, S. Cisternino et al., "Immune quiescence of the brain is set by astroglial connexin 43," *Journal of Neuroscience*, vol. 35, no. 10, pp. 4427–4439, 2015.

[65] C. A. Whittaker and R. O. Hynes, "Distribution and evolution of von Willebrand/integrin A domains: widely dispersed domains with roles in cell adhesion and elsewhere," *Molecular Biology of the Cell*, vol. 13, no. 10, pp. 3369–3387, 2002.

[66] A. Naba, K. R. Clauser, S. Hoersch, H. Liu, S. A. Carr, and R. O. Hynes, "The matrisome: *in silico* definition and *in vivo* characterization by proteomics of normal and tumor extracellular matrices," *Molecular & Cellular Proteomics*, vol. 11, no. 4, article M111 014647, 2012.

[67] K. Markoullis, I. Sargiannidou, N. Schiza et al., "Gap junction pathology in multiple sclerosis lesions and normal-appearing white matter," *Acta Neuropathologica*, vol. 123, no. 6, pp. 873–886, 2012.

[68] K. Masaki, S. O. Suzuki, T. Matsushita et al., "Connexin 43 astrocytopathy linked to rapidly progressive multiple sclerosis and neuromyelitis optica," *PLoS One*, vol. 8, no. 8, article e72919, 2013.

[69] L. A. B. Elias, D. D. Wang, and A. R. Kriegstein, "Gap junction adhesion is necessary for radial migration in the neocortex," *Nature*, vol. 448, no. 7156, pp. 901–907, 2007.

[70] L. A. B. Elias, M. Turmaine, J. G. Parnavelas, and A. R. Kriegstein, "Connexin 43 mediates the tangential to radial migratory switch in ventrally derived cortical interneurons," *Journal of Neuroscience*, vol. 30, no. 20, pp. 7072–7077, 2010.

[71] A. Alonso, E. Reinz, J. W. Jenne et al., "Reorganization of gap junctions after focused ultrasound blood-brain barrier opening in the rat brain," *Journal of Cerebral Blood Flow & Metabolism*, vol. 30, no. 7, pp. 1394–1402, 2010.

[72] X. Li, C. Olson, S. Lu et al., "Neuronal connexin36 association with zonula occludens-1 protein (ZO-1) in mouse brain and interaction with the first PDZ domain of ZO-1," *European Journal of Neuroscience*, vol. 19, no. 8, pp. 2132–2146, 2004.

[73] S. J. Mulligan and B. A. MacVicar, "Calcium transients in astrocyte endfeet cause cerebrovascular constrictions," *Nature*, vol. 431, no. 7005, pp. 195–199, 2004.

[74] M. Zonta, M. C. Angulo, S. Gobbo et al., "Neuron-to-astrocyte signaling is central to the dynamic control of brain microcirculation," *Nature Neuroscience*, vol. 6, no. 1, pp. 43–50, 2003.

[75] M. A. Retamal, N. Froger, N. Palacios-Prado et al., "Cx43 hemichannels and gap junction channels in astrocytes are regulated oppositely by proinflammatory cytokines released from activated microglia," *Journal of Neuroscience*, vol. 27, no. 50, pp. 13781–13792, 2007.

[76] M. A. Retamal, K. A. Schalper, K. F. Shoji, M. V. L. Bennett, and J. C. Saez, "Opening of connexin 43 hemichannels is increased by lowering intracellular redox potential," *Proceedings of the National Academy of Sciences of the United States of America*, vol. 104, no. 20, pp. 8322–8327, 2007.

[77] M. De Bocka, M. Culot, N. Wang et al., "Low extracellular Ca^{2+} conditions induce an increase in brain endothelial permeability that involves intercellular Ca^{2+} waves," *Brain Research*, vol. 1487, pp. 78–87, 2012.

[78] W. H. Evans and L. Leybaert, "Mimetic peptides as blockers of connexin channel-facilitated intercellular communication," *Cell Communication & Adhesion*, vol. 14, no. 6, pp. 265–273, 2007.

[79] J. Kang, N. Kang, D. Lovatt et al., "Connexin 43 hemichannels are permeable to ATP," *Journal of Neuroscience*, vol. 28, no. 18, pp. 4702–4711, 2008.

[80] K. Braet, W. Vandamme, P. E. Martin, W. H. Evans, and L. Leybaert, "Photoliberating inositol-1,4,5-trisphosphate triggers ATP release that is blocked by the connexin mimetic peptide gap 26," *Cell Calcium*, vol. 33, no. 1, pp. 37–48, 2003.

[81] K. Braet, S. Aspeslagh, W. Vandamme et al., "Pharmacological sensitivity of ATP release triggered by photoliberation of inositol-1,4,5-trisphosphate and zero extracellular calcium in brain endothelial cells," *Journal of Cellular Physiology*, vol. 197, no. 2, pp. 205–213, 2003.

[82] W. Vandamme, K. Braet, L. Cabooter, and L. Leybaert, "Tumour necrosis factor alpha inhibits purinergic calcium signalling in blood-brain barrier endothelial cells," *Journal of Neurochemistry*, vol. 88, no. 2, pp. 411–421, 2004.

[83] H. K. Eltzschig, T. Eckle, A. Mager et al., "ATP release from activated neutrophils occurs via connexin 43 and modulates adenosine-dependent endothelial cell function," *Circulation Research*, vol. 99, no. 10, pp. 1100–1108, 2006.

[84] E. Decrock, E. de Vuyst, M. Vinken et al., "Connexin 43 hemichannels contribute to the propagation of apoptotic cell death in a rat C6 glioma cell model," *Cell Death and Differentiation*, vol. 16, no. 1, pp. 151–163, 2009.

[85] T. Constantinou, F. Baumann, M. D. Lacher, S. Saurer, R. Friis, and A. Dharmarajan, "SFRP-4 abrogates Wnt-3a-induced β-catenin and Akt/PKB signalling and reverses a Wnt-3a-imposed inhibition of *in vitro* mammary differentiation," *Journal of Molecular Signaling*, vol. 3, p. 10, 2008.

[86] L. Liu, W. Wan, S. Xia, B. Kalionis, and Y. Li, "Dysfunctional Wnt/β-catenin signaling contributes to blood–brain barrier breakdown in Alzheimer's disease," *Neurochemistry International*, vol. 75, pp. 19–25, 2014.

[87] B. Obermeier, R. Daneman, and R. M. Ransohoff, "Development, maintenance and disruption of the blood-brain barrier," *Nature Medicine*, vol. 19, no. 12, pp. 1584–1596, 2013.

[88] E. Brand-Schieber, P. Werner, D. A. Iacobas et al., "Connexin43, the major gap junction protein of astrocytes, is down-regulated in inflamed white matter in an animal model of multiple sclerosis," *Journal of Neuroscience Research*, vol. 80, no. 6, pp. 798–808, 2005.

[89] E. A. Eugenin, D. Basilio, J. C. Sáez et al., "The role of gap junction channels during physiologic and pathologic conditions of the human central nervous system," *Journal of Neuroimmune Pharmacology*, vol. 7, no. 3, pp. 499–518, 2012.

[90] K. Markoullis, I. Sargiannidou, C. Gardner, A. Hadjisavvas, R. Reynolds, and K. A. Kleopa, "Disruption of oligodendrocyte gap junctions in experimental autoimmune encephalomyelitis," *Glia*, vol. 60, no. 7, pp. 1053–1066, 2012.

[91] S. E. Lutz, C. S. Raine, and C. F. Brosnan, "Loss of astrocyte connexins 43 and 30 does not significantly alter susceptibility

or severity of acute experimental autoimmune encephalomyelitis in mice," *Journal of Neuroimmunology*, vol. 245, no. 1-2, pp. 8–14, 2012.

[92] J. D. Huber, K. A. Witt, S. Hom, R. D. Egleton, K. S. Mark, and T. P. Davis, "Inflammatory pain alters blood-brain barrier permeability and tight junctional protein expression," *American Journal of Physiology-Heart and Circulatory Physiology*, vol. 280, no. 3, pp. H1241–H1248, 2001.

[93] H.-S. Choi, D. H. Roh, S. Y. Yoon et al., "The role of spinal interleukin-1β and astrocyte connexin 43 in the development of mirror-image pain in an inflammatory pain model," *Experimental Neurology*, vol. 287, pp. 1–13, 2017.

[94] G. Chen, C. K. Park, R. G. Xie, T. Berta, M. Nedergaard, and R. R. Ji, "Connexin-43 induces chemokine release from spinal cord astrocytes to maintain late-phase neuropathic pain in mice," *Brain*, vol. 137, no. 8, pp. 2193–2209, 2014.

[95] C. A. Lee-Kubli, M. Ingves, K. W. Henry et al., "Analysis of the behavioral, cellular and molecular characteristics of pain in severe rodent spinal cord injury," *Experimental Neurology*, vol. 278, pp. 91–104, 2016.

[96] M. J. Chen, B. Kress, X. Han et al., "Astrocytic CX43 hemichannels and gap junctions play a crucial role in development of chronic neuropathic pain following spinal cord injury," *Glia*, vol. 60, no. 11, pp. 1660–1670, 2012.

[97] Z. Zhou, X. Wei, J. Xiang et al., "Protection of erythropoietin against ischemic neurovascular unit injuries through the effects of connexin43," *Biochemical and Biophysical Research Communications*, vol. 458, no. 3, pp. 656–662, 2015.

[98] T. Nakase, S. Fushiki, and C. C. G. Naus, "Astrocytic gap junctions composed of connexin 43 reduce apoptotic neuronal damage in cerebral ischemia," *Stroke*, vol. 34, no. 8, pp. 1987–1993, 2003.

[99] N. M. Kerr, C. S. Johnson, C. F. de Souza et al., "Immunolocalization of gap junction protein connexin43 (GJA1) in the human retina and optic nerve," *Investigative Ophthalmology & Visual Science*, vol. 51, no. 8, pp. 1028–1034, 2010.

[100] J. A. Orellana, P. J. Sáez, K. F. Shoji et al., "Modulation of brain hemichannels and gap junction channels by pro-inflammatory agents and their possible role in neurodegeneration," *Antioxidants & Redox Signaling*, vol. 11, no. 2, pp. 369–399, 2009.

[101] N. N. Osborne, R. J. Casson, J. P. M. Wood, G. Chidlow, M. Graham, and J. Melena, "Retinal ischemia: mechanisms of damage and potential therapeutic strategies," *Progress in Retinal and Eye Research*, vol. 23, no. 1, pp. 91–147, 2004.

[102] A. Rodriguez-Sinovas, A. Cabestrero, D. Lopez et al., "The modulatory effects of connexin 43 on cell death/survival beyond cell coupling," *Progress in Biophysics and Molecular Biology*, vol. 94, no. 1-2, pp. 219–232, 2007.

[103] C. Kaur, V. Sivakumar, Y. Zhang, and E. A. Ling, "Hypoxia-induced astrocytic reaction and increased vascular permeability in the rat cerebellum," *Glia*, vol. 54, no. 8, pp. 826–839, 2006.

[104] W. D. Dietrich, O. Alonso, and M. Halley, "Early microvascular and neuronal consequences of traumatic brain injury: a light and electron microscopic study in rats," *Journal of Neurotrauma*, vol. 11, no. 3, pp. 289–301, 1994.

[105] A. Hirano, T. Kawanami, and J. F. Llena, "Electron microscopy of the blood-brain barrier in disease," *Microscopy Research & Technique*, vol. 27, no. 6, pp. 543–556, 1994.

[106] A. Rami, T. Volkmann, and J. Winckler, "Effective reduction of neuronal death by inhibiting gap junctional intercellular communication in a rodent model of global transient cerebral ischemia," *Experimental Neurology*, vol. 170, no. 2, pp. 297–304, 2001.

[107] J. O. Davidson, C. R. Green, L. F. B. Nicholson et al., "Connexin hemichannel blockade improves outcomes in a model of fetal ischemia," *Annals of Neurology*, vol. 71, no. 1, pp. 121–132, 2012.

[108] A. C. Wilson, L. Clemente, T. Liu, R. L. Bowen, S. V. Meethal, and C. S. Atwood, "Reproductive hormones regulate the selective permeability of the blood-brain barrier," *Biochimica et Biophysica Acta (BBA) - Molecular Basis of Disease*, vol. 1782, no. 6, pp. 401–407, 2008.

[109] M. P. Mattson, "Cellular actions of beta-amyloid precursor protein and its soluble and fibrillogenic derivatives," *Physiological Reviews*, vol. 77, no. 4, pp. 1081–1132, 1997.

[110] N. J. Haughey and M. P. Mattson, "Alzheimer's amyloid β-peptide enhances ATP/gap junction-mediated calcium-wave propagation in astrocytes," *NeuroMolecular Medicine*, vol. 3, no. 3, pp. 173–180, 2003.

[111] C. Yi, P. Ezan, P. Fernández et al., "Inhibition of glial hemichannels by boldine treatment reduces neuronal suffering in a murine model of Alzheimer's disease," *Glia*, vol. 65, no. 10, pp. 1607–1625, 2017.

[112] C. Yi, X. Mei, P. Ezan et al., "Astroglial connexin43 contributes to neuronal suffering in a mouse model of Alzheimer's disease," *Cell Death & Differentiation*, vol. 23, no. 10, pp. 1691–1701, 2016.

[113] X. Mei, P. Ezan, C. Giaume, and A. Koulakoff, "Astroglial connexin immunoreactivity is specifically altered at β-amyloid plaques in β-amyloid precursor protein/presenilin1 mice," *Neuroscience*, vol. 171, no. 1, pp. 92–105, 2010.

[114] H. Takeuchi, H. Mizoguchi, Y. Doi et al., "Blockade of gap junction hemichannel suppresses disease progression in mouse models of amyotrophic lateral sclerosis and Alzheimer's disease," *PLoS One*, vol. 6, no. 6, article e21108, 2011.

[115] L. P. Cacheaux, S. Ivens, Y. David et al., "Transcriptome profiling reveals TGF-β signaling involvement in epileptogenesis," *Journal of Neuroscience*, vol. 29, no. 28, pp. 8927–8935, 2009.

[116] R. Kovacs, U. Heinemann, and C. Steinhauser, "Mechanisms underlying blood-brain barrier dysfunction in brain pathology and epileptogenesis: role of astroglia," *Epilepsia*, vol. 53, Supplement 6, pp. 53–59, 2012.

[117] Y. David, L. P. Cacheaux, S. Ivens et al., "Astrocytic dysfunction in epileptogenesis: consequence of altered potassium and glutamate homeostasis?," *The Journal of Neuroscience*, vol. 29, no. 34, pp. 10588–10599, 2009.

[118] Z. Gajda, E. Hermesz, E. Gyengesi, Z. Szupera, and M. Szente, "The functional significance of gap junction channels in the epileptogenicity and seizure susceptibility of juvenile rats," *Epilepsia*, vol. 47, no. 6, pp. 1009–1022, 2006.

[119] M. Samoilova, K. Wentlandt, Y. Adamchik, A. A. Velumian, and P. L. Carlen, "Connexin 43 mimetic peptides inhibit spontaneous epileptiform activity in organotypic hippocampal slice cultures," *Experimental Neurology*, vol. 210, no. 2, pp. 762–775, 2008.

[120] M. A. Cosenza, M.-L. Zhao, Q. Si, and S. C. Lee, "Human brain parenchymal microglia express CD14 and CD45 and

are productively infected by HIV-1 in HIV-1 encephalitis," *Brain Pathology*, vol. 12, no. 4, pp. 442–455, 2002.

[121] E. A. Eugenin and J. W. Berman, "Gap junctions mediate human immunodeficiency virus-bystander killing in astrocytes," *The Journal of Neuroscience*, vol. 27, no. 47, pp. 12844–12850, 2007.

[122] M. J. Churchill, S. L. Wesselingh, D. Cowley et al., "Extensive astrocyte infection is prominent in human immunodeficiency virus-associated dementia," *Annals of Neurology*, vol. 66, no. 2, pp. 253–258, 2009.

[123] E. A. Eugenin, J. E. Clements, M. C. Zink, and J. W. Berman, "Human immunodeficiency virus infection of human astrocytes disrupts blood-brain barrier integrity by a gap junction-dependent mechanism," *Journal of Neuroscience*, vol. 31, no. 26, pp. 9456–9465, 2011.

[124] J. Z. Zhou and J. X. Jiang, "Gap junction and hemichannel-independent actions of connexins on cell and tissue functions–an update," *FEBS Letters*, vol. 588, no. 8, pp. 1186–1192, 2014.

[125] M. Vinken, E. Decrock, L. Leybaert et al., "Non-channel functions of connexins in cell growth and cell death," *Biochimica et Biophysica Acta (BBA) - Biomembranes*, vol. 1818, no. 8, pp. 2002–2008, 2012.

[126] R. Yamasaki, H. Lu, O. Butovsky et al., "Differential roles of microglia and monocytes in the inflamed central nervous system," *Journal of Experimental Medicine*, vol. 211, no. 8, pp. 1533–1549, 2014.

8

Molecular Mechanisms of Oxytocin Signaling at the Synaptic Connection

Jan Bakos,[1,2] **Annamaria Srancikova**,[1] **Tomas Havranek**,[1] **and Zuzana Bacova**[1]

[1]*Institute of Experimental Endocrinology, Biomedical Research Center, Slovak Academy of Sciences, Bratislava, Slovakia*
[2]*Institute of Physiology, Faculty of Medicine, Comenius University, Bratislava, Slovakia*

Correspondence should be addressed to Jan Bakos; j.bakos@savba.sk

Academic Editor: Victor Anggono

Aberrant regulation of oxytocin signaling is associated with the etiology of neurodevelopmental disorders. Synaptic dysfunctions in neurodevelopmental disorders are becoming increasingly known, and their pathogenic mechanisms could be a target of potential therapeutic intervention. Therefore, it is important to pay attention to the role of oxytocin and its receptor in synapse structure, function, and neuron connectivity. An early alteration in oxytocin signaling may disturb neuronal maturation and may have short-term and long-term pathological consequences. At the molecular level, neurodevelopmental disorders include alterations in cytoskeletal rearrangement and neuritogenesis resulting in a diversity of synaptopathies. The presence of oxytocin receptors in the presynaptic and postsynaptic membranes and the direct effects of oxytocin on neuronal excitability by regulating the activity of ion channels in the cell membrane implicate that alterations in oxytocin signaling could be involved in synaptopathies. The ability of oxytocin to modulate neurogenesis, synaptic plasticity, and certain parameters of cytoskeletal arrangement is discussed in the present review.

1. Introduction

Although it has been known for a long time that oxytocin exerts modulatory effects on synaptic activity, recent studies have produced many important findings related to the neuron and glial cell structure, development, and functionality. In a broader sense, oxytocin is one of the most studied molecules in the context of brain development and social behavior. Oxytocin acts on oxytocin and partially on vasopressin receptors; therefore, regardless of focus on the oxytocin system, it is important to keep in mind the significant receptor cross-reactivity for their endogenous ligands [1, 2]. Functional oxytocin receptors have been recently discovered at neural progenitor cells which implies that they could be associated with cell fate selection [3]. Furthermore, oxytocin plays a role in the early development of neurons and participates in synapse formation [4]. Oxytocin-producing cells appear during the early phase of the brain development [5], and their maturation, particularly their ability to produce oxytocin, may influence the formation of neural circuits [6].

With regard to the defects in oxytocin signaling, there is a whole spectrum of neurodevelopmental disorders frequently associated with them, which include autism; therefore, it is increasingly important to pay attention to the role of oxytocin and its receptor in synapse structure, function, and neuron connectivity. An early alteration in oxytocin signaling may disturb neuronal maturation and may have short-term and long-term pathological consequences [7]. At the cell and molecular level, autism is a heterogeneous disorder, and its pathology includes alterations in cytoskeletal rearrangement, neuritogenesis, and elongation of axons and dendrites resulting in a diversity of synaptopathies [8]. In particular, impaired synapse formation results in disrupted neuronal connectivity and circuit stabilization which in turn can explain the pathogenesis of the disease [9]. Given the growing prevalence of autism, identification of risk factors and therapeutic interventions is a key factor of the relevant objectives of the current neurobiology research. The ability of oxytocin to modulate neurogenesis, synaptic plasticity, and certain parameters of cytoskeletal arrangement is discussed in the following review.

2. Oxytocin Receptors in Neurons

It is well known that receptors for neuropeptides are found heterogeneously distributed throughout the brain and may be expressed on cell bodies, dendrites, and axon terminals [10]. Oxytocin receptors are distributed in all brain regions, and oxytocin-producing neurons project from the hypothalamus to various brain areas including the limbic regions and brain cortex [11]. Oxytocin receptors are among the group of G protein-coupled receptors. Different intracellular pathways are activated by oxytocin according to the specific G proteins that they activate [2]. In neurons, an oxytocin receptor is coupled to $G_{\alpha i}$ and $G_{\alpha q}$, with protein kinase C/phospholipase Cβ as downstream effectors, rather than cAMP [12].

Modern techniques allow for specifically tracing and optogenetically stimulating oxytocin receptor-expressing neurons in different brain regions in order to observe the effects on thirst-related neural circuits or social behavior-related circuits [13, 14]. A recent study has discovered that oxytocin promotes the survival and maturation of newborn neurons in the hippocampus via its receptor [15]. Stimulation of neurogenesis in the hippocampus by oxytocin has been observed in previous studies [16]. This finding could be extended to other brain areas as one study has already proved neurogenesis in oxytocin-containing neurons in the hypothalamus [17]. Moreover, oxytocin may affect expression of neurotrophic factors such as the brain-derived neurotrophic factor (BDNF) and the nerve growth factor (NGF), which contribute to neural plasticity [18]. In the following study, we have observed that oxytocin affects the expression of neuron and glial markers in the brain [19]. Therefore, it can be suggested that the oxytocin system is involved in the regulation of development of neuronal precursor cells in the brain. This is in line with the recent study suggesting the role of oxytocin in neural progenitors [3]. The authors concluded that exposure to oxytocin increases generation of neurons and decreases production of oligodendrocytes and astrocytes [3]. It is generally accepted that oxytocin receptors are localized in neurons and glial cells as well; however, the majority of studies are focused on the effects of oxytocin on excitability of the neuron cell membrane [20].

Neurons constantly undergo structural and functional alterations as part of a process called synaptic plasticity; therefore, there is no doubt that oxytocin could affect synaptic activity at many levels of regulation. A recent study has demonstrated that the oxytocin receptor mRNA could be detected during mouse embryonal development in both sexes, although females appear to have more of the oxytocin receptor mRNA than males [21]. These differences between males and females may relate to hormonal differences, which alter oxytocin signaling. These findings are especially important in the context of development of neural circuits and their potential alterations. It is necessary to emphasize that some studies suggest that oxytocin inhibits fetal neurons resulting in the switch of GABAergic neurons from excitatory to inhibitory [22, 23]. Oxytocin receptors in neurons could represent a critical factor in organizing neural circuitry and the development of social behavior.

3. The Role of Oxytocin in Neural Circuits

Balance between excitation and inhibition is an important feature of neuronal circuits. Oxytocin can directly increase neuronal excitability by regulating the activity of ion channels in the membrane and thus modulating synaptic transmission [24]. However, the extent of oxytocin action depends on the brain region, type of neurons, and their initial membrane excitability. Over the past decade, both *in vivo* and *in vitro* studies have made the progress from investigating electrical spiking activity of the oxytocin neurons ranging from the hypothalamus, the hippocampus, and the amygdala to the spinal cord [25–27]. Originally, even though electrical properties of oxytocin-producing neurons have been mostly related to parturition and/or lactation, nowadays it is clear that the wide spectrum of physiological functions including analgesia and regulation of behavior is associated with oxytocin. Indeed, oxytocin actions on synaptic transmission in the adult brain are often specific in the context of social communication [28]. Oxytocin induces excitation of neurons in the amygdala, [29] and it could be suggested that together with the effects on hippocampal formation, oxytocin is involved in information processing in limbic circuits and plays a role in memory and learning regulation [30]. Furthermore, many studies have implicated oxytocin with anxiolytic effects in the limbic areas and prefrontal cortex [31]. Nevertheless, in contrast to previous studies, it has been found that oxytocin produces antinociception in part by reducing excitatory neurotransmitter release [32]. These authors explain their findings by oxytocin modulation of high voltage-gated calcium channels, primarily of the N-type, to reduce presynaptic glutamate release [33]. Many studies claim that oxytocin released from the hypothalamus is distributed through oxytocin-containing fibers to the spinal cord and has stress-inducing analgesic effects [34, 35]. In a broader sense, neuropeptide modulation of GABA and glutamate synaptic actions are complex and require knowledge of the cell type, brain region, composition of synaptic membrane, and coupling of receptors to ion channels. In the case of oxytocin, it is important to consider the effects of oxytocin on both oxytocin and vasopressin receptors. It might be especially important to know how balanced these receptors are in the synaptic cleft.

4. Presynaptic Modulation by Oxytocin

Presynaptic oxytocin receptors were described in the 1980s by Audigier and Barberis [36], and at that time, there were already speculations on how oxytocin could affect neurotransmission [37]. These authors [36] isolated synaptic plasma membranes and proved that they contain binding sites for oxytocin and vasopressin. Since that time, the presence and functionality of oxytocin receptors at the synapse have been repeatedly proved in many areas of the central and peripheral nervous systems. Activation of the oxytocin receptor on the presynaptic membrane, resulting in an increase in intracellular calcium concentration, may increase the secretion of the neurotransmitter into the synaptic cleft. Oxytocin stimulates the increase of calcium through two major mechanisms (Figure 1). First is through $G_{\alpha q}$-mediated activation of the

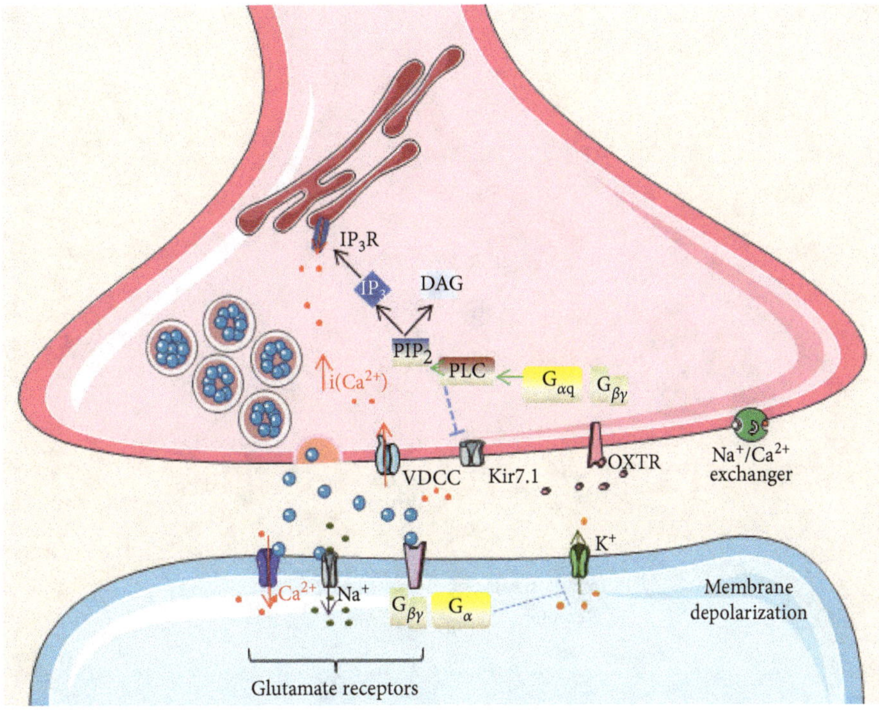

FIGURE 1: Presynaptic G protein-coupled oxytocin receptors modulate membrane polarity. OXTR: oxytocin receptor; VDCC: voltage-dependent calcium channels; PIP_2: phosphatidylinositol biphosphate; IP_3: inositol 1,4,5-trisphosphate; DAG: diacylglycerol.

phospholipase C, which by the action of inositol-triphosphate binding on inositol 1,4,5-trisphosphate receptor (IP_3R) induces release of calcium from intracellular sources [38]. Second is through inhibition of the potassium Kir7.1 channels, which induces plasma membrane depolarization and calcium entry through the voltage-dependent calcium channel [39, 40]. Another mechanism on how oxytocin may induce membrane depolarization on presynaptic membranes is through activation of Na^+/Ca^{2+} exchanger and the opening of a nonselective cation channel [41]. The activation of the Na^+/Ca^{2+} exchanger by G protein-coupled receptors has been suggested in different hypothalamic systems [42, 43].

4.1. Excitatory Synapse. Modulation of excitatory synaptic transmission by the action of oxytocin on its receptors is complex and may differ in various parts of the brain. A recent study has demonstrated that the activation of presynaptic oxytocin receptors enhances the release of depolarization-evoked glutamate in the hippocampus [44]. Nevertheless, other brain regions are also the target of oxytocin effects. It has been demonstrated that the activation of oxytocin receptors facilitates glutamatergic synaptic transmission in the spinal cord [45]. These authors explained their findings in the way that oxytocin acts on presynaptic membrane of subpopulation of glutamatergic neurons and as a result of this action promotes release of the neurotransmitter. This release of glutamate results in excitation of GABAergic neurons and when connected to further neurons transmits inhibitory message on them. This complicated concept is used in current studies for explanation of the nociceptive effects of oxytocin. Nevertheless, it is likely that interneurons in the spinal cord may use oxytocin as a neurotransmitter. It also means that synaptic contacts with neurons in the second or third order could be under a different oxytocin modulation. Contradictory to the results that describe the enhancement of excitatory synaptic transmission, there are also suggestions that oxytocin works against glutamate release from the presynaptic membrane. It has been revealed that dendritically released oxytocin decreases evoked excitatory synaptic transmission by inhibiting glutamate release from the presynaptic terminals [46]. The authors of this study explain the effect of oxytocin by evidence of modulation of voltage-dependent calcium channels, mainly N-type and to a lesser extent P/Q-type channels, located on glutamatergic terminals. This concept suggests the existence of two-way communication between the presynaptic terminal and the postsynaptic synaptic membrane. Although in our study we did not distinguish between presynaptic/postsynaptic actions of oxytocin, we confirmed that oxytocin acts via a mechanism involving the N-type channels and P/Q-type channels inducing neurite outgrowth [47]. It is widely accepted that the presynaptic effect of oxytocin is dependent on extracellular calcium [48]. Furthermore, oxytocin receptors were found at the so-called putative excitatory synapses, both at presynaptic and postsynaptic terminals and at inhibitory synapses as well [49]. Taken together, the results of the available studies are not conclusive leaving a room for various interpretations. Therefore, more studies can bring more specific data on oxytocin action in excitatory synapse.

4.2. Inhibitory Synapse. The active role of oxytocin in inhibitory synapses could also be a matter of discussion. Some studies explain the role oxytocin in inhibitory terminals in the way that oxytocin acts via presynaptic activation of

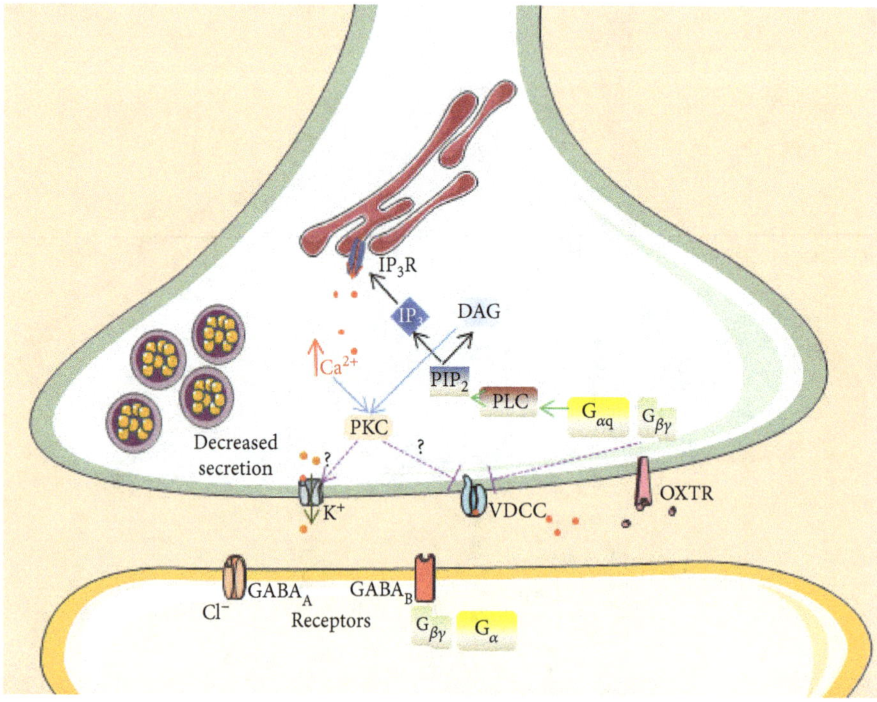

FIGURE 2: Presynaptic G protein-coupled oxytocin receptors modulate neurotransmitter release. OXTR: Oxytocin receptor; VDCC: voltage-dependent calcium channels; PIP_2: phosphatidylinositol biphosphate; IP_3: inositol 1,4,5-trisphosphate; DAG: diacylglycerol; GABA: γ-aminobutyric acid receptor.

oxytocin receptors resulting in a decrease of GABAergic transmitter release [49]. In this study, the authors suggest that the predominant effect of oxytocin modulation is to reduce inhibitory transmission without directly affecting excitation. The pathways responsible for the decrease of GABA secretion (Figure 2) include the inhibition of voltage-dependent calcium channels by protein kinase C and/or calcium-dependent potassium channels [50]. This conclusion is supported by other studies in different brain areas: the auditory cortex, piriform cortex, hypothalamus, and hippocampus [51, 52]. Conversely, another study has suggested that oxytocin depresses spontaneously occurring GABA receptor-mediated inhibitory potential by acting presynaptically in the olfactory blub [53]. This is supported by the inhibitory effects of oxytocin on different sets of interneurons *in vitro* [54]. Taken together, the activity of oxytocin on its receptors at the presynaptic membrane depends on the neuron type and brain area and most likely also on the complex presynaptic inputs including astrocyte-originated transmission [55].

5. Postsynaptic Modulation by Oxytocin

Regulation of postsynaptic membrane potential represents a significant part of oxytocin's contribution to the modulation of synaptic function. Oxytocin can directly act via oxytocin receptors on postsynaptic neurons in order to alter the activity of neural circuits which regulate social behaviors [56, 57]. Yao et al. [56] discovered the presence of oxytocin receptors in a special subpopulation of neurons in the amygdala which express the steroid-converting enzyme aromatase. This finding has extended the knowledge of oxytocin receptor stimulation to specific female-evoked neural responses and behaviors in the male mouse. The effect of oxytocin on membrane excitability of rat dorsal root ganglion neurons has also been investigated [58]. The authors found that oxytocin significantly decreased the amplitude of the depolarization and number of action potentials induced by acid stimuli. In this context, the authors also stressed the role of vasopressin receptor V1a. Another recent study has demonstrated that oxytocin enhances the frequency of spontaneous inhibitory postsynaptic currents [59]. It is relevant to note that the authors also suggest that both V1a and oxytocin receptors play an important role. Another study has found that oxytocin induces an increase in intracellular calcium on the postsynaptic membrane, which consequently depresses inhibitory synaptic transmission [60]. Oxytocin affects the spontaneous rate of inhibitory and excitatory postsynaptic currents in the olfactory cortex as well [28]. It has been found that oxytocin depolarizes interneurons and enhances synaptic transmission in the hippocampal area CA1 [27]. Other electrophysiological studies have proved that stimulation of oxytocin receptors reduces spontaneous firing yet enhances excitatory postsynaptic potential onto pyramidal cells in the hippocampus [52].

6. The Oxytocin Receptors in the Glial Cells

Glial cells and in particular astrocytes have been identified as targets of oxytocin action. Studies using autoradiography have proved the presence of oxytocin-binding sites located on both soma and processes of astrocyte-like types of cells [61]. Other studies have produced evidence on the effects of oxytocin on astrocytoma cell lines [62, 63], implicating that oxytocin receptors could modulate cellular growth. One study has shown that stimulation of astrocytic oxytocin receptors results in the release of calcium from intracellular stores [64]. The functional aspects of oxytocin receptors were revealed in astrocytes by electrophysiological experiments which proved that oxytocin evokes depolarization of astrocytic membrane potential, and in the context of suckling, it could induce retraction of astrocyte processes [65]. This phenomenon is particularly important to keep in mind in the context of astrocytic participation in neuronal activity. Astroglial-neuronal interactions however are very complex, and in the view of synaptic connectivity, astrocytic transformations are related to the number of synapses. It has been repeatedly demonstrated that the astrocyte oxytocin receptor is coupled to a G protein-coupled receptor and increases intracellular calcium concentration mobilized from IP_3-sensitive stores [61, 66].

7. The Formation and Stability of the Synapse

A recent study has directly shown that oxytocin affects the number of synapses [4]. This study has suggested that the number of excitatory presynapses is increased in cultures from oxytocin receptor knockout mice, whereas the number of inhibitory presynapses is slightly decreased. Moreover, the authors proved that oxytocin exposure of cultured mouse hippocampal glutamatergic neurons caused altered neuronal dendrite complexity and altered numbers of excitatory synapses. Another study found a decreased ratio of GABAergic versus total presynapses in hippocampal neurons cultured from oxytocin receptor knockout mice [67]. In the context of synapse formation, it is important to take into account as well the effects of oxytocin on neurofilaments. It has been demonstrated that oxytocin promotes the formation of filamentous actin (F-actin) networks on the membrane in the cells of the brain cortex [55]. Furthermore, in our study, we have found increased expression of the actin-binding protein drebrin and the intermediate filament vimentin in response to oxytocin [68]. Thus, oxytocin contributes to the regulation of expression of cytoskeletal proteins associated with neurite growth *in vitro*. Taken from a structural point of view, it is important to emphasize that oxytocin receptor knockout mice suffer from reduction of postsynaptic density protein 95 [69]. It implies that oxytocin receptors can be related to the regulation of synapse scaffolding proteins. This conclusion is supported also by our results on the effects of oxytocin on the SHANK family of scaffolding proteins [47]. Higher dendritic complexity has been observed under the effect of oxytocin [70]. Oxytocin has been found to phosphorylate cAMP-responsive element-binding protein (CREB) [30] and other CREB-regulated genes [71]. This could be a regulatory pathway to many scaffolding proteins, cytoskeleton rearrangement, and synapse formation. Oxytocin signaling has developmental dynamics [11], and therefore, it is important to note that early phases of neuronal development are crucial for functionality of mature oxytocin receptor system. Nevertheless, oxytocin receptors have different brain regional localization. A recent study has especially stressed the distribution of oxytocin receptors in the brain cortex [72]. This could be important for cortical organization and the establishment of synapses and neural circuits for complex social behaviors.

8. Future Outlook

Even though the mechanisms are far from clear, promising results on the use of oxytocin have been produced by some research groups. One recent study has revealed that early oxytocin treatment could be an effective strategy for the treatment of neurodevelopmental diseases such as Prader-Willi syndrome and autism spectrum disorders [73]. Mutations of the Magel2 gene have been described in patients with autism and a loss of Magel2 is also associated with Prader-Willi syndrome. In general, behavioral and psychiatric disturbances beginning in early childhood are observed in affected individuals [74, 75]. The pathophysiological mechanism is the object of intensive research, and many studies are focusing on the developmental aspects of the oxytocin system. The research presented by Schaller et al. [76] has shown that the hypothalamus of the neonatal Magel2-deficient mouse had significantly lower levels of oxytocin, and oxytocin administration reversed the feeding difficulties in Magel2-deficient murine pups. Furthermore, it has been confirmed that oxytocin plays an important role in the onset of feeding. In mice, Magel2 is highly expressed in postmitotic hypothalamic neurons from early embryogenesis, and it occurs in the highest expression levels in the suprachiasmatic (SCN), the paraventricular (PVN), and supraoptic (SON) nuclei, in particular in vasopressin-positive neurons in the adult brain [77, 78]. It should be emphasized that the developmental effects of oxytocin in the regulation of feeding behavior are different from the studies involving the acute effects of oxytocin on food intake. Oxytocin was found to reduce feeding in animals; nevertheless, its anorexigenic effect depends on the dosage, method of administration, and diet composition [79].

Oxytocin administration in the first postnatal week was sufficient to prevent deficits in social behavior and learning abilities in Magel2-deficient mice. It seems that the impact of oxytocin on the developing brain around the time of birth has long-term consequences on behavior and on cognition. The research revealed that an oxytocin administration in Magel2-deficient mice acts directly on oxytocin-binding sites in brain structures and partially on oxytocin neurons, resulting in the release of endogenous oxytocin and suppressing the accumulation of oxytocin-intermediate forms in oxytocin neurons [76]. The effect of oxytocin on cognition during development has been confirmed in another recent study [80]. These authors have shown that oxytocin influences primate infant cognitive abilities. Moreover, yet another study has clinically proved beneficial effects of continual oxytocin administration on the social symptoms in patients with autism [81]. Nevertheless, the use of oxytocin and its analogs is still under intense debate, and numerous clinical trials of oxytocin in autism spectrum disorders are ongoing [82]. In the context of neurodevelopmental disorders, a therapeutic strategy could include some specific small-size neuropeptides. It seems very likely that one of the factors which plays a role in the pathogenesis of autism is the oxytocin receptor system especially in early development. As mentioned earlier, oxytocin affects the expression of neuron and glial markers in the brain [19], and it appears to be a relevant factor for the regulation of scaffolding proteins as well [47]. It has been suggested that oxytocin could be effective in the early treatment of neurodevelopmental diseases [83]. Development of the oxytocin system is essential for the early postnatal life of mammals; therefore, oxytocin is required in critical windows of time that play a pivotal role in brain development [84]. Indeed, it has been demonstrated that oxytocin receptors are associated with timing of the switch of GABAergic neurotransmission from excitatory to inhibitory during development of the nervous system [85]. Leonzino et al. have shown that the GABA switch is delayed in the absence of oxytocin receptor expression via a mechanism involving a chloride transporter. In this context, it is important to note that it has been recently shown that oxytocin exerts an early and cell-type-specific "priming" effect on developing excitatory neurons [4]. Therefore, it can be concluded that neuronal wiring is influenced by the action of oxytocin. Recent findings could be particularly important for the understanding of pathological processes of neurodevelopmental diseases and their compensation by early treatment.

Conflicts of Interest

The authors declare no conflict of interest.

Acknowledgments

This work was supported by the Project 2/0116/16 of the Grant Agency of the Ministry of Education and Slovak Academy of Sciences (VEGA) and by the Slovak Research and Development Agency Projects APVV-15-205 and APVV-15-0045.

References

[1] A. Schorscher-Petcu, S. Sotocinal, S. Ciura et al., "Oxytocin-induced analgesia and scratching are mediated by the vasopressin-1A receptor in the mouse," *The Journal of Neuroscience*, vol. 30, no. 24, pp. 8274–8284, 2010.

[2] R. Stoop, "Neuromodulation by oxytocin and vasopressin," *Neuron*, vol. 76, no. 1, pp. 142–159, 2012.

[3] A. Palanisamy, R. Kannappan, Z. Xu et al., "Oxytocin alters cell fate selection of rat neural progenitor cells *in vitro*," *PLoS One*, vol. 13, no. 1, article e0191160, 2018.

[4] S. Ripamonti, M. C. Ambrozkiewicz, F. Guzzi et al., "Transient oxytocin signaling primes the development and function of excitatory hippocampal neurons," *eLife*, vol. 6, article e22466, 2017.

[5] E. Madarász, Z. Környci, D. A. Poulain, and D. T. Theodosis, "Development of oxytocinergic neurons in monolayer cultures derived from embryonic, fetal and postnatal rat hypothalami," *Journal of Neuroendocrinology*, vol. 4, no. 4, pp. 433–439, 1992.

[6] J. Bakos, M. Zatkova, Z. Bacova, and D. Ostatnikova, "The role of hypothalamic neuropeptides in neurogenesis and neuritogenesis," *Neural Plasticity*, vol. 2016, Article ID 3276383, 10 pages, 2016.

[7] F. Muscatelli, M. G. Desarménien, V. Matarazzo, and V. Grinevich, "Oxytocin signaling in the early life of mammals: link to neurodevelopmental disorders associated with ASD," *Current Topics in Behavioral Neurosciences*, 2017.

[8] J. Bakos, Z. Bacova, S. G. Grant, A. M. Castejon, and D. Ostatnikova, "Are molecules involved in neuritogenesis and axon guidance related to autism pathogenesis?," *Neuromolecular Medicine*, vol. 17, no. 3, pp. 297–304, 2015.

[9] M. Zatkova, J. Bakos, J. Hodosy, and D. Ostatnikova, "Synapse alterations in autism: review of animal model findings," *Biomedical Papers*, vol. 160, no. 2, pp. 201–210, 2016.

[10] A. N. van den Pol, "Neuropeptide transmission in brain circuits," *Neuron*, vol. 76, no. 1, pp. 98–115, 2012.

[11] V. Grinevich, M. G. Desarménien, B. Chini, M. Tauber, and F. Muscatelli, "Ontogenesis of oxytocin pathways in the mammalian brain: late maturation and psychosocial disorders," *Frontiers in Neuroanatomy*, vol. 8, p. 164, 2015.

[12] G. Gimpl and F. Fahrenholz, "The oxytocin receptor system: structure, function, and regulation," *Physiological Reviews*, vol. 81, no. 2, pp. 629–683, 2001.

[13] P. J. Ryan, S. I. Ross, C. A. Campos, V. A. Derkach, and R. D. Palmiter, "Oxytocin-receptor-expressing neurons in the parabrachial nucleus regulate fluid intake," *Nature Neuroscience*, vol. 20, no. 12, pp. 1722–1733, 2017.

[14] T. Raam, K. M. McAvoy, A. Besnard, A. H. Veenema, and A. Sahay, "Hippocampal oxytocin receptors are necessary for discrimination of social stimuli," *Nature Communications*, vol. 8, no. 1, p. 2001, 2017.

[15] Y. T. Lin, C. C. Chen, C. C. Huang, K. Nishimori, and K. S. Hsu, "Oxytocin stimulates hippocampal neurogenesis via oxytocin receptor expressed in CA3 pyramidal neurons," *Nature Communications*, vol. 8, no. 1, p. 537, 2017.

[16] B. Leuner, J. M. Caponiti, and E. Gould, "Oxytocin stimulates adult neurogenesis even under conditions of stress and elevated glucocorticoids," *Hippocampus*, vol. 22, no. 4, pp. 861–868, 2012.

[17] A. D. Raymond, N. N. A. Kucherepa, K. R. S. Fisher, W. G. Halina, and G. D. Partlow, "Neurogenesis of oxytocin-containing neurons in the paraventricular nucleus (PVN) of the female pig in 3 reproductive states: puberty gilts, adult gilts and lactating sows," *Brain Research*, vol. 1102, no. 1, pp. 44–51, 2006.

[18] T. Havranek, M. Zatkova, Z. Lestanova et al., "Intracerebroventricular oxytocin administration in rats enhances object recognition and increases expression of neurotrophins, microtubule-associated protein 2, and synapsin I," *Journal of Neuroscience Research*, vol. 93, no. 6, pp. 893–901, 2015.

[19] T. Havránek, Z. Lešťanová, B. Mravec, V. Štrbák, J. Bakoš, and Z. Bačová, "Oxytocin modulates expression of neuron and glial markers in the rat hippocampus," *Folia Biologica*, vol. 63, no. 3, pp. 91–97, 2017.

[20] D. Huber, P. Veinante, and R. Stoop, "Vasopressin and oxytocin excite distinct neuronal populations in the central amygdala," *Science*, vol. 308, no. 5719, pp. 245–248, 2005.

[21] S. Tamborski, E. M. Mintz, and H. K. Caldwell, "Sex differences in the embryonic development of the central oxytocin system in mice," *Journal of Neuroendocrinology*, vol. 28, no. 4, 2016.

[22] R. Tyzio, R. Cossart, I. Khalilov et al., "Maternal oxytocin triggers a transient inhibitory switch in GABA signaling in the fetal brain during delivery," *Science*, vol. 314, no. 5806, pp. 1788–1792, 2006.

[23] R. Tyzio, R. Nardou, D. C. Ferrari et al., "Oxytocin-mediated GABA inhibition during delivery attenuates autism pathogenesis in rodent offspring," *Science*, vol. 343, no. 6171, pp. 675–679, 2014.

[24] Y. H. Jo, M. E. Stoeckel, M. J. Freund-Mercier, and R. Schlichter, "Oxytocin modulates glutamatergic synaptic transmission between cultured neonatal spinal cord dorsal horn neurons," *The Journal of Neuroscience*, vol. 18, no. 7, pp. 2377–2386, 1998.

[25] D. Viviani, T. Terrettaz, F. Magara, and R. Stoop, "Oxytocin enhances the inhibitory effects of diazepam in the rat central medial amygdala," *Neuropharmacology*, vol. 58, no. 1, pp. 62–68, 2010.

[26] H. S. Knobloch, A. Charlet, L. C. Hoffmann et al., "Evoked axonal oxytocin release in the central amygdala attenuates fear response," *Neuron*, vol. 73, no. 3, pp. 553–566, 2012.

[27] S. W. Harden and C. J. Frazier, "Oxytocin depolarizes fast-spiking hilar interneurons and induces GABA release onto mossy cells of the rat dentate gyrus," *Hippocampus*, vol. 26, no. 9, pp. 1124–1139, 2016.

[28] L. L. Oettl, N. Ravi, M. Schneider et al., "Oxytocin enhances social recognition by modulating cortical control of early olfactory processing," *Neuron*, vol. 90, no. 3, pp. 609–621, 2016.

[29] M. G. Terenzi and C. D. Ingram, "Oxytocin-induced excitation of neurones in the rat central and medial amygdaloid nuclei," *Neuroscience*, vol. 134, no. 1, pp. 345–354, 2005.

[30] K. Tomizawa, N. Iga, Y. F. Lu et al., "Oxytocin improves long-lasting spatial memory during motherhood through MAP kinase cascade," *Nature Neuroscience*, vol. 6, no. 4, pp. 384–390, 2003.

[31] I. D. Neumann and R. Landgraf, "Balance of brain oxytocin and vasopressin: implications for anxiety, depression, and social behaviors," *Trends in Neurosciences*, vol. 35, no. 11, pp. 649–659, 2012.

[32] S. Hobo, K. Hayashida, and J. C. Eisenach, "Oxytocin inhibits the membrane depolarization-induced increase in intracellular calcium in capsaicin sensitive sensory neurons: a peripheral mechanism of analgesic action," *Anesthesia and Analgesia*, vol. 114, no. 2, pp. 442–449, 2012.

[33] M. Hirasawa, S. B. Kombian, and Q. J. Pittman, "Oxytocin retrogradely inhibits evoked, but not miniature, EPSCs in the rat supraoptic nucleus: role of N- and P/Q-type calcium channels," *The Journal of Physiology*, vol. 532, no. 3, pp. 595–607, 2001.

[34] D. A. Robinson, F. Wei, G. D. Wang et al., "Oxytocin mediates stress-induced analgesia in adult mice," *The Journal of Physiology*, vol. 540, no. 2, pp. 593–606, 2002.

[35] M. Condés-Lara, N. Marina González, G. Martínez-Lorenzana, O. Luis Delgado, and M. José Freund-Mercier, "Actions of oxytocin and interactions with glutamate on spontaneous and evoked dorsal spinal cord neuronal activities," *Brain Research*, vol. 976, no. 1, pp. 75–81, 2003.

[36] S. Audigier and C. Barberis, "Pharmacological characterization of two specific binding sites for neurohypophyseal hormones in hippocampal synaptic plasma membranes of the rat," *The EMBO Journal*, vol. 4, no. 6, pp. 1407–1412, 1985.

[37] R. M. Buijs, "Vasopressin and oxytocin—their role in neurotransmission," *Pharmacology & Therapeutics*, vol. 22, no. 1, pp. 127–141, 1983.

[38] R. C. Lambert, G. Dayanithi, F. C. Moos, and P. Richard, "A rise in the intracellular Ca2+ concentration of isolated rat supraoptic cells in response to oxytocin," *The Journal of Physiology*, vol. 478, no. 2, pp. 275–287, 1994.

[39] Y. Osako, T. Otsuka, M. Taniguchi, T. Oka, and H. Kaba, "Oxytocin enhances presynaptic and postsynaptic glutamatergic transmission between rat olfactory bulb neurones in culture," *Neuroscience Letters*, vol. 299, no. 1-2, pp. 65–68, 2001.

[40] N. York, P. Halbach, M. A. Chiu, I. M. Bird, D. A. M. Pillers, and B. R. Pattnaik, "Oxytocin (OXT)-stimulated inhibition of Kir7.1 activity is through PIP_2-dependent Ca^{2+} response of the oxytocin receptor in the retinal pigment epithelium in vitro," *Cellular Signalling*, vol. 37, pp. 93–102, 2017.

[41] Y. Yao, L. Y. Fu, X. Zhang, and A. N. van den Pol, "Vasopressin and oxytocin excite MCH neurons, but not other lateral hypothalamic GABA neurons," *American Journal of Physiology. Regulatory, Integrative and Comparative Physiology*, vol. 302, no. 7, pp. R815–R824, 2012.

[42] D. Burdakov, B. Liss, and F. M. Ashcroft, "Orexin excites GABAergic neurons of the arcuate nucleus by activating the sodium–calcium exchanger," *The Journal of Neuroscience*, vol. 23, no. 12, pp. 4951–4957, 2003.

[43] R. Parmentier, S. Kolbaev, B. P. Klyuch et al., "Excitation of histaminergic tuberomamillary neurons by thyrotropin-releasing hormone," *The Journal of Neuroscience*, vol. 29, no. 14, pp. 4471–4483, 2009.

[44] J. Mairesse, E. Gatta, M. L. Reynaert et al., "Activation of presynaptic oxytocin receptors enhances glutamate release in the ventral hippocampus of prenatally restraint stressed rats," *Psychoneuroendocrinology*, vol. 62, pp. 36–46, 2015.

[45] J. D. Breton, P. Veinante, S. Uhl-Bronner et al., "Oxytocin-induced antinociception in the spinal cord is mediated by a subpopulation of glutamatergic neurons in lamina I-II which amplify GABAergic inhibition," *Molecular Pain*, vol. 4, 2008.

[46] S. B. Kombian, M. Hirasawa, D. Mouginot, and Q. J. Pittman, "Chapter 18 modulation of synaptic transmission by oxytocin and vasopressin in the supraoptic nucleus," *Progress in Brain Research*, vol. 139, pp. 235–246, 2002.

[47] M. Zatkova, A. Reichova, Z. Bacova, V. Strbak, A. Kiss, and J. Bakos, "Neurite outgrowth stimulated by oxytocin is modulated by inhibition of the calcium voltage-gated channels," *Cellular and Molecular Neurobiology*, vol. 38, no. 1, pp. 371–378, 2018.

[48] M. Raggenbass, "Vasopressin- and oxytocin-induced activity in the central nervous system: electrophysiological studies using in-vitro systems," *Progress in Neurobiology*, vol. 64, no. 3, pp. 307–326, 2001.

[49] M. Mitre, B. J. Marlin, J. K. Schiavo et al., "A distributed network for social cognition enriched for oxytocin receptors," *The Journal of Neuroscience*, vol. 36, no. 8, pp. 2517–2535, 2016.

[50] I. Kruglikov and B. Rudy, "Perisomatic GABA release and thalamocortical integration onto neocortical excitatory cells are regulated by neuromodulators," *Neuron*, vol. 58, no. 6, pp. 911–924, 2008.

[51] B. J. Marlin, M. Mitre, J. A. D'amour, M. V. Chao, and R. C. Froemke, "Oxytocin enables maternal behaviour by balancing

cortical inhibition," *Nature*, vol. 520, no. 7548, pp. 499–504, 2015.

[52] S. F. Owen, S. N. Tuncdemir, P. L. Bader, N. N. Tirko, G. Fishell, and R. W. Tsien, "Oxytocin enhances hippocampal spike transmission by modulating fast-spiking interneurons," *Nature*, vol. 500, no. 7463, pp. 458–462, 2013.

[53] Y. Osako, T. Otsuka, M. Taniguchi, T. Oka, and H. Kaba, "Oxytocin depresses spontaneous γ-aminobutyric acid-ergic inhibitory postsynaptic currents in cultured mitral cells of the rat olfactory bulb by a presynaptic mechanism," *Neuroscience Letters*, vol. 289, no. 1, pp. 25–28, 2000.

[54] P. Maier, M. E. Kaiser, V. Grinevich, A. Draguhn, and M. Both, "Differential effects of oxytocin on mouse hippocampal oscillations *in vitro*," *The European Journal of Neuroscience*, vol. 44, no. 11, pp. 2885–2898, 2016.

[55] Y. F. Wang and G. I. Hatton, "Mechanisms underlying oxytocin-induced excitation of supraoptic neurons: prostaglandin mediation of actin polymerization," *Journal of Neurophysiology*, vol. 95, no. 6, pp. 3933–3947, 2006.

[56] S. Yao, J. Bergan, A. Lanjuin, and C. Dulac, "Oxytocin signaling in the medial amygdala is required for sex discrimination of social cues," *eLife*, vol. 6, article e31373, 2017.

[57] M. Nakajima, A. Görlich, and N. Heintz, "Oxytocin modulates female sociosexual behavior through a specific class of prefrontal cortical interneurons," *Cell*, vol. 159, no. 2, pp. 295–305, 2014.

[58] F. Qiu, C. Y. Qiu, H. Cai et al., "Oxytocin inhibits the activity of acid-sensing ion channels through the vasopressin, V_{1A} receptor in primary sensory neurons," *British Journal of Pharmacology*, vol. 171, no. 12, pp. 3065–3076, 2014.

[59] L. J. Wrobel, I. Reymond-Marron, A. Dupré, and M. Raggenbass, "Oxytocin and vasopressin enhance synaptic transmission in the hypoglossal motor nucleus of young rats by acting on distinct receptor types," *Neuroscience*, vol. 165, no. 3, pp. 723–735, 2010.

[60] A. B. Brussaard, J. Wossink, J. C. Lodder, and K. S. Kits, "Progesterone-metabolite prevents protein kinase C-dependent modulation of γ-aminobutyric acid type a receptors in oxytocin neurons," *Proceedings of the National Academy of Sciences of the United States of America*, vol. 97, no. 7, pp. 3625–3630, 2000.

[61] D. di Scala-Guenot and M. T. Strosser, "Oxytocin receptors on cultured astroglial cells. Regulation by a guanine-nucleotide-binding protein and effect of Mg^{2+}," *The Biochemical Journal*, vol. 284, no. 2, pp. 499–505, 1992.

[62] P. Cassoni, A. Sapino, A. Stella, N. Fortunati, and G. Bussolati, "Presence and significance of oxytocin receptors in human neuroblastomas and glial tumors," *International Journal of Cancer*, vol. 77, no. 5, pp. 695–700, 1998.

[63] J. Bakos, V. Strbak, N. Ratulovska, and Z. Bacova, "Effect of oxytocin on neuroblastoma cell viability and growth," *Cellular and Molecular Neurobiology*, vol. 32, no. 5, pp. 891–896, 2012.

[64] J. Kuo, O. R. Hariri, and P. Micevych, "An interaction of oxytocin receptors with metabotropic glutamate receptors in hypothalamic astrocytes," *Journal of Neuroendocrinology*, vol. 21, no. 12, pp. 1001–1006, 2009.

[65] P. Wang, D. Qin, and Y. F. Wang, "Oxytocin rapidly changes astrocytic GFAP plasticity by differentially modulating the expressions of pERK 1/2 and protein kinase a," *Frontiers in Molecular Neuroscience*, vol. 10, p. 262, 2017.

[66] D. di Scala-Guenot and M. T. Strosser, "Oxytocin receptors on cultured astroglial cells. Kinetic and pharmacological characterization of oxytocin-binding sites on intact hypothalamic and hippocampic cells from foetal rat brain," *The Biochemical Journal*, vol. 284, no. 2, pp. 491–497, 1992.

[67] M. Sala, D. Braida, D. Lentini et al., "Pharmacologic rescue of impaired cognitive flexibility, social deficits, increased aggression, and seizure susceptibility in oxytocin receptor null mice: a neurobehavioral model of autism," *Biological Psychiatry*, vol. 69, no. 9, pp. 875–882, 2011.

[68] Z. Lestanova, Z. Bacova, A. Kiss, T. Havranek, V. Strbak, and J. Bakos, "Oxytocin increases neurite length and expression of cytoskeletal proteins associated with neuronal growth," *Journal of Molecular Neuroscience*, vol. 59, no. 2, pp. 184–192, 2016.

[69] S. Miyazaki, Y. Hiraoka, S. Hidema, and K. Nishimori, "Prenatal minocycline treatment alters synaptic protein expression, and rescues reduced mother call rate in oxytocin receptor-knockout mice," *Biochemical and Biophysical Research Communications*, vol. 472, no. 2, pp. 319–323, 2016.

[70] D. I. Sánchez-Vidaña, N.-M. J. Chan, A. H. L. Chan et al., "Repeated treatment with oxytocin promotes hippocampal cell proliferation, dendritic maturation and affects socio-emotional behavior," *Neuroscience*, vol. 333, pp. 65–77, 2016.

[71] B. Jurek, D. A. Slattery, Y. Hiraoka et al., "Oxytocin regulates stress-induced *Crf* gene transcription through CREB-regulated transcription coactivator 3," *The Journal of Neuroscience*, vol. 35, no. 35, pp. 12248–12260, 2015.

[72] A. Duchemin, A. M. H. Seelke, T. C. Simmons, S. M. Freeman, and K. L. Bales, "Localization of oxytocin receptors in the prairie vole (*Microtus ochrogaster*) neocortex," *Neuroscience*, vol. 348, pp. 201–211, 2017.

[73] H. Meziane, F. Schaller, S. Bauer et al., "An early postnatal oxytocin treatment prevents social and learning deficits in adult mice deficient for *Magel2*, a gene involved in Prader-Willi syndrome and autism," *Biological Psychiatry*, vol. 78, no. 2, pp. 85–94, 2015.

[74] S. B. Cassidy and D. J. Driscoll, "Prader–Willi syndrome," *European Journal of Human Genetics*, vol. 17, no. 1, pp. 3–13, 2009.

[75] J. Chevalere, V. Postal, J. Jauregui, P. Copet, V. Laurier, and D. Thuilleaux, "Assessment of executive functions in Prader-Willi syndrome and relationship with intellectual level," *Journal of Applied Research in Intellectual Disabilities*, vol. 26, no. 4, pp. 309–318, 2013.

[76] F. Schaller, F. Watrin, R. Sturny, A. Massacrier, P. Szepetowski, and F. Muscatelli, "A single postnatal injection of oxytocin rescues the lethal feeding behaviour in mouse newborns deficient for the imprinted *Magel2* gene," *Human Molecular Genetics*, vol. 19, no. 24, pp. 4895–4905, 2010.

[77] S. Lee, C. L. Walker, and R. Wevrick, "Prader-Willi syndrome transcripts are expressed in phenotypically significant regions of the developing mouse brain," *Gene Expression Patterns*, vol. 3, no. 5, pp. 599–609, 2003.

[78] K. F. Tacer and P. R. Potts, "Cellular and disease functions of the Prader-Willi syndrome gene *MAGEL2*," *The Biochemical Journal*, vol. 474, no. 13, pp. 2177–2190, 2017.

[79] M. Leslie, P. Silva, Y. Paloyelis, J. Blevins, and J. Treasure, "A systematic review and quantitative meta-analysis of oxytocin's effects on feeding," *Journal of Neuroendocrinology*, 2018.

[80] E. A. Simpson, A. Paukner, V. Sclafani, S. S. K. Kaburu, S. J. Suomi, and P. F. Ferrari, "Acute oxytocin improves memory and gaze following in male but not female nursery-reared

infant macaques," *Psychopharmacology*, vol. 234, no. 3, pp. 497–506, 2017.

[81] T. Watanabe, M. Kuroda, H. Kuwabara et al., "Clinical and neural effects of six-week administration of oxytocin on core symptoms of autism," *Brain*, vol. 138, no. 11, pp. 3400–3412, 2015.

[82] L. J. Young and C. E. Barrett, "Neuroscience. Can oxytocin treat autism?," *Science*, vol. 347, no. 6224, pp. 825-826, 2015.

[83] M. Tauber, K. Boulanouar, G. Diene et al., "The use of oxytocin to improve feeding and social skills in infants with Prader-Willi syndrome," *Pediatrics*, vol. 139, no. 2, article e20162976, 2017.

[84] S. Sannino, B. Chini, and V. Grinevich, "Lifespan oxytocin signaling: maturation, flexibility, and stability in newborn, adolescent, and aged brain," *Developmental Neurobiology*, vol. 77, no. 2, pp. 158–168, 2017.

[85] M. Leonzino, M. Busnelli, F. Antonucci, C. Verderio, M. Mazzanti, and B. Chini, "The timing of the excitatory-to-inhibitory GABA switch is regulated by the oxytocin receptor via KCC2," *Cell Reports*, vol. 15, no. 1, pp. 96–103, 2016.

9

Changes to Neural Activation Patterns (c-fos Labeling) in Chinchilla Auditory Midbrain following Neonatal Exposure to an Enhanced Sound Environment

Lisa M. D'Alessandro[1,2,3] **and Robert V. Harrison**[1,2,3,4]

[1]*Department of Physiology, University of Toronto, Toronto, Canada M5S 1A8*
[2]*Institute of Biomaterials & Biomedical Engineering, University of Toronto, Toronto, Canada M5S 3G9*
[3]*The Auditory Science Laboratory, Program in Neurosciences and Mental Health, The Hospital for Sick Children, Toronto, Canada M5G 1X8*
[4]*Department of Otolaryngology-Head and Neck Surgery, University of Toronto, Toronto, Canada M5G 2N2*

Correspondence should be addressed to Robert V. Harrison; rvh@sickkids.ca

Academic Editor: Clive R. Bramham

Sensory brain regions show neuroplastic changes following deficits or experimental augmentation of peripheral input during a neonatal period. We have previously shown reorganization of cortical tonotopic maps after neonatal cochlear lesions or exposure to an enhanced acoustic environment. Such experiments probe the cortex and show reorganization, but it is unclear if such changes are intrinsically cortical or reflect projections from modified subcortical regions. Here, we ask whether an enhanced neonatal acoustic environment can induce midbrain (inferior colliculus (IC)) changes. Neonatal chinchillas were chronically exposed to a 70 dB SPL narrowband (2 ± 0.25 kHz) sound stimulus for 4 weeks. In line with previous studies, we hypothesized that such exposure would induce widening of the 2 kHz tonotopic map region in IC. To probe c-fos expression in IC (central nucleus), sound-exposed and nonexposed animals were stimulated with a 2 kHz stimulus for 90 minutes. In sound-exposed subjects, we find no change in the width of the 2 kHz tonotopic region; thus, our hypothesis is not supported. However, we observed a significant increase in the number of c-fos-labeled neurons over a broad region of best frequencies. These data suggest that neonatal sound exposure can modify midbrain regions and thus change the way neurons in IC respond to sound stimulation.

1. Introduction

The objective of this study is to examine the effects of a frequency-enhanced neonatal acoustic environment on c-fos expression patterns in the auditory midbrain (inferior colliculus). Many studies have revealed alterations in sensory cortical representation after deafferentation or enhanced sensory stimulation. Seminal work on such neuroplasticity has been made in visual cortex [1, 2], in somatosensory cortex [3], and in auditory cortex [4]. However, a question that arises is whether such plasticity is intrinsically cortical or whether it reflects, wholly or partially, reorganization at subcortical levels. In the auditory system of the cat, we have reported extensive reorganization of cortical tonotopic maps after neonatal cochlear hair cell lesions [5] and subsequently established that thalamic areas were similarly reorganized [6]. We have also observed tonotopic map changes in the inferior colliculus (IC) of the chinchilla auditory midbrain as a result of neonatal partial cochlear deafferentation [7]. In experiments where neonatal manipulations are made to the auditory system (either by sound deprivation or by augmentation), it is important to consider whether the experimental animal is altricious (born with an immature inner ear) or precocious (with hearing present at birth). In altricious rodent species, studies have revealed midbrain plasticity after augmented auditory stimulation during a neonatal

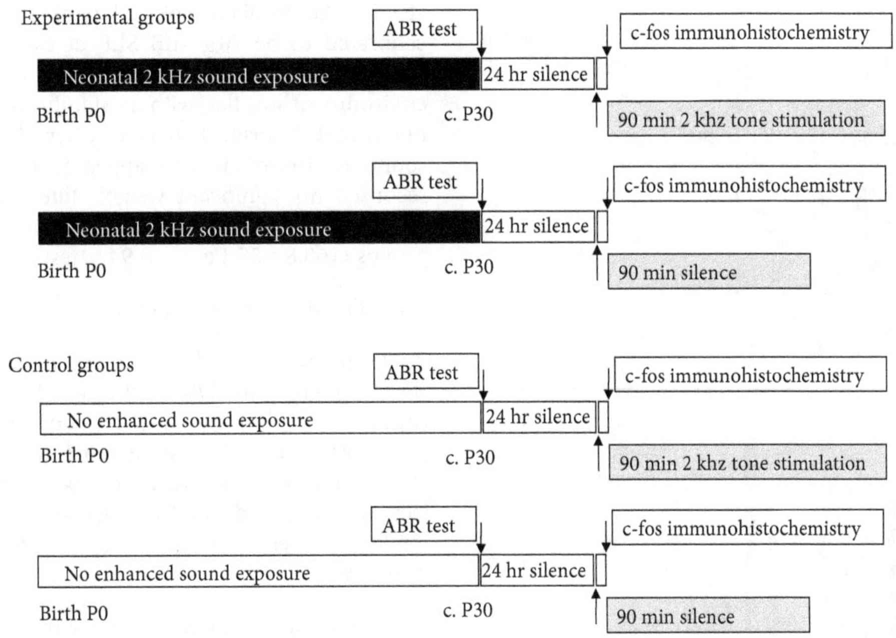

FIGURE 1: Experimental timelines for experimental neonatal sound-exposed groups and nonexposed controls.

period [8–14]. However, in precocious species such as the chinchilla (and humans), it remains unclear whether an enhanced acoustic environment in a neonatal period can induce neuroplastic change at the level of the auditory midbrain. We address this question in the present study. Newborn chinchilla pups are exposed to a 70 dB SPL narrowband (2 ± 0.25 kHz) sound stimulus for 4 weeks, and midbrain (IC; central nucleus) neural activity patterns are assessed using c-fos labeling techniques.

c-fos immunohistochemistry has been used to study neural activation patterns in a variety of brain regions following brief periods of enhanced sensory stimulation (e.g., [15–19]). In the auditory brain, c-fos labeling studies have been used in a range of species (cat [20], mouse [21], rat [22, 23], gerbil [24], and bat [25]), and we have previously reported on a successful c-fos protocol for the chinchilla [26]. We have shown that chronic stimulation with a tonal stimulus results in a band (sheet) of c-fos-labeled neurons in IC that corresponds to the tonotopic map functionally verified using single-unit electrophysiological recordings [26]. In the present study, we have used this c-fos expression method to reveal possible neuroplasticity in the IC of neonatal chinchillas exposed to a 70 dB SPL narrowband (2 ± 0.25 kHz) sound stimulus for 4 weeks. We compare the pattern and number of c-fos-labeled neurons in exposed subjects with age-matched control subjects. Based on previous studies that report neural overrepresentation of areas related to exposure stimuli, we hypothesize that our sound exposure will cause widening of the 2 kHz tonotopic map region in IC.

2. Materials and Methods

2.1. Overview of Experimental Protocol. Our aim is to examine the effects of a tone-enhanced acoustic environment on c-fos expression patterns in IC (central nucleus) of the chinchilla. The experimental protocols are summarized in Figures 1 and 2. For the main experimental group (upper panel of Figure 1), experimental subjects were placed in a 2 kHz frequency-augmented sound environment from birth (P0) for about 30 days (27–34-day range). At the end of this period, auditory brainstem responses (ABRs) to click stimuli were recorded to confirm normal hearing thresholds. This testing was carried out under anesthesia (ketamine 15 mg/kg, i.p.; xylazine 2.5 mg/kg, i.p.). In comparing ABR thresholds across frequency between sound-enriched and control animals, we have found and previously reported [27] no significant differences between enriched and control animals. Animals were kept overnight in a sound-attenuating booth. Subjects (unanesthetized) then either received a 90 min period of 2 kHz tone bursts (500 ms; 100 ms rise/fall) or remained in silence (second panel in Figure 1). There are two age-matched control groups with no neonatal sound augmentation (lower panels of Figure 1). The procedures for assessing neural activity with c-fos labeling were identical for all groups. Animals were anaesthetized (ketamine 15 mg/kg, i.p.; xylazine 2.5 mg/kg, i.p.) and perfused (transcardiac) for brain tissue fixation. IC specimens were processed to reveal c-fos protein expression in any activated neurons in IC. Cell count data were quantified as outlined in Figure 2.

2.2. Subjects. Twenty chinchillas (*Chinchilla laniger*; 10 females, 10 males) were obtained either on the day of birth (P0) or one day later (Roseneath Chinchilla, Ontario, Canada). Subjects were included in the study when auditory brainstem response (ABR) thresholds to broadband (47 μs click) stimuli were <35 dB SPL. This initial screening was carried out in the anesthetized animal (ketamine 15 mg/kg, i.p.; xylazine 2.5 mg/kg, i.p.). Animals were randomly assigned to four groups (5 subjects in each) as outlined in Figure 1. There are two sound-exposed groups, where subjects were

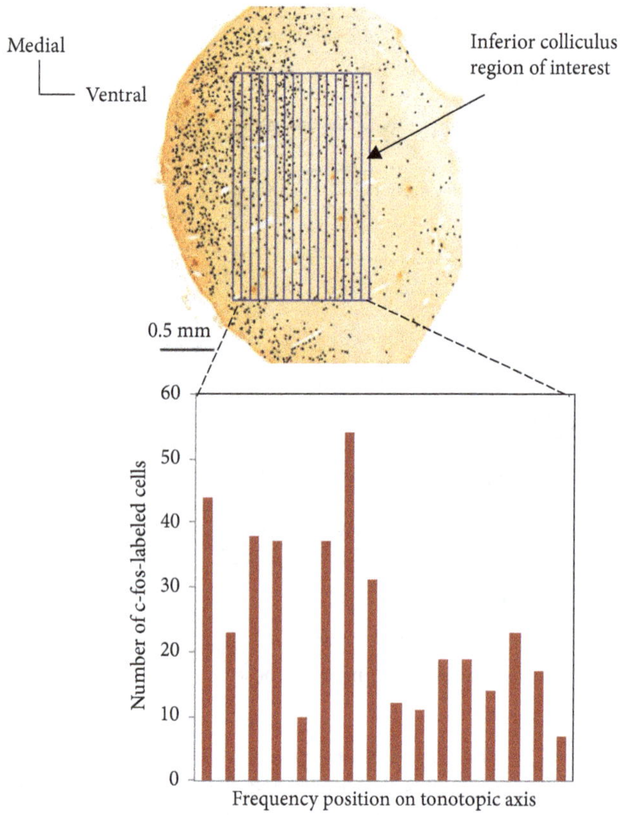

Figure 2: Quantification of c-fos immunolabeling results. The region of interest corresponds approximately to central nucleus of inferior colliculus. Scale bar 500 μm. This is a representative sample from a subject stimulated for 90 min with a 2 kHz tone burst. The grid is superimposed to obtain cell counts shown in the lower bar graph. This upper histology image is reproduced from a methods description paper ([26]; fig. 4) with permission.

placed in an enhanced auditory environment for 27–34 days (average 30 days) and then either were stimulated with a 90 min period of 2 kHz tone bursts or received no further sound stimulation. There are two control groups, where subjects experienced no enhanced auditory environment and then had either a 90 min period of 2 kHz tone bursts (to induce frequency bands of fos-labeled cells) or no sound stimulation. Data from these two control groups were reported in a methods paper describing our c-fos labeling technique [26]. That previous publication has no scientific overlap with the present study. Some of the illustrative histological sections and control data have been reproduced or adapted in the present paper with permission (as stated in the figure legends). All procedures were approved under The Hospital for Sick Children Animal Care Committee protocols, following guidelines of the Canadian Council on Animal Care (CCAC).

2.3. Neonatal Sound Exposure. A pulsed (500 ms; 20 ms rise/fall; 1 s duty cycle) narrowband (2 ± 0.25 kHz) acoustic signal was presented continuously for c. 30 days in free field (Sony Micro Hi-Fi, CMT BX20i, coupled to Sony transducer Model #SS-CBX20, Miniato, Tokyo, Japan). The acoustic signal was calibrated to be 70 ± 5 dB SLP at ear level of the subject. Otherwise, the frequency spectrum of the ambient sound environment was flat, with no significant peaks. Animals did not exhibit abnormal behaviour when placed in this enhanced sound environment, and appeared to feed normally. We recorded no significant weight difference between control (mean ± SD; 169.9 ± 40.5 g) and neonatally sound-exposed groups (168.8 ± 35.1 g; $p = 0.94$, t-test).

2.4. c-fos Immunohistochemistry

2.4.1. Acoustic Stimulation to Induce Tonotopic Frequency Bands of Labeled Cells in IC. Based on studies by others (in mouse: [21]; in rat: [17]) and our work in the chinchilla [26]), we used a 90-minute tonal stimulation duration to elicit tonotopic bands of c-fos-labeled neurons in IC. Subjects were exposed to a 2 kHz gated (100 ms rise/fall) signal for 90 minutes, calibrated to be 60 ± 5 dB SPL at the level of the ear.

2.4.2. Histology Protocol. Following the end of the 90-minute period of stimulation (or silence for controls), subjects were perfused transcardially with saline, then with fixative (4% paraformaldehyde in 0.1 M phosphate buffer (PB) at 4°C). Whole brains were removed and kept overnight at 4°C in fixative. Coronal slices (40 μm) were cut with a vibratome and treated to visualize the c-fos antigen. Sections were rinsed in PB (pH 7.4), incubated in 0.3% H_2O_2, rinsed in PB, incubated for 1 hr in blocking solution (0.1% bovine serum albumin; 0.2% Triton X-100; 2% goat serum in 0.1 M PB), and then further incubated for 48 hrs at 4°C in primary antibody (rabbit anti-Fos polyclonal IgG; diluted 1 : 500 in blocking solution). Sections were rinsed in PB, incubated for 1.5–2 hrs in biotinylated secondary antibody (goat anti-rabbit IgG; diluted 1 : 100 in blocking solution) at room temperature, then rinsed in PB, and reacted with ABC (Avidin-Biotin Complex in blocking solution, 1 : 50). Sections were incubated for 8 minutes in a 3,3′-diaminobenzidine (DAB) solution (0.05%); then, 0.001% H_2O_2 was added to reveal staining. Sections were rinsed with PB, mounted on gelatinized slides, dried, dehydrated through graded alcohol rinses, and cover-slipped.

2.4.3. Image Analysis. Each midbrain IC was digitally imaged at 7x magnification using Mirax Scan™. Images were then analyzed using ImageJ™ as follows. Thresholds were selected that best captured the pattern of c-fos-labeled neurons across the entire colliculus. As illustrated in Figure 2, we defined a region of interest (ROI) that corresponds approximately to central nucleus of IC. By rotation of each specimen image, the axis of the labeled cell region was vertically positioned to align with the ROI grid. Thus, the ROI consisted of a series of contiguous, equal-sized rectangles that lay 200–400 μm away from the dorsal and ventral edges of the colliculus and that are approximately parallel to the isofrequency tonotopic bands in IC. For each colliculus, we counted the number of labeled cells in each column of the ROI using a custom-made macro and present the data in histogram form. In Figures 3, 4, and 5, we scale the

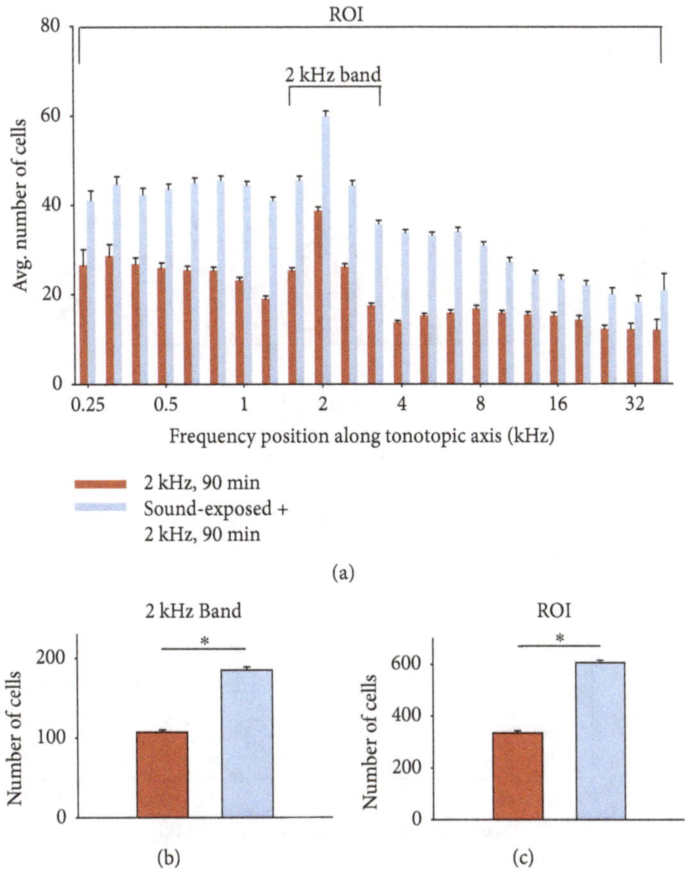

Figure 3: (a) Red bars (158 samples from 5 subjects) show average cell counts for subjects not reared with neonatal sound augmentation, but heard only the 2 kHz, 90 min probe. Average cell counts from subjects reared in the augmented acoustic environment, who then heard the 2 kHz, 90 min probe, are indicated in blue (194 samples from 5 subjects). One coronal slice produces 2 samples. Error bars show SEM. The difference in cell counts (b) within the 2 kHz band and (c) over the entire region of interest (ROI) are significant, $^*p < 0.001$.

histogram abscissae to represent frequency position along the tonotopic axis of IC [26].

3. Results

The qualitative examples in Figure 6 show typical patterns of c-fos labeling in the IC for the four experimental conditions. Figure 6(a) shows c-fos labeling in IC following only 90 min of 2 kHz pure-tone sound stimulation, in a subject with no enhanced neonatal acoustic exposure. Note the labelling reveals a 2 kHz tonotopic band (between the arrows) as well as other background neural activation. Figure 6(b) is from an animal reared for 4 weeks in the enhanced sound environment and is further stimulated with 2 kHz tone bursts for 90 min. Here, c-fos labeling shows the 2 kHz tonotopic band as well as an increase in c-fos-labelled cells over a broad range of the inferior colliculus. Compare this background activity with Figure 6(a) that had no enhanced neonatal exposure. Figure 6(c) shows the typical low level of c-fos labelling in a subject with no sound exposure and no 90 min 2 kHz probe tone, and Figure 6(d) shows the IC of a subject reared for 4 weeks in the enhanced sound environmental and then had 90 minutes of silence before c-fos staining.

The effects of neonatal sound exposure on the activity patterns in IC (i.e., a comparison of the subject groups (a) and (b) of Figure 6) are shown in Figure 3. Here, quantification of cell counts from all subjects has been analyzed as described in Figure 2. There is a significant increase in both the numbers of c-fos-labeled cells both in the 2 kHz tonotopic band (3B) and over the entire region of interest (3C) compared with control subjects who were not reared in the enhanced sound enhancement ($p < 0.001$; data values are listed in Table 1).

Our original hypothesis was that the 2 kHz neonatal exposure would result in an enhanced midbrain neural representation of the 2 kHz tonotopic band. However, we report no difference in the width of the 2 kHz band. Our analysis of IC frequency bandwidth and experimental comparison is shown in Figure 4. The width of the 2 kHz tonotopic representation is measured as the distance between the two troughs, that is, regions of decreased neural labelling adjacent to the excited region.

The significant difference observed between the neonatal-exposed subjects and the nonexposed group (Figure 3; Table 1) is the overall increase in c-fos-labeled activity. Both groups have received the final 2 kHz "probe" stimulus before the activity is assessed. The neonatally sound-exposed subjects have in effect received 2 "treatments," that is, the early sound exposure, and the 90 min period of 2 kHz tone bursts. To determine if the increase in c-fos-labeled neurons was due

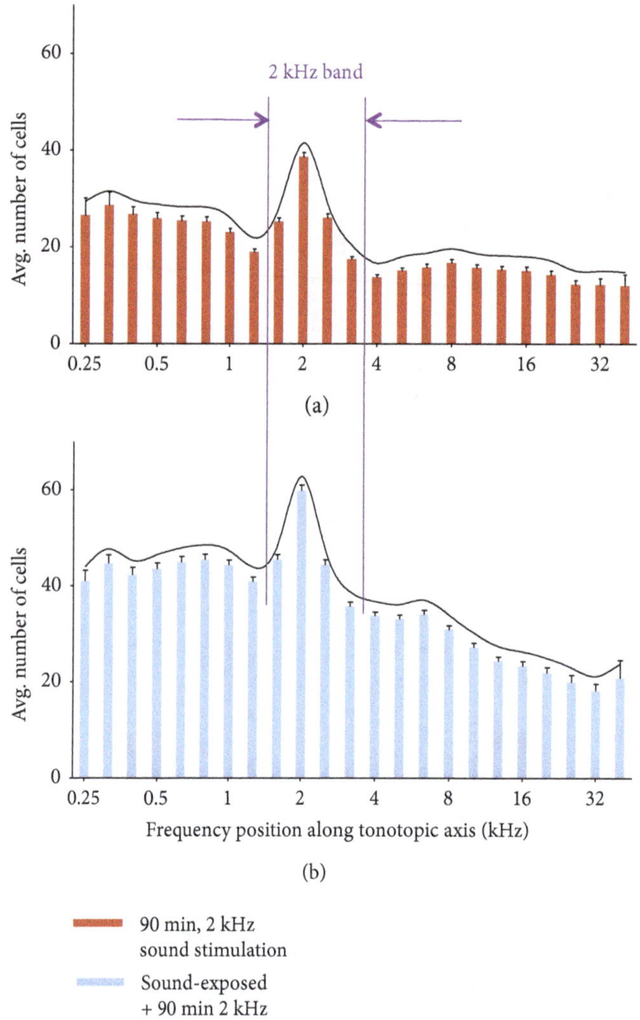

FIGURE 4: Comparison of the width of the 2 kHz tonotopic band in IC between subjects with neonatal 2 kHz sound exposure (b) and nonexposed controls (a). There is no significant difference in bandwidth between control (a) and sound-exposed (b) subjects. The upper graph has been adapted from a previously published methods description ([21]; fig. 3) with permission .

to sound exposure alone, we conducted a separate set of experiments in which subjects were exposed to the enhanced sound environment, then received no additional probe sound stimulation. Qualitative data are shown in Figures 6(c) and 6(d); note that there are no labelled tonotopic bands. Data quantification is illustrated in Figure 5. There is no difference in the number of labelled neurons either in the (estimated) 2 kHz band region or over the entire region of interest. These results suggest that there is no effect of sound exposure alone on basal levels of c-fos active cells but that the IC appears primed to be more generally active to subsequent acoustic stimulation.

4. Discussion

We have previously demonstrated a viable c-fos labelling protocol for the chinchilla [26]. We use this method here to study neuroplastic change in sound frequency representation in IC following rearing in an enhanced acoustic environment. Our focus on the midbrain is because so much evidence of developmental plasticity changes have reported on cortical reorganization, with little regard to possible subcortical plasticity.

Neonatal subjects reared for 4 weeks with a moderately intense 2 kHz sound exposure stimulus, then probed with a 90 min 2 kHz tone burst, and exhibited a significant increase in the number of c-fos-labeled neurons over the entire region of interest studied, including in the 2 kHz tonotopic band. We had hypothesized a widening of the 2 kHz tonotopic band, in line with other demonstrations of overrepresentation in neural areas correlated to exposure stimulus characteristics. However, we did not observe a change in the width of the 2 kHz band. This finding is important. At the cortical level in a precocious animal model, developmental plasticity results in considerable neural reorganization. At the auditory midbrain level, this window of developmental plasticity may well be closed.

However, we do observe subtle changes to stimulus activity levels in IC. In the subjects exposed to the neonatal 4-week enhanced sound stimulus and with no further probe

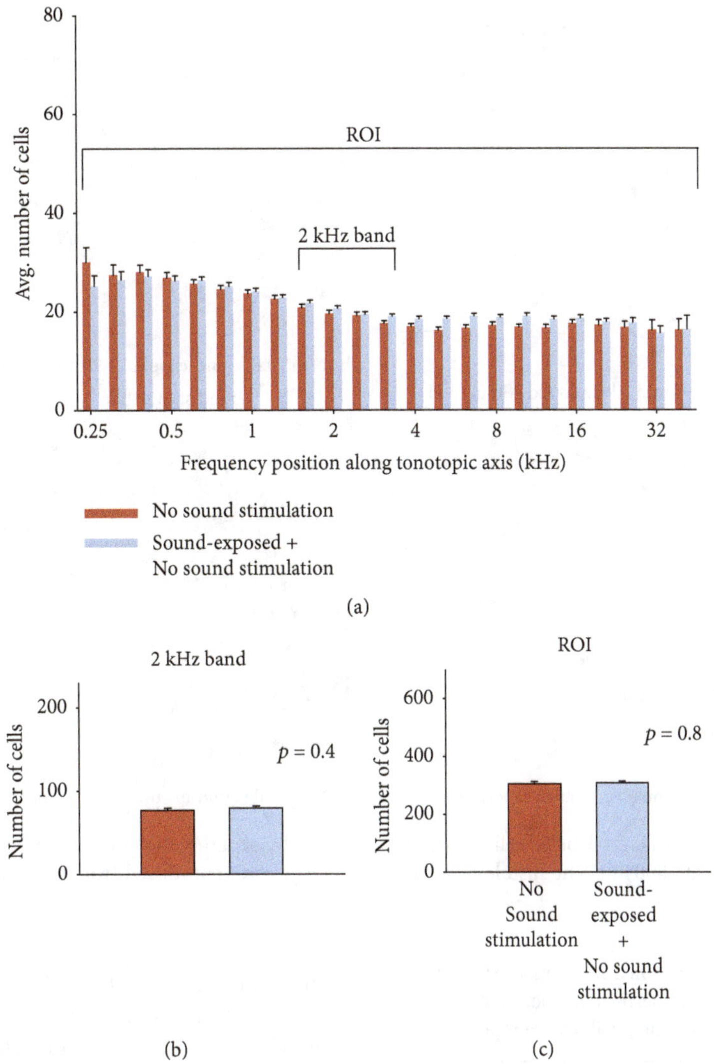

FIGURE 5: (a) Data in red show average counts of c-fos labeled neurons for subjects who received neither the 4-week sound exposure from birth stimulus nor subsequent 2 kHz tone stimulation (199 samples from 5 subjects). Data for subjects having the neonatal exposure and then no additional sound stimulation are plotted in blue (249 samples from 5 subjects). Error bars show SEM. There is no significant difference in cell count in the estimated 2 kHz region (b) or over the entire region of interest (ROI; c). In (a), the "No Sound Stim" control data (red) has been reproduced from a previously published methods paper ([26]; fig. 3) with permission.

sound stimulation, the c-fos expression patterns are no different from (age-matched) control animals having no experimental sound exposures. This is illustrated in Figure 5. These results suggest that the 4-week neonatal sound-exposure stimulus does not affect basal levels of neural activity as reflected in c-fos expression. Of interest, the data suggest a form of sensitization; that sound exposure alters how neurons in inferior colliculus respond to a subsequent somewhat prolonged (90 min) presentation of a pure-tone sound stimulus.

4.1. Use of c-fos Labeling Methodology. We sought a method to reveal global neural activation patterns in IC following experimental neonatal sound exposure. We selected c-fos immunohistochemistry from other immediate early genes for several reasons. First, basal expression levels of this protein are relatively low, allowing us to observe possible increases in neural activity following neonatal rearing in an enhanced sound environment. An alternative, the protein product of the NGFI-A immediate early gene, for example, is expressed at high basal activity levels [28]. Secondly, the c-fos protein is localized to the cell nucleus; thus, each instance of c-fos labeling indicates that that neuron has recently been activated. Various studies have used c-fos expression to examine how sensory stimulation can change neural activity patterns. In somatosensory cortex, vibrissae stimulation has been shown to increase c-fos expression in barrel cortex [16, 18]. In visual cortex, various studies have used c-fos labeling to explore light-induced neuroplastic change (e.g., [15, 19]). In the auditory system, midbrain changes to tonotopic maps have been demonstrated using c-fos methods (mouse: [21]; rat: [17]). A number of studies,

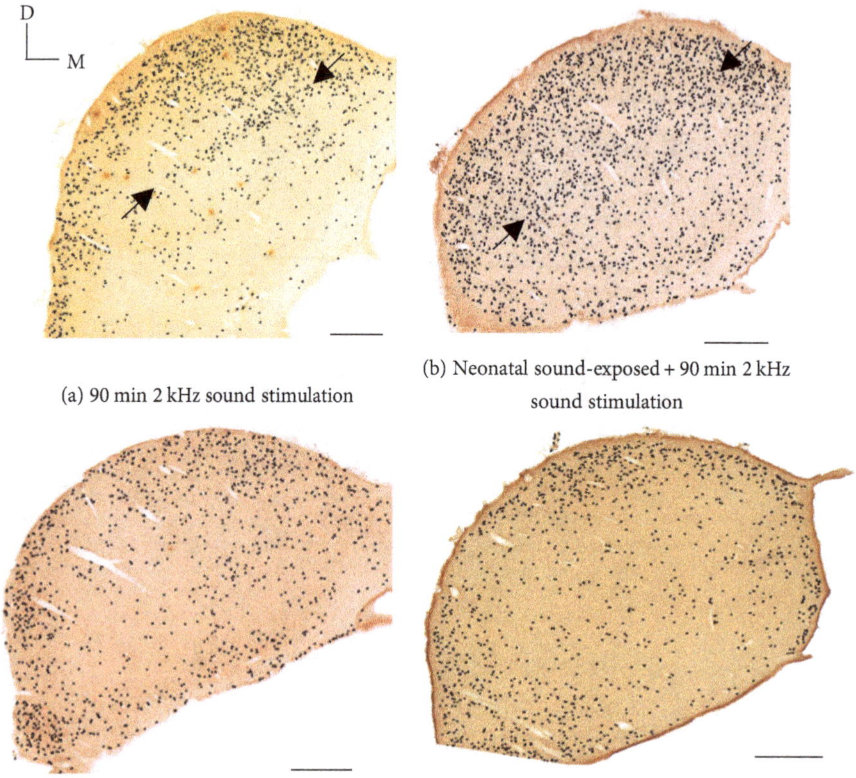

(a) 90 min 2 kHz sound stimulation

(b) Neonatal sound-exposed + 90 min 2 kHz sound stimulation

(c) Control: no sound exposure

(d) Neonatal sound-exposed + no sound stimulation

Figure 6: Representative patterning of c-fos-labeled cells in inferior colliculus by experimental group. Where present, arrows denote bands of labeled neurons. Scale bars indicate 500 μm. The histology sections (a) and (c) are reproduced from a previously published methods paper ([26]; fig. 1) with permission.

Table 1: Average counts of c-fos-labelled neurons (±SEM) by the experimental group. t-tests were performed between pairs of groups, as indicated; the corresponding p values are reported.

Experimental group	Number of cells: 2 kHz band		Number of cells: ROI	
2 kHz, 90 min	106.9 ± 3.0	$p < 0.001$	334.0 ± 9.4	$p < 0.001$
Sound-exposed + 2 kHz, 90 min	184.9 ± 3.8		604.6 ± 10.3	
No sound	76.2 ± 2.8	$p = 0.4$	306.1 ± 7.7	$p = 0.8$
Sound-exposed + no sound	79.2 ± 2.1		309.0 ± 6.3	

including our own, report on the neural representation of sound frequency in IC following postnatal sound exposure using electrophysiological methods (e.g., [10–14, 26, 29]). However, the advantage of using c-fos immunolabeling is that it allows visualization of global neural activity patterns with cellular resolution.

4.2. IC Activity Patterns following Neonatal Sound Exposure. In regard to our neonatal sound exposure (2 kHz narrow-band signal for 30 days at 70 dB SPL), one obvious question is whether it causes damage at the level of the cochlea. We suggest not because with a similar exposure, we have previously reported no change to ABR audiograms or to cochlear hair cell integrity as shown by scanning electron microscopy [27]. However, recent studies on noise exposure in rodent models have revealed inner hair cell synaptopathy and related spiral ganglion cell degeneration [30, 31]. These changes are not revealed by any monitoring of audiometric thresholds and have thus led to the notion of "hidden hearing loss." Our own cochlear histology with scanning microscopy cannot detect synaptic pathology. So it is possible that the IC changes we observe may not be intrinsically midbrain but have some peripheral origin. An added point of interest is that Hickox and Liberman's group has linked noise-induced synaptopathy with tinnitus generation and hyperacusis [32]. A general sensitization of IC neural activity such as we demonstrate here is in-line, albeit tentatively, with a neural substrate for hyperacusis.

Subjects having the sound-exposure stimulus for 4 weeks and then no additional sound stimulation did not exhibit c-fos expression patterns that differed from age-matched controls (Figures 6(c) and 6(d); Figure 5). These results imply that sound exposure does not change basal levels of neural activity in inferior colliculus. Sound-exposed subjects who subsequently heard the 90 min 2 kHz tone burst exhibited increased c-fos expression levels, both near the 2 kHz region of interest and over a broad frequency range of inferior colliculus (Figures 6(b) and 3). Taken together, these data suggest that the sound-exposure stimulus alters the way in which neurons respond to a subsequent presentation of a sound stimulus, of sufficient duration, in the frequency range of the sound exposure stimulus (90 min 2 kHz tone burst).

Our main experimental finding is well captured in Figure 3. These data show that early sound-exposure stimulus alters the way in which neurons in IC respond to a subsequent presentation of a sound stimulus, and suggest a form of global sensitization. Our results resemble in some ways receptive field sensitization patterns in auditory cortex reported by Bakin and Weinberger and Weinberger [33, 34]. In their work on receptive field plasticity in auditory cortex, guinea pigs were subjected to various "sensitization training" stimulation paradigms, such that overall, subjects heard tone bursts at 80 dB for approximately 50 minutes. This sensitization training resulted in a broad, nonspecific increase in response across auditory cortical receptive fields; response changes were seen across a wide range of best frequencies up to 30 kHz [33]. Essentially, these sensitization results provide an example of pure-tone stimulation affecting change across a broad tonotopic frequency region and are an interesting comparison for the results presented herein.

The following question might be posed. Does the significant increase in the number of c-fos-labelled neurons, over a broad tonotopic frequency range in sound-exposed subjects, produce some change in hearing function? The answer has to be speculative, because we are far from understanding the exact relationship between neural activity patterns and perceived sounds. With that said, if we assume the pattern of excitation (across a broad tonotopic array) in IC is the direct substrate for higher-level sound processing, then the general increase in activity might translate into increase in loudness perception. This might perhaps contribute to some degree of hyperacusis. Secondly, if the general level of excitability is increased across all tonotopic areas, this might be considered "noise" in relation to a more specific coded sound signal. We could speculate that this would reduce the signal to noise in a neural representation of an acoustic signal. At an extreme, if this enhancement of IC neural activity is spontaneous and sustained (and perceived), it might contribute to some (broadband) tinnitus sensation.

In summary, the data presented here suggest that persistent exposure to an abnormal sound environment during an early postnatal period can alter neural activity patterns to sound in later life. Our data show such changes at the auditory midbrain level, but does not preclude the possibility of sensitization at brainstem or even cochlear levels of the system.

Conflicts of Interest

The authors declare that they have no conflicts of interest.

Acknowledgments

This study was funded by the Canadian Institute of Health Research (CIHR), the Canadian Natural Sciences and Engineering Research Council (NSERC), and an Ontario Graduate Scholarship (OGS).

References

[1] T. N. Wiesel and D. H. Hubel, "Comparison of the effects of unilateral and bilateral eye closure on cortical unit responses in kittens," *Journal of Neurophysiology*, vol. 28, no. 6, pp. 1029–1040, 1965.

[2] T. N. Wiesel and D. H. Hubel, "Single-cell responses in striate cortex of kittens deprived of vision in one eye," *Journal of Neurophysiology*, vol. 26, no. 6, pp. 1003–1017, 1963.

[3] D. D. Rasmusson, "Reorganization of raccoon somatosensory cortex following removal of the fifth digit," *The Journal of Comparative Neurology*, vol. 205, no. 4, pp. 313–326, 1982.

[4] D. Robertson and D. R. Irvine, "Plasticity of frequency organization in auditory cortex of guinea pigs with partial unilateral deafness," *The Journal of Comparative Neurology*, vol. 282, no. 3, pp. 456–471, 1989.

[5] R. V. Harrison, A. Nagasawa, D. W. Smith, S. Stanton, and R. J. Mount, "Reorganization of auditory cortex after neonatal high frequency cochlear hearing loss," *Hearing Research*, vol. 54, no. 1, pp. 11–19, 1991.

[6] S. G. Stanton and R. V. Harrison, "Projections from the medial geniculate body to primary auditory cortex in neonatally deafened cats," *The Journal of Comparative Neurology*, vol. 426, no. 1, pp. 117–129, 2000.

[7] R. V. Harrison, D. Ibrahim, and R. J. Mount, "Plasticity of tonotopic maps in auditory midbrain following partial cochlear damage in the developing chinchilla," *Experimental Brain Research*, vol. 123, no. 4, pp. 449–460, 1998.

[8] Z. Bureš, J. Bartošová, J. Lindovský, T. Chumak, J. Popelář, and J. Syka, "Acoustical enrichment during early postnatal development changes response properties of inferior colliculus neurons in rats," *The European Journal of Neuroscience*, vol. 40, no. 11, pp. 3674–3683, 2014.

[9] H. P. Lu, J. Syka, T. W. Chiu, and P. W. Poon, "Prolonged sound exposure has different effects on increasing neuronal size in the auditory cortex and brainstem," *Hearing Research*, vol. 314, pp. 42–50, 2014.

[10] A. Miyakawa, R. Gibboni, and S. Bao, "Repeated exposure to a tone transiently alters spectral tuning bandwidth of neurons in the central nucleus of inferior colliculus in juvenile rats," *Neuroscience*, vol. 230, pp. 114–120, 2013.

[11] D. L. Oliver, M. A. Izquierdo, and M. S. Malmierca, "Persistent effects of early augmented acoustic environment on the auditory brainstem," *Neuroscience*, vol. 184, pp. 75–87, 2011.

[12] P. W. Poon and X. Chen, "Postnatal exposure to tones alters the tuning characteristics of inferior collicular neurons in the rat," *Brain Research*, vol. 585, no. 1-2, pp. 391–394, 1992.

[13] D. H. Sanes and M. Constantine-Paton, "The sharpening of frequency tuning curves requires patterned activity during development in the mouse, mus musculus," *The Journal of Neuroscience*, vol. 5, no. 5, pp. 1152–1166, 1985.

[14] X. Yu, D. H. Sanes, O. Aristizabal, Y. Z. Wadghiri, and D. H. Turnbull, "Large-scale reorganization of the tonotopic map in mouse auditory midbrain revealed by MRI," *Proceedings of the National Academy of Sciences of the United States of America*, vol. 104, no. 29, pp. 12193–12198, 2007.

[15] C. J. Beaver, D. E. Mitchell, and H. A. Robertson, "Immunohistochemical study of the pattern of rapid expression of C-fos protein in the visual cortex of dark-reared kittens following initial exposure to light," *The Journal of Comparative Neurology*, vol. 333, no. 4, pp. 469–484, 1993.

[16] R. K. Filipkowski, M. Rydz, B. Berdel, J. Morys, and L. Kaczmarek, "Tactile experience induces c-fos expression in rat barrel cortex," *Learning & Memory*, vol. 7, no. 2, pp. 116–122, 2000.

[17] H. P. Lu, S. T. Chen, and P. W. Poon, "Nuclear size of c-fos expression at the auditory brainstem is related to the time-varying nature of the acoustic stimuli," *Neuroscience Letters*, vol. 451, no. 2, pp. 139–143, 2009.

[18] K. J. Mack and P. A. Mack, "Induction of transcription factors in somatosensory cortex after tactile stimulation," *Brain Research Molecular Brain Research*, vol. 12, no. 1-3, pp. 141–147, 1992.

[19] K. M. Rosen, M. A. McCormack, L. Villa-Komaroff, and G. D. Mower, "Brief visual experience induces immediate early gene expression in the cat visual cortex," *Proceedings of the National Academy of Sciences of the United States of America*, vol. 89, no. 12, pp. 5437–5441, 1992.

[20] J. C. Adams, "Sound stimulation induces Fos-related antigens in cells with common morphological properties throughout the auditory brainstem," *The Journal of Comparative Neurology*, vol. 361, no. 4, pp. 645–668, 1995.

[21] M. C. Brown and T. S. Liu, "Fos-like immunoreactivity in central auditory neurons of the mouse," *The Journal of Comparative Neurology*, vol. 357, no. 1, pp. 85–97, 1995.

[22] E. Friauf, "Tonotopic order in the adult and developing auditory system of the rat as shown by c-fos immunocytochemistry," *The European Journal of Neuroscience*, vol. 4, no. 9, pp. 798–812, 1992.

[23] M. Nakamura, S. K. Rosahl, E. Alkahlout, G. F. Walter, and M. M. Samii, "Electrical stimulation of the cochlear nerve in rats: analysis of c-fos expression in auditory brainstem nuclei," *Brain Research*, vol. 1031, no. 1, pp. 39–55, 2005.

[24] H. Scheich and W. Zuschratter, "Mapping of stimulus features and meaning in gerbil auditory cortex with 2-deoxyglucose and c-fos antibodies," *Behavioural Brain Research*, vol. 66, no. 1-2, pp. 195–205, 1995.

[25] Y. Qian and P. H. Jen, "Fos-like immunoreactivity elicited by sound stimulation in the auditory neurons of the big brown bat *eptesicus fuscus*," *Brain Research*, vol. 664, no. 1-2, pp. 241–246, 1994.

[26] L. M. D'Alessandro and R. V. Harrison, "Excitatory and inhibitory tonotopic bands in chinchilla inferior colliculus revealed by c-fos immuno-labeling," *Hearing Research*, vol. 316, pp. 122–128, 2014.

[27] L. M. D'Alessandro and R. V. Harrison, "Midbrain frequency representation following moderately intense neonatal sound exposure in a precocious animal model (*Chinchilla laniger*)," *Neural Plasticity*, vol. 2016, Article ID 3734646, 11 pages, 2016.

[28] L. Kaczmarek and A. Chaudhuri, "Sensory regulation of immediate-early gene expression in mammalian visual cortex: implications for functional mapping and neural plasticity," *Brain Research. Brain Research Reviews*, vol. 23, no. 3, pp. 237–256, 1997.

[29] D. R. Moore and L. M. Aitkin, "Rearing in an acoustically unusual environment—effects on neural auditory responses," *Neuroscience Letters*, vol. 1, no. 1, pp. 29–34, 1975.

[30] S. G. Kujawa and M. C. Liberman, "Adding insult to injury: cochlear nerve degeneration after "temporary" noise-induced hearing loss," *The Journal of Neuroscience*, vol. 29, no. 45, pp. 14077–14085, 2009.

[31] S. G. Kujawa and M. C. Liberman, "Synaptopathy in the noise-exposed and aging cochlea: primary neural degeneration in acquired sensorineural hearing loss," *Hearing Research*, vol. 330, Part B, pp. 191–199, 2015.

[32] A. E. Hickox and M. C. Liberman, "Is noise-induced cochlear neuropathy key to the generation of hyperacusis or tinnitus?," *Journal of Neurophysiology*, vol. 111, no. 3, pp. 552–564, 2014.

[33] J. S. Bakin and N. M. Weinberger, "Classical conditioning induces CS-specific receptive field plasticity in the auditory cortex of the guinea pig," *Brain Research*, vol. 536, no. 1-2, pp. 271–286, 1990.

[34] N. M. Weinberger, "Dynamic regulation of receptive fields and maps in the adult sensory cortex," *Annual Review of Neuroscience*, vol. 18, no. 1, pp. 129–158, 1995.

10

Comparison of Acceptable Noise Level Generated using Different Transducers and Response Modes

Liang Xia,[1] Jingchun He,[2] Yuanyuan Sun,[1] Yi Chen,[1] Qiong Luo,[1] Haibo Shi,[1] Yanmei Feng,[1] and Shankai Yin[1]

[1]*Department of Otolaryngology, Shanghai Jiao Tong University Affiliated Sixth People's Hospital, No. 600, Yishan Road, Xuhui District, Shanghai 200233, China*
[2]*Department of Otolaryngology, Shanghai Jiao Tong University Affiliated Xinhua Hospital, No. 1665, Kongjiang Road, Yangpu District, Shanghai 200092, China*

Correspondence should be addressed to Haibo Shi; haibo99@hotmail.com and Yanmei Feng; feng.yanmei@126.com

Academic Editor: Geng-lin Li

The acceptable noise level (ANL) was defined by subtracting the background noise level (BNL) from the most comfortable listening level (MCL) (ANL = MCL − BNL). This study compared the ANL obtained through different methods in 20 Chinese subjects with normal hearing. ANL was tested with Mandarin speech materials using a loudspeaker or earphones, with each subject tested by himself or by the audiologist. The presentation and response modes were as follows: (1) loudspeaker with self-adjusted noise levels using audiometer controls (LS method); (2) loudspeaker with the subject signaling the audiologist to adjust speech and noise levels (LA method); (3) earphones with self-adjusted noise levels using audiometer controls (ES method); and (4) earphones with the subject signaling the audiologist to adjust speech and noise levels (EA method). ANL was calculated from three measurements with each method. There was no significant difference in the ANL obtained through different presentation modes or response modes sound. The correlations between ANL, MCL, and BNL obtained from each two methods were significant. In conclusion, the ANL in normal-hearing Mandarin listeners may not be affected by presentation modes such as a loudspeaker or earphones nor is it affected by self-adjusted or audiologist-adjusted response modes. Earphone audiometry is as reliable as sound field audiometry and provides an easy and convenient way to measure ANL.

1. Introduction

The acceptable noise level (ANL) test was developed to quantify the critical amount of background noise that subjects could accept while listening to speech [1–6]. ANL is defined as the lowest signal-to-noise ratio (SNR) that a subject could accept when the target speech was presented at the most comfortable listening level (MCL) [6, 7]. ANL is derived by subtracting the background noise level (BNL) that the subject can accept from the MCL. A low ANL indicates that a subject has a high tolerance for background noises, while a subject with high ANL has low tolerance for background noises [7]. According to Nabelek et al. [8], subjects with an ANL below 7 dB are likely to become successful full-time hearing aid users, while subjects with an ANL above 13 dB are likely to become unsuccessful hearing aids users occasionally or not at all. Previous studies have shown that there is a large variation in ANL across normal-hearing subjects [1, 7, 9–13]. This variation seems unrelated to age [1, 11], gender [14], middle-ear function [15], hearing sensitivity [1, 7, 9, 15, 16], outer hair cell function [15], and efferent pathways utilizing the medial olivocochlear bundle [15]. However, it was influenced by speech materials, noise materials, presentation mode, instructions, and working memory capacity [17].

Several types of sensors have been used to present the ANL signal. In most studies, the sound signal was presented in the sound field through a loudspeaker [18]. However, some studies presented the signals used to measure ANL through an earphone [1]. Olsen and Brännström [17] indicated that the values of ANL obtained from an earphone or loudspeaker may be different. If transducers other than a loudspeaker were used, the ANL data for the specific transducer should be considered. Clinically, audiologists may use ANL data obtained from different transducers. Although most audiologists use a loudspeaker to do ANL, some audiologists could do ANL with earphone when the loudspeaker is not available and predict the ANL results with loudspeaker from the ANL results with earphone. Therefore, it is necessary to contrast different sound presentation modes in ANL tests.

On the other hand, Brannstrom et al. [11] suggested that ANL might be influenced by extrinsic factors such as examiner attitude, instructions, and/or cultural differences in the acceptability of background noise. In most ANL tests, the subject signals the experimenter to adjust the sound volume. However, Nabelek et al. [1] directed subjects to adjust the levels by themselves with visual feedback from the audiometer. The main difference between self-adjusted and audiologist-adjusted measurements is the method to determine the MCL and BNL intensity. During the self-adjusted method, the subjects will determine the MCL and BNL by adjusting the sound levels using the control buttons. During the audiologist-adjusted method, the subjects tell the audiologist the optimal intensity and the maximum intensity signal as the noise level changes continuously; however, there could be a time lag or bias of intensity during this period which can produce differences between the final results and the subjects' true results on ANL tests.

To identify factors that may influence ANL values, this study proposed to investigate and compare the test results of ANL measured through a loudspeaker or earphones and further compared the effect of the self-adjusted or audiologist-adjusted testing method.

2. Methods

The program was approved by the Ethics Committee of Shanghai Jiao Tong University Affiliated Sixth People's Hospital. All participants provided written informed consent prior to the study's commencement.

2.1. Subjects. This study was conducted in twenty adults (10 male, 10 female) with normal hearing whose native language was Mandarin. Their ages ranged from 21 to 30 years and they were all university students. The criterion for normal hearing sensitivity was pure-tone air conduction thresholds for each ear less than or equal to 15 dB HL at each frequency from 0.25 to 8 kHz with an octave step. The subjects reported no recent otologic problems, such as ear infection, draining ears, otalgia, or surgery on or in the ears during the past eight weeks. The equipment set-ups were calibrated before the study started.

2.2. Materials. The test used Mandarin-acceptable noise level material established by Chen et al. [18]. The materials were *The Spring Festival of Beijing* which was chosen from the official textbooks for primary school. The noise signal used to measure BNL was the 12 multitalker babbles routinely used for ANL tests [18]. The ANL signals were a speech signal in one channel and a noise signal in the other channel. In each test condition, the MCL and BNL were tested three measurements, and the average of three measurements for each individual was used as the MCL and BNL of the subjects, and the MCL and BNL of each group were the average values of all the subjects.

2.3. Stimuli and Procedure. In sound field audiometry, listeners were tested individually in an audiometric booth that met ANSI standards for ambient noise levels (ANSI, S 3.1-1991). All the stimuli were generated from a compact disc player and delivered via a clinical audiometer (GN Otometrics, Taastrup, Denmark) connected to a calibrated loudspeaker (GSI) located in a sound-proof room. Both speech and noise were presented from the loudspeaker at zero degrees azimuth 1.5 m away from the subjects. The calibration tone was a 1 kHz pure tone. When calibrating, the two channels were calibrated, respectively, and the readout of the VU table on the audiometer panel should be adjusted to 0. The output levels of the speech stimuli and background noise were calibrated at the position occupied by the listener.

In earphone audiometry, listeners were tested individually in an audiometric booth that met ANSI standards for ambient noise levels (ANSI, S 3.1-1991). All the stimuli were generated from a compact disc player and delivered via clinical audiometer (GN Otometrics, Taastrup, Denmark) connected to a calibrated earphone (Sennheiser HDA 200 circumaural earphones). The calibration tone was a 1 kHz pure tone. The output levels of the speech stimuli and background noise were calibrated using B&K 4134 pressure microphone and B&K 4153 simulation ear. When calibrating, the two channels were calibrated, respectively, and the readout of the VU table on the audiometer panel should be adjusted to 0.

2.4. The Procedure for Audiologist-Adjusted ANL Tests. Both written and oral instructions were given prior to ANL testing. The instructions were Chinese versions of the English instructions. If the subjects had any doubts, the instructions were clarified. Examples of speech and noise were then presented. Subjects' ANLs were obtained as described previously [18].

The initial stimulus level for each repetition was 30 dB HL for both speech and noise signals, and a 2 dB step size was used for all adjustments for both MCL and BNL. Audiologists increased the sound volume until the speech signal became too loud, then decreased it until it became too soft, and finally the subject selected the sound volume that was the most comfortable listening level. The verbal and written instructions for determining the MCL were as follows:

You will listen to a story through a loudspeaker or earphones. After a few moments, select the sound volume level for the story that is most comfortable for you, as if listening to a radio. Hand motions will allow you to signal the audiologist to adjust the signal level up (thumbs up) or down (thumbs down) or to stop adjustments (flat palm; this means that you feel the current level is the most comfortable for you).

Then, BNL was established by adding a noise signal as the speech signal and the subject was instructed to repeat a similar procedure; the speech signal remained fixed at

TABLE 1: The mean and standard error (SE) of MCL, BNL, and ANL obtained from the three repeated measurements in different methods. MCL: most comfortable listening level; BNL: background noise level; ANL: acceptable noise level; LS: measured through loudspeaker with self-adjusted levels using audiometer controls; LA: measured through loudspeaker with the subject signaling the audiologist to adjust the levels of speech and noise; ES: measured through earphones with self-adjusted levels using audiometer controls; EA: measured through earphones with the subject signaling the audiologist to adjust the levels of speech and noise.

Values	Method	1st measurement		2nd measurement		3rd measurement	
		Mean	SE	Mean	SE	Mean	SE
MCL (dB HL)	LS	35.9	1.54	37.2	1.36	37.4	1.37
	LA	38.1	1.61	38.1	1.32	38.6	1.16
	ES	43.3	1.85	43.8	1.83	45.2	2.01
	EA	44.8	1.45	45.2	1.49	43.8	1.65
BNL (dB HL)	LS	35.8	1.73	37.6	1.46	38.5	1.51
	LA	38.2	1.50	38.7	1.42	39.3	1.23
	ES	43.0	2.02	43.9	1.83	45.5	2.21
	EA	44.2	1.39	45.6	1.72	44.2	1.73
ANL (dB)	LS	0.1	0.76	−0.4	0.54	−1.1	0.62
	LA	−0.1	0.72	−0.6	0.56	−0.9	0.62
	ES	0.4	0.83	−0.1	0.49	−0.3	0.84
	EA	0.6	0.56	−0.5	0.78	−0.4	0.55

the previously established MCL and the subject increased the sound volume of the noise until it became too loud, then decreased it until the speech became very clear, and finally the subject selected the sound volume that he or she could tolerate without becoming tense or tired while following the speech signal for a long period of time. The subject reported when the BNL had been found. The verbal and written instructions for determining the BNL were as follows [18]:

You will now listen to the same story with background noise. After you have listened to this for a few moments, select the maximum level of background noise which you would be willing to tolerate without becoming tense or tired while following the story. Hand motions will also allow you to signal the investigator to adjust the signal level.

2.5. The Procedure of Self-Adjusted ANL Tests. The main steps were the same as those of the audiologist-guided test. After brief instructions to the subjects, they conducted the ANL test by themselves. Instructions for the self-adjusted ANL test were as follows:

You will listen to a story through a loudspeaker or earphones. After a few moments, select the sound volume level for the story that is most comfortable for you, as if you were listening to a radio. You do not need signal the audiologist to adjust the signal level up (thumbs up) or down (thumbs down) or to stop adjustments (flat palm, meaning that you feel the current level is the most comfortable for you). You should regulate the sound volume of sound though the clinical audiometer. When the MCL was found, the multitalker babble was introduced from the loudspeaker or earphones at 30 dB HL. You will now listen to the same story with background noise. After you have listened to this for a few moments, select the maximum level of the background noise which you would be willing to tolerate without becoming tense or tired while following the story. You should regulate the sound volume of the sound though the clinical audiometer too. Both the sound volume level of the 12-talker babble or story are increased in 2 dB steps.

The MCL and BNL were measured three times with a 30 min gap between two measurements. The ANL from each measurement was obtained by subtracting the BNL from the MCL (ANL = MCL − BNL) for each participant and each experimental condition. The average of the three measurements was used to calculate ANL.

2.6. Statistical Analysis. All the statistical analyses were performed using SPSS version 20.0 (IBM Corp., Armonk, NY, USA). Descriptive statistics were calculated for the MCL, BNL, and ANL. The values of different measurements in the same method were compared by paired *t*-test. Pearson's correlation coefficient was used to evaluate the relationship between ANL, MCL, and BNL among three measurements in each condition. Two-way repeated measures analyses of variance (ANOVA) were used to assess the effects of MCL, BNL, and ANL within each method; Pearson's correlation coefficient was used to examine the relationship between the results of ANL and MCL and between ANL and BNL in each method. Correlations between ANL, MCL, and BNL in each method were investigated by Pearson's correlation. The significance level was set at $p < 0.05$.

3. Results

3.1. MCL, BNL, and ANL Obtained from the Three Measurements with Different Methods. The means and standard error of MCL, BNL, and ANL obtained from the three measurements in different methods are listed in Table 1. The MCL and BNL increased with an increasing number of repetitions in the LS, LA, and ES methods, but the ANL decreased with increasing number of measurements in the LS, LA, and ES methods. However, in the EA method, the MCL and BNL increased first and then decreased with

Table 2: The paired t-tests for MCL, BNL, and ANL obtained from the three measurements in different methods. The significance level was set at $p < 0.05$.

Values	Method	1st versus 2nd measurement t	1st versus 2nd measurement p value	1st versus 3rd measurement t	1st versus 3rd measurement p value	2nd versus 3rd measurement t	2nd versus 3rd measurement p value
MCL (dB HL)	LS	−1.488	0.153	−1.510	0.148	−0.261	0.797
	LA	−0.469	0.645	1.070	0.298	1.889	0.074
	ES	−0.553	0.587	−1.594	0.127	−1.730	0.100
	EA	−0.469	0.645	1.070	0.298	1.889	0.074
BNL (dB HL)	LS	−1.616	0.122	−2.236	0.038*	−1.917	0.070
	LA	−0.592	0.561	−1.291	0.212	−1.301	0.209
	ES	−0.785	0.442	−1.724	0.101	−1.875	0.076
	EA	−1.453	0.163	0.000	1.000	1.759	0.095
ANL (dB)	LS	0.773	0.449	2.698	0.014*	1.437	0.167
	LA	1.045	0.309	1.506	0.148	0.825	0.419
	ES	0.815	0.425	0.941	0.358	0.335	0.741
	EA	2.604	0.017*	2.517	0.021*	−0.252	0.804

*Values were significantly different from each other.

Table 3: Values of the mean, standard error (SE), and range for MCL, BNL, and ANL averaged across all the subjects for each method. The significance level was set at $p < 0.05$.

Method	MCL value (dB HL) Mean	MCL SE	MCL Range	BNL value (dB HL) Mean	BNL SE	BNL Range	ANL value (dB) Mean	ANL SE	ANL Range
LS	36.83*	1.33	25.33~48.00	37.30**	1.47	27.33~55.33	−0.47	0.57	−7.33~3.33
LA	38.27*	1.32	29.33~50.00	38.27**	1.32	30.00~54.67	−0.53	0.58	−4.67~4.00
ES	44.10*	1.81	31.33~60.67	44.13#	1.91	29.33~64.00	0.00	0.63	−4.67~6.00
EA	44.60*	1.45	36.67~58.67	44.67#	1.54	35.33~63.33	−0.10	0.60	−5.33~4.00

*Values of MCL were significantly different from each other. **Values of BNL were significantly different between the ES and EA methods. #Values of BNL were significantly different between the LS and LA methods.

increasing number of repetitions; the ANL decreased first and then increased with increasing number of repetitions. The statistical results comparing the values obtained from the three measurements by paired t-tests within each method are shown in Table 2. The significant difference did not exist in most situations except the BNL in the first measurement versus the third measurement with the LS method, ANL in the first measurement versus the second measurement with the EA method, and ANL in the first measurement versus the third measurement with the LS and EA methods.

The correlations of ANL, MCL, and BNL among three measurements within each method indicated that the correlation coefficient of ANL, MCL, and BNL between any two measurements was significant for each method. The range of correlation coefficients was 0.548 to 0.951 with all $p < 0.05$.

Table 4: The correlations between MCL and ANL and between BNL and ANL within each method. The significance level was set at $p < 0.05$.

Method	MCL-ANL r	MCL-ANL p value	BNL-ANL r	BNL-ANL p value
LS	−0.033	0.890	−0.4173	0.067
LA	0.207	0.381	0.207	0.327
ES	0.038	0.875	0.298	0.202
EA	0.075	0.753	0.325	0.162

3.2. MCL, BNL, and ANL Averaged from the Three Measurements with Different Methods. MCL, BNL, and ANL values averaged across three repeated measurements were calculated for the four test methods and were shown in Table 3. A two-way repeated measurement analysis of variance was used to assess the effects of different test methods of on MCL, BNL, and ANL. The dependent variable was MCL, BNL, or ANL. The within-subject factor was response modes, with two levels (self-adjusted or audiologist-adjusted), and the between-subject factor was presentation modes, with two factors (loudspeaker or earphones). First, the results show that the main effect of response modes and presentation modes was statistically significant for MCL (response modes [$F = 4.364$; $p = 0.043$] and presentation modes [$F = 10.875$; $p = 0.002$]). However, the interaction effect of response modes × presentation modes was not significant [$F = 1.017$; $p = 0.320$]. These outcomes indicated

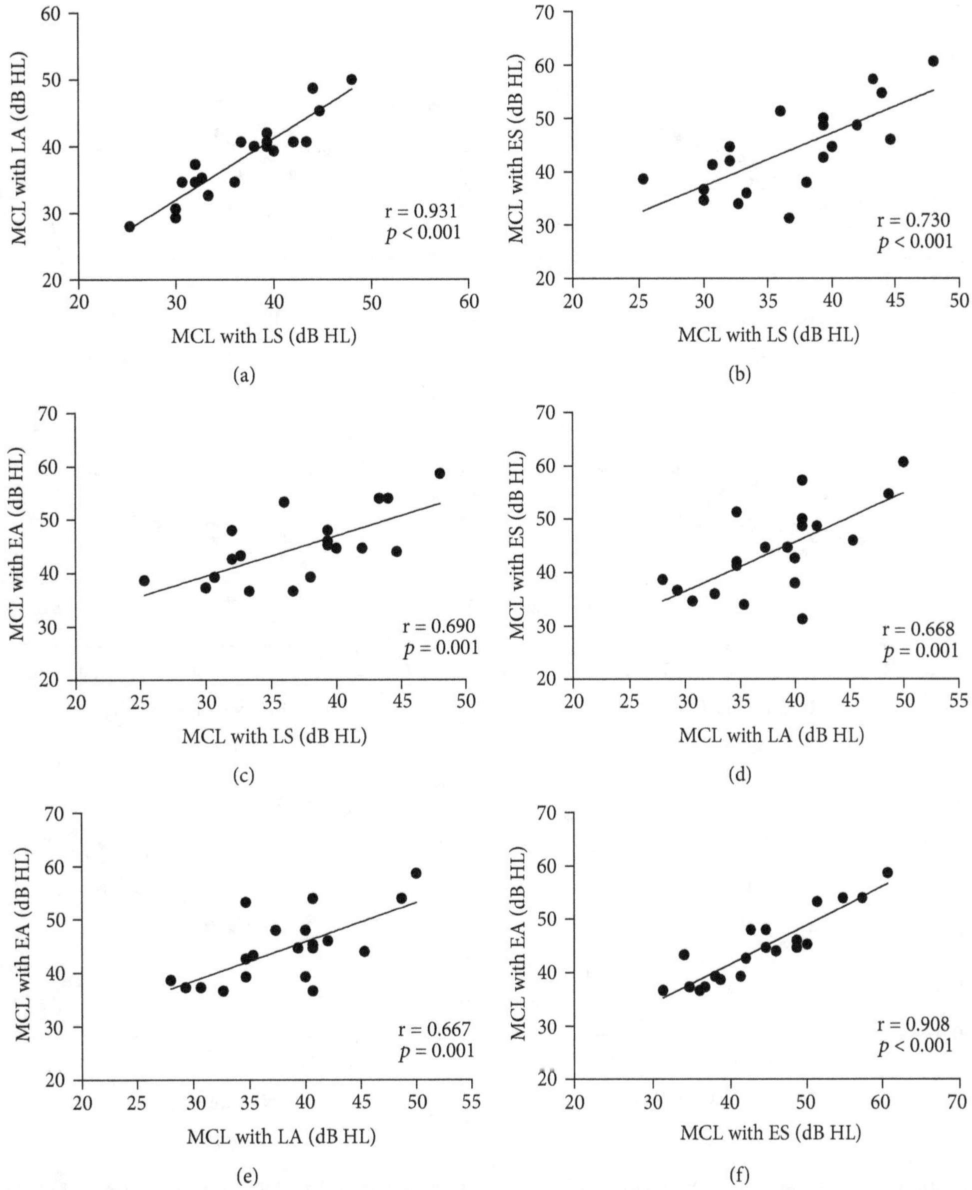

FIGURE 1: The correlations for MCL between each two methods. A: LS and LA; B: LS and ES; C: LS and EA; D: LA and ES; E: LA and EA; F: ES and EA. The significance level was set $p < 0.05$.

that the MCL was affected by response modes and presentation modes. Second, the results show that the main effect of response modes and presentation modes was different in BNL (response modes [$F = 3.759$; $p = 0.060$] and presentation modes [$F = 8.660$; $p = 0.006$]); the interaction effect of response modes × presentation modes was also not significant ($F = 0.787$; $p = 0.381$). The results indicated that the presentation modes may impact BNL, unlike the response modes. The analysis revealed that the main effect of response modes and presentation modes was not statistically significant for ANL (response modes [$F = 0.191$; $p = 0.665$] and presentation modes [$F = 0.302$; $p = 0.586$]); the interaction effect of response modes × presentation modes was also not significant ($F = 0.008$; $p = 0.931$). Both response modes and presentation modes did not affect ANL values. This showed that the ANL values of different response modes do not change with presentation modes because all the differences for interaction effects are not significant.

3.3. Correlations between MCL and ANL and between BNL and ANL within Each Method. Pearson correlation coefficients were used to observe the relationship between the MCL and ANL and between the BNL and ANL for each test situation. The correlations between MCL-ANL and between BNL-ANL within each method were not significant: coefficients are shown in Table 4.

3.4. Correlations of MCL, BNL, and ANL among Each Method. The correlation results of MCL, BNL, and ANL among each method are displayed in Figures 1, 2, and 3, respectively, and all correlations were significant. The correlations of MCL, BNL, and ANL between any two methods

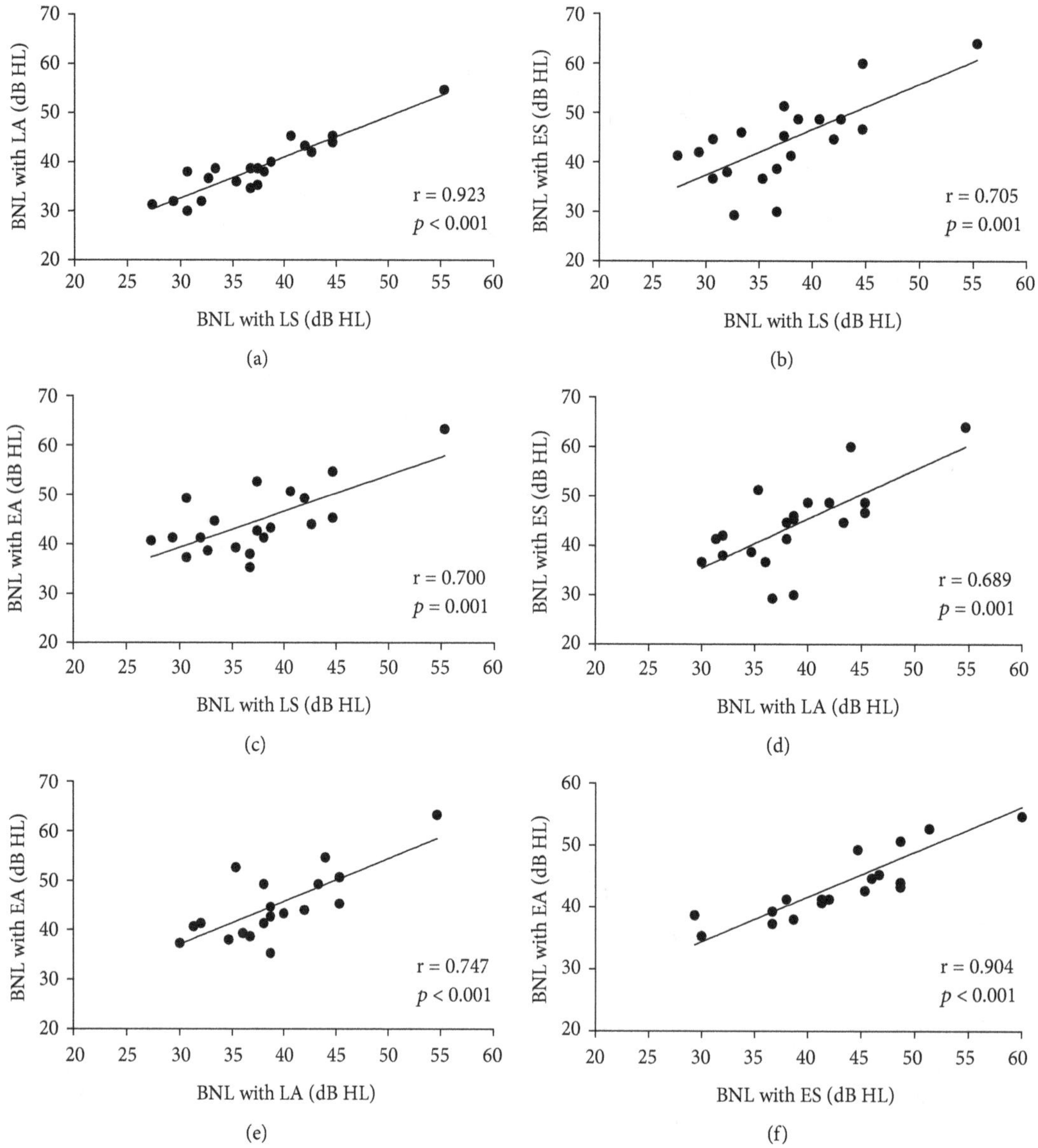

FIGURE 2: The correlations for BNL between each two methods. A: LS and LA; B: LS and ES; C: LS and EA; D: LA and ES; E: LA and EA; F: ES and EA. The significance level was set $p < 0.05$.

were strongly correlated in this study. Correlation coefficients ranged from 0.667 to 0.931; $p \leq 0.001$.

4. Discussion

This study compared the MCL, BNL, and ANL obtained with the LS, LA, ES, and EA methods in subjects with hearing in normal range. The results initially suggest that the values of MCL and BNL increased and the values of ANL decreased with an increasing number of measurements, except in the EA method. Although ANL value tended to decrease, showing a potential learning effect during this test, and tolerance may influence the ANL tests, the difference of MCL, BNL and ANL values obtained from different measurements within each method was not statistically significant in most situations. And our study also shows that the correlations between ANL, MCL, and BNL obtained from both methods and both measurements were significant. This indicated that the repeatability of the ANL test method was credible. Previous studies [18–21] showed that the Pearson correlations suggested significant correlations between ANL and MCL with a LA method, but the correlations of the current study suggested that ANL values were reliable across testing methods; there were no correlations between ANL and BNL or between ANL and MCL in either method. This means that the ANL did not change with MCL or BNL. ANL may be an intrinsic property for every subject and MCL or BNL could affect ANL in different methods.

The main purpose of this study was to compare the acceptable noise level obtained with a loudspeaker or earphones in Chinese subjects with normal hearing. Clinically, the application of the loudspeaker and earphones is different. Sound field audiometry is used to evaluate the auditory function of the subject in a sound field using the loudspeaker.

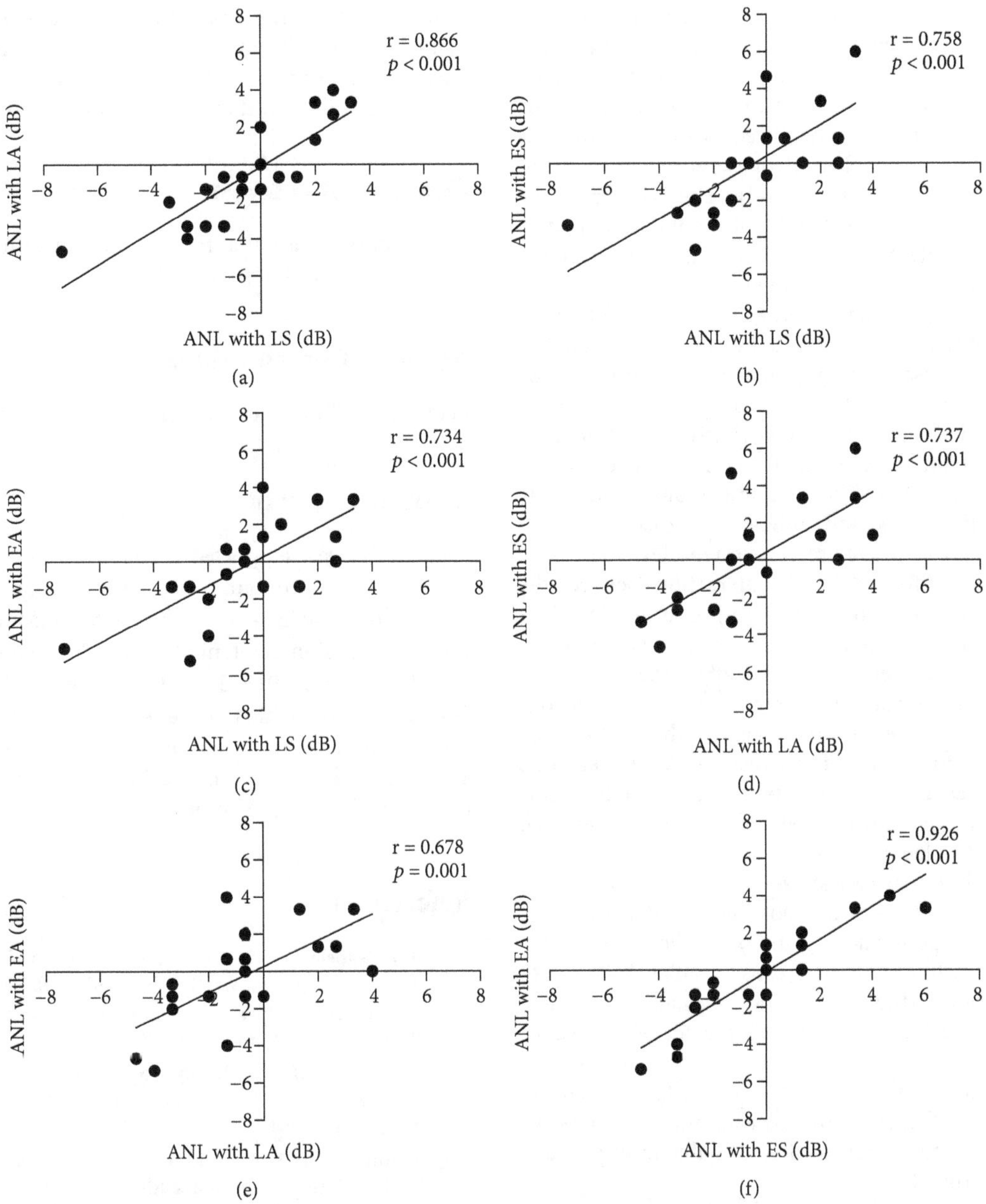

FIGURE 3: The correlations for ANL between each two methods. A: LS and LA; B: LS and ES; C: LS and EA; D: LA and ES; E: LA and EA; F: ES and EA. The significance level was set $p < 0.05$.

Sound field audiometry has incomparable superiority compared with earphones in children's pure-tone threshold audiometry, hearing aid matching, and evaluation of cochlear implants [22]. When evaluating the effect of the hearing aid, earphones and loudspeakers can be used for the unaided ear, while the patient wearing a hearing aid must be carried out in the sound field through a loudspeaker. Moreover, the results obtained with sound field measurements are more realistic than earphone audiometry. However, sound field audiometry can be easily affected by room size and layout. If the room is too small, subjects may consider it depressing. The capacity for noise isolation and absorption is also important in sound field audiometry. Taken together, the sound field audiometry standards are strict, and the actual operation is complicated. Therefore, it is necessary to conduct ANL testing with earphones and to compare these results with those obtained from earphones and loudspeaker. The results of this study suggest that ANL obtained with earphones is comparable to that obtained with a loudspeaker. Therefore, the hardware requirements and the complexity of the operation could be reduced, which is beneficial to the popularization of ANL tests. For those which do not have sound field conditions and those who are not suitable for sound field audiometry, the ANL obtained from earphones could be used as a reference to that obtained with a loudspeaker in a sound field.

The second main finding of this study compared the acceptable noise level with self-adjusted and audiologist-adjusted levels obtained in Chinese subjects with normal hearing. The ANL tests assess the subject's ability to accept noise, and the researchers speculate that acceptance of noise may be an intrinsic property of an individual [1]. The loci of control and self-control seem to influence acceptable noise levels [23]. The concept of locus of control was proposed by Rotter [24] and refers to a generalized expectation that the results of events are controlled by oneself (internal control) or external forces (external control). The former is the responsibility for the inherent traits of the individual (such as ability and effort), while the latter is the responsibility attributed to factors beyond their own (such as environmental factors and luck). Garstecki and Erler [25] found that the locus of control tends to be external in women, who are less likely to accept the use of hearing aid. Cox et al. [26] reported that personality characteristic had an impact on the assessment of their hearing aid in a subjective questionnaire. Patients with a high locus of external control are less suited to the noise environment. The ANL test results in our study showed that self-adjusted and audiologist-adjusted tests did not differ in the two types of presentation modes. There were also no significant differences in the interactions between the different presentation modes and response modes. Our results indicated that response modes as factors of external control and internal control may not affect the ANL tests, and the locus of control theory is not consistent with our results. This may be because the subjects who participated were not uniform in personality characteristic. If the subjects were grouped according to their personality characteristic, the ANL tests in our study may be different. Future research requires more detailed analysis.

This study has some weaknesses. First, the age of subjects was 20 to 30, so it is not possible to extrapolate the results to all age populations. Moreover, the younger age of the subjects in this study may cause smaller ANL values than seen in other studies. Secondly, the subjects in this study had a good education, and the influence of knowledge level was not studied in previous studies. Thirdly, our results are from subjects with normal hearing. This conclusion remains to be confirmed in the hearing-impaired subjects. Obviously, larger studies are needed to enable multiple variables to be controlled.

However, our research has several protective measures to minimize other potential limitations. When the same audiologist tested three measurements for the subjects, it is impossible for the audiologist to be completely blind to the previous ANL results. Therefore, we attempted to surmount this limitation by ensuring that there was a minimum of a 30 min gap between the two measurements and scheduling the audiologist to perform at least three further measurements on other subjects before repeating the test on that subject again. Moreover, each subject had at least a 30 min gap between each ANL test in each of the four methods, so that the learning effect had less impact on results.

5. Conclusion

In conclusion, ANL results obtained through a loudspeaker or earphones with the sound levels adjusted by the subjects themselves or by the audiologist are comparable. The results of correlation relationship for ANL under different methods could provide us the possibility of predicting one measurement based on the other. Clinically, the audiologist could select the appropriate method to conduct the ANL tests according to the facilities and the subjects' conditions.

Conflicts of Interest

The authors declare that there is no competing interest relevant to the publication of this paper.

Authors' Contributions

Liang Xia and Jingchun He contributed equally to this paper.

Acknowledgments

This study was supported by grants from the State Key Development Program for Basic Research of China (Grant no. 2014CB541705), the Shanghai Municipal Education Commission/Gaofeng Clinical Medicine Grant Support (Grant no. 20152526), the National Natural Science Foundation of China (Grant no. 81771015), and the Three-year Action Program on Promotion of Clinical Skills/Clinical Innovation for Municipal Hospitals (Grant no. 16CR4027A) to Yanmei Feng.

References

[1] A. K. Nabelek, F. M. Tucker, and T. R. Letowski, "Toleration of background noises: relationship with patterns of hearing aid use by elderly persons," *Journal of Speech and Hearing Research*, vol. 34, no. 3, pp. 679–685, 1991.

[2] K. L. Recker and C. Micheyl, "Speech intelligibility as a cue for acceptable noise levels," *Ear and Hearing*, vol. 38, no. 4, pp. 465–474, 2017.

[3] K. Jonas Brannstrom and S. O. Olsen, "The acceptable noise level and the pure-tone audiogram," *American Journal of Audiology*, vol. 26, no. 1, pp. 80–87, 2017.

[4] H. C. Ho, Y. H. Wu, S. H. Hsiao, E. Stangl, E. J. Lentz, and R. A. Bentler, "The equivalence of acceptable noise level (ANL) with English, Mandarin, and non-semantic speech: a study across the U.S. and Taiwan," *International Journal of Audiology*, vol. 52, no. 2, pp. 83–91, 2012.

[5] E. M. Adams, S. Gordon-Hickey, R. E. Moore, and H. Morlas, "Effects of reverberation on acceptable noise level measurements in younger and older adults," *International Journal of Audiology*, vol. 49, no. 11, pp. 832–838, 2010.

[6] Y. H. Wu, H. C. Ho, S. H. Hsiao, R. B. Brummet, and O. Chipara, "Predicting three-month and 12-month post-fitting real-world hearing-aid outcome using pre-fitting acceptable noise level (ANL)," *International Journal of Audiology*, vol. 55, no. 5, pp. 285–294, 2016.

[7] A. K. Nabelek, J. W. Tampas, and S. B. Burchfield, "Comparison of speech perception in background noise with acceptance of background noise in aided and unaided conditions," *Journal of Speech, Language, and Hearing Research*, vol. 47, no. 5, pp. 1001–1011, 2004.

[8] A. K. Nabelek, M. C. Freyaldenhoven, J. W. Tampas, S. B. Burchfield, and R. A. Muenchen, "Acceptable noise level as a predictor of hearing aid use," *Journal of the American Academy of Audiology*, vol. 17, no. 9, pp. 626–639, 2006.

[9] M. C. Freyaldenhoven, D. Fisher Smiley, R. A. Muenchen, and T. N. Konrad, "Acceptable noise level: reliability measures and comparison to preference for background sounds," *Journal of the American Academy of Audiology*, vol. 17, no. 9, pp. 640–648, 2006.

[10] S. O. Olsen, L. H. Nielsen, J. Lantz, and K. J. Brännström, "Acceptable noise level: repeatability with Danish and non-semantic speech materials for adults with normal hearing," *International Journal of Audiology*, vol. 51, no. 7, pp. 557–563, 2012.

[11] K. Jonas Brännström, J. Lantz, L. H. Nielsen, and S. Ø. Olsen, "Acceptable noise level with Danish, Swedish, and non-semantic speech materials," *International Journal of Audiology*, vol. 51, no. 3, pp. 146–156, 2011.

[12] K. J. Brännström, E. Zunic, A. Borovac, and T. Ibertsson, "Acceptance of background noise, working memory capacity, and auditory evoked potentials in subjects with normal hearing," *Journal of the American Academy of Audiology*, vol. 23, no. 7, pp. 542–552, 2012.

[13] K. J. Brännström, L. Holm, T. Kastberg, and S. Ø. Olsen, "The acceptable noise level: the effect of repeated measurements," *International Journal of Audiology*, vol. 53, no. 1, pp. 21–29, 2013.

[14] D. S. Rogers, A. W. Harkrider, S. B. Burchfield, and A. K. Nabelek, "The influence of listener's gender on the acceptance of background noise," *Journal of the American Academy of Audiology*, vol. 14, no. 7, pp. 372–82; quiz 401, 2003.

[15] A. W. Harkrider and S. B. Smith, "Acceptable noise level, phoneme recognition in noise, and measures of auditory efferent activity," *Journal of the American Academy of Audiology*, vol. 16, no. 8, pp. 530–545, 2005.

[16] S. Gordon-Hickey and R. E. Moore, "Influence of music and music preference on acceptable noise levels in listeners with normal hearing," *Journal of the American Academy of Audiology*, vol. 18, no. 5, pp. 417–427, 2007.

[17] S. Ø. Olsen and K. J. Brännström, "Does the acceptable noise level (ANL) predict hearing-aid use?," *International Journal of Audiology*, vol. 53, no. 1, pp. 2–20, 2013.

[18] J. Chen, H. Zhang, P. N. Plyler, W. Cao, and J. Chen, "Development and evaluation of the Mandarin speech signal content on the acceptable noise level test in listeners with normal hearing in mainland China," *International Journal of Audiology*, vol. 50, no. 6, pp. 354–360, 2011.

[19] C. A. Franklin Jr, J. W. Thelin, A. K. Nabelek, and S. B. Burchfield, "The effect of speech presentation level on acceptance of background noise in listeners with normal hearing," *Journal of the American Academy of Audiology*, vol. 17, no. 2, pp. 141–146, 2006.

[20] A. W. Harkrider and J. W. Tampas, "Differences in responses from the cochleae and central nervous systems of females with low versus high acceptable noise levels," *Journal of the American Academy of Audiology*, vol. 17, no. 9, pp. 667–676, 2006.

[21] M. C. Freyaldenhoven, P. N. Plyler, J. W. Thelin, and M. S. Hedrick, "The effects of speech presentation level on acceptance of noise in listeners with normal and impaired hearing," *Journal of Speech Language and Hearing Research*, vol. 50, no. 4, p. 878, 2007.

[22] G. Walker, H. Dillon, and D. Byme, "Sound field audiometry: recommended stimuli and procedures," *Ear and Hearing*, vol. 5, no. 1, pp. 13–21, 1984.

[23] A. C. Nichols and S. Gordon-Hickey, "The relationship of locus of control, self-control, and acceptable noise levels for young listeners with normal hearing," *International Journal of Audiology*, vol. 51, no. 4, pp. 353–359, 2012.

[24] J. B. Rotter, "Internal versus external control of reinforcement: a case history of a variable," *American Psychologist*, vol. 45, no. 4, pp. 489–493, 1990.

[25] D. C. Garstecki and S. F. Erler, "Hearing loss, control, and demographic factors influencing hearing aid use among older adults," *Journal of Speech, Language, and Hearing Research*, vol. 41, no. 3, pp. 527–537, 1998.

[26] R. M. Cox, G. C. Alexander, and G. Gray, "Personality and the subjective assessment of hearing aids," *Journal of the American Academy of Audiology*, vol. 10, no. 1, pp. 1–13, 1999.

11

Roles of Gasotransmitters in Synaptic Plasticity and Neuropsychiatric Conditions

Ulfuara Shefa,[1] Dokyoung Kim,[1,2] Min-Sik Kim,[3] Na Young Jeong,[4] and Junyang Jung[1,2,5]

[1]Department of Biomedical Science, Graduate School, Kyung Hee University, 26 Kyungheedae-ro, Dongdaemun-gu, Seoul 02447, Republic of Korea
[2]Department of Anatomy and Neurobiology, College of Medicine, Kyung Hee University, 26 Kyungheedae-ro, Dongdaemun-gu, Seoul 02447, Republic of Korea
[3]Department of Applied Chemistry, College of Applied Science, Kyung Hee University, Deogyeong-daero, Giheung-gu, Yongin-si, Gyeonggi-do 17104, Republic of Korea
[4]Department of Anatomy and Cell Biology, College of Medicine, Dong-A University, 32 Daesingongwon-ro, Seo-gu, Busan 49201, Republic of Korea
[5]East-West Medical Research Institute, Kyung Hee University, 26 Kyungheedae-ro, Dongdaemun-gu, 13 Seoul 02447, Republic of Korea

Correspondence should be addressed to Junyang Jung; jjung@khu.ac.kr

Academic Editor: Steven W. Johnson

Synaptic plasticity is important for maintaining normal neuronal activity and proper neuronal functioning in the nervous system. It is crucial for regulating synaptic transmission or electrical signal transduction to neuronal networks, for sharing essential information among neurons, and for maintaining homeostasis in the body. Moreover, changes in synaptic or neural plasticity are associated with many neuropsychiatric conditions, such as schizophrenia (SCZ), bipolar disorder (BP), major depressive disorder (MDD), and Alzheimer's disease (AD). The improper maintenance of neural plasticity causes incorrect neurotransmitter transmission, which can also cause neuropsychiatric conditions. Gas neurotransmitters (gasotransmitters), such as hydrogen sulfide (H_2S), nitric oxide (NO), and carbon monoxide (CO), play roles in maintaining synaptic plasticity and in helping to restore such plasticity in the neuronal architecture in the central nervous system (CNS). Indeed, the upregulation or downregulation of these gasotransmitters may cause neuropsychiatric conditions, and their amelioration may restore synaptic plasticity and proper neuronal functioning and thereby improve such conditions. Understanding the specific molecular mechanisms underpinning these effects can help identify ways to treat these neuropsychiatric conditions.

1. Introduction

The polish psychologist Konorski (1948) first used the term "synaptic plasticity" to describe consistent and activity-dependent changes in synaptic strength [1]. Synaptic plasticity is an experience-dependent change in synaptic strength [2]. Changes in synaptic strength are essential for information storage during memory formation [3], and recent work has revealed that synaptic plasticity also plays roles in other adaptive responses, including mood stability, drug addiction, and chronic pain [4]. The mechanisms underpinning synaptic plasticity are broadly linked to long-term memory. Synapse modifications are commonly monitored by two important phenomena: long-term potentiation (LTP) and long-term depression (LTD), which cause an increase or a reduction in synaptic strength, respectively. LTP and LTD also have roles in memory and learning [1]. Neurotransmitters are the chemical messengers that activate, amplify, and harmonize signals between neurons and other cells in the body. Neuronal functions rely on a balance between the number of relevant excitatory and inhibitory processes, which may happen individually or concomitantly [5].

The gas neurotransmitters (gasotransmitters) in our body include hydrogen sulfide (H_2S), nitric oxide (NO), and carbon monoxide (CO); they play essential roles in normal physiology and under pathological conditions. H_2S is a member of the gasotransmitter family that is associated with the maintenance of neuronal plasticity, excitability, and the central nervous system (CNS) [6]. *N*-Methyl-D-aspartate (NMDA) receptors are targets of H_2S in the brain; H_2S potentiates the activity of NMDA receptors and facilitates the induction of hippocampal LTP [7]. Hence, a recent study demonstrated that H_2S could reduce NMDA receptor-mediated currents in pyramidal neurons of the Cornu Ammonis (CA3) region of neonatal hippocampal slices [6]. NO is a ubiquitous signaling molecule in the brain as well as in other organs in the body, and many reviews have described its role in retrograde signaling [8], cellular function, synaptic plasticity [9], development, excitotoxicity, blood flow, and mental health [10]. NO inhibits the activity of NMDA receptors and thereby reduces the effects of glutamate and induces changes in neural transmission. A reduction in NMDA receptor (NMDAR) expression is associated with the change in synaptic plasticity driven by the age-related conditions in sensory input, demonstrating age-related impairment in the function of the NMDAR/NO signaling pathway in the CNS [11]. Physiologically, CO is generated by two heme oxygenases, hemeoxygenase-1 (HO-1) and hemeoxygenase-2 (HO-2), which catalyze the catabolism of heme groups [12]. HO-2 is concentrated in hippocampal pyramidal cells; therefore, CO might be a candidate retrograde messenger for LTP as the HO inhibitor zinc protoporphyrin IX (Znpp-9) blocks the induction of LTP in hippocampal slices [13].

In this review, we will briefly describe the role of synaptic plasticity in normal neuronal functioning or homeostasis and examine how alterations in neural plasticity hamper the release and signaling of neurotransmitters, such as H_2S, NO, and CO, to cause neuropsychiatric conditions, such as major depressive disorder (MDD), schizophrenia (SCZ), bipolar disorder (BD), and Alzheimer's disease (AD). We will also address how the upregulation or downregulation of these gasotransmitters affects disease progression. Finally, we will discuss therapeutic options and how, by understanding the pathways through which alterations in neural plasticity cause disorders, we can target the responsible molecules to prevent these neuropsychiatric conditions.

2. Synaptic Plasticity and Its Neurobiology

Synaptic plasticity in the mature nervous system includes structural and morphological modifications, such as dendritic spine growth and synaptogenesis [14]. These modifications are the cellular response to the changes in neuronal activity that are thought to be responsible for learning and memory [15]. The mitochondria present in axonal terminals and the dendrites of neurons play important roles in synaptic activity [16].

Various neurotransmitter receptors are functionally linked with protein kinases as well as other G-proteins that modulate cascades of molecules which in turn maintain essential cellular functions [17]. As an example, the mitogen-activated protein kinase- (MAPK-) related pathway activates transcription factors associated with learning, memory, and cell proliferation as well as apoptosis. This pathway intricates extracellular stimuli via the phosphorylation of c-Jun *N*-terminal kinase (JNK), extracellular signal-regulated kinase (ERK), and P38 as well as other kinases. Similarly, the MAPK-involved pathway and $3'$-$5'$-cyclic adenosine monophosphate- (cAMP-) associated pathway are also jointed to activate neurotransmitter receptors as well as modulate cellular functions via the activation of protein kinase A (PKA), exchange protein stimulated by cAMP (EPAC), and other molecules [18]. Modifications of the MAPK-and c-AMP-related signaling pathways may affect intracellular Ca^{2+} levels, neurotransmitter receptors, transcription factors, and the cross link between signaling pathways as well as other biological functions which is essential for neuroplasticity [19].

Structurally, synaptic plasticity involves the insertion into or the removal of α-amino-3-hydroxy-5-methyl-isoxazole-4-propanoic acid (AMPA) receptors from the postsynaptic membrane and the enlargement or shrinkage of the dendritic spines where most excitatory synapses (~90%) are located [20]. Functionally, synaptic plasticity is regarded as the LTP or LTD of synaptic strength, demonstrating changes in conductance via AMPA receptors (AMPARs) in the postsynaptic membrane. During the period of plasticity, NMDAR activation allows calcium ions (Ca^{2+}) to cross the postsynaptic membrane and initiate intracellular signaling cascades (Figure 1). These cascades trigger gene transcription, AMPAR trafficking via action dynamics, reorganization of the cytoskeleton, and enlargement or elimination of dendritic spines. The integrity of the synaptic structure, AMPAR trafficking, and dendritic spine dynamics are all pivotal for generating lasting synaptic plasticity changes (Figure 1) [20].

On the neurobiological level, learning and memory depend on regulated signaling processes at synapses as well as synaptic communication between neurons and other cellular partners. Molecular-level plasticity can be driven by increased expression of plasticity-related genes, such as brain-derived neurotrophic factor (BDNF), calcium/calmodulin kinase II (CaMKII), and cyclic AMP (cAMP) response element binding (CREB) protein, as well as by enhanced surface expression of glutamatergic AMPARs and NMDARs. The neurotrophin BDNF and its signaling partners are the main regulators of synaptic plasticity, a biological process that regulates synaptic strength via neuronal activity [21]. Different neuromodulatory factors affect neuronal plasticity such as BDNF which may serve as a real mediator rather than simply a modulator of synaptic plasticity and synaptic communication [21]. Moreover, BDNF and neurotransmitter signaling cascades can work together in close temporal association to induce immediate and guided effects on synaptic plasticity [22]. However, more attention has been given to BDNF because specifically interfering with BDNF-related signaling is a key strategy for initiating neuronal and functionally restorative treatments for neurological and psychiatric disorders [23].

AMPARs and NMDARs are the receptors that synergize at postsynaptic terminals to facilitate different forms

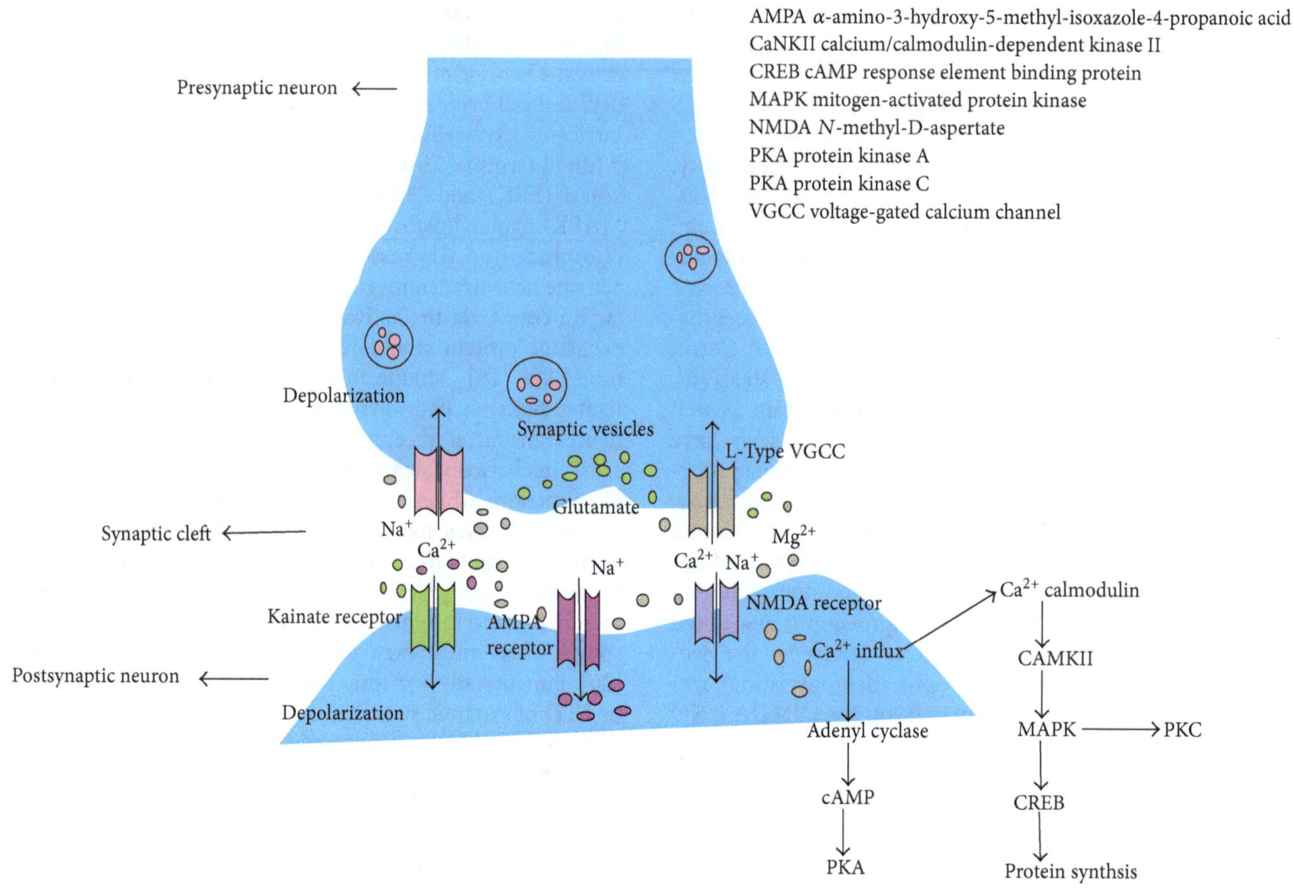

FIGURE 1: Transmission of signals through the synaptic junctions. Signals or impulses at the presynaptic terminal trigger the release of glutamate that binds to glutamate receptors at the postsynaptic membrane. Activation of α-amino-3-hydroxy-5-methyl-isoxazole-4-propanoic acid (AMPA) as well as kainate receptors which subsequently transport sodium ions that trigger postsynaptic depolarization. As membrane potential changes, it initiates the release of magnesium ions which blocks *N*-methyl-D-aspartate (NMDA) receptors. Influx of calcium via NMDA channels sets off a chain of events which establish long-term potentiation. Kainate receptors at the presynaptic end also seem to facilitate synaptic transmission at particular synapses by accumulating neurotransmitter release.

of synaptic plasticity (Figure 1). Constant activation of AMPARs by a series of impulses arriving at presynaptic terminals leads to depolarization of the presynaptic membrane, which removes the magnesium ions (Mg^{2+}) that are obstructed at NMDARs [24]. Hence, consistent with the Hebb hypothesis, the simultaneous excitation of pre- and postsynaptic neurons expedites the gating of NMDA channels and strengthens the synapse. This is a crucial feature of NMDA channels that is specifically associated with synaptic plasticity and its high permeability to calcium. Consequently, the second messenger calcium modulates a battery of signaling pathways and the responses that collectively elicit synaptic modification [25]. NMDARs are also involved in synaptic plasticity, but the situation is far more complex, as many forms of LTP are imparted by diverse inputs in various neurons. One intriguing case is that of activity-dependent synaptic plasticity, which is stimulated by presynaptic NMDA channels. In the lateral nucleus of the amygdala, neuronal activity induces a form of LTP that requires NMDARs but is independent of postsynaptic activity [26]. These observations suggest that NMDA functions, which are critical for learning and memory, are not limited to postsynaptic terminals [25].

Voltage-gated calcium channels (VGCCs) play roles in signal transduction between neurons as well as in various forms of synaptic plasticity. Interestingly, patients with AD express higher levels of L-type VGCC in the hippocampus compared with control subjects [27]. Activity-dependent neuroplastic mechanisms in the hippocampus that are fundamental to learning and memory, such as LTP, can be altered by the preceding synaptic activity. The concept of neuroplasticity has been implicated in various neurological and psychiatric diseases and conditions, including AD, depression, SCZ, aging, epilepsy, neurodevelopmental disorders, metabolic disorders, and neuroinflammation, such as multiple sclerosis (MS) [28].

In summary, various receptors and ion channels regulate synaptic plasticity, proper neural functioning, and neural homeostasis.

3. Gasotransmitters (H_2S, NO, and CO) in the Nervous System

Three main gasotransmitters that play crucial physiological roles in the body were discovered recently: H_2S,

CO, and NO. These gasotransmitters also have pathologic functions [29].

3.1. H_2S. H_2S is an essential signaling molecule with many homeostatic functions, such as neurotransmission and neuromodulation; it is also associated with learning, memory, and nociception [29]. *In vivo*, five enzymes are associated with H_2S synthesis: cystathionine β-synthase (CBS), 3-mercaptopyruvate sulfurtransferase (3-MST), cystathionine γ-lyase (CSE), cysteine aminotransferase (CAT), and D-amino acid oxidase (DAAO) [30]. CBS is thought to be the major H_2S-producing enzyme in the brain [31].

Novel signaling molecules linked to polysulfide (H_2S_n) such as hydrogen persulfide and trisulfide (H_2S_2 and H_2S_3) help maintain neuronal transmission, vascular tone, cytoprotection, inflammation, and oxygen-sensing. A recent study reported that H_2S_2, H_2S_3, and H_2S are generated by 3-MST [32]. H_2S_2 and H_2S_3 are also produced via an interaction between H_2S and NO. H_2S_n performs additional physiological functions, such as stimulating transient receptor potential ankyrin 1 (TRPA1) channels to impart Ca^{2+} influx in astrocytes [33, 34] and dorsal root ganglion (DRG) neurons [35]. Additionally, H_2S_2 along with H_2S_3 shields neuronal cells from oxidative as well as carbonyl stresses through exerting reduced synthesis of glutathione, which is dependent on the nuclear factor erythroid 2-related factor 2 (Nrf2) [36]. Hylin and Wood demonstrated that cysteine residues in proteins can be persulfurated in the presence of 3-mercaptopyruvate (3-MP), a substrate of 3-MST [37]. Another potential mechanism of persulfuration involves H_2S_2 and H_2S_3 generated by 3-MST, which promptly interact with free cysteine and glutathione (GSH) to generate cysteine-persulfide (Cys-SSH) and glutathione-persulfide (GSSH) and also react with the cysteine residues in proteins to produce persulfurated proteins. Alternatively, 3-MST can transfer sulfur from 3-MP to cysteine, GSH, H_2S, and cysteine residues to generate Cys-SSH, GSSH, H_2S_2, and persulfurated proteins. It is possible that these pathways proceed together to generate persulfurated species [38].

H_2S accelerates the initiation of hippocampal LTP, which is a synaptic model of memory development, by increasing the function of NMDARs [7]. CBS is expressed in the brain, and the neuronal activity of H_2S stimulates the flow of Ca^{2+} between astrocytes and neurons to adjust synaptic function [39]. The responses of astrocytes to H_2S are suppressed by wide-spectrum transient receptor potential (TRP) channel blockers, lanthanide ions (La^{3+}), gadolinium ion (Gd^{3+}), and ruthenium red (RR). In a 2013 study, Kimura et al. showed that polysulfide induces Ca^{2+} inflow by stimulating transitory receptor potential TRPA1 channels in rat astrocytes [33]. The optimum activity was imparted at 0.5 μM, which is 1/130 of the concentration of H_2S needed to obtain feedback of similar magnitude. Additionally, TRPA1-specific agonists, allyl isothiocyanate, and cinnamaldehyde induced Ca^{2+} inflow, whereas responses to polysulfides were suppressed by the TRAP1-specific inhibitors HC-030031 and AP-18 as well as by TRAP1-specific small interfering RNA (siRNA). This study demonstrated that polysulfides are required for the H_2S-derived signaling molecules that activate TRP channels in the brain [33].

Kimura demonstrated that exogenous H_2S expedites the induction of hippocampal LTP by increasing NMDAR activity [40]. For example, an H_2S donor enhanced NMDAR-mediated currents in the entorhinal cortex and the potentiating effect of exogenous H_2S on NMDAR-dependent LTP has been revealed that physiological role of endogenous sulfhydration in plasticity [41]. Another recent study identified a crucial role for activity-dependent sulfhydration in D-serine-dependent synaptic plasticity. Specifically, neuronal activity facilitated H_2S production and sulfhydrated serine racemase (SR) formation, and use of an H_2S donor enhanced hippocampal D-serine availability, expedited hippocampal LTP via a D-serine-dependent pathway, and slowed age-related LTP impairment [41]. In this study, H_2S levels and SR sulfhydration were reduced significantly in aged rats. As H_2S is an important reducing agent, these changes restored D-serine levels in the hippocampus of aged rats and replenished the deficits in D-serine-dependent plasticity. Additionally, endogenous H_2S signals protected against the age-associated impairment of synaptic plasticity [41]. The results of this study suggest that H_2S-linked sulfhydration plays an essential role in D-serine-dependent synaptic plasticity, probably by regulating SR activation. Therefore, therapies that involve inhaled H_2S or compounds that moderately raise brain H_2S levels may be effective for the treatment of age-associated memory impairment [41].

3.2. NO. NO is regarded as a chemical transmitter which has essential functions in the mammalian central as well as peripheral nervous system [42]. NO is a gaseous molecule that can passively cross cell membranes via diffusion. It is generated by the conversion of the amino acid L-arginine into L-citrulline via the enzyme NO synthase (NOS) and inducible NOS (iNOS). Constitutive nitric oxide synthase (cNOS), or type I, is the neuronal NOS (nNOS), and it is expressed at high levels in the brain, especially in the cortex [43]. Additionally, type III or endothelial NOS (eNOS) is expressed in the endothelium. cNOS generates low levels of NO (nM range) for a short duration (seconds–minutes) under regular physiological conditions because it needs to bind to calmodulin, which occurs only while local calcium levels are increased [43].

NO is the second mediator that can activate NMDARs, which are a subtype of glutamatergic receptors [44]. NMDARs are related to the NO system. NMDAR activation persistently enhances the activity of neuronal nitric oxide synthase (nNOS) in the neuronal cytoplasm. It then catalyzes the generation of endogenous NO from L-arginine followed by the enhanced release of NO from neurons [45, 46]. Activation of these receptors by glutamate stimulates the calcium influx into cells and the generation of NO by NOS, which rapidly stimulates guanylate cyclase and increases cyclic guanosine monophosphate (cGMP) synthesis [47]. The concentration of NO reflects glutamatergic neurotransmission [48]. Hence, other glutamate receptors, such as AMPA, can also produce NO; this pathway modulates the release of glutamate and dopamine. AMPARs are important ion channels that have four subunits that operate like NMDARs, such as Glu1–4 or GluA-D [49]. Nevertheless, AMPAR trafficking, expression, and S-nitrosylation activity are maintained by NO. An ATPase named *N*-ethylmaleimide-sensitive factor (NSF) is enriched in neurons which binds with GluR2, stabilizing or recycling AMPARs with postsynaptic membranes [50]. Physiologically, synaptic NSF is S-nitrosylated by endogenous, neuronally derived NO in the mouse brain. Activation of NMDAR increases the binding of NSF to GluR2, as well as the surface insertion of GluR2. Together, these studies revealed a NO-sensitive pathway involving NMDARs and AMPARs. In particular, NMDARs stimulate NO generation, which enhances NSF S-nitrosylation, stimulates its association with GluR2, and increases the surface expression of GluR2-containing AMPARs. However, the direct S-nitrosylation activity of AMPARs has not been studied [50]. Additionally, NO is associated with the storage, uptake, and release of mediators, such as acetylcholine, noradrenaline, gamma amino butyric acid (GABA), taurine, and a glycine [51]. NO can stimulate its own extrasynaptic receptors, which are located some distance from sites of NO synthesis. In addition, NO is associated with the process of development of the nervous system [8]. For example, nNOS-containing neurons actively participate in the rostral path of neuroblast migration, which involves new synaptic connections and influences neurogenesis [52]. Astrocyte migration is also regulated by the release of NO under the actions of iNOS. NO is also recognized as critical for the formation of synapses and the growth of nerve fibers [53].

3.3. CO. CO is a new gaseous neuromodulatory agent that functions as a neurotransmitter or neuromodulator [54]. CO is produced during heme metabolism by HO-1 and HO-2; HO-1 is an inducible enzyme, and HO-2 is constitutively expressed. HO is the enzyme responsible for CO synthesis *in vivo*; it catalyzes the metabolism of heme to biliverdin, free iron, and CO [55]. There are three distinct HO isoforms: HO-1, HO-2, and HO-3. Of these, HO-1 and HO-2 are the most studied and best known [56] and are expressed in many tissues, including neural tissue [57]. The CO generated from heme by HO stimulates soluble guanylate cyclase activity, which promotes an increase in cGMP in neurons as well as cardiovascular functions [58]. CO may also have involved in biological activities via alternative pathways, such as the activation of cyclooxygenase, which participates in fever generation by acting on the CNS [54]. In the CNS, the CO/heme oxygenase axis plays a vital role in processes associated with cytoprotection, vasomodulation, neuroinflammation, cell death, metabolism, and cellular redox responses [59]. CO was first recognized as a neurotransmitter by Verma et al. [60]. Their research led to broad investigations into CO, heme oxygenase, and the exogenous administration of CO as a method of imparting neuroprotection and regulating tissue homeostasis in response to pathophysiological conditions, such as cerebral ischemia, cerebrovasodilation, and neurodegenerative diseases [61]. In neurons, CO-induced cGMP generation helps protect from cell death, and NO signaling is associated with the anti-inflammatory effects of CO in microglia [62].

Semiquantitative cytokine profiling of cell lysates and conditioned culture medium demonstrated increased vascular endothelial growth factor (VEGF) levels in CO-treated cultures (cell lysates) compared with controls. This is consistent with other experiments describing that CO increases VEGF levels in astrocytes and cardiomyocytes [63]. Surprisingly, a decrease in neurotrophin-3 and an increase in neurotrophin-4 levels were found in lysates from cells treated with CO. Although no studies have assessed the effects of CO treatment on neurotrophin-3 and neurotrophin-4, both neurotrophins are associated with neuronal growth and synapse formation, maturation, and plasticity. Additionally, neurotrophin-3 is expressed in neural stem cells (NSCs), and it stimulates neuronal differentiation and survival [62].

In conclusion, various gasotransmitters, such as H_2S, NO, and CO, have potential roles in maintaining synaptic plasticity in the nervous system.

4. Role of Gasotransmitters in Neuropsychiatric Disease

4.1. MDD. MDD is a lifelong catastrophic mental disorder with high rates of morbidity and mortality [64]. The lifelong chronic–recurrent persistence of MDD is associated with very high economic and social burdens [65]. It is expected to be the second leading cause of disability worldwide by the World Health Organization (WHO) by 2020 [66]. The two gasotransmitters such as H_2S and NO are found to have some functions in MDD.

4.1.1. MDD and H_2S. H_2S is a toxic gas characterized by the smell of rotten eggs. Physiological concentrations of H_2S selectively increase NMDAR-induced responses as well as the advantageous induction of LTP [7]. One study demonstrated that H_2S can help maintain amygdala-dependent emotional memory by increasing the function of GluN2B-expressing NMDARs in the amygdala of rats [67]. Pathophysiological concentrations (200 pM) of sodium hydrogen sulfate (NaHS), an H_2S donor, stimulates seizure-like events in rats *in vivo* and *in vitro*, which may be due to increased neuronal excitation [68]. Previous studies indicated that H_2S might improve depressive and anxiety-related behaviors in nonstressed rats and mice, but the effects of H_2S on MDD animal models and the potential mechanism behind these effects are unknown [69]. To understand the actions and underlying mechanisms of H_2S related to depressive-like behavior, a recent study (intraperitoneally) injected the H_2S donor NaHS or administered inhaled H_2S in a chronic unpredictable mild stress (CUMS) model. The role of the mechanistic target of rapamycin (mTOR) signaling pathway and glutamate receptors (Figure 2) in the antidepressant effects of H_2S was evaluated [70]. The results indicated that a deficiency in endogenous H_2S in the hippocampus is responsible for the abnormal behaviors associated with CUMS, whereas enhancing hippocampal H_2S levels by the administration of NaHS or inhalation of H_2S could correct the depressive-like behaviors of rats within a few hours. This suggests that H_2S could function as a rapid-onset antidepressant. Additionally, H_2S could counteract the loss of

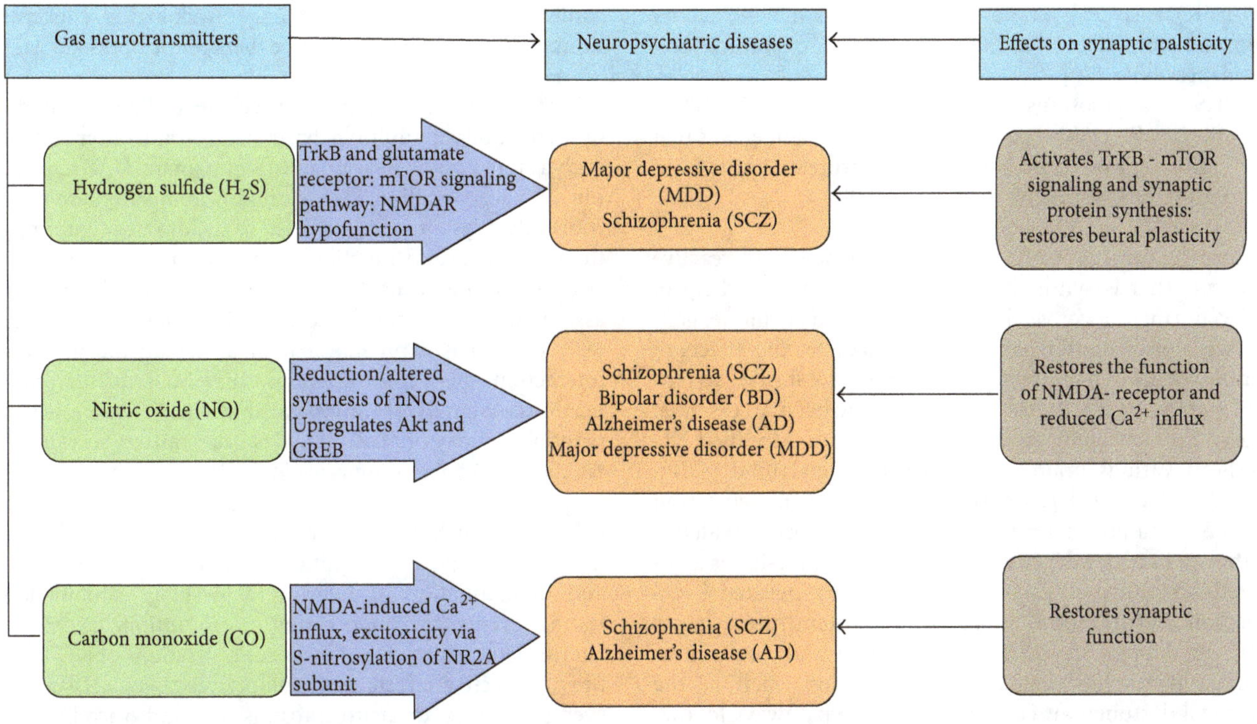

FIGURE 2: Role of gas neurotransmitters in neuropsychiatric diseases. The three gas neurotransmitters such as hydrogen sulfide (H_2S), nitric oxide (NO), and carbon dioxide (CO) have a role in neuropsychiatric conditions such as major depressive disorder (MDD), schizophrenia (SCZ), bipolar disorder (BD), and Alzheimer's disease (AD) to maintain proper synaptic plasticity as well as neural homeostasis. H_2S has a role in tropomyosin receptor kinase B (TrKB) and glutamate as well as mechanistic targets of rapamycin (mTOR) signaling pathways, and it activates the TrKB-mTOR signaling pathway as well as synaptic protein in MDD. NO has a role in the regulation of altered synthesis of nNOS as well as upregulates Akt and cyclic AMP (cAMP) response element binding (CREB) protein which restores function in *N*-methyl-D aspartate (NMDA) receptor and reduces Ca^{2+} influx in schizophrenia, MDD, and AD. CO has a role in NMDA-induced calcium ion (Ca^{2+}) influx or excitotoxicity via S-nitrosylation of antiglutamate receptor NMDAR2A (NR2A) subunit and restores synaptic function in AD and SCZ. However, these gas neurotransmitters work on various ways to maintain or restore synaptic plasticity in these neuropsychiatric diseases.

dendritic spines in the hippocampus that is associated with CUMS [70].

BDNF induces traditional antidepressant actions, and BDNF deletion in the hippocampus weakens antidepressant behavioral responses [71]. Some studies demonstrated that H_2S reversed the decrease in tropomyosin receptor kinase B (TrKB) receptors induced by CUMS, demonstrating the pivotal role of neurotrophic signaling in the antidepressant effects of H_2S. These findings are consistent with observations that H_2S exerted neuroprotective effects against formaldehyde-induced toxicity in PC12 cells via the BDNF–TrKB pathway [72]. This suggests that the synaptogenesis induced by glutamate receptor activation requires the release of BDNF to activate TrKB-mTOR signaling and synaptic protein synthesis (Figure 2). In another study, it was unclear whether the peripheral effects of H_2S played a role in the antidepressant responses; thus, additional studies are needed [70]. Nevertheless, this study also demonstrated that the acute application of H_2S, via either the H_2S donor NaHS or H_2S gas inhalation, induced robust antidepressant effects that were mediated by activation of the mechanistic target of rapamycin complex 1 (mTORC1) signaling pathway followed by the enhanced synthesis of synaptic proteins containing postsynaptic density protein 95 (PSD95) and synaptophysin. H_2S also increases the levels of TrKB receptors, which further increases the activity of the GluR1 and GluR2 subunits of AMPARs. An improved understanding of the roles of H_2S could provide insight into potential therapeutic interventions for depression [70].

Ketamine is a noncompetitive blocker of NMDAR that also stimulates the mTOR signaling pathway and subsequently increases the synthesis of the proteins involved in synapses to induce fast-acting antidepressant effects [73]. A study on ketamine-induced antidepressant effects provided an opportunity to explore the ability of new antidepressants with rapid-acting effects to provide sustained relief and fewer side effects. Various studies have demonstrated a link between H_2S and the mTOR signaling pathway. A recent study demonstrated that H_2S could decrease smoking-induced autophagic cell death by activating mTOR [74]. A novel H_2S-releasing molecule GYY4137 (water-soluble, slow-releasing H_2S donor) likely protected against high glucose-induced cytotoxicity by activating the mTOR signaling pathway in H9C2 (embryonic cardiomyocyte cell line) cells [75]. Additionally, H_2S ameliorated hepatic ischemia/reperfusion injury by stimulating phosphorylation of the pyruvate dehydrogenase kinase 1 (PDK-1)/Akt (protein kinase B)/mTOR/70 kDa ribosomal protein S6 kinase (p70S6K) axis [76]. The effects of H_2S on mTOR activation are consistent with the mechanism of rapid-onset antidepressants [70].

H_2S is a gasotransmitter that activates the TrKB or mTOR signaling pathways to exert antidepressant effects that are indirectly associated with synaptic protein synthesis or restoration of synaptic plasticity in MDD.

4.1.2. MDD and NO. NO is a highly diffusible and reactive molecule that is synthesized and released with the help of NOSs during the conversion of arginine into citrulline, generating NO in the process [77]. NO mediates the effects of various neurotransmitters, such as norepinephrine, serotonin, glutamate, and dopamine, and thereby plays an essential role in the neurobiology of major depression. Modified NO levels in various brain regions, cerebrospinal fluid (CSF), blood, and exhaled gas have been reported in depression [78]. A meta-analysis revealed disorders in neurooxidative pathways in major depression [79]. Major depression is associated with nitrosative stress, as marked by elevated iNOS function and nitration, as well as by protein nitrosylation [80]. In depression, both neurooxidative and neuronitrative pathways may cause neuroprogression, such as the neuronal dysfunctions caused by oxidative pathways following enhanced neurotoxicity and cytotoxicity, disorders in synaptic plasticity, and reduced neuroprotection [81].

Postmortem studies of patients with MDD revealed reduced neuronal NO synthase levels in the locus coeruleus and a lower number of density of NO synthase-immunoreactive neurons in the hypothalamic nuclei of patients compared with healthy controls [82]. When peripheral NO levels were measured in MDD, some studies reported increased levels [83], whereas other studies found no change [84]. In medication-free depression, various studies found reduced NO levels [85]. In MDD, NO levels were reduced in drug-free patients experiencing depressive episodes in one study [85], but they were either increased or unchanged in another study [84]. Lu et al. demonstrated that NO levels were much higher in MDD patients but then decreased after antidepressant treatment. In the same study, the levels of amino acids, such as citrulline and arginine, were estimated as an index of NO synthesis [78]. In another study, elevated plasma NO levels were reported in male rat models of chronic and unpredictable stress as well as in first-episode MDD patients [86]. The plasma levels of NO metabolites, such as nitrite and nitrate, which reflect plasma NO levels, are also increased in depression [84]. One study described that elevated plasma NO levels in melancholic MDD patients are persistent [78]. This is consistent with previous reports, which also found increased NO plasma levels in MDD patients [87]. Additionally, the elevated NO plasma levels may be associated with suicide attempts in these patients. Modified glutamatergic and decreased GABAergic activity and NO neurotransmission were reported in various brain systems in depression, and this may have a critical effect on the neuronal functions associated with stress responses and mood maintenance [78].

NO is an essential gasotransmitter for neuronal homeostasis, and its upregulation is linked with MDD found in some studies above. Maintaining physiological concentrations of NO could be an effective therapeutic option in MDD.

4.2. SCZ. SCZ is a complex psychiatric illness caused by dysregulation of multiple brain neurotransmitter systems, such as those involving dopamine, glutamate, GABA, serotonin, and acetylcholine. Hence, modifications to these neurotransmitter systems [88] have led to hypotheses centering on the expression and functions of neurotransmitter receptors as critical elements of the pathophysiology of this condition; assimilation of signaling mediated by various neurotransmitter receptors is a pivotal step in achieving the functional interactions of receptor activation [89]. Subsequently, modifications of signal integration pathways may have a role to the pathophysiology of SCZ [88]. Gasotransmitters such as H_2S, NO, and CO have some roles in SCZ.

4.2.1. SCZ and NO. NO is associated with synaptic plasticity, neural plasticity, and cognition [90]. It bolsters the survival and differentiation of neurons as well as exhibits long-lasting events by maintaining transcription factors and altering gene expression. Lower concentrations of NO induce neuroprotective effects and support physiological signaling events, leading to neurotransmission and vasodilatation. In contrast, higher concentrations promote inflammatory effects and are neurotoxic [91]. It was hypothesized that NO could act as a retrograde messenger at synapses, transmitting signals from target neurons back to the synapses and maintaining synaptic plasticity. These same characteristics also allow NO to signal to any local compartment and to cells with defective synaptic activity and NOS expression [92]. Recent evidence revealed roles for NO and related molecules in the pathogenesis of SCZ. Changes in various effects of NO in CNS development may result in neurodevelopmental changes involved in SCZ [92]. NO is associated with many processes in the brain, such as the maintenance of synaptic plasticity, the release of mediators, and the development of nervous tissue [93].

Russian scientists Averbukh et al. (1966) and Bulba et al. (1968) first hypothesized that NO was involved in the onset of SCZ [94]. Studies reporting elevated levels of NO in the postmortem brain tissue [95] and plasma [96] of patients with SCZ also support a link between NOS activity and SCZ. The amount of nNOS differs in patients with SCZ and healthy controls [97]; yet, this issue is conflicted. The nNOS levels in the cortex of the cerebelli of patients with SCZ did not differ from the levels found in those of healthy controls in a study performed by Doyle and Slater in 1995 [98]. In another study, enhanced NO synthase activity was detected in Purkinje cells and the dentate nucleus of patients with SCZ but not with depression [99]. However, data regarding the presence of NOS in the neocortex are inconsistent [100]. Although the upregulated expression of nNOS was reported in the prefrontal cortex in SCZ [100], contrasting data have also been published. Striking data were carried out in the period of investigations of neurons of hypothalamus. The downregulation of nNOS-containing neurons was reported in the periventricular nucleus of patients with SCZ and affective disorders [101]. It was reported that NO in the hypothalamus maintains the synthesis and release of the hormones that maintain the hypothalamic–pituitary–adrenal system (HPAS), including oxytocin, vasopressin, and corticoliberin. The altered production and release of these peptides leads to hyperactivation of HPAS in patients with SCZ [102].

NO levels have also been measured in biological fluids from SCZ patients. The level of NOS and its metabolites in the blood of patients with SCZ and depression has been assessed in many studies, and the results are conflicting [92]. A meta-analysis performed by Maia-de-Oliveira et al. found no significant difference in the NO levels of patients with SCZ and healthy controls. However, higher levels of NO were found in patients treated with antipsychotics, highlighting the influence of these drugs on the metabolism of NOS [103]. Therefore, the enhanced formation of NO does not seem to be caused by NMDARs. This suggests that AMPARs likely play an important role, especially as they are expressed at high levels in patients with SCZ [104]. The subsequent release of NO results in disturbed synaptogenesis and synaptic remodeling as well as in synaptic membrane modification [105].

Antipsychotics modify NO metabolism in the brain. For example, haloperidol suppresses nNOS activity [106]. Hence, the long-term administration of this drug results in nNOS hyperactivity in the striatum of rats [107]. The authors of this study demonstrated that late modification of nNOS activity in the neostriatum during antipsychotic treatment plays an important role in the pathogenesis of late dyskinesia. It is worth repeating that nNOS activity is higher in the plasma of patients with SCZ receiving antipsychotics compared with healthy controls [103]. These studies call into question the influence of nNOS activity in the brains of patients with SCZ [108]. The effects of antipsychotics on other NOS isoforms have also been studied. Clozapine can prevent iNOS activity and reduce microglial inflammation and NO levels in the brain [109]. The effects of antipsychotics on NO metabolism restore the normal function of NMDARs [92].

In summary, SCZ is a neuropsychiatric disorder in which normal synaptic plasticity is hampered. NO plays important roles in maintaining synaptic functions and synaptic plasticity in account of maintaining proper neuronal functioning.

4.2.2. SCZ, H_2S, and CO. CBS-derived H_2S is needed for amygdalar synaptic plasticity and fear conditioning in rats. In particular, inhibiting the function of amygdalar CBS prevented activity-stimulated H_2S production, blocked LTP initiation, and altered cued fear memory in rats [110]. Treatment with an H_2S donor corrected the LTP and memory impairments caused via CBS inhibition. This CBS inhibition was related to the maintenance of NMDAR function, as the NMDAR-supported synaptic response was lower when CBS was inhibited and the use of a H_2S donor increased the amplitude of the NMDAR EPSPs (5-enolpyruvylshikimate-3-phosphate) to a level comparable to those of the normal controls. This suggests that H_2S homeostasis in the brain is critical for the generation of synaptic plasticity and memory. S-Adenosylmethionine (SAM) stimulates CBS activity; it combines with the regulatory C-terminal domain of CBS to activate the generation of endogenous H_2S. Nevertheless, the mechanisms by which CBS inhibition alters amygdalar synaptic plasticity and memory require further investigation. Activation of NMDAR modulates synaptic plasticity, learning, and memory, and NMDAR hypofunction (Figure 2) was linked to cognitive deficits in aging as well as other psychiatric disorders, such as SCZ [110].

One study showed that prenatal exposure to CO leads to a variety of neurological effects. Lower concentrations of CO lead to a variety of neurobehavioral disorders in rat offspring. Prenatal CO exposure also hampers various neurotransmitters in the growing brains of male rats; low concentrations altered the mesolimbic dopaminergic function and sexual behavior [111]. Changes in cerebellar catecholamines linked these changes to deficits in motor test performance, learning, and memory, as determined by the reduced total GABA content in the cerebelli of 10-day-old rats exposed to CO prenatally. This suggests that GABAergic neurons may have a specific role in CO toxicity. Another study demonstrated that GABAergic neurons may be specifically vulnerable to CO toxicity. Therefore, GABA signaling is modified in neurological disorders, such as SCZ [111]. HO-1 expression in SCZ can be increased by oxidative and inflammatory stimuli [112]. The selective overexpression of HO-1 in the astrocytes of transgenic mice resulted in oxidative stress, lower neuronal reelin content, increased dopamine and serotonin concentrations in the basal ganglia, decreased D1 receptor binding in the nucleus acumens, and altered hippocampal cytoarchitectures. These pathological changes were related to enhanced co-motor activity and reduced proton pump inhibitors but did not affect anxiety or motor balance [113].

H_2S and CO have a potential role in neuronal homeostasis, and maintaining proper amounts of these gasotransmitters is a crucial factor in case of SCZ.

4.3. BD. BD is a severe neuropsychiatric condition that results in repeated episodes of mania, which are pathologically energized states characterized by poor judgment, euphoria, irritability, and in depressive episodes, which are characterized by dispiriting moods, decreased energy, volitional states, and decreased cognitive capacity [114]. The gasotransmitter NO is related to the BD which is briefly discussed below.

4.3.1. BD and NO. Modified NO signaling, which directly affects neurotransmitter release and synaptic plasticity cascades, has been demonstrated in BD. Lithium maintains NO levels in preclinical models. However, the effects of lithium ion NO levels have not been studied in humans [115]. Upregulated NO levels were reported during various mood states [116], particularly depressive episodes [117]. The NO pathway is particularly important in neuropsychiatric disorders. Altered NO levels affect neurotransmitter release [90] and synaptic plasticity [118]. High concentrations of NO have dose-dependent neurotoxic effects, whereas physiological concentrations play neuromodulatory and neuroprotective roles [91]. The neuroprotective effects of NO include reducing Ca^{2+} influx and subsequent cell death (Figure 2) [119]. Additionally, NO upregulates the expression of the neuroprotective proteins Akt and CREB (Figure 2) [120] and the potent antioxidant bilirubin [121].

NO effects are persistent with neuroprotective as well as neurotrophic roles of lithium [122]. Lithium is the standard and first-line treatment option for BD [123]. Its mechanism of action is complex and involves multiple intracellular signaling pathways. Various animal studies have revealed that lithium maintains central and peripheral NO levels [124] and significantly increases NO levels in BD depression after 6 weeks of treatment. However, there was no marked difference in NO levels between unmedicated BD patients and matched healthy controls [122]. These experiments suggest that NO levels may be maintained by lithium in humans. Along these lines, an increasing body of preclinical evidence suggests that lithium can directly target NO signaling [124]. For example, lithium upregulates *NOS* messenger RNA (mRNA) expression in glial cultured cells [125], the hypothalamus [126], and the hippocampus [127] and also increases cortical NO metabolites in rodents. Other preclinical studies showed that lithium reduces NO metabolites [128] in rat neural tissues [129]. The upregulated NO levels were not associated with clinical improvement, increasing the possibility that the effects of lithium ion NO may be an epiphenomenon or an intermediate pathway for the antidepressant effect [115].

In a recent study, the plasma NO levels in BD patients did not differ from those of healthy controls [115]. In terms of mood disorders, studies on NO have yielded mixed results. At the same time, several studies reported enhanced NO levels in BD [116], and another study that analyzed NO levels during a depressive episode in BD [117] showed elevated NO metabolite levels in subjects with BD receiving multiple medications that can influence NO [103]. The fact that the sample contained drug-free patients with a short duration of illness means that it is possible that NO plays a more important role in BD late in the course of the illness, after patients have been exposed to chronic insults such as repetitive episodes, medications, and comorbidities. Additionally, the number of previous mood episodes was positively correlated with NO levels in BD [130]. These studies may support a crucial role for NO signaling in the trophic and neuroprotective effects of lithium in BD and other neuropsychiatric disorders [115].

In conclusion, the gasotransmitter NO plays a pivotal role in maintaining neural plasticity and proper neuronal functioning in the service of preserving the activity of the CNS in BD.

4.4. AD. AD is characterized by the loss of neurons and synapses in the hippocampus, cerebral cortex, and subcortical regions, as well as the formation of amyloid beta (Aβ) plaques and neurofibrillary lesions. The main protein component of plaques is amyloid-β, which is derived from the proteolytic cleavage of amyloid precursor protein (APP). Mutations associated with early-onset of familial AD increase Aβ production. Aβ isolated directly from human AD brains caused impaired synaptic plasticity and memory in rodents [131]. Synaptic activity and chronic sleep restriction increase the amount of Aβ in brain and intestinal fluid, as well as plaque formation in APP transgenic mice [132]. AD is related with some gasotransmitters such as CO and NO, which is discussed briefly in the following subsections.

4.4.1. AD and CO. As discussed above, mammalian tissues express two isoforms of heme oxygenase: HO-1 and HO-2. The third isoform, HO-3, is a retrotransposition of the *HO-2* gene and is only found in rats [133]. The basal expression of HO-1 in the normal brain is restricted to small groups of scattered neurons and neuroglia [134], whereas HO-2 is more broadly expressed across the neuraxis [60]. HO-1 is a 32 kDa protein that catalyzes the breakdown of heme to free iron, CO, and biliverdin. In "stressed" astroglia, HO-1 hyperactivity stimulates mitochondrial iron sequestration and macroautophagy, which may be responsible for the pathological iron accumulation and bioenergetic failure observed in AD as well as in other neurodevelopmental conditions. The expression of glial HO-1 may also affect neuroplasticity and cell survival by modulating the brain sterol metabolism and the proteasomal deterioration of neurotoxic proteins [135].

HO-1 immunoreactivity in glia increases progressively as aging progresses in the normal human brain [136]. HO-1 deteriorates as neural tissue senesces, which may be responsible for the biogenesis of the corpora amylacea and glycoprotein-rich inclusions generally encountered in aging mammalian cells [137]. The number of glial fibrillary acid protein- (GFAP-) positive astrocytes that express HO-1 is increased significantly in the hippocampus and cerebral cortex of patients with AD compared with age-matched, nondemented controls. An excessive increase in glial HO-1 levels is already apparent in the brains of subjects with mild cognitive impairment (MCI), which is a common precursor or indication of incipient AD [138]. In the temporal cortex of patients with MCI, the number of astrocytes with immunoreactivity for HO-1 is related to the degree of neurofibrillary pathology and also the reductions in scores on tests of global cognition, episodic memory, semantic memory, and working memory. Similarly, HO-1 expression in astroglia is associated with lower scores for global cognition, perceptual speed, and semantic memory.

Elevated CO is found in the above studies in AD, and regulating physiological levels of CO could be a therapeutic option in case of AD.

4.4.2. AD and NO. Deficits in synaptic plasticity are increasingly recognized as causes of memory loss in AD [139]. However, the early mechanisms driving synaptic pathophysiology are poorly understood. Short-term plasticity and long-term plasticity are calcium-dependent processes that can be altered by second messengers, such as NO. NO is produced by NOS via NMDAR-mediated calcium entry [140]. NO signaling is involved in neurodegenerative diseases via the formation of reactive nitrogen species and cGMP signaling cascades [141]. NO also has neuroprotective effects, as shown in AD mouse models in which it reduces cell loss and tau pathology [142]. In AD models, NO can be altered via various mechanisms. For example, the NMDAR-mediated calcium entry that activates NOS is augmented by abnormal ryanodine receptor- (RyR-) mediated calcium-induced calcium release [143]. NOS protein levels and RyR levels are also increased in both AD mouse models and human AD brains [144]. In presynaptic AD mice, these conditions that amplify NO levels occur alongside exaggerated hippocampal synaptic depression. These deficits occur when homeostasis is challenged, such as in the presence of reduced RyR-calcium release. Although the hippocampal network and cognitive performance appear normal, they clearly are not [145].

In one study, the primary site of NO regulation in 3×-Tg-AD mice was the presynaptic terminals, where it increased evoked and spontaneous vesicle release, as determined by PPF assays and spontaneous vesicle-release properties [146]. In this study, NO could increase transmitter release via cGMP signaling as well as the S-nitrosylation of synaptic proteins, which increases the presynaptic binding of syntaxin to VAMP and SNAPZS [147]. NO also alters the magnitude of vesicular release by converting reserve pool vesicles into easily releasable vesicles [148]. NO can also increase RyR channel opening, possibly via S-nitrosylation. The opposing interactions between enhanced RyR-calcium signaling and increased nNOS expression in AD neurons can sustain enhanced NO production or synthesis and also increase presynaptic gain. Postsynaptically, the neuroprotective characteristics of NO curb the excessive NMDAR-induced calcium influx and excitotoxicity by causing S-nitrosylation of the antiglutamate receptor NMDAR2A (NR2A) subunit (Figure 2). At the same time, the S-nitrosylation of caspase-3, -8, and -9 decreases apoptosis. The enhanced nNOS levels and NO activity in AD brains may have a neuroprotective role, as demonstrated by the selectively spared NOS-positive neurons in AD. Hence, constant increases in NO have harmful effects, such as oxidative stress, the fragmentation loss of synaptic functioning, and apoptosis [141].

In summary, AD is a major neuropsychiatric disorder, and the regulation of NO is essential for maintaining proper neuronal functioning and synaptic plasticity in the CNS during AD.

5. Future Directions

Gasotransmitters are the essential molecules that help regulate synaptic and neuroplasticity in the CNS. Three gas neurotransmitters, H_2S, NO, and CO, were discussed briefly. These gasotransmitters are related to neuropsychiatric conditions. For example, H_2S downregulation was involved with the progression of MDD in one study, but the molecular mechanisms by which reduced H_2S levels lead to MDD need to be studied further [69, 70]. In terms of other gasotransmitters, higher NO levels were reported in the postmortem brains of SCZ patients [103]; thus, downregulation or modified regulation could be a therapeutic option for treating SCZ. NO levels are also altered in BD patients, and this could facilitate the identification of therapies to treat these neuropsychiatric conditions. Additionally, increased levels of HO-1 or CO were observed in AD patients, which highlights how gasotransmitters may be involved with neuropsychiatric conditions and how regulating these gasotransmitters could help treat these disorders.

6. Conclusion

Maintaining synaptic plasticity is crucial for regulating neuronal health and homeostasis. Neuronal functioning declines over time or under stressful conditions whereas many reactive species can lead to different neuropsychiatric conditions, such as SCZ, MDD, BD, and AD. Several gasotransmitters, such as H_2S, NO, and CO, balance synaptic plasticity when the normal condition is altered directly or indirectly. However, as the mechanisms or pathways through which they act are poorly understood, further studies are needed. Because the up- or downregulation of these gasotransmitters is responsible for causing the pathological conditions that lead to neuropsychiatric diseases, the normalization of their levels could exert protective effects. Hence, ensuring that the levels of these gasotransmitters are appropriate could help in the treatment of neuropsychiatric conditions. Moreover, improvements in our understanding of these pathways may lead to the identification of new therapeutic options for these neuropsychiatric conditions.

Abbreviations

AD: Alzheimer's disease
AMPA: α-Amino-3-hydroxy-5-methyl-isoxazole-4-propanoic acid
AMPARs: α-Amino-3-hydroxy-5-methyl-isoxazole-4-propanoic acid receptors
$A\beta$: Amyloid beta
APP: Amyloid precursor protein
BD: Bipolar disorder
BDNF: Brain derivative neurotrophic factor
CA3: Cornu Ammonis 3
CaMKII: Calcium/calmodulin-dependent kinase II
CREB: Cyclic AMP response element binding protein
CO: Carbon monoxide
Ca^{2+}: Calcium ion
CBS: Cystathionine β-synthase
CSE: Cystathionine γ-lyase
CAT: Cysteine aminotransferase
cGMP: Cyclic guanosine monophosphate
cAMP: Cyclic adenosine monophosphate
CUMS: Chronic unpredictable mild stress
DAAO: D-Amino acid oxidase
DRG: Dorsal root ganglion
ERK: Extracellular signal-regulated kinase
EPAC: Exchange protein stimulated by cAMP
GABA: Gamma amino butyric acid
GFAP: Glial fibrillary acid protein
GSH: Glutathione
GSSH: Glutathione persulfide
H_2S_n: Polysulfide
H_2S: Hydrogen sulfide
HO-1: Hemeoxygenase-1
HO-2: Hemeoxygenase-2
HO-3: Hemeoxygenase-3
HPAS: Hypothalamic–pituitary–adrenal system
JNK: C-Jun *N*-terminal kinase
LTP: Long-term potentiation

LTD: Long-term depression
MDD: Major depressive disorder
MAPK: Mitogen-activated protein kinases
3-MST: 3-Mercaptopyruvate sulfurtransferase
mTOR: Mechanistic target of rapamycin
mRNA: Messenger ribonucleic acid
MCI: Mild cognitive impairment
NMDA: *N*-Methyl-D-aspartate
NMDARs: *N*-Methyl-D-aspartate receptors
NO: Nitric oxide
NOS: Nitric oxide synthase
NaHS: Sodium hydrogen sulfate
NSCs: Neural stem cells
Nrf2: Nuclear factor erythroid 2-related factor 2
PKA: Protein kinase A
RyR: Ryanodine receptor
SCZ: Schizophrenia
SSRIs: Serotonin reuptake inhibitors
SAM: S-Adenosylmethionine
siRNA: Small interfering RNA
TrkB: Tropomyosin receptor kinase B
TRPA1: Transient receptor potential ankyrin 1
VGCC: Voltage-gated calcium channels
VEGF: Vascular endothelial growth factor
WHO: World Health Organization.

Conflicts of Interest

The authors reported no potential conflict of interests.

Acknowledgments

This work was supported by the Basic Science Research Program through the National Research Foundation of Korea (NRF) funded by the Ministry of Science, ICT and Future Planning (2018R1A2B6001123).

References

[1] A. Kumar, "Long-term potentiation at CA3–CA1 hippocampal synapses with special emphasis on aging, disease, and stress," *Frontiers in Aging Neuroscience*, vol. 3, pp. 1–20, 2011.

[2] T. V. P. Bliss and G. L. Collingridge, "A synaptic model of memory: long-term potentiation in the hippocampus," *Nature*, vol. 361, no. 6407, pp. 31–39, 1993.

[3] C. R. Bramham and E. Messaoudi, "BDNF function in adult synaptic plasticity: the synaptic consolidation hypothesis," *Progress in Neurobiology*, vol. 76, no. 2, pp. 99–125, 2005.

[4] R. C. Malenka and M. F. Bear, "LTP and LTD: an embarrassment of riches," *Neuron*, vol. 44, no. 1, pp. 5–21, 2004.

[5] E. P. Rico, D. B. Rosemberg, K. J. Seibt, K. M. Capiotti, R. S. Da Silva, and C. D. Bonan, "Zebrafish neurotransmitter systems as potential pharmacological and toxicological targets," *Neurotoxicology and Teratology*, vol. 33, no. 6, pp. 608–617, 2011.

[6] A. V. Yakovlev, E. D. Kurmasheva, R. Giniatullin, I. Khalilov, and G. F. Sitdikova, "Hydrogen sulfide inhibits giant depolarizing potentials and abolishes epileptiform activity of neonatal rat hippocampal slices," *Neuroscience*, vol. 340, pp. 153–165, 2017.

[7] K. Abe and H. Kimura, "The possible role of hydrogen sulfide as an endogenous neuromodulator," *Journal of Neuroscience*, vol. 16, no. 3, pp. 1066–1071, 1996.

[8] N. Hardingham, J. Dachtler, and K. Fox, "The role of nitric oxide in pre-synaptic plasticity and homeostasis," *Frontiers in Cellular Neuroscience*, vol. 7, pp. 1–19, 2013.

[9] C. Hölscher, "Nitric oxide, the enigmatic neuronal messenger: its role in synaptic plasticity," *Trends in Neurosciences*, vol. 20, no. 7, pp. 298–303, 1997.

[10] J. R. Steinert, T. Chernova, and I. D. Forsythe, "Nitric oxide signaling in brain function, dysfunction, and dementia," *The Neuroscientist*, vol. 16, no. 4, pp. 435–452, 2010.

[11] J. Jung, C. Na, and Y. Huh, "Alterations in nitric oxide synthase in the aged CNS," *Oxidative Medicine and Cellular Longevity*, vol. 2012, Article ID 718976, 7 pages, 2012.

[12] K. D. Poss and S. Tonegawa, "Reduced stress defense in heme oxygenase 1-deficient cells," *Proceedings of the National Academy of Sciences of the United States of America*, vol. 94, no. 20, pp. 10925–10930, 1997.

[13] C. F. Stevens and Y. Wang, "Reversal of long-term potentiation by inhibitors of haem oxygenase," *Nature*, vol. 364, no. 6433, pp. 147–149, 1993.

[14] M. P. Mattson, "Mitochondrial regulation of neuronal plasticity," *Neurochemical Research*, vol. 32, no. 4-5, pp. 707–715, 2007.

[15] H. J. Carlisle and M. B. Kennedy, "Spine architecture and synaptic plasticity," *Trends in Neurosciences*, vol. 28, no. 4, pp. 182–187, 2005.

[16] V. Todorova and A. Blokland, "Mitochondria and synaptic plasticity in the mature and aging nervous system," *Current Neuropharmacology*, vol. 15, no. 1, pp. 166–173, 2017.

[17] D. Mauceri, F. Gardoni, E. Marcello, and M. Di Luca, "Dual role of CaMKII-dependent SAP97 phosphorylation in mediating trafficking and insertion of NMDA receptor subunit NR2A," *Journal of Neurochemistry*, vol. 100, no. 4, pp. 1032–1046, 2007.

[18] X. Cheng, Z. Ji, T. Tsalkova, and F. Mei, "Epac and PKA: a tale of two intracellular cAMP receptors," *Acta Biochimica et Biophysica Sinica*, vol. 40, no. 7, pp. 651–662, 2008.

[19] A. A. Reichenberg, "The assessment of neuropsychological functioning in schizophrenia," *Dialogues in Clinical Neuroscience*, vol. 12, no. 3, pp. 383–392, 2010.

[20] V. M. Ho, J.-A. Lee, and K. C. Martin, "The cell biology of synaptic plasticity," *Science*, vol. 334, no. 6056, pp. 623–628, 2011.

[21] H. Park and M. Poo, "Neurotrophin regulation of neural circuit development and function," *Nature Reviews Neuroscience*, vol. 14, no. 1, pp. 7–23, 2013.

[22] M. Sasi, B. Vignoli, M. Canossa, and R. Blum, "Neurobiology of local and intercellular BDNF signaling," *Pflügers Archiv - European Journal of Physiology*, vol. 469, no. 5-6, pp. 593–610, 2017.

[23] B. Lu, G. Nagappan, X. Guan, P. J. Nathan, and P. Wren, "BDNF-based synaptic repair as a disease-modifying strategy for neurodegenerative diseases," *Nature Reviews Neuroscience*, vol. 14, no. 6, pp. 401–416, 2013.

[24] N. W. Daw, P. S. G. Stein, and K. Fox, "The role of NMDA receptors in information processing," *Annual Review of Neuroscience*, vol. 16, no. 1, pp. 207–222, 1993.

[25] G. Voglis and N. Tavernarakis, "The role of synaptic ion channels in synaptic plasticity," *EMBO Reports*, vol. 7, no. 11, pp. 1104–1110, 2006.

[26] Y. Humeau, H. Shaban, S. Bissière, and A. Lüthi, "Presynaptic induction of heterosynaptic associative plasticity in the mammalian brain," *Nature*, vol. 426, no. 6968, pp. 841–845, 2003.

[27] A. L. Coon, D. R. Wallace, C. F. Mactutus, and R. M. Booze, "L-type calcium channels in the hippocampus and cerebellum of Alzheimer's disease brain tissue," *Neurobiology of Aging*, vol. 20, no. 6, pp. 597–603, 1999.

[28] T. Novkovic, T. Mittmann, and D. Manahan-Vaughan, "BDNF contributes to the facilitation of hippocampal synaptic plasticity and learning enabled by environmental enrichment," *Hippocampus*, vol. 25, no. 1, pp. 1–15, 2015.

[29] U. Shefa, S. G. Yeo, M. S. Kim et al., "Role of gasotransmitters in oxidative stresses, neuroinflammation, and neuronal repair," *BioMed Research International*, vol. 2017, Article ID 1689341, 15 pages, 2017.

[30] N. Shibuya, S. Koike, M. Tanaka et al., "A novel pathway for the production of hydrogen sulfide from D-cysteine in mammalian cells," *Nature Communications*, vol. 4, p. 1366, 2013.

[31] M. Lee, C. Schwab, S. Yu, E. McGeer, and P. L. McGeer, "Astrocytes produce the antiinflammatory and neuroprotective agent hydrogen sulfide," *Neurobiology of Aging*, vol. 30, no. 10, pp. 1523–1534, 2009.

[32] M. S. Vandiver, B. D. Paul, R. Xu et al., "Sulfhydration mediates neuroprotective actions of parkin," *Nature Communications*, vol. 4, p. 1626, 2013.

[33] Y. Kimura, Y. Mikami, K. Osumi, M. Tsugane, J. Oka, and H. Kimura, "Polysulfides are possible H_2S-derived signaling molecules in rat brain," *The FASEB Journal*, vol. 27, no. 6, pp. 2451–2457, 2013.

[34] S. Koike, K. Kawamura, Y. Kimura, N. Shibuya, H. Kimura, and Y. Ogasawara, "Analysis of endogenous H_2S and H_2S_n in mouse brain by high-performance liquid chromatography with fluorescence and tandem mass spectrometric detection," *Free Radical Biology & Medicine*, vol. 113, pp. 355–362, 2017.

[35] Y. Hatakeyama, K. Takahashi, M. Tominaga, H. Kimura, and T. Ohta, "Polysulfide evokes acute pain through the activation of nociceptive TRPA1 in mouse sensory neurons," *Molecular Pain*, vol. 11, no. 1, p. 24, 2015.

[36] Y. Kimura, Y. Toyofuku, S. Koike et al., "Identification of H_2S_3 and H_2S produced by 3-mercaptopyruvate sulfurtransferase in the brain," *Scientific Reports*, vol. 5, no. 1, article 14774, 2015.

[37] J. W. Hylin and J. L. Wood, "Enzymatic formation of polysulfides from mercaptopyruvate," *The Journal of Biological Chemistry*, vol. 234, no. 8, pp. 2141–2144, 1959.

[38] Y. Kimura, S. Koike, N. Shibuya, D. Lefer, Y. Ogasawara, and H. Kimura, "3-Mercaptopyruvate sulfurtransferase produces potential redox regulators cysteine- and glutathione-persulfide (Cys-SSH and GSSH) together with signaling molecules H_2S_2, H_2S_3 and H_2S," *Scientific Reports*, vol. 7, no. 1, article 10459, 2017.

[39] Y. Nagai, M. Tsugane, J.-I. Oka, and H. Kimura, "Hydrogen sulfide induces calcium waves in astrocytes," *The FASEB Journal*, vol. 18, no. 3, pp. 557–559, 2004.

[40] H. Kimura, "Hydrogen sulfide induces cyclic AMP and modulates the NMDA receptor," *Biochemical and Biophysical Research Communications*, vol. 267, no. 1, pp. 129–133, 2000.

[41] Y.-L. Li, P.-F. Wu, J.-G. Chen et al., "Activity-dependent sulfhydration signal controls N-methyl-D-aspartate subtype glutamate receptor-dependent synaptic plasticity *via* increasing d-serine availability," *Antioxidants & Redox Signaling*, vol. 27, no. 7, pp. 398–414, 2017.

[42] J. Garthwaite, "From synaptically localized to volume transmission by nitric oxide," *The Journal of Physiology*, vol. 594, no. 1, pp. 9–18, 2016.

[43] J. Prickaerts, N. P. Van Goethem, W. Gulisano, E. K. Argyrousi, A. Palmeri, and D. Puzzo, "Physiological and pathological processes of synaptic plasticity and memory in drug discovery: do not forget the dose-response curve," *European Journal of Pharmacology*, vol. 817, pp. 59–70, 2017.

[44] K. E. Hoque, R. P. Indorkar, S. Sammut, and A. R. West, "Impact of dopamine–glutamate interactions on striatal neuronal nitric oxide synthase activity," *Psychopharmacology*, vol. 207, no. 4, pp. 571–581, 2010.

[45] J. Garthwaite, S. L. Charles, and R. Chess-Williams, "Endothelium-derived relaxing factor release on activation of NMDA receptors suggests role as intercellular messenger in the brain," *Nature*, vol. 336, no. 6197, pp. 385–388, 1988.

[46] D. S. Bredt and S. H. Snyder, "Nitric oxide, a novel neuronal messenger," *Neuron*, vol. 8, no. 1, pp. 3–11, 1992.

[47] E. Szabadits, C. Cserép, A. Szőnyi et al., "NMDA receptors in hippocampal GABAergic synapses and their role in nitric oxide signaling," *Journal of Neuroscience*, vol. 31, no. 16, pp. 5893–5904, 2011.

[48] G. K. Kolluru, X. Shen, S. C. Bir, and C. G. Kevil, "Hydrogen sulfide chemical biology: pathophysiological roles and detection," *Nitric Oxide*, vol. 35, pp. 5–20, 2013.

[49] R. Dingledine, K. Borges, D. Bowie, and S. F. Traynelis, "The glutamate receptor ion channels," *Pharmacological Reviews*, vol. 51, no. 1, pp. 7–61, 1999.

[50] J. Q. Wang, X.-P. Chu, M.-L. Guo et al., "Modulation of ionotropic glutamate receptors and acid-sensing ion channels by nitric oxide," *Frontiers in Physiology*, vol. 3, pp. 1–6, 2012.

[51] B. H. Tan, P. T. H. Wong, and J. S. Bian, "Hydrogen sulfide: a novel signaling molecule in the central nervous system," *Neurochemistry International*, vol. 56, no. 1, pp. 3–10, 2010.

[52] J. Blasko, K. Fabianova, M. Martoncikova, D. Sopkova, and E. Racekova, "Immunohistochemical evidence for the presence of synaptic connections of nitrergic neurons in the rat rostral migratory stream," *Cellular and Molecular Neurobiology*, vol. 33, no. 6, pp. 753–757, 2013.

[53] R. M. Cooke, R. Mistry, R. A. J. Challiss, and V. A. Straub, "Nitric oxide synthesis and cGMP production is important for neurite growth and synapse remodeling after axotomy," *Journal of Neuroscience*, vol. 33, no. 13, pp. 5626–5637, 2013.

[54] A. A. Steiner, E. Colombari, and L. G. S. Branco, "Carbon monoxide as a novel mediator of the febrile response in the central nervous system," *American Journal of Physiology-Regulatory, Integrative and Comparative Physiology*, vol. 277, no. 2, pp. R499–R507, 1999.

[55] M. D. Maines, "Carbon monoxide: an emerging regulator of cGMP in the brain," *Molecular and Cellular Neuroscience*, vol. 4, no. 5, pp. 389–397, 1993.

[56] J. F. Ewing and M. D. Maines, "In situ hybridization and immunohistochemical localization of heme oxygenase-2 mRNA and protein in normal rat brain: differential distribution of isozyme 1 and 2," *Molecular and Cellular Neuroscience*, vol. 3, no. 6, pp. 559–570, 1992.

[57] G. S. Marks, J. F. Brien, K. Nakatsu, and B. E. McLaughlin, "Does carbon monoxide have a physiological function?," *Trends in Pharmacological Sciences*, vol. 12, no. 5, pp. 185–188, 1991.

[58] T. Morita, M. A. Perrella, M.-E. Lee, and S. Kourembanas, "Smooth muscle cell-derived carbon monoxide is a regulator of vascular cGMP," *Proceedings of the National Academy of Sciences of the United States of America*, vol. 92, no. 5, pp. 1475–1479, 1995.

[59] C. S. F. Queiroga, A. Vercelli, and H. L. A. Vieira, "Carbon monoxide and the CNS: challenges and achievements," *British Journal of Pharmacology*, vol. 172, no. 6, pp. 1533–1545, 2015.

[60] A. Verma, D. J. Hirsch, C. E. Glatt, G. V. Ronnett, and S. H. Snyder, "Carbon monoxide: a putative neural messenger," *Science*, vol. 259, no. 5093, pp. 381–384, 1993.

[61] S.-Y. Hung, H.-C. Liou, K.-H. Kang, R.-M. Wu, C.-C. Wen, and W.-M. Fu, "Overexpression of heme oxygenase-1 protects dopaminergic neurons against 1-methyl-4-phenylpyridinium-induced neurotoxicity," *Molecular Pharmacology*, vol. 74, no. 6, pp. 1564–1575, 2008.

[62] N. Dreyer-Andersen, A. S. Almeida, P. Jensen et al., "Intermittent, low dose carbon monoxide exposure enhances survival and dopaminergic differentiation of human neural stem cells," *PLoS One*, vol. 13, no. 1, article e0191207, 2018.

[63] Y. K. Choi, C.-K. Kim, H. Lee et al., "Carbon monoxide promotes VEGF expression by increasing HIF-1α protein level via two distinct mechanisms, translational activation and stabilization of HIF-1α protein," *Journal of Biological Chemistry*, vol. 285, no. 42, pp. 32116–32125, 2010.

[64] R. C. Kessler, P. Berglund, O. Demler et al., "The epidemiology of major depressive disorder: results from the National Comorbidity Survey Replication (NCS-R)," *JAMA*, vol. 289, no. 23, pp. 3095–3105, 2003.

[65] M. Miret, J. L. Ayuso-Mateos, J. Sanchez-Moreno, and E. Vieta, "Depressive disorders and suicide: epidemiology, risk factors, and burden," *Neuroscience & Biobehavioral Reviews*, vol. 37, no. 10, pp. 2372–2374, 2013.

[66] C. J. L. Murray and A. D. Lopez, "Alternative projections of mortality and disability by cause 1990–2020: Global Burden of Disease Study," *The Lancet*, vol. 349, no. 9064, pp. 1498–1504, 1997.

[67] C.-M. Wang, Y.-J. Yang, J.-T. Zhang et al., "Regulation of emotional memory by hydrogen sulfide: role of GluN2B-containing NMDA receptor in the amygdala," *Journal of Neurochemistry*, vol. 132, no. 1, pp. 124–134, 2015.

[68] Y. Luo, P. F. Wu, J. Zhou et al., "Aggravation of seizure-like events by hydrogen sulfide: involvement of multiple targets that control neuronal excitability," *CNS Neuroscience & Therapeutics*, vol. 20, no. 5, pp. 411–419, 2014.

[69] W.-L. Chen, B. Xie, C. Zhang et al., "Antidepressant-like and anxiolytic-like effects of hydrogen sulfide in behavioral models of depression and anxiety," *Behavioural Pharmacology*, vol. 24, no. 7, pp. 590–597, 2013.

[70] X.-Y. Hou, Z.-L. Hu, D.-Z. Zhang et al., "Rapid antidepressant effect of hydrogen sulfide: evidence for activation of mTORC1-TrkB-AMPA receptor pathways," *Antioxidants & Redox Signaling*, vol. 27, no. 8, pp. 472–488, 2017.

[71] L. M. Monteggia, M. Barrot, C. M. Powell et al., "Essential role of brain-derived neurotrophic factor in adult hippocampal function," *Proceedings of the National Academy of Sciences of the United States of America*, vol. 101, no. 29, pp. 10827–10832, 2004.

[72] J.-M. Jiang, C.-F. Zhou, S.-L. Gao et al., "BDNF-TrkB pathway mediates neuroprotection of hydrogen sulfide against formaldehyde-induced toxicity to PC12 cells," *PLoS One*, vol. 10, no. 3, article e0119478, 2015.

[73] N. Li, B. Lee, R.-J. Liu et al., "mTOR-dependent synapse formation underlies the rapid antidepressant effects of NMDA antagonists," *Science*, vol. 329, no. 5994, pp. 959–964, 2010.

[74] X. Zhou, G. An, and J. Chen, "Hydrogen sulfide improves left ventricular function in smoking rats via regulation of apoptosis and autophagy," *Apoptosis*, vol. 19, no. 6, pp. 998–1005, 2014.

[75] W. Wei, X. Hu, X. Zhuang, L. Liao, and W. Li, "GYY4137, a novel hydrogen sulfide-releasing molecule, likely protects against high glucose-induced cytotoxicity by activation of the AMPK/mTOR signal pathway in H9c2 cells," *Molecular and Cellular Biochemistry*, vol. 389, no. 1-2, pp. 249–256, 2014.

[76] S. Shimada, M. Fukai, K. Wakayama et al., "Hydrogen sulfide augments survival signals in warm ischemia and reperfusion of the mouse liver," *Surgery Today*, vol. 45, no. 7, pp. 892–903, 2015.

[77] O. W. Griffith and D. J. Stuehr, "Nitric oxide synthases: properties and catalytic mechanism," *Annual Review of Physiology*, vol. 57, no. 1, pp. 707–734, 1995.

[78] Y.-R. Lu, Y. Zhang, Y.-B. Rao et al., "The changes in and relationship between plasma nitric oxide and corticotropin-releasing hormone in patients with major depressive disorder," *Clinical and Experimental Pharmacology and Physiology*, vol. 45, no. 1, pp. 10–15, 2018.

[79] T. Liu, S. Zhong, X. Liao et al., "A meta-analysis of oxidative stress markers in depression," *PLoS One*, vol. 10, no. 10, article e0138904, 2015.

[80] P. Gałecki, E. Gałecka, M. Maes et al., "The expression of genes encoding for COX-2, MPO, iNOS, and sPLA2-IIA in patients with recurrent depressive disorder," *Journal of Affective Disorders*, vol. 138, no. 3, pp. 360–366, 2012.

[81] B. Kanchanatawan, S. Tangwongchai, A. Sughondhabhirom et al., "Add-on treatment with curcumin has antidepressive effects in Thai patients with major depression: results of a randomized double-blind placebo-controlled study," *Neurotoxicity Research*, vol. 33, no. 3, pp. 621–633, 2018.

[82] H. G. Bernstein, A. Heinemann, D. Krell et al., "Hypothalamic nitric oxide synthase in affective disorder: focus on the suprachiasmatic nucleus," *Cellular and Molecular Biology*, vol. 51, no. 3, pp. 279–284, 2005.

[83] E. Suzuki, G. Yagi, T. Nakaki, S. Kanba, and M. Asai, "Elevated plasma nitrate levels in depressive states," *Journal of Affective Disorders*, vol. 63, no. 1–3, pp. 221–224, 2001.

[84] Y.-K. Kim, J.-W. Paik, S.-W. Lee, D. Yoon, C. Han, and B.-H. Lee, "Increased plasma nitric oxide level associated with suicide attempt in depressive patients," *Progress in Neuro-Psychopharmacology and Biological Psychiatry*, vol. 30, no. 6, pp. 1091–1096, 2006.

[85] R. G. García, J. G. Zarruk, C. Barrera et al., "Plasma nitrate levels and flow-mediated vasodilation in untreated major depression," *Psychosomatic Medicine*, vol. 73, no. 4, pp. 344–349, 2011.

[86] Y.-R. Lu, X. Y. Fu, L. G. Shi et al., "Decreased plasma neuroactive amino acids and increased nitric oxide levels in

melancholic major depressive disorder," *BMC Psychiatry*, vol. 14, no. 1, p. 123, 2014.

[87] S.-F. Gao, Y.-R. Lu, L.-G. Shi et al., "Nitric oxide synthase and nitric oxide alterations in chronically stressed rats: a model for nitric oxide in major depressive disorder," *Psychoneuroendocrinology*, vol. 47, pp. 136–140, 2014.

[88] A. J. Funk, R. E. McCullumsmith, V. Haroutunian, and J. H. Meador-Woodruff, "Abnormal activity of the MAPK- and cAMP-associated signaling pathways in frontal cortical areas in postmortem brain in schizophrenia," *Neuropsychopharmacology*, vol. 37, no. 4, pp. 896–905, 2012.

[89] D. W. Volk, S. M. Eggan, and D. A. Lewis, "Alterations in metabotropic glutamate receptor 1α and regulator of G protein signaling 4 in the prefrontal cortex in schizophrenia," *American Journal of Psychiatry*, vol. 167, no. 12, pp. 1489–1498, 2010.

[90] H. Prast and A. Philippu, "Nitric oxide as modulator of neuronal function," *Progress in Neurobiology*, vol. 64, no. 1, pp. 51–68, 2001.

[91] V. Calabrese, C. Mancuso, M. Calvani, E. Rizzarelli, D. A. Butterfield, and A. M. Giuffrida Stella, "Nitric oxide in the central nervous system: neuroprotection versus neurotoxicity," *Nature Reviews Neuroscience*, vol. 8, no. 10, pp. 766–775, 2007.

[92] R. F. Nasyrova, D. V. Ivashchenko, M. V. Ivanov, and N. G. Neznanov, "Role of nitric oxide and related molecules in schizophrenia pathogenesis: biochemical, genetic and clinical aspects," *Frontiers in Physiology*, vol. 6, pp. 1–16, 2015.

[93] S. M. Gibbs, "Regulation of neuronal proliferation and differentiation by nitric oxide," *Molecular Neurobiology*, vol. 27, no. 2, pp. 107–120, 2003.

[94] M. L. Averbukh, A. F. Kas'ko, E. S. Nikolenko, and I. I. Rybas, "On the diagnostic significance of Black's reaction in psychiatric patients," *Laboratornoe Delo*, vol. 5, pp. 289–291, 1965.

[95] J. K. Yao, S. Leonard, and R. D. Reddy, "Increased nitric oxide radicals in postmortem brain from patients with schizophrenia," *Schizophrenia Bulletin*, vol. 30, no. 4, pp. 923–934, 2004.

[96] M. Zhang, Z. Zhao, L. He, and C. Wan, "A meta-analysis of oxidative stress markers in schizophrenia," *Science China Life Sciences*, vol. 53, no. 1, pp. 112–124, 2010.

[97] O. Akyol, S. Zoroglu, F. Armutcu, S. Sahin, and A. Gurel, "Nitric oxide as a physiopathological factor in neuropsychiatric disorders," *In vivo*, vol. 18, no. 3, pp. 377–390, 2004.

[98] C. A. Doyle and P. Slater, "Application of [^{3}H] l-N^G-nitro-arginine labelling to measure cerebellar nitric oxide synthase in patients with schizophrenia," *Neuroscience Letters*, vol. 202, no. 1-2, pp. 49–52, 1995.

[99] S. Bhattacharjee and W. J. Lukiw, "Alzheimer's disease and the microbiome," *Frontiers in Cellular Neuroscience*, vol. 7, pp. 1–4, 2013.

[100] H. Baba, T. Suzuki, H. Arai, and P. C. Emson, "Expression of nNOS and soluble guanylate cyclase in schizophrenic brain," *Neuroreport*, vol. 15, no. 4, pp. 677–680, 2004.

[101] H.-G. Bernstein, A. Stanarius, B. Baumann et al., "Nitric oxide synthase-containing neurons in the human hypothalamus: reduced number of immunoreactive cells in the paraventricular nucleus of depressive patients and schizophrenics," *Neuroscience*, vol. 83, no. 3, pp. 867–875, 1998.

[102] M. C. M. Ryan, N. Sharifi, R. Condren, and J. H. Thakore, "Evidence of basal pituitary–adrenal overactivity in first episode, drug naïve patients with schizophrenia," *Psychoneuroendocrinology*, vol. 29, no. 8, pp. 1065–1070, 2004.

[103] J. P. Maia-de-Oliveira, C. Trzesniak, I. R. Oliveira et al., "Nitric oxide plasma/serum levels in patients with schizophrenia: a systematic review and meta-analysis," *Revista Brasileira de Psiquiatria*, vol. 34, pp. 149–162, 2012.

[104] K. Tanda, A. Nishi, N. Matsuo et al., "Abnormal social behavior, hyperactivity, impaired remote spatial memory, and increased D1-mediated dopaminergic signaling in neuronal nitric oxide synthase knockout mice," *Molecular Brain*, vol. 2, no. 1, p. 19, 2009.

[105] C. R. Sunico, F. Portillo, D. González-Forero, and B. Moreno-López, "Nitric oxide-directed synaptic remodeling in the adult mammal CNS," *Journal of Neuroscience*, vol. 25, no. 6, pp. 1448–1458, 2005.

[106] X. R. Zhang, Y. X. Wang, Z. J. Zhang, L. Li, and G. P. Reynolds, "The effect of chronic antipsychotic drug on hypothalamic expression of neural nitric oxide synthase and dopamine D2 receptor in the male rat," *PLoS One*, vol. 7, no. 4, article e33247, 2012.

[107] Y.-S. Lau, E. Petroske, G. E. Meredith, and J. Q. Wang, "Elevated neuronal nitric oxide synthase expression in chronic haloperidol-treated rats," *Neuropharmacology*, vol. 45, no. 7, pp. 986–994, 2003.

[108] F. I. Tarazi, K. Zhang, and R. J. Baldessarini, "Long-term effects of newer antipsychotic drugs on neuronal nitric oxide synthase in rat brain," *Nitric Oxide*, vol. 7, no. 4, pp. 297–300, 2002.

[109] B. M. M. Ribeiro, M. R. S. do Carmo, R. S. Freire et al., "Evidences for a progressive microglial activation and increase in iNOS expression in rats submitted to a neurodevelopmental model of schizophrenia: reversal by clozapine," *Schizophrenia Research*, vol. 151, no. 1–3, pp. 12–19, 2013.

[110] H. B. Chen, W. N. Wu, W. Wang et al., "Cystathionine-β-synthase-derived hydrogen sulfide is required for amygdalar long-term potentiation and cued fear memory in rats," *Pharmacology Biochemistry and Behavior*, vol. 155, pp. 16–23, 2017.

[111] J. F. Trentini, J. T. O'Neill, S. Poluch, and S. L. Juliano, "Prenatal carbon monoxide impairs migration of interneurons into the cerebral cortex," *Neurotoxicology*, vol. 53, pp. 31–44, 2016.

[112] S. Prabakaran, J. E. Swatton, M. M. Ryan et al., "Mitochondrial dysfunction in schizophrenia: evidence for compromised brain metabolism and oxidative stress," *Molecular Psychiatry*, vol. 9, no. 7, pp. 684–697, 2004.

[113] X.-Q. Song, L.-X. Lv, W.-Q. Li, Y.-H. Hao, and J.-P. Zhao, "The interaction of nuclear factor-kappa B and cytokines is associated with schizophrenia," *Biological Psychiatry*, vol. 65, no. 6, pp. 481–488, 2009.

[114] C. J. L. Murray and A. D. Lopez, "Evidence-based health policy–lessons from the global burden of disease study," *Science*, vol. 274, no. 5288, pp. 740–743, 1996.

[115] R. T. de Sousa, M. V. Zanetti, G. F. Busatto et al., "Lithium increases nitric oxide levels in subjects with bipolar disorder during depressive episodes," *Journal of Psychiatric Research*, vol. 55, pp. 96–100, 2014.

[116] A. C. Andreazza, M. Kauer-Sant'Anna, B. N. Frey et al., "Oxidative stress markers in bipolar disorder: a meta-analysis," *Journal of Affective Disorders*, vol. 111, no. 2-3, pp. 135–144, 2008.

[117] S. Selek, H. A. Savas, H. S. Gergerlioglu, F. Bulbul, E. Uz, and M. Yumru, "The course of nitric oxide and superoxide dismutase during treatment of bipolar depressive episode," *Journal of Affective Disorders*, vol. 107, no. 1-3, pp. 89–94, 2008.

[118] C. L. M. Bon and J. Garthwaite, "On the role of nitric oxide in hippocampal long-term potentiation," *Journal of Neuroscience*, vol. 23, no. 5, pp. 1941–1948, 2003.

[119] L. Liu and J. S. Stamler, "NO: an inhibitor of cell death," *Cell Death & Differentiation*, vol. 6, no. 10, pp. 937–942, 1999.

[120] A. Riccio, R. S. Alvania, B. E. Lonze et al., "A nitric oxide signaling pathway controls CREB-mediated gene expression in neurons," *Molecular Cell*, vol. 21, no. 2, pp. 283–294, 2006.

[121] O. Sergent, B. Griffon, I. Morel et al., "Effect of nitric oxide on iron-mediated oxidative stress in primary rat hepatocyte culture," *Hepatology*, vol. 25, no. 1, pp. 122–127, 1997.

[122] R. T. de Sousa, M. T. van de Bilt, B. S. Diniz et al., "Lithium increases plasma brain-derived neurotrophic factor in acute bipolar mania: a preliminary 4-week study," *Neuroscience Letters*, vol. 494, no. 1, pp. 54–56, 2011.

[123] T. Bschor and M. Bauer, "Efficacy and mechanisms of action of lithium augmentation in refractory major depression," *Current Pharmaceutical Design*, vol. 12, no. 23, pp. 2985–2992, 2006.

[124] M. Ghasemi and A. R. Dehpour, "The NMDA receptor/nitric oxide pathway: a target for the therapeutic and toxic effects of lithium," *Trends in Pharmacological Sciences*, vol. 32, no. 7, pp. 420–434, 2011.

[125] D. L. Feinstein, "Potentiation of astroglial nitric oxide synthase type-2 expression by lithium chloride," *Journal of Neurochemistry*, vol. 71, no. 2, pp. 883–886, 1998.

[126] H. Anai, Y. Ueta, R. Serino, M. Nomura, Y. Nakashima, and H. Yamashita, "Activation of hypothalamic neuronal nitric oxide synthase in lithium-induced diabetes insipidus rats," *Psychoneuroendocrinology*, vol. 26, no. 2, pp. 109–120, 2001.

[127] G. Bagetta, M. T. Corasaniti, G. Melino, A. M. Paoletti, A. Finazziagro, and G. Nistico, "Lithium and tacrine increase the expression of nitric oxide synthase mRNA in the hippocampus of rat," *Biochemical and Biophysical Research Communications*, vol. 197, no. 3, pp. 1132–1139, 1993.

[128] B. H. Harvey, M. E. Carstens, and J. J. F. Taljaard, "Evidence that lithium induces a glutamatergic: nitric oxide-mediated response in rat brain," *Neurochemical Research*, vol. 19, no. 4, pp. 469–474, 1994.

[129] P. Bhalla, N. Singla, and D. K. Dhawan, "Potential of lithium to reduce aluminium-induced cytotoxic effects in rat brain," *Biometals*, vol. 23, no. 2, pp. 197–206, 2010.

[130] H. A. Savas, H. S. Gergerlioglu, F. Armutcu et al., "Elevated serum nitric oxide and superoxide dismutase in euthymic bipolar patients: impact of past episodes," *The World Journal of Biological Psychiatry*, vol. 7, no. 1, pp. 51–55, 2006.

[131] M. Van Spronsen and C. C. Hoogenraad, "Synapse pathology in psychiatric and neurologic disease," *Current Neurology and Neuroscience Reports*, vol. 10, no. 3, pp. 207–214, 2010.

[132] J. E. Kang, M. M. Lim, R. J. Bateman et al., "Amyloid-beta dynamics are regulated by orexin and the sleep-wake cycle," *Science*, vol. 326, no. 5955, pp. 1005–1007, 2009.

[133] G. Scapagnini, V. D'Agata, V. Calabrese et al., "Gene expression profiles of heme oxygenase isoforms in the rat brain," *Brain Research*, vol. 954, no. 1, pp. 51–59, 2002.

[134] D. E. Barañano and S. H. Snyder, "Neural roles for heme oxygenase: contrasts to nitric oxide synthase," *Proceedings of the National Academy of Sciences of the United States of America*, vol. 98, no. 20, pp. 10996–11002, 2001.

[135] H. M. Schipper and W. Song, "A heme oxygenase-1 transducer model of degenerative and developmental brain disorders," *International Journal of Molecular Sciences*, vol. 16, no. 12, pp. 5400–5419, 2015.

[136] W. Hirose, K. Ikematsu, and R. Tsuda, "Age-associated increases in heme oxygenase-1 and ferritin immunoreactivity in the autopsied brain," *Legal Medicine*, vol. 5, pp. S360–S366, 2003.

[137] W. Song, H. Zukor, A. Liberman et al., "Astroglial heme oxygenase-1 and the origin of corpora amylacea in aging and degenerating neural tissues," *Experimental Neurology*, vol. 254, pp. 78–89, 2014.

[138] H. M. Schipper, W. Song, H. Zukor, J. R. Hascalovici, and D. Zeligman, "Heme oxygenase-1 and neurodegeneration: expanding frontiers of engagement," *Journal of Neurochemistry*, vol. 110, no. 2, pp. 469–485, 2009.

[139] R. Nisticò, V. Cavallucci, S. Piccinin et al., "Insulin receptor β-subunit haploinsufficiency impairs hippocampal late-phase LTP and recognition memory," *Neuromolecular Medicine*, vol. 14, no. 4, pp. 262–269, 2012.

[140] J. Garthwaite, "Concepts of neural nitric oxide-mediated transmission," *European Journal of Neuroscience*, vol. 27, no. 11, pp. 2783–2802, 2008.

[141] Q.-F. Zhao, J.-T. Yu, and L. Tan, "S-Nitrosylation in Alzheimer's disease," *Molecular Neurobiology*, vol. 51, no. 1, pp. 268–280, 2015.

[142] D. M. Wilcock, M. R. Lewis, W. E. van Nostrand et al., "Progression of amyloid pathology to Alzheimer's disease pathology in an amyloid precursor protein transgenic mouse model by removal of nitric oxide synthase 2," *Journal of Neuroscience*, vol. 28, no. 7, pp. 1537–1545, 2008.

[143] I. Goussakov, M. B. Miller, and G. E. Stutzmann, "NMDA-mediated Ca^{2+} influx drives aberrant ryanodine receptor activation in dendrites of young Alzheimer's disease mice," *Journal of Neuroscience*, vol. 30, no. 36, pp. 12128–12137, 2010.

[144] D. Shilling, M. Muller, H. Takano et al., "Suppression of InsP3 receptor-mediated Ca^{2+} signaling alleviates mutant presenilin-linked familial Alzheimer's disease pathogenesis," *Journal of Neuroscience*, vol. 34, no. 20, pp. 6910–6923, 2014.

[145] S. Chakroborty and G. E. Stutzmann, "Early calcium dysregulation in Alzheimer's disease: setting the stage for synaptic dysfunction," *Science China Life Sciences*, vol. 54, no. 8, pp. 752–762, 2011.

[146] S. Chakroborty, J. Kim, C. Schneider, A. R. West, and G. E. Stutzmann, "Nitric oxide signaling is recruited as a compensatory mechanism for sustaining synaptic plasticity in Alzheimer's disease mice," *Journal of Neuroscience*, vol. 35, no. 17, pp. 6893–6902, 2015.

[147] Z. J. Palmer, R. R. Duncan, J. R. Johnson et al., "S-Nitrosylation of syntaxin 1 at Cys145 is a regulatory switch controlling Munc18-1 binding," *Biochemical Journal*, vol. 413, no. 3, pp. 479–491, 2008.

[148] A. Ratnayaka, V. Marra, D. Bush, J. J. Burden, T. Branco, and K. Staras, "Recruitment of resting vesicles into recycling pools supports NMDA receptor-dependent synaptic potentiation in cultured hippocampal neurons," *The Journal of Physiology*, vol. 590, no. 7, pp. 1585–1597, 2012.

12

Hydromechanical Structure of the Cochlea Supports the Backward Traveling Wave in the Cochlea *In Vivo*

Fangyi Chen,[1,2] Dingjun Zha,[2,3] Xiaojie Yang,[1] Allyn Hubbard,[4] and Alfred Nuttall[2,5]

[1]*Department of Biomedical Engineering, Southern University of Science and Technology, Shenzhen, Guangdong 518055, China*
[2]*Oregon Hearing Research Center, Department of Otolaryngology and Head and Neck Surgery, Oregon Health and Science University, Portland, OR 97239, USA*
[3]*Department of Otolaryngology-Head and Neck Surgery, Xijing Hospital, Fourth Military Medical University, Xi'an, Shaanxi 710032, China*
[4]*Department of Electrical & Computer Engineering, Boston University, Boston, MA 02215, USA*
[5]*Kresge Hearing Research Institute, The University of Michigan, Ann Arbor, MI 48109, USA*

Correspondence should be addressed to Fangyi Chen; chenfy@sustc.edu.cn and Dingjun Zha; zhadjun@fmmu.edu.cn

Academic Editor: Jian Wang

The discovery that an apparent forward-propagating otoacoustic emission (OAE) induced basilar membrane vibration has created a serious debate in the field of cochlear mechanics. The traditional theory predicts that OAE will propagate to the ear canal via a backward traveling wave on the basilar membrane, while the opponent theory proposed that the OAE will reach the ear canal via a compression wave. Although accepted by most people, the basic phenomenon of the backward traveling wave theory has not been experimentally demonstrated. In this study, for the first time, we showed the backward traveling wave by measuring the phase spectra of the basilar membrane vibration at multiple longitudinal locations of the basal turn of the cochlea. A local vibration source with a unique and precise location on the cochlear partition was created to avoid the ambiguity of the vibration source in most previous studies. We also measured the vibration pattern at different places of a mechanical cochlear model. A slow backward traveling wave pattern was demonstrated by the time-domain sequence of the measured data. In addition to the wave propagation study, a transmission line mathematical model was used to interpret why no tonotopicity was observed in the backward traveling wave.

1. Introduction

Ears not only hear sound but also generate sound, which is called the otoacoustic emission (OAE) and was discovered in 1978 [1]. There are currently two competing theories established to explain the propagation of sound from the place where it is produced inside the cochlea towards the exit of the cochlea. The backward traveling wave theory, which postulates that OAE-induced waves travel slowly along the basilar membrane (BM), is widely accepted as an explanation of the propagation of the OAE [1, 2]. However, this predominant backward slow-wave theory cannot explain some experimental phenomena [3–6] favoring the fast compression wave theory that would exist in the lymph fluids surrounding the BM. In the compression wave theory, the slow-speed propagation of the backward transversal wave motion of the BM is replaced by a fast-fluidic compression wave and experimental time/phase differences are accounted for by mechanisms independent of the wave. To date, it is still an open question about the OAE path. Resolving this question is important because the OAE has become a useful and noninvasive clinical tool for hearing screening. To utilize the OAE for more precise diagnoses, it is necessary to understand how it propagates backward to the ear canal. In relation to the backward propagation of the OAE, von Békésy discovered that the wave on the BM always traveled from the base to the apex, even the stimulus (the stapes vibration) was placed at the apex of the cochlea. This so-called paradoxical wave was a hurdle that prevented people from believing that the OAE can propagate along the BM backward at the time when OAE was just discovered. In a few years since then, the seeming contradiction to the paradoxical phenomena was explained by stating that the vibration source of OAE was on the BM rather than in the fluid by the stapes as in the paradoxical wave. Hence, the theory of backward traveling wave was widely accepted.

One critical issue that causes the uncertainty in determining the wave propagation mechanism is that the actual location of the OAE source is uncertain. Most of the previous studies used nonlinear, intrinsic vibration to the organ of Corti to generate organ vibration at the intermodulation frequency of two tones. This intrinsic vibration initializes the backward wave propagation, but the spatial location of the vibration along the BM is still debated. This caused the analysis of the experimental data to be difficult because the generation mechanism of the OAE is complicated [2], and the origin of the OAE could be multiple sites. Although the width and location of the generation site are so important, they cannot be ascertained. The uncertainty of the source location also makes it difficult to estimate the wave propagation speed, which is a critical data for distinguishing the propagation forms and testing which theory explains the sound propagation mechanisms. Such an uncertainty has often resulted in interpretations of the same experimental results [6–8] using both competing theories. Thus, it is critical to study the backward wave propagation from a vibration source at a unique and precise location in the cochlea.

In addition, although as a widely accepted theory, the backward traveling wave theory has not been validated directly using an experiment where the vibration on the BM is measured [3]. The evidence used to support this theory is mostly from mathematical modeling [7, 9–14] and indirect measurements [15, 16]. Attempts have been made to experimentally generate local vibration on the BM via optical [17] and direct mechanical [18] methods but with limited success. The optical method [17] does not provide enough mechanical vibration until the light is strong enough to cause damage to the organ of Corti. The mechanical stimulation in Richter et al. [18] did provide an accurate vibration source with enough energy, but the hemicochlea preparation in this study destroyed the integrity of the basic hydromechanical structure of the cochlea. Also, the poor sensitivity (~10 nm) of the vibration measurement method limited its capability to detect the small vibration on the BM.

Since the hypothesized backward traveling wave is a transverse vibration on the BM, these indirect measurements [15, 16] have also been criticized to not truly represent the BM vibration [19, 20]. Moreover, other structures (e.g., tectorial membrane and Reissner's membrane) in the cochlea have also been suggested to be capable of supporting wave propagation inside the cochlea [21, 22], but their contribution to the cochlear mechanical dynamics has not been thoroughly studied and determined. Therefore, a direct measurement of the BM vibration using an experiment is necessary to determine the wave propagation mechanism of OAE in cochlea.

In the present study, we designed a novel method using a mechanical/piezoelectric stimulator to drive the BM at a precisely known location; thus, the location of the vibration source initiating the backward wave was accurately known. The BM vibration was then directly measured at multiple locations in an *in vivo* cochlear preparation. We found that the phase of the measured BM motion showed a consistent lag with the increase of the distance from the vibration source. The speed of the wave propagation was shown in the order of tens of meters per second, much less than the speed of a compression wave in water. This study, for the first time, used directly an experiment to prove that there was a slow backward traveling wave on the BM of the cochlea *in vivo*. The computer simulation of the experimental results in a mechanical model, termed "artificial cochlea," also confirmed that the hydromechanical structure of the cochlea supported the backward traveling wave.

2. Methods

2.1. Specimens. A total of 6 young guinea pigs weighted at 250 g–400 g were used in this study. After an animal was anesthetized by intramuscular injection of a mixture of ketamine (30 mg/kg) and xylazine (20 mg/kg), the temporal bone was opened using the dorsal-ventricle approach as described by Zheng et al. [23]. During the experiment, the animal was anesthetized with regular supplements of anesthetics. Tracheotomy was performed, and a ventilation tube was inserted into the trachea for natural breathing. The guinea pig's head was then mounted on a heated head holder. A surgical operation was performed to expose the left bulla, which was then opened for access to the cochlea. During the experiment, the core temperature of the animal was maintained at 37°C-38°C by a heating blanket and a rectal thermometer, which was controlled by a servo temperature controller (FHC, Bowdoinham, ME, USA) [23]. After the bulla was opened to expose the cochlea, an oblong window of about 2 mm long and 0.5 mm wide was opened on the bony wall at the cochlear basal turn to expose the BM. As shown in Figure 1(a), the basal turn of the cochlea was cut to open and the BM was exposed over almost the whole basal turn. Reflective beads assigned names of basal, middle, and apical were placed on the BM along the longitudinal direction. The tip of stimulator touched the BM at the apical end of the basal turn and delivered the vibration to initiate the backward wave. The wave propagation along the BM was recorded by focusing the laser of the vibrometer onto the reflective beads.

In the preparation, the joint between the incus and stapes was dislocated so that the middle ear chain was disrupted, significantly reducing any possible middle-ear-conducted acoustic stimulation. The ossicular dislocation was done because the piezo stack used to stimulate the BM also radiates acoustic energy. This sound will propagate to the adjacent tympanic membrane, initiating a normal acoustic stimulus to the cochlea and thus producing a forward traveling wave in the cochlea if the ossicular chain is intact. That forward traveling wave would interfere with the backward wave initiated by the stimulation probe on the BM. The fluid level of the perilymph in the scala tympani was carefully lowered using cotton wicks so that only a very small amount of fluid (~30 μm thick based on visual comparison with the

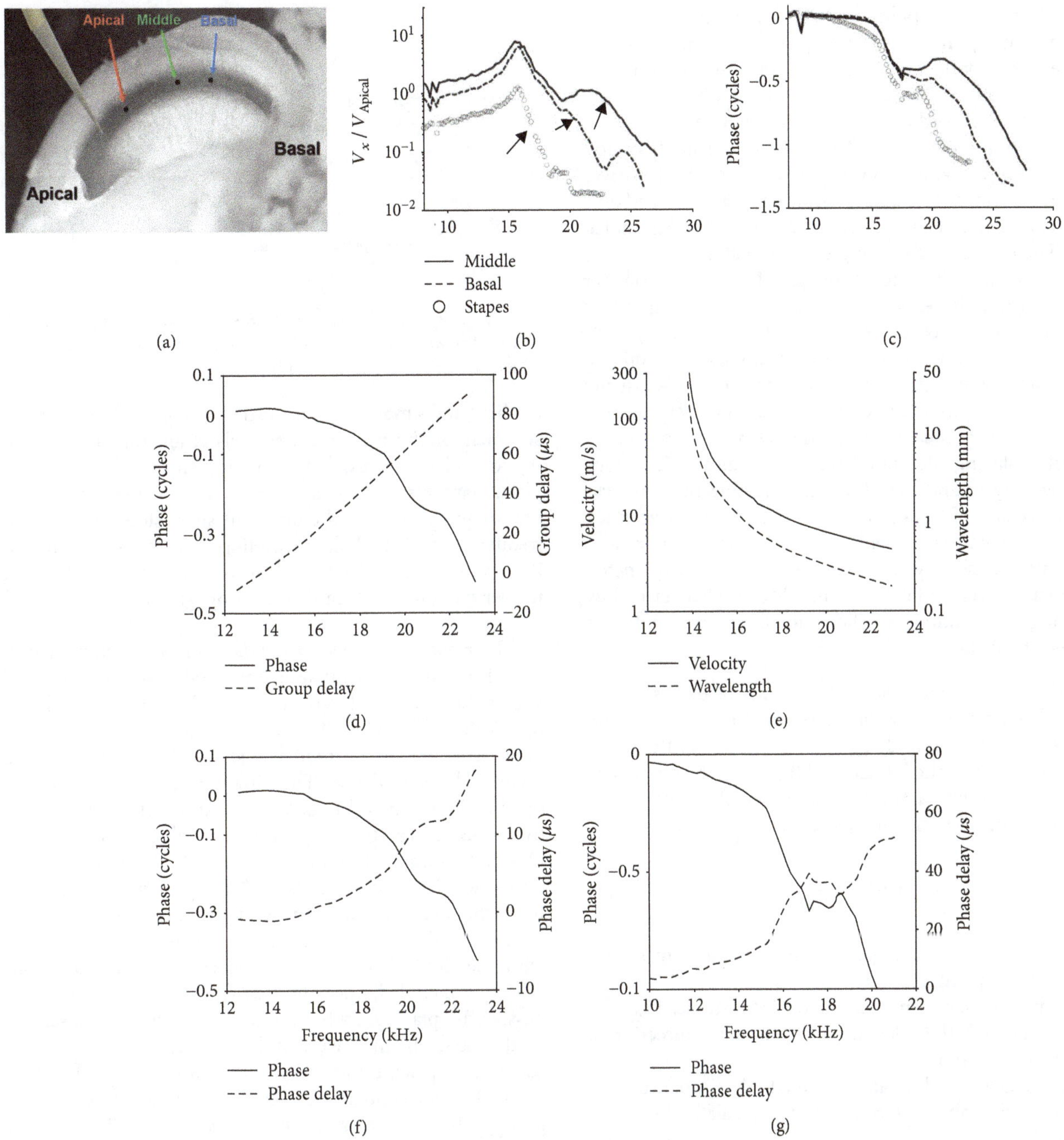

FIGURE 1: BM and stapes vibration spectra induced by a point stimulation of the BM. (a) The opened cochlea with stimulator and reflective beads in place. The stimulator probe is a blunt pipette driven by a piezoelectric stack. Reflective beads are placed on the BM, labeled as apical, middle, or basal, in the direction away from the stimulator. A bead was also placed on the stapes for recording its vibration. Vibration amplitude (b) and phase (c) of the middle (solid), basal (dash), and the stapes (circle) beads, relative to that of the apical bead. (d) Phase difference (solid) between the middle and basal beads and the calculated group delay (dash). (e) Wave velocity and the wavelength, calculated from the phase difference in D. The negative delay value at lower frequencies (<14 kHz) in both (d) and (e) is likely due to a local disturbance, such as the local reflection with the insertion of the stimulator. The wave speed is high at lower frequencies, and the distance between these two beads is small. Both effects make it vulnerable to the disturbance. For a wider range, apical to stapes, this small negative delay is absent (g). (f) Phase difference (solid) between the middle and basal beads and the calculated phase delay (dash). (g) Phase of the stapes vibration (solid) relative to the apical bead and the calculated phase delay (dash).

known diameter of the probe tip) was left to moisten the exposed BM.

The study was approved by the Institutional Animal Care and Use Committee of Oregon Health and Science University.

2.2. Piezo Stimulator Design and Mounting. The accurate location of the vibration source was a problem in almost all of the previous studies designed to measure the backward wave propagation in the cochlea. In our study, the direct mechanical driving method was adopted with a different design. The tip of a pulled pipette when heated with an electrical cautery, melted into a sphere of about 50 μm in diameter. This rounded tip was appropriate in size compared to the BM width for the delivery of a local vibration. Then a ~2 cm piece from the tip end of the pipette was cut off and attached to a piezo stack (AE0203D04F from Thorlabs, Newton, New Jersey) using cyanoacrylate cement. The driver was then cemented onto a steel bar, which was mounted on a micromanipulator. Figure 2 shows a view of the assembled probe. The overall size of the piezo stimulator allowed it to fit under the objective lens of the laser Doppler vibrometer (LDV). During the experiment, the piezo stimulator was advanced in about a 60-degree (relative to the horizon) angle by the micromanipulator into the opened scala tympani and to get contact with the BM by the tip. This process is visually guided under a surgical microscope. Careful attention was taken to avoid significant deformation or perforation on the BM. After placing the stimulator, the surgical microscope was moved away and the LDV with the objective lens was then moved in for vibration measurement. The piezo stack and the steel bar were held in such a way as to reduce interference caused by the laser beam of the velocimeter. The contact of the probe tip to the BM was also verified by measuring the vibration of the bead that is closest to the probe on the BM.

2.3. Calculation of the Delays. Two kinds of delays, group delay and phase delay, were calculated from the phase spectra in this study. The group delay is the derivative of the phase difference. To avoid the influence of the noise, the phase data was firstly fitted with a 4th-order polynomial to smooth the curve before performing the differentiation.

$$\text{Group delay} = -\frac{d\varphi}{2\pi df}, \tag{1}$$

where d is the differential operator, φ is the phase in radius, and f is the frequency.

Group delay has been used in most OAE studies [2, 5, 15, 16, 24] to quantify the delay for determining the direction of the wave propagation.

Besides group delay, another method to quantify the delay from the phase response is to calculate the phase delay by

$$\text{Phase delay} = -\frac{\varphi}{2\pi f}. \tag{2}$$

This method has been adopted in previous studies by Ren and his colleagues [3–6, 17, 19].

2.4. The Mechanical Cochlear Model. In this study, a mechanical model of the cochlea was used to verify the backward wave propagation. This mechanical device consisted of a fluid channel, a membrane section, and an artificial BM to simulate the basic hydromechanical structure of the cochlea [25]. The artificial BM was constructed from a polymer membrane with 32 copper beams deposited on it. The lengths of the copper slots increased gradually from one (basal) end to the other (apical) and resulted in a stiffness gradient for simulating that in the cochlea. Vibration measurement on this mechanical model demonstrated the traveling wave-like features, that is, tonotopicity, the frequency-to-place map, unsymmetrical filtering (the shallow slope at the low-frequency side of the peak but steep slope at the high-frequency side), and slow traveling wave phase. Therefore, it is a valid model of the cochlear hydromechanical structure for verifying the backward wave propagation.

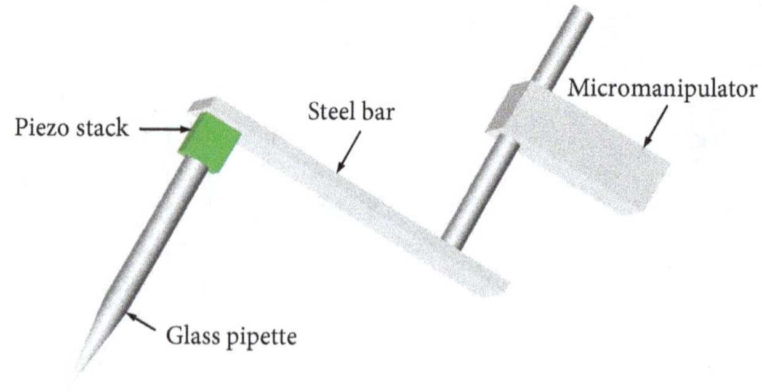

Figure 2: Construction of the piezo stimulator. Glass pipette with melted tip was glued on a piezo stack and then on a steel bar, which was fixed on a micromanipulator.

2.5. Transmission Line Model of the Cochlea. A mathematical model, lumped transmission line model, was created and simulated in a circuit simulator LTSPICE (Linear Technology, Milpitas, CA) based on acoustic-electrical analogy. The basic structure of the model is shown in Figure 3(a) and reviewed by Ni et al. [26]. This circuit model was firstly developed by Peterson and Bogert [27] and represented the basic hydromechanical property of the cochlea. Rather than a one-dimensional structure, our model includes a two-dimensional matrix of mass and dampers to represent the fluid channel. The cochlear partition was modeled as 400 sections of dampened mass-spring resonators and coupled with the fluid channel. No active component (outer hair cell) was included since the experimental preparation was passive. By placing a vibration source at the very basal end of the fluid channel, we simulated the stapes driving the cochlea; by placing the source inside a more apical section on the BM, we simulated the backward wave case where the glass probe stimulates the BM directly. The BM stiffness was taken from Puria and Steele [28], and the cochlear tonotopicity was taken from Greenwood [29].

3. Results

3.1. In Vivo Data Demonstrated a Slow Backward Wave on the BM. For this experiment, the cochlea of a young guinea pig was surgically exposed and the basal turn of the cochlea was widely opened. Reflective beads were placed on the BM at different longitudinal locations and on the head of stapes, as shown in Figure 1(a). In a typical experiment, vibration spectra were measured from three beads (named apical, middle, and basal, according to their relative longitudinal locations) and from the stapes. Vibration spectra measured at the middle and basal beads were scaled by the spectra measured at the apical bead, the closest one to the vibration

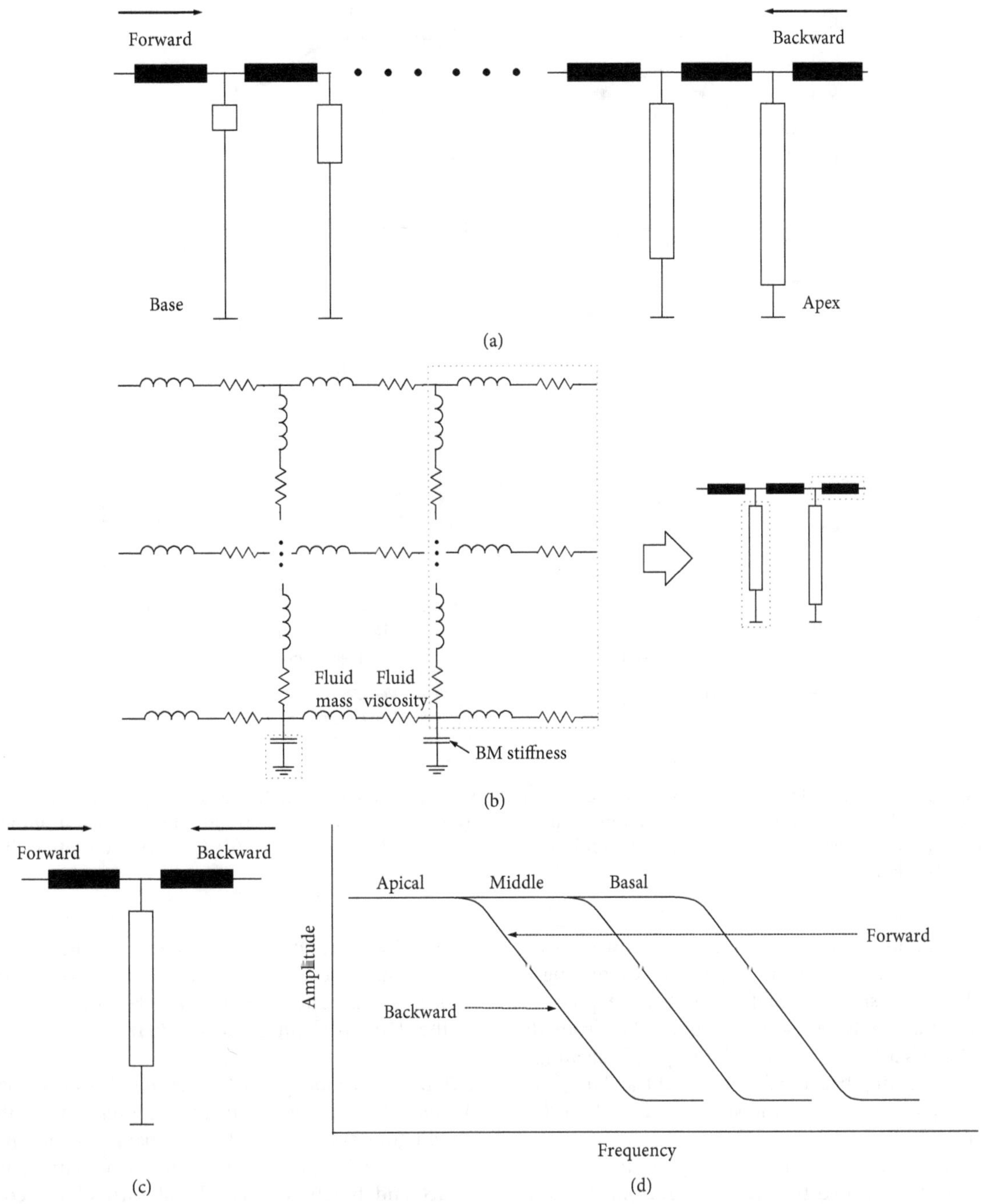

FIGURE 3: Model of the cochlear passive hydromechanical structure. (a) Schematic of the model structure. The thick solid lines represent the fluid channel and the open rectangles represent the cochlear partition, or simply BM. In this lumped model, the fluid channel and the cochlear partition (or simply BM) were divided into a series of sections. The rectangle is wider and shorter at the base and thinner and longer at the apex, representing the BM stiffness gradient: stiffer at the base and softer at the apex. (b) Circuit analogy of each section. The fluid mass is analogous to a series of inductors; the fluid viscosity is analogous to a series of resistors; the stiffness of the partition is analogous to a capacitor. (c) At each section, the forward and backward waves experience the same low-pass filtering. (d) Schematic shows the low-pass filters that the traveling wave experiences during the forward and backward propagation. Note that the forward direction is towards the low frequency. The roll-off frequency at the basal, middle, and apical locations decreases.

source, in order to calculate the transfer functions. Figure 1(b) shows the amplitude responses. In this plot, the amplitude of all the transfer functions demonstrated peaks at about 16 kHz and a gradually decreasing roll-off frequency in the direction away from the stimulus. This peak is likely due to the standing wave that was introduced by inserting the probe. In absolute units, the maximum vibration velocity magnitudes are 1.3 mm/s, which correspond to a displacement of 12 nm at the 16 kHz peak of the middle location response. As indicated by the arrows in Figure 1(b), in addition to the 16 kHz peak and the roll-off after, the amplitude responses showed higher-frequency roll-offs from about

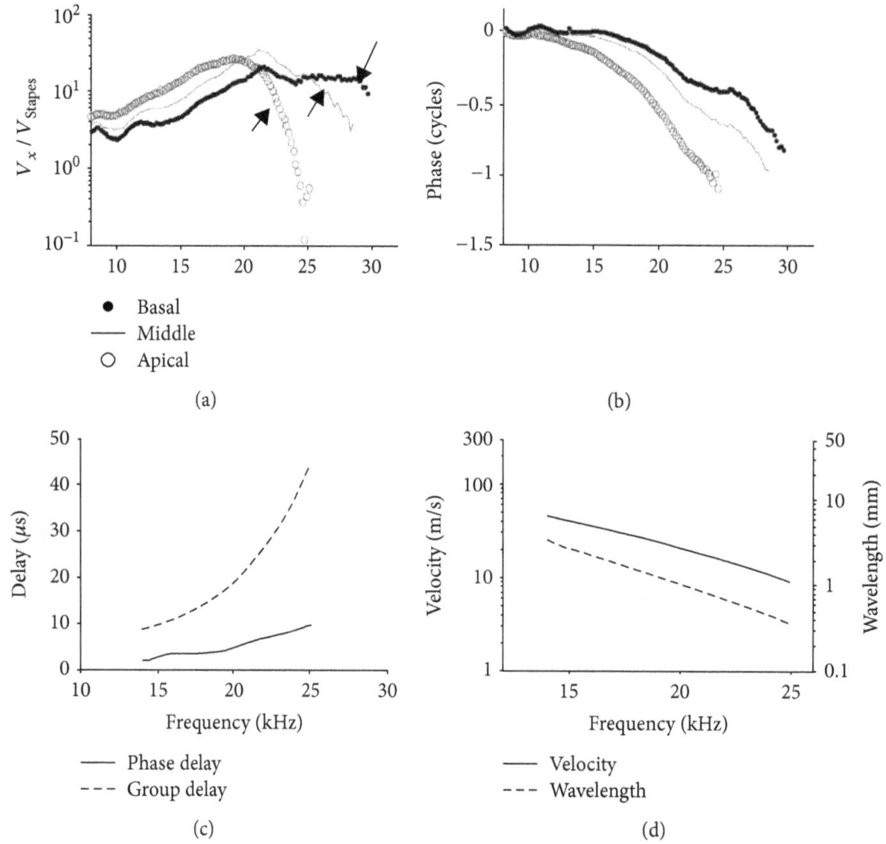

FIGURE 4: BM responses induced by normal acoustic stimulation at the ear drum. Vibration amplitude (a) and phase (b) of the beads on the BM. They are labeled as basal (dotted), middle (solid line), and apical (open cycle). Arrows in (a) indicates the roll-off of the amplitude responses. (c) Calculated phase and group delay between basal (dotted) and middle (solid line). (d) Calculated velocity (solid line) and wavelength (dashed line).

23 kHz for the middle location to about 20 kHz for the basal location and about 17 kHz at the stapes. Corresponding to the gradually decreasing roll-off frequencies, the phase of the spectra demonstrates a significant phase lag from the middle to the basal bead and then the stapes, indicating a slow wave propagating backward in the cochlea. The phase lag from the apical location to the stapes is more than one cycle (Figure 1(c)).

Phase difference between two neighboring—middle and basal—beads was used to calculate values of the wave propagation parameters: delay, wave velocity, and wavelength. The phase data were smoothed and fitted with polynomial before calculating the delay and velocity, as stated in Methods. The group delay between the middle and basal beads gradually increased with an increasing vibration frequency. It amounted to 62 μs at 20 kHz (Figure 1(d)). Correspondingly, the wave velocity and wavelength decreased. The wave velocity was about 6.4 m/s at 20 kHz for the distance of 400 μm between the two beads (Figure 1(e)).

Another method used to estimate the delay from the phase response was to calculate the phase delay. In Figure 1(f), we show that the phase delay value also increases with increasing frequencies but was smaller than the group delay, about 10 μs at 20 kHz. This resulted in a higher estimated speed of 38 m/s, as compared with using group delay. However, both speed values were much smaller than the estimated compression wave speed of approximately 1500 m/s. The calculated phase delay from the apical bead to the stapes is about 40 μs at 20 kHz.

3.2. BM Vibrations from Conventional Acoustic Stimulation Validated the Preparation. In this preparation, the sound-conduction system (i.e., the tympanic membrane and the ossicular chain) inside the middle ear was maintained to be intact and functional. The basal turn of the cochlea was widely opened, and the fluid at the scala tympani of the basal turn was maintained only at a level to moisten the BM. The cochlea thus became a single-channel hydrodynamic structure. To verify that this single-channel preparation preserved the forward traveling wave feature of the normal cochlea, the BM vibration was measured at the same longitudinal locations under normal acoustic conditions, that is, the sound was delivered to the ear drum. Rather than scaled by the vibration spectrum of the apical bead, here, the vibration spectra of three beads were scaled by the stapes vibration to obtain the forward cochlear-transfer functions. The amplitude plotted in Figure 4(a) shows a tonotopic map. The vibration spectrum rolled off at 28 kHz at the basal location; it rolled off at about 25 kHz at the middle location and at about 20 kHz at the apical location. Correspondingly, the phase

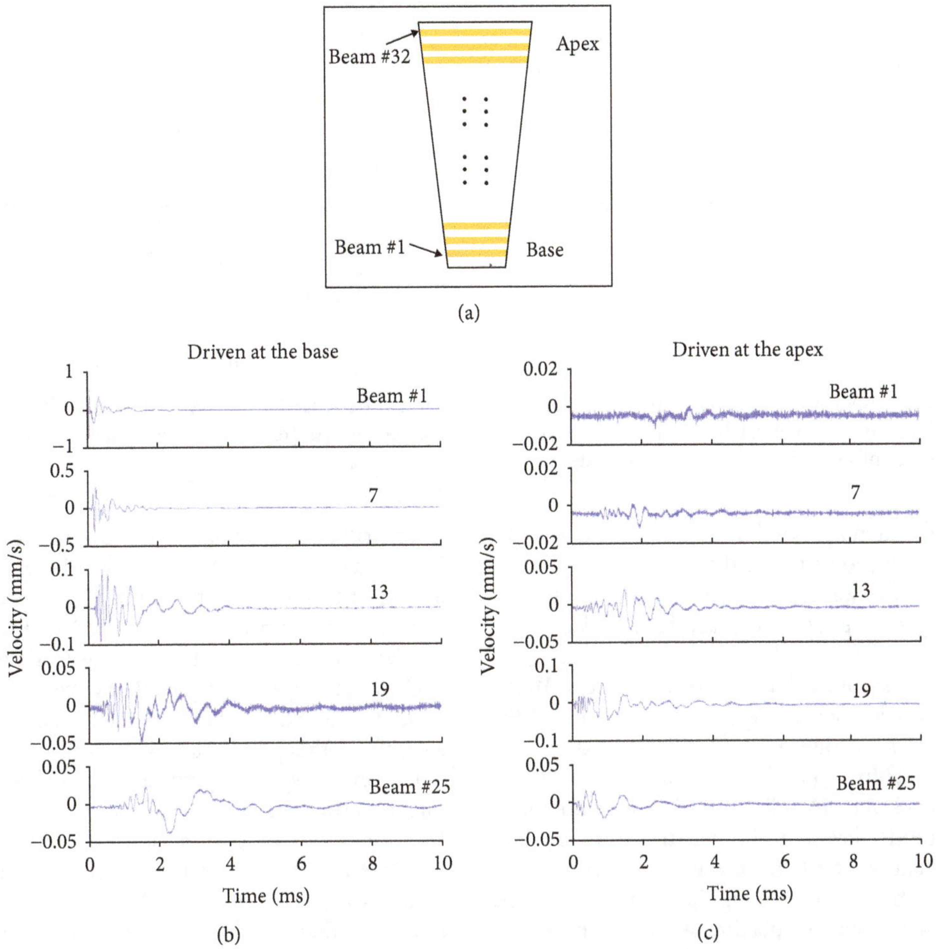

FIGURE 5: Vibration responses of a mechanical model of the cochlea. (a) Schematic view of the artificial BM. The length of the copper beam varies from 4 mm at the base (narrower) to 8 mm at the apex (wider). A total of 32 beams are placed on a membrane. The distance between beam #1 and #32 is about 20 mm. (b) BM vibration of the model while it was driven at the base, the narrowest, and thus the stiffest end. The driver was placed on the membrane right next to beam #1 at the base. Note that the scale of y-axis decreases from the top to the bottom, showing that the vibration amplitude was attenuated during the propagation. (c) BM vibration while it was driven at the apex. The driver was placed on the membrane at beam #29, close to the apex.

plotted in Figure 4(b) shows gradually the increasing phase lag from the basal to the middle and then to the apical locations. These are expected traveling wave-like features under conventional acoustic stimulation. The phase and group delay increased with the increasing frequency (Figure 4(c)). The phase delay amounted to about 1/5 of the group delay, similar to what they were in the backward direction as shown in Figures 1(d) and 1(f). The velocity and wavelength decreased with the increasing frequency (Figure 4(d)). The velocity ranged from about 10 m/s to 40 m/s. Correspondingly, the wavelength ranged from 0.3 mm to 2 mm. The trend and the values of the delay, velocity, and the wavelength all indicated a slow forward traveling wave. This experimentally verifies the wave propagation function of the single-channel cochlea.

3.3. Forward and Backward Traveling Waves Were Observed in the Mechanical Model of the Cochlea. To better understand the role of the hydromechanical structure of the cochlea in the backward wave propagation, we studied a mechanical model of the cochlea. This artificial device was composed of a fluid channel to simulate the scala vestibuli and a membrane to simulate the BM. Figure 5(a) shows the top schematic view of the device. Thirty-two copper beams are deposited on a membrane to form an artificial BM. The beam length varies gradually from beam #1 to beam #32, simulating the BM stiffness gradient from the base to the apex. The single fluid channel is underneath the BM (detailed construction of the device can be found in Chen et al. [25]). In a previous study, we showed that this hydromechanical structure could demonstrate cochlea-like features and its capability to support the forward cochlear traveling wave [25].

Figure 5(b) shows the time-domain response of the beam vibration, when the artificial cochlea was driven at the base, just before beam #1. About 1 ms delay was demonstrated between the onset responses of beam #1 and beam #25. The distance of these two beams was about 15 mm, so the speed of the wave propagation was about 15 m/s. Figure 5(c) shows the results when the device was driven at the apex, on Beam #32. A clear

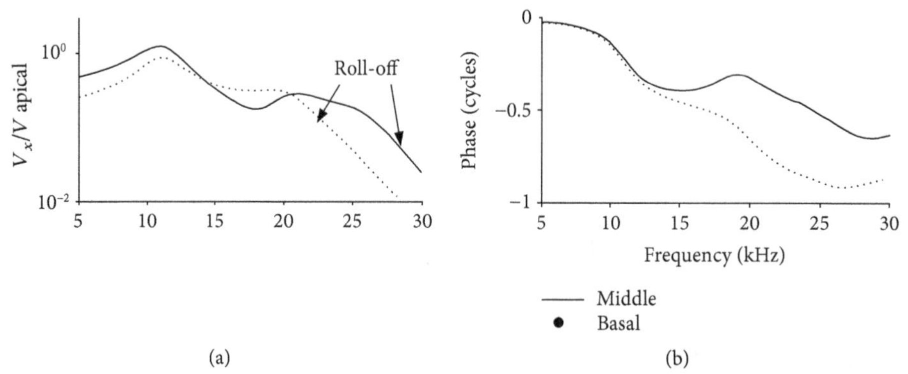

Figure 6: BM vibration responses of a mathematical model of the cochlea under backward driving. (a) Amplitude responses of BM vibration at two longitudinal locations. Solid line, labeled as middle, is at a more apical location; dotted line, labeled as basal, is at a more basal location. The arrows marked the roll-off points. (b) Phase responses.

backward delay was demonstrated in the plots. The amount of the delay was similar to its forward counterpart and so as the speed. This slow wave propagation implies that a backward traveling wave exists in this artificial device.

3.4. Simulation Results from a Mathematical Cochlear Model Where a Point Vibration Source Reproduced Features of the Experimental Data. In addition to the *in vivo* data and the experimental results from the mechanical model, we also studied the backward traveling wave in a mathematical model. This model has a traditional transmission line structure for simulating the hydromechanical structure of the cochlea. With this model, we simulated the backward responses. This was done by placing a vibration source at about 1/3 of the length of the cochlear model from the base and computing the BM vibration responses at more basal places towards to the stapes. BM vibration at three locations was computed to simulate the measured results at the apical, middle, and basal beads. As in the experimental results, the vibration spectra of the middle and basal beads were scaled by that of the apical bead, as shown in Figure 6. Features in the experimental results, as shown in Figures 1(b) and 1(c), were also demonstrated in the simulation results. The spectra can be viewed at two different frequency ranges. At lower frequencies (about <15 kHz), the amplitude response in Figure 6(a) shows a peak at about 12 kHz for both middle and basal locations. Correspondingly, the phase plotted in Figure 6(b) shows a steep roll off at the peak frequency. This could be due to reflection between the point source and the stapes. At frequencies lower than the peak, the phase responses of both locations almost overlap. This can be interpreted as a fast traveling wave at lower frequencies. The amplitude response rolled off at about 25 kHz for the middle location and at about 20 kHz for the basal location. Correspondingly, the phase response showed a clear delay from the middle to the basal location. This indicates a slow backward wave.

4. Discussion

4.1. Direction of the Wave Propagation. It has been hypothesized [1] that the OAE, generated as vibration at the organ of Corti, will propagate backward toward the stapes via a traveling wave on the BM. Although this theory is widely accepted and used to interpret the OAEs [2], the backward traveling wave has never been demonstrated with direct evidence of the BM vibration. Analysis of the OAE phase [9, 15] and cochlear microphonic signal that were measured at the round window [16] was used as indirect evidence of backward propagation. In this present study, the organ of Corti was set into vibration at a specific point location. This produced the first directly observed *in vivo* backward wave propagating on the BM. The phase plotted in Figure 1(c) has a gradual increase of phase lag at the vibration spectra measured at the apical (used as the reference; not shown) to the middle, the basal bead, and then the stapes. The velocity and delay calculated from the phase plot were within the same order of magnitude of their forward counterpart (Figure 4). These results are also evidence of a slow transverse wave propagating backward on the BM. In addition, we found a slow reverse wave propagation in a mechanical model of the cochlea (Figure 5). Since the cochlea prepared through the surgical procedure became a passive one (surgical damage removes the amplification by cochlear outer hair cells), this wave propagation appears to be a fundamental property of the hydromechanical structure of the cochlea. The artificial cochlea, which mimics the basic hydromechanical structure of the cochlea, confirms and supports the essential nature of the slow transverse waves, that is, they exhibit bidirectional propagation.

4.2. Interpretation of No Tonotopicity in Backward Wave Propagation. Although the experimental results in Figure 1 demonstrated the correct phase in reverse propagation, the amplitude response did not show the expected cochlear tonotopicity: the peak-frequency-to-place map [29]. In contrast, there was a slight inversion or reversal of the map, that is, the roll-off frequency is higher at the more apical location and lower at the more basal location. These seemly controversial reverse wave features are simulated by the transmission line model of the cochlea, as shown schematically in Figure 3.

The hydromechanical theory of the cochlea asserts that tonotopicity is achieved with the combination of fluid coupling in the scalae and a local resonance at the BM, the so-called critical-layer resonance [30]. For a passive cochlea, as used in this study, the hydromechanical structure is the dominant contributor [31]. The passive responses lack sharp tuning and diminish at high frequencies. Therefore, the local resonance is simplified in the model to a capacitor because the resonator is stiffness dominant at the lower frequencies. Acoustic energy in the fluid couples to the BM, whose stiffness decreases from the base to the apex.

Although the stiffness gradient is the most important feature for the tonotopicity [32], a small amount of frequency selectivity can be achieved without it. This process is most easily explained with an electric circuit analogy. The cochlear hydromechanical structure is analogous to a lossy transmission line, as originally proposed by Zwislocki [31]. In a lumped model, the cochlea is divided into a series of connected repeating sections (Figure 3(a)). At each section (Figure 3(b)), the fluid coupling effect was modeled as a series of inductors and resistors, representing the fluid mass and viscosity, respectively [33]; the mechanical impedance of the cochlear partition was modeled as a capacitor, representing the stiffness of the BM. Although the BM is usually modeled as a second-order resonator to account for the sharp tuning of the cochlea, generality is maintained with the simplification to a spring (capacitor in a circuit analogy) to model the passive responses. This simplification is fundamental to Zwislocki's transmission line theory [31] to interpret the passive vibration data observed by von Békésy [34]. With this simplification, the propagation of the BM vibration was described using a wave equation [31]. Each section of the structure applies a low-pass filtering effect onto the vibration of the BM, attenuating the high-frequency components and producing propagation delay. Vibration, originated from either a basal or apical location, will experience the same low-pass filtering sections (Figure 3(c)), but from different directions. Therefore, the high-frequency components of the BM vibration are continuously attenuated, and the phase delay is continuously accumulated during the propagation, no matter which end the wave originates.

Figure 3(d) explains why no cochlear tonotopicity is achieved in reverse propagation. In the forward direction, the stiffness of the cochlear partition decreases in the direction of the propagation. Therefore, the roll-off frequency of the low-pass filtering, implemented by the fluid mass and the stiffness of the partition, becomes lower and lower. Therefore, the high-frequency components of the traveling wave are cut off gradually during the propagation, resulting in the passive cochlear tonotopicity. In the reverse direction, the traveling wave encounters the low-pass section with the lowest roll-off first. Most of the high-frequency components are attenuated at this early section. During the propagation, although the traveling wave will still experience low-pass sections, its already low-passed components will not be further cut off because the roll-off frequencies of the later sections are all higher. The result is that no clear tonotopicity is produced, but the high-frequency components are still slightly attenuated along the direction of propagation.

Despite the significant difference in the amplitude responses, the transmission line-like structure of the cochlea produces a propagation delay in the direction of away from the vibration source, no matter where the vibration source is located. This is shown in both the experimental data in Figure 1(c) and the simulation results in Figure 6(b).

4.3. Validation of the Preparation. Since we opened the cochlea widely and drained the fluid in the scala tympani at the base, we need to ensure that this preparation can still support the wave propagation as a normal cochlea. The single-channel preparation for the measurement of basilar membrane vibration has been used previously [35, 36] and has theoretically been proven to be able to produce forward traveling wave features [37]. LePage [36] used a capacitive probe to measure the BM motion, which required the fluid in the scala tympani to be removed. It was shown that the BM vibration showed similar responses as its dual-channel counterpart. The acoustic driving results in Figure 4 also showed traveling wave features. Therefore, this preparation still maintains the basic hydromechanical structure of the cochlea. The *in vivo* physiological environment in the cochlea is maintained stably so that the mechanical properties provided by the cellular structure of the organ of Corti do not deteriorate during the experiments. Although this preparation is designed to verify the backward traveling wave, it does not preclude the existence of the compression wave, as the intact scala vestibule can still support the compression wave propagation. The open channel at the scala tympani could influence the speed of the compression wave. However, this influence is minimal considering that the speed of the compression wave is two orders of magnitude higher than that of the traveling wave. The BM vibration measurement method used in this study is also essentially the same as that used by He et al. and Ren et al. [3–5]. Therefore, if the compression wave does exist in this preparation, we should be able to observe its effect, as a transverse wave in the forward direction in our experiments.

To ensure that the vibration source in this study is on the BM, we drained the perilymph at the opened portion of the scala tympani and then maintained the fluid at a very low level (~30 μm) with a cotton wick. According to the current theory, it is the vibration generated in the organ of Corti on the BM that initiates the backward traveling wave. The OAE is also generated in the organ of Corti. The stimulus in the fluid may result in a similar effect as the stimulation by the stapes, producing a forward wave. This phenomenon has been demonstrated by von Békésy [38] and termed as the *paradoxical wave*, where even if the stapes is placed at the apex of the cochlea, a forward traveling wave was still observed, moving towards the source.

4.4. Passive or Active Preparation. In this study, the extensive surgery on the cochlea resulted in a loss of sensitivity, so that the preparation was essentially passive. Although loss of cochlear amplification would influence the generation of the OAE, the passive preparation is an advantage in studying the wave propagation. The wave propagation inside the cochlea is mostly determined by the hydromechanical structure, and our preparation preserves the basic hydromechanical components of the cochlea.

The advantage in the use of the passive preparation is that it avoids any phase delay introduced by the active tuning of the cochlea. In a sensitive preparation, active tuning of the cochlea contributes strongly to the measured group delay [20]. Tuning-induced group delay is primarily responsible for the enhancement of the propagation delay in the forward-propagation condition, because the tuning frequency of the cochlea decreases in the forward direction and this frequency gradient produces a phase lag in the same direction. In a sensitive cochlea, artificially driven to produce a backward wave, tuning-induced forward delay may mask the possible backward traveling wave delay. The propagation delay increases while traveling away from the source. However, the tuning delay is determined by the cochlear frequency map and it always increases from the base to the apex, no matter where the source is. Therefore, in the measured phase responses in a backward-traveling-wave study, there are two components that can contribute oppositely to the total delay. This tuning-induced delay could be one way to explain the results of He et al., Ren et al., and Ren [3–6], in which the measured phase delay increased from the base to the apex and thus indicated the absence of a detectable backward traveling wave. In those experiments, however, a very sensitive preparation was usually required by the vibration-source-generation method (acoustically produced distortion product or electrically stimulated emission). The tuning delay may be significant, especially when the vibration at two close locations is compared to determine the direction of the wave propagation [3]. In their study, the measurement range was narrow, and thus, the propagation delay was relatively small, compared to the tuning delay.

5. Conclusions

In this study, we investigated the backward wave propagation inside the cochlea. By creating a vibration source at a precise location, we avoided the uncertainty of the place where the vibration was originated in most previous studies. With measurements at multiple longitudinal locations along the cochlea, we, for the first time, demonstrated a slow backward traveling wave towards the stapes. This result was also confirmed in a mechanical model of the cochlea and interpreted with a traditional transmission line mathematical model.

Conflicts of Interest

The authors declare that they have no conflicts of interest.

Authors' Contributions

Fangyi Chen and Dingjun Zha designed the experiments; Fangyi Chen analyzed the data; Fangyi Chen, Xiaojie Yang, Allyn Hubbard, and Alfred Nuttall wrote the paper; and all authors helped with the manuscript preparation and revision.

Acknowledgments

The authors would like to thank Drs. Egbert DeBoer, Anders Fridberger, and Sripriya Ramamoorthy for their comments on the manuscript. This work was funded by the National Natural Science Foundation of China (Grant nos. 81470701 and 81771882), the Fundamental Research (Discipline Layout) Foundation from Shenzhen Committee of Science, Technology and Innovation (Grant no. JCYJ20170817111912585), and Deafness Research Foundation for Fangyi Chen; the National Natural Science Foundation of China (Grant nos. 81271077 and 81470695) for Dingjun Zha; and NIDCDR01 (Grant nos. DC000141 and DC010399) for Alfred Nuttall.

References

[1] D. T. Kemp, "Stimulated acoustic emissions from within the human auditory system," *The Journal of the Acoustical Society of America*, vol. 64, no. 5, pp. 1386–1391, 1978.

[2] C. A. Shera and J. J. Guinan Jr, "Evoked otoacoustic emissions arise by two fundamentally different mechanisms: a taxonomy for mammalian OAEs," *The Journal of the Acoustical Society of America*, vol. 105, no. 2, pp. 782–798, 1999.

[3] W. He, A. Fridberger, E. Porsov, K. Grosh, and T. Ren, "Reverse wave propagation in the cochlea," *Proceedings of the National Academy of Sciences of the United States of America*, vol. 105, no. 7, pp. 2729–2733, 2008.

[4] W. He, A. Fridberger, E. Porsov, and T. Ren, "Fast reverse propagation of sound in the living cochlea," *Biophysical Journal*, vol. 98, no. 11, pp. 2497–2505, 2010.

[5] T. Ren, W. He, M. Scott, and A. L. Nuttall, "Group delay of acoustic emissions in the ear," *Journal of Neurophysiology*, vol. 96, no. 5, pp. 2785–2791, 2006.

[6] T. Ren, "Reverse propagation of sound in the gerbil cochlea," *Nature Neuroscience*, vol. 7, no. 4, pp. 333-334, 2004.

[7] C. A. Shera, A. Tubis, and C. L. Talmadge, *Four Counter-Arguments for Slow-Wave OAEs in 9th International Symposium*, A. L. Nuttall, Ed., pp. 449–457, 2015.

[8] H. Zhang and D. C. Mountain, *Concepts and Challenges in the Biophysics of Hearing*, N. P. Cooper and D. T. Kemp, Eds., World Scientific, Singapore, 2009.

[9] E. de Boer, J. Zheng, E. Porsov, and A. L. Nuttall, "Inverted direction of wave propagation (IDWP) in the cochlea," *The Journal of the Acoustical Society of America*, vol. 123, no. 3, pp. 1513–1521, 2008.

[10] Y. Li and K. Grosh, "Direction of wave propagation in the cochlea for internally excited basilar membrane," *The Journal of the Acoustical Society of America*, vol. 131, no. 6, pp. 4710–4721, 2012.

[11] C. A. Shera, "Mechanisms of mammalian otoacoustic emission and their implications for the clinical utility of otoacoustic emissions," *Ear and Hearing*, vol. 25, no. 2, pp. 86–97, 2004.

[12] A. Vetešník and A. W. Gummer, "Transmission of cochlear distortion products as slow waves: a comparison of experimental and model data," *The Journal of the Acoustical Society of America*, vol. 131, no. 5, pp. 3914–3934, 2012.

[13] R. Sisto, A. Moleti, T. Botti, D. Bertaccini, and C. A. Shera, "Distortion products and backward-traveling waves in nonlinear active models of the cochlea," *The Journal of the Acoustical Society of America*, vol. 129, no. 5, pp. 3141–3152, 2011.

[14] S. J. Elliott, G. Ni, B. R. Mace, and B. Lineton, "A wave finite element analysis of the passive cochlea," *The Journal of the Acoustical Society of America*, vol. 133, no. 3, pp. 1535–1545, 2013.

[15] W. Dong and E. S. Olson, "Supporting evidence for reverse cochlear traveling waves," *The Journal of the Acoustical Society of America*, vol. 123, no. 1, pp. 222–240, 2008.

[16] S. W. F. Meenderink and M. van der Heijden, "Reverse cochlear propagation in the intact cochlea of the gerbil: evidence for slow traveling waves," *Journal of Neurophysiology*, vol. 103, no. 3, pp. 1448–1455, 2010.

[17] A. Fridberger and T. Ren, "Local mechanical stimulation of the hearing organ by laser irradiation," *Neuroreport*, vol. 17, no. 1, pp. 33–37, 2006.

[18] C.-P. Richter, B. N. Evans, R. Edge, and P. Dallos, "Basilar membrane vibration in the gerbil hemicochlea," *Journal of Neurophysiology*, vol. 79, no. 5, pp. 2255–2264, 1998.

[19] T. Ren and E. Porsov, "Reverse propagation of sounds in the intact cochlea," *Journal of Neurophysiology*, vol. 104, no. 6, p. 3732, 2010.

[20] M. A. Ruggero and A. N. Temchin, "Similarity of traveling-wave delays in the hearing organs of humans and other tetrapods," *Journal of the Association for Research in Otolaryngology*, vol. 8, no. 2, pp. 153–166, 2007.

[21] R. Ghaffari, A. J. Aranyosi, and D. M. Freeman, "Longitudinally propagating traveling waves of the mammalian tectorial membrane," *Proceedings of the National Academy of Sciences of the United States of America*, vol. 104, no. 42, pp. 16510–16515, 2007.

[22] T. Reichenbach, A. Stefanovic, F. Nin, and A. J. Hudspeth, "Waves on Reissner's membrane: a mechanism for the propagation of otoacoustic emissions from the cochlea," *Cell Reports*, vol. 1, no. 4, pp. 374–384, 2012.

[23] J. Zheng, N. Deo, Y. Zou, K. Grosh, and A. L. Nuttall, "Chlorpromazine alters cochlear mechanics and amplification: in vivo evidence for a role of stiffness modulation in the organ of Corti," *Journal of Neurophysiology*, vol. 97, no. 2, pp. 994–1004, 2007.

[24] M. A. Ruggero, "Comparison of group delays of 2f1–f2 distortion product otoacoustic emissions and cochlear travel times," *Acoustics Research Letters Online*, vol. 5, no. 4, pp. 143–147, 2004.

[25] F. Chen, H. I. Cohen, T. G. Bifano et al., "A hydromechanical biomimetic cochlea: experiments and models," *The Journal of the Acoustical Society of America*, vol. 119, no. 1, pp. 394–405, 2006.

[26] G. Ni, S. J. Elliott, M. Ayat, and P. D. Teal, "Modelling cochlear mechanics," *BioMed Research International*, vol. 2014, no. 7, Article ID 150637, 42 pages, 2014.

[27] L. C. Peterson and B. P. Bogert, "A dynamical theory of the cochlea," *The Journal of the Acoustical Society of America*, vol. 22, no. 3, pp. 369–381, 1950.

[28] S. Puria and C. R. Steele, *The Senses: A Comprehensive Reference*, A. I. Bassbaum, A. Kaneko, G. M. Shepherd, and G. Westheimer, Eds., vol. 3, Ch. Audition, Academic Press, 2008.

[29] D. D. Greenwood, "A cochlear frequency-position function for several species—29 years later," *The Journal of the Acoustical Society of America*, vol. 87, no. 6, pp. 2592–2605, 1990.

[30] J. Lighthill, "Energy flow in the cochlea," *Journal of Fluid Mechanics*, vol. 106, no. 1, pp. 149–213, 1981.

[31] J. Zwislocki, "Theory of the acoustical action of the cochlea," *The Journal of the Acoustical Society of America*, vol. 22, no. 6, pp. 778–784, 1950.

[32] G. Ni, L. Sun, and S. J. Elliott, "A linearly tapered box model of the cochlea," *The Journal of the Acoustical Society of America*, vol. 141, no. 3, pp. 1793–1803, 2017.

[33] G. Ni and S. J. Elliott, "Comparing methods of modeling near field fluid coupling in the cochlea," *The Journal of the Acoustical Society of America*, vol. 137, no. 3, pp. 1309–1317, 2015.

[34] G. V. Békésy, "The variation of phase along the basilar membrane with sinusoidal vibrations," *The Journal of the Acoustical Society of America*, vol. 19, no. 3, pp. 452–460, 1947.

[35] J. P. Wilson and J. R. Johnstone, "Basilar membrane and middle-ear vibration in guinea pig measured by capacitive probe," *The Journal of the Acoustical Society of America*, vol. 57, no. 3, pp. 705–723, 1975.

[36] E. L. LePage, "The application of a capacitive probe technique for direct observation of electromechanical processes in the guinea pig cochlea," *The Journal of the Acoustical Society of America*, vol. 82, no. 1, pp. 126–138, 1987.

[37] R. Patuzzi, "Springer Handbook of Auditory Research," in *The Cochlea*, P. Dallos, Ed., vol. 8, Springer, New York, 1996.

[38] G. v. Békésy, "Paradoxical direction of wave travel along the cochlear partition," *The Journal of the Acoustical Society of America*, vol. 27, no. 1, pp. 137–145, 1955.

13

Cholinergic Mechanisms of Target Oddball Stimuli Detection: The Late "P300-Like" Event-Related Potential in Rats

A. Ahnaou, R. Biermans, and W. H. I. M. Drinkenburg

Department of Neuroscience, Janssen Research & Development, Janssen Pharmaceutica NV, Turnhoutseweg 30, 2340 Beerse, Belgium

Correspondence should be addressed to A. Ahnaou; aahnaou@its.jnj.com

Academic Editor: Malgorzata Kossut

Event-related potentials (ERPs) and oscillations (EROs) provide powerful tools for studying the brain's synaptic function underlying information processing. The P300 component of ERPs indexing attention and working memory shows abnormal amplitude and latency in neurological and psychiatric diseases that are sensitive to pharmacological agents. In the active auditory oddball discriminant paradigm, behavior and auditory-evoked potentials (AEPs) were simultaneously recorded in awake rats to investigate whether P300-like potentials generated in rats responding to rare target oddball tones are sensitive to subcutaneous modulation of the cholinergic tone by donepezil (1 mg/kg) and scopolamine (0.64 mg/kg). After operant training, rats consistently discriminate rare target auditory stimuli from frequent irrelevant nontarget auditory stimuli by a higher level of correct lever presses (i.e., accuracy) in target trials associated with a food reward. Donepezil attenuated the disruptive effect of scopolamine on the level of accuracy and premature responses in target trials. Larger P300-like peaks with early and late components were revealed in correct rare target stimuli trials as compared to frequent tones. Donepezil enhanced the peak amplitude of the P300-like component to target stimuli and evoked slow theta and gamma oscillations, whereas scopolamine altered the amplitude of the P300-like component and EROs to target stimuli. Pretreatment with donepezil attenuated effects of scopolamine on the peak amplitude of the P300-like component and on EROs. This study provides evidence that AEP P300-like responses can be elicited by rats engaged in attentive and memory processing of target stimuli and outline the relevance of the cholinergic system in stimulus discrimination processing. The findings highlight the sensitivity of this translational index for investigating brain circuits and/or novel pharmacological agents, which modulate cholinergic transmission associated with increased allocation of attentional resources.

1. Introduction

Despite the recent flurry of research efforts in contemporary cognitive neuroscience, there remains a need to identify an early biomarker with high sensitivity and specificity for cognitive impairments. Many cognitive functions are unique to humans and cannot be addressed in experimental animals whilst cognitive paradigms and models must have translational validity to be of use in drug discovery. Animal models are often discussed regarding face, constructive, and predictive validity criteria, and the better an animal model fulfils these criteria, the more successful the translation of preclinical data to clinical applications is likely to be. Despite the availability of some level of face and construct validity for assays and disease models used in cognition research, the critical feature for drug discovery is the predictive validity [1–3]. Ideal animal models of cognition should provide a prediction of the specific conditions for which compounds would be most useful and could be combined with toxicology and safety pharmacology models to estimate the therapeutic effect [4]. A recent promising project seeking to develop new ways to classify mental disorders proposes a new research domain criteria (RDoC) approach that may facilitate translational research. Focus on brain neuronal circuits and connectivity is a promising approach to provide a closer link between animal models and the disorders they model [5–9].

Cognition refers to mental processes that are involved in gaining knowledge and comprehension such as problem-solving and decision-making, attention, memory and working memory, judgment, evaluation, and production of language. Neurons do not generally act in isolation but act as synchronized and rhythmically active assemblies to encode, transmit, and modulate information underpinning cognitive function under normal or evoked modalities. Thus, cognition can better be understood in terms of complex disparate networks operating over multiple temporal scales and incorporating diverse dimensions. Changes in the pattern of synaptic weights underlie the efficacy of communication neuronal ensembles and the process of long-term potentiation (LTP), an electrophysiological basic correlate of learning and memory [10–13]. Although mostly studied in hippocampal and neocortex animal preparations [14–16], rapid visual or auditory tetanus stimuli elicited changes in amplitude of event-related potentials (ERPs) recorded from the scalp of adult humans that are suggestive of LTP-like characteristics that are seen in experimental animals [17–19]. ERP components are voltage changes in the electroencephalographic activity that are specifically linked to a physical or mental stimulus, which provide a direct window into the brain mechanisms that are reflected in performance measures during attention processing paradigms in normal and disease conditions [20–23]. The temporal encoding of information is essential for synaptic plasticity, and the temporal immediacy of ERPs is advantageous in the study of memory encoding and retrieval processes.

In the oddball discrimination-task paradigm, the evoked ERP waveforms defined by their polarity and latency reflect a cascade of information processing of a stimuli that are functionally specified to attentional and memory mechanisms. The early P1-N1-P2 complex component reflects a preattentional response following the initial memory encoding of the stimulus characteristics [24, 25], whereas the N2 and P300 components are only elicited following selective attentional allocation to target stimuli [26]. The P300 or (P3) peak is a scalp positivity bioelectric ERP correlate that is elicited by low-probability task-relevant stimuli during stimulus classification tasks in auditory, visual, and somatosensory modalities. It occurs at approximately 300 ms after stimuli onset in humans. In rodents, there is a reduced latency of this signal due to the shorter distance that the signal must travel in the smaller brain of rodents. It can be classed as an "endogenous" component in the sense that it relies on the processing of the stimulus context and the levels of attention and arousal [23, 26, 27]. Following an initial sensory processing, an attention-driven comparison process evaluates the representation of the previous event in the working memory. The P300 peak amplitude and latency are modulated by a variety of factors, including subjective probability, stimulus saliency, availability of attentional resources, and it appears to be generated by a network of neural regions; the inferotemporal, perirhinal, prefrontal, cingulate, superior temporal, and parietal cortices, as well as the hippocampus.

The ERP P300 component is regarded as a neurophysiological indicator of cognitive processing of a stimulus [27]. In neurological and psychiatric disorders, a key prerequisite would be a biomarker that can reliably predict a transition and progression of the disease and facilitate early pharmacological intervention. Several neurological and psychiatric studies demonstrate the links between memory and cognitive impairments and negative changes observed in P300 peak latency and amplitude. P300 has emerged as a viable endophenotype for schizophrenia and may provide a robust marker for illness progression in an individual patient considered at risk of developing schizophrenia [28–30]. P300 peak delayed latency can serve to produce biomarkers of mild cognitive impairments [31, 32], predictive measure of brain amyloid load in preclinical Alzheimer's disease [33], and dementia and its progression [34, 35].

The P300 component amplitude is thought to be related to the processing and brain activity involved in the working memory. The most common theory is the context updating theory, which reflects the information processing involved when incoming information is integrated with a memory representation of a stimulus and the context with which it occurs. The latency with which the P300 wave occurs is thought to be negatively correlated to mental function. The latency shows the processing time needed before a response can be generated; hence, the later appearance of the peak shows a direct link to slowing of cognitive function [26]. Patients that have a damage in the temporoparietal junction have the auditory P300 response eliminated, which suggests that this neocortical region is potentially critical in the generation or propagation of the scalp P300 [36].

In addition to ERP waveforms, event-related oscillations (EROs) synchrony quantifies the time-locked change in the power of the EEG spectral contents associated with the event-related trials. Oscillations can be evoked (phase-locked to the stimulus) or induced (nonphase-locked to the stimulus). Functionally, EROs are not yet fully understood, as complex and integrative brain functions seem to rely on the superimposition of several oscillations [36]. Neuronal oscillations play a fundamental role in linking and coordinating interlinked and overlapping cerebral regions. Oscillatory rhythms in the theta and gamma frequency ranges are related to episodic memory and are widely used to monitor oscillations driven by hippocampal regions in coordination with the frontal cortical areas. Additionally, various neuromodulators such as the neurotransmitter acetylcholine (ACh) play key roles in influencing cognitive performance. For instance, the prefrontal cortex (PFC) and hippocampus receive a rich cholinergic input and are also heavily innervated by serotonergic, dopaminergic, noradrenergic, and histaminergic neurons [37]. Cholinergic transmission is the main target for most of the current symptomatic therapies in neurodegenerative diseases, in the form of ACh esterase (AChE) inhibitors such as donepezil. The pharmacological model based on scopolamine, which temporarily blocks muscarinic cholinergic receptors in the brain, is widely regarded as a standard model for investigating cognitive deficits and may be useful in the search for improved procognitive drugs. Despite the peripheral side effects that occur at higher doses of scopolamine, the primary effects on stimulus discrimination and attention make this compound good for pharmacological validation of the two-tone discrimination task.

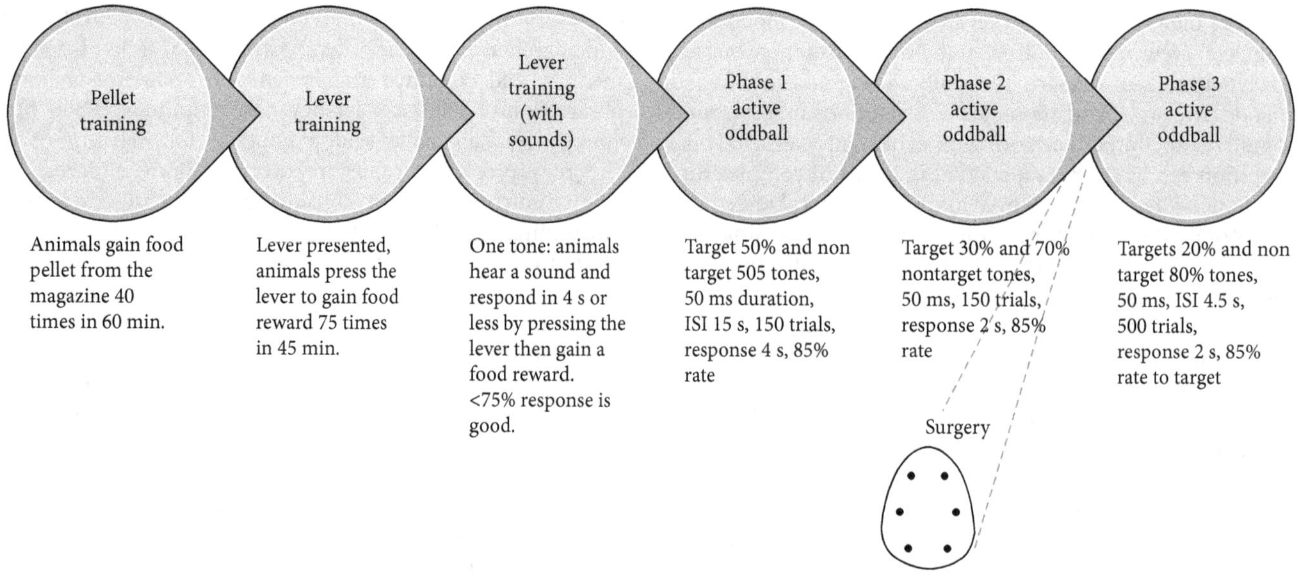

Figure 1: Schematic presentation of different phases of the active oddball discriminant task. Animals had to correctly respond to infrequent target (oddball) tones whilst correctly ignoring frequent standard tones. The criteria for good behavioral performance was >80% response to target and <20% response to standard tones. Epidural electrodes implanted in the rats recorded continuous EEG from specific brain areas (frontal, parietal, and occipital).

Over the last decade, animal models of the long-latency ERP P300 component have been developed in cats [38] and non-human primates [39]. In rodents, studies using the passive oddball, where animals do not require extensive training, revealed late positive potentials in the mouse [40] and rat cortex [41–43]. In the active oddball paradigm, late positive components with peak latency at approximately 200–500 ms were identified in electrodes overlying cortical, hippocampal, and nucleus accumbens- and amygdala-recording sites [43, 44]. This was clearly identified in rats that paid attention to target stimuli in the active oddball, whereas it was not revealed in animals not performing in the passive oddball paradigm [41, 45]. In addition, the rat's ERP P300-like response was sensitive to pharmacological modulation of the cholinergic tone [46], which is consistent with changes observed in healthy human studies because of diminished cholinergic neurotransmission by scopolamine or a selective muscarinic receptor antagonist [47, 48].

Donepezil has been shown to attenuate scopolamine-induced reduction of the P300 amplitude, which is consistent with the modulation of P300 by donepezil in AD Alzheimer's patients [49]. It is important to note that the translational ability of the rat P300-like response to human P300 responses depends not on the polarity of the component, but on the location of the source of the activity and the morphological properties of its surrounding tissue, which are key to determining the cortical polarity of an ERP component [50]. Habituation during tasks has not been found to be a problem, with the P300-like response not changing dramatically for the number of trials required to obtain stable EEG averages [51].

The present study used an active oddball paradigm to demonstrate that P300-like responses and related EROS could be generated in rats under baseline conditions and to confirm that this P300-like response of attentive and memory processing is sensitive to modulation of cholinergic neurotransmission.

2. Materials and Methods

2.1. Animal Husbandry. All experimental procedures were conducted in strict accordance with the guidelines of the Association for Assessment and Accreditation of Laboratory Animal Care International (AAALAC) and with the European Communities Council Directive of 24th November 1986 (86/609/EEC) and were approved by the local ethical committee. The experiments were carried out on male adult Long-Evans rats (Harlan, Netherlands), weighing 300 g at the time of surgery and were housed in full-view Plexiglas (25 × 33 × 18 cm) individually ventilated cages (IVCs). All rats were provided with a microchip for identification and maintained under controlled environmental conditions, temperature 22°C ± 2°C, and humidity 60%, in a reverse 12-hour light-dark cycle (lights off at 07 : 00, lights on at 19 : 00). All experiments were conducted during the dark phase of the circadian rhythm. Once animals were fully grown, they were placed on a food-restricted diet of 20 g on nontask days and 15 g on task days, with water ad libitum and food available ad libitum on weekends, removed 24 h before the next training or test session. Weights of the animals were regularly monitored.

2.2. Two-Tone Auditory Discrimination Task (TTADT) Training. The training protocol is presented in Figure 1. In brief, animals first receive two to three food dispenser and magazine training sessions (operant box, Med Associates). The rats could explore the chamber, approach the food magazine, and eat the dustless precision pellets (BIOSERV,

Frenchtown, NJ, USA). Magazine training sessions lasted for 60 min or until 40 pellets in the tray had been consumed, whichever occurred first (Figure 1). In the next session, rats were trained to press a lever for the food pellets reward under a fixed ratio-1 schedule of reinforcement. One tone (8 kHz target tone) was then presented, and animals were required to hear the tone and respond by lever pressing within 4 s to gain the food reward. A response of >75% within 4 s was considered and failure to press the lever within 4 s resulted in a timeout period of 15 s with house light off if they lever-pressed in the interstimulus interval (ISI) to discourage this behavior. If animals had a low number of lever presses in the ISI, then they progressed onto the active oddball phase 1. A total of 150 trials were presented to the animal in a 50/50 probability of occurrence for target tones (8 kHz) and nontarget tones (4 kHz) at 90 dB, 20 ms. Response to the target tone by pressing the lever within 4 s resulted in a food pellet reward, which would be a correct target trial. No reward was given for a lever press on the standard tone. Animals were required to have a response rate of ≥85% to the target tone with a standard response at ≤50%. Animals then progressed to phase 2, with the probability of a target tone reduced to 30%, and response to this target tone reduced to 2 s. Progression criteria were the same as for phase 1. Phase 3 had 500 trials, 20% probability of target tone, with 4.5 s ISI, and a response within 2 s of the target tone. After the training sessions, animals were chronically implanted with 6 epidural electrodes in the fronto-parieto-occipital areas.

2.3. Surgical Procedure. The surgery was performed as previously described [52]. Briefly, animals were equipped with 6 active electrodes over the right and left hemispheres (auditory cortex: ±2 mm posterior to Bregma and ±2 mm lateral to the midline; parietal cortex: −3 mm posterior to Bregma and ±4 mm lateral to the midline; and the occipital cortex −6.5 mm posterior to Bregma and ±4 mm lateral to the midline) and referenced to the ground electrode placed on the cerebellum. Electrodes were connected to a pin with a small insert and fitted into a 10-hole connector. The whole assembly was fixed with dental cement to the cranium.

2.4. Two-Tone Auditory Discrimination Task (TTADT) under Pharmacological Procedure. After a two-week recovery period, animals were placed in the operant box and connected to a wire to enable EEG recording. Animals were presented with one to two sessions of phase 3 training under the same conditions as before (500 trials, 20% probability of target tone, with 4.5 s ISI, and response within 2 s to target tones). Simultaneous EEG and behavioral response measurements started first with a silent recording run followed by a baseline recording run carried out during the task performance with nontarget and target tones. Continuous EEG were acquired at 2 kHz sample rate with an input range of ±500 mV through a Biosemi ActiveTwo system (Biosemi, Amsterdam, Netherlands) referenced to the CMS-DRL ground.

Afterwards, animals received combined pharmacological treatments with an interval of 30 min between both injections (group 1: vehicle + vehicle; group 2: donepezil + vehicle; group 3: vehicle + scopolamine; and group 4: donepezil + scopolamine). The postdrug run of 250 trials and behavioral recordings run started 30 min later.

Auditory stimuli were generated with a custom program written in LabVIEW, and sound stimuli were delivered through a speaker mounted above the floor of the experimental box. Sound intensity was calibrated with a sound meter 80 dB SPL in different locations of the recording box. In this active oddball paradigm, two stimulus conditions (target and nontarget) were pseudo-randomly presented with the restriction that consecutive target tones were separated by at least three nontarget tones. Continuous EEG were acquired at 2 kHz sample rate with an input range of ±500 mV through a Biosemi ActiveTwo system (Biosemi, Amsterdam, Netherlands) referenced to the CMS-DRL ground.

2.5. Data Analysis

2.5.1. Behavioral Analysis. Scores were determined for correct target and correct nontarget trials, and numbers of premature responses (pressing lever during ITI) were used to calculate the percentage of responses. A full correct response was deemed as the rat responding to the target tone within 2 sec and gaining the food reward. Incomplete responses occurred if the animal had pressed the lever but failed to gain the food reward, and incorrect responses were considered.

2.5.2. EEG Analysis. The peak amplitudes of the ERP waveforms and EROs were computed in artefact-free EG intervals, which were bandpass-filtered using a zero-phase lag filter with a 48 dB/octave roll-off. Stimulus-locked trials were extracted for all instances where there was a correct behavioral response for each of the two experimental conditions (nontarget and rare target stimuli), with each trial comprising up to 800 ms of data and − 100 ms prestimulus. The response window for correct responses on the target trials was 200–500 ms. A semi-automated algorithm was used to select discernable ERP peaks, which were baseline-corrected using the 100 ms prestimulus interval. Waveform averages were generated for correct target and correct nontarget trials for each animal, and grand average AEP waveforms for each of the components were computed across groups. The peak amplitudes and latencies of the P300-like components were calculated for each rat and condition. Additionally, event-related oscillations (EROs) were computed using the multitaper Morlet wavelet analysis, which offers superior time resolution to identify rapid changes in spectral components locked to stimuli during performance in the discriminant behavioral task. Trial-by-trial time-frequency decomposition was applied in the frequency range of 1–50 Hz (0.25 Hz steps). Wavelet transformation was applied to each single trial. The absolute power for each single trial wavelet cycle was then computed by taking the square of the magnitude of the complex valued for each trial, and these were then averaged across all trials to produce a resultant EROS that was termed event-induced oscillations per electrode site per subject.

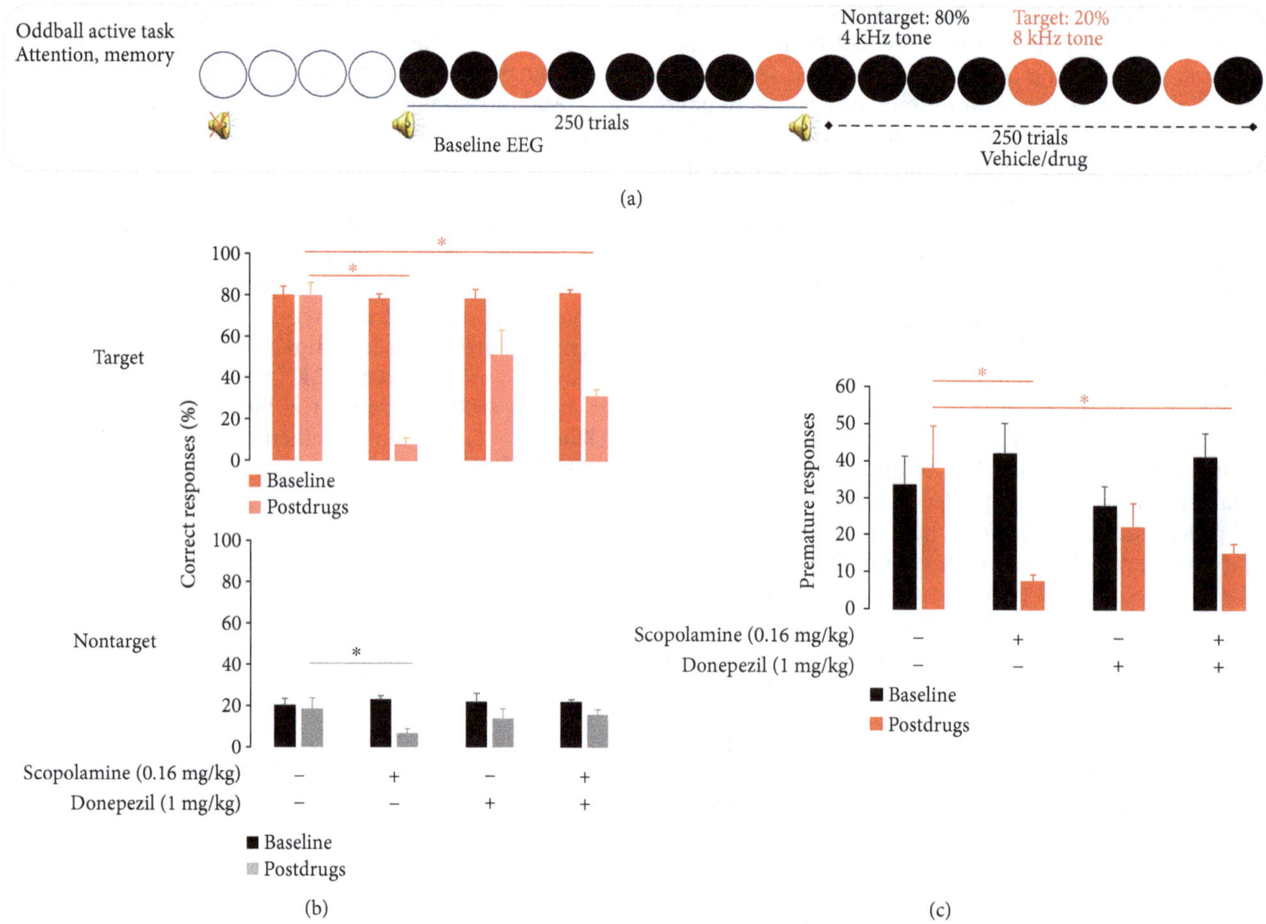

FIGURE 2: (a) Schematic presentation of the auditory active oddball protocol. The experiment started with a baseline run of 250 trials (20% oddball), followed by the administration of either vehicle or donepezil. Afterwards, scopolamine or vehicle was administered and the postdrug run continued with 250 trials (20% oddball). All recordings were carried out during the dark phase of the circadian rhythm. (b) Behavioral correct response during baseline and following pharmacological treatment in animals performing an auditory discrimination cognitive task to nontarget and target stimuli. (c) Behavioral premature response during baseline and following pharmacological treatment. Data are presented as mean ± SEM behavioral response baseline condition for each treatment group and to vehicle ($n = 8$), scopolamine ($n = 5$), donepezil ($n = 7$), and donepezil + scopolamine ($n = 10$). * indicates significance difference from vehicle treatment.

2.6. Drugs. Donepezil (Ningbo Distant Chemicals Co., Ltd, China) and scopolamine (Enzo Life Sciences International Inc., USA) were dissolved in sterile 0.9% saline solution and were administered subcutaneously (sc) in a volume of 10 ml/kg body weight. Saline was administered in control groups. Donepezil (1.0 mg/kg) and scopolamine (0.16 mg/kg) were administered at the doses that showed efficacy in neurophysiological and behavioral studies in rodents [53, 54]. In reversal pharmacological conditions, donepezil was given 30 min prior to scopolamine.

2.7. Statistical Analysis. Behavioral and AEP P300 amplitude and latency data were analyzed independently using a repeated-measures one-way ANOVA test. Scores for correct target and nontarget trials, number of premature responses, waveform peaks, and latencies were presented as mean ± SEM, and statistical analyses were performed using the SPSS program. If significant, Tukey's HSD post hoc analysis was performed. The P300 amplitude was determined as the highest peak between 200 and 500 ms, and latency was defined as the time lag between the onsets of stimuli to the P300-like peak amplitude.

3. Results

3.1. Behavioral Response

3.1.1. Correct Lever Press Responses to Target versus Nontarget Auditory Tones. Animals that followed all phases of the active oddball discriminant task (Figure 2(a)) showed high behavioral performance as animals markedly discriminated between target and nontarget tones by higher levels of correct pressing of the lever in target trials (≥80%) and lower level for incorrect lever presses (≤20%). Behavioral quantification of animals' ability to discriminate between target and nontarget tones is shown in Figures 2(b) and 2(c). In the vehicle condition, rats correctly responded with a lever press in 80% ± 6% for target trials (baseline

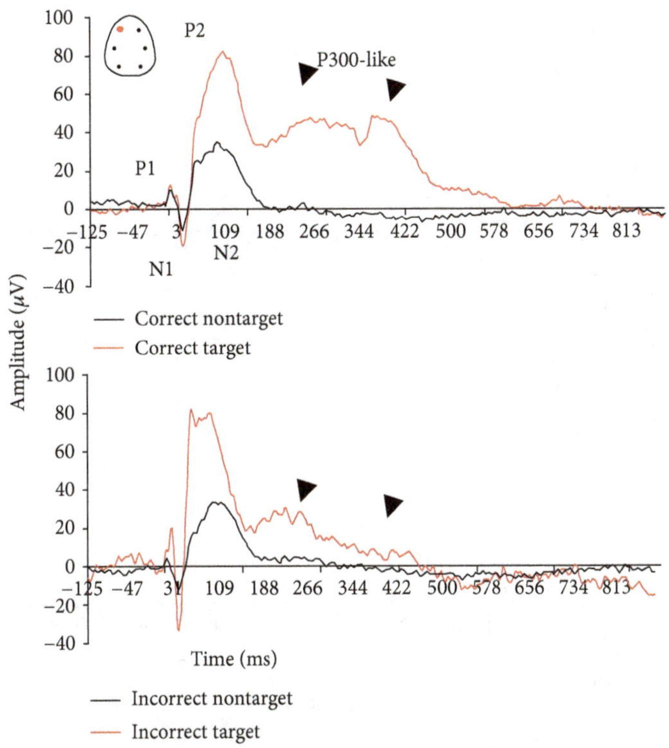

FIGURE 3: Grand average auditory-evoked waveforms recorded from the frontal left electrodes in rats performing in the auditory oddball discrimination task. Auditory potentials to target tone (red curve) stimuli consist of early positive (P1) and negative components (N1) and a late positive component (P300-like), which is preceded by a negative component (N2). In the late P300-like component, we could distinguish early and late positive waves occurring between 200 and 500 ms after target stimuli onset. Those components were smaller in AEPs to nontarget stimuli (black curve), and no P300 response was revealed by nontarget stimuli. This grand averaged waveform was calculated for all animals.

80% ± 4%), whereas correct lever presses were seen in 18% ± 5% for nontarget trials (baseline 20% ± 3%).

There was a treatment effect $F(3, 32) = 20.8$, $p < 0.0001$. When compared with vehicle, animals treated with scopolamine showed a significant decrease in behavioral performance as they correctly responded with a lever press in 7% ± 3% for target trials (baseline 78% ± 2%) and responses to the nontarget tones in 7% ± 2% (baseline 23% ± 3%). Donepezil reduced the correct responses to target tones with a lever press in 51% ± 12% of target trials (baseline 78% ± 4%), and although it reduced the responses to nontarget tone trials in 14% ± 5% (baseline 22% ± 1%), this was not statistically significant. In the combined pharmacological treatment group (Figure 2(b)), donepezil attenuated scopolamine-induced impairments in behavioral performance as animals treated with both drugs correctly responded with a lever press in 31% ± 3% for target trials (baseline 81% ± 2%) and responses to nontarget tones in 16% ± 3% (baseline 22% ± 1%) ($p < 0.0001$, resp.).

3.1.2. Premature Lever Press Responses. Assessment of behavioral performance showed that the vehicle had no effects on premature lever press scores in 38.1 ± 11 (baseline: 33.4 ± 7.8) (Figure 2(c)). In pharmacologically challenged animals, there was a treatment effect $F(3, 32) = 3.21$, $p = 0.03$). When compared with vehicle, scopolamine significantly decreased premature lever press responses in 7.7 ± 1.5 (baseline: 41.9 ± 8.2) ($p = 0.005$). Donepezil had a slight effect on premature lever press responses 22.2 ± 6.3 (baseline: 27.9 ± 5.5), whereas a significant reduction in premature lever press responses was found in the combined pharmacological treatment in 15.2 ± 2.6 (baseline: 41.0 ± 6.4) ($p = 0.02$).

3.2. ERP Response

3.2.1. P300-Like Amplitude and Latencies. The active oddball AEP paradigm allowed the assessment of both preattention and attention-relevant cortical responses in rats performing a discriminant auditory task. All AEP responses presented here were derived from the frontal left electrode only. Under baseline conditions, rats that discriminate between stimulus tones showed complex components (P1, N1, P2, N2, and P300-like) in all AEP responses (Figure 3). The difference in the amplitude response to target versus nontarget tones is consistent with the ability to allocate attention resources required to discriminate and process target rare from nontarget stimulus tones. Animals that paid attention to the target stimuli generated two positive deflections between 200 and 500 ms after the onset of the tone stimuli, suggestive of early and late P300-like components (Figure 3).

P300-like responses revealed significantly larger peak amplitudes in target trials compared to nontarget trials in baseline and vehicle conditions (Figures 3 and 4). There

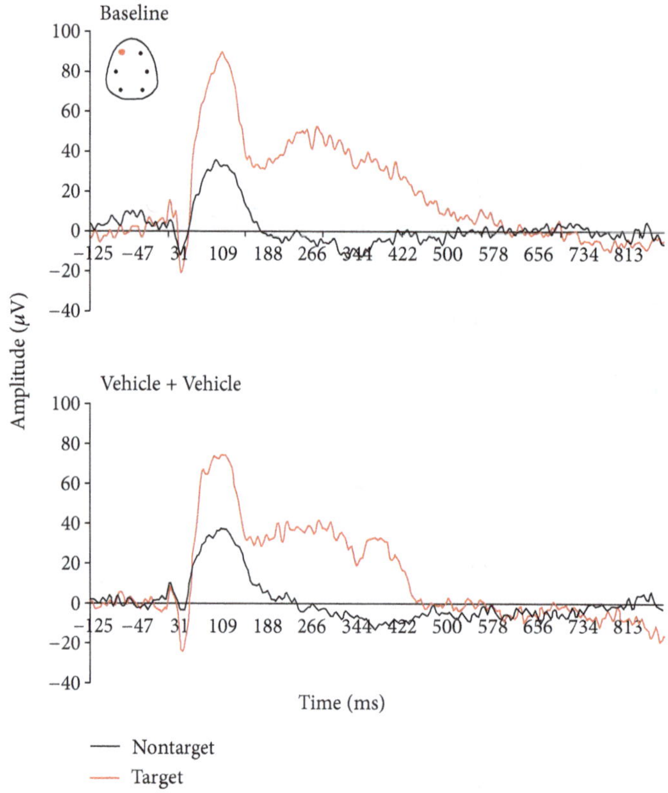

FIGURE 4: Grand average auditory-evoked waveforms recorded from the frontal left electrodes in rats performing an auditory discrimination task under baseline and following subcutaneous administration of vehicle ($n = 8$). Auditory potentials to target tones stimuli (red curves) showed similar evoked waveforms in both conditions.

was a treatment effect at the amplitude of the P-300 like response ($F(3, 25) = 3.91$, $p = 0.02$). When compared to the vehicle condition, scopolamine consistently disrupted the AEP response to rare target stimuli and P300-like peak responses ($p = 0.003$) (Figures 5 and 6). No significant effect at the latency to apparent P300-like amplitude was observed (Figure 6).

In donepezil-treated animals, a slight enhancement of the P300-like amplitude was observed (Figures 6 and 7). In the combined pharmacologically treated animals, donepezil slightly attenuated scopolamine-induced disruptive effects on complex components ($p = 0.04$) (Figures 6 and 8). No treatment effect on peak latency was observed in target trials ($F(3, 25) = 1.6$, $p = 0.2$).

3.3. EROS Response. The frontal P300-like response of the vehicle-treated animals performing the auditory discrimination cognitive task emerged with an event increase in cortical theta rhythm (Figure 9). The target stimuli did result in significantly more activation compared to nontarget stimuli. Scopolamine was associated with enhanced delta oscillatory rhythm (1–4 Hz) and alpha peak activity around 10 Hz to both target and nontarget stimuli. Donepezil elicited prominent increases in the slow theta (4–6 Hz) and beta-gamma oscillatory rhythms (12–40 Hz) observed at about 50 ms particularly for target stimuli. When combined, donepezil attenuated the effects of scopolamine on slow delta.

4. Discussion

In this active oddball study, rats could reach high performance levels after training to correctly respond by lever press after correct discrimination of target from nontarget tones. Task-relevant target tones evoked P300-like responses in animals that paid attention and reacted on the correct target stimuli, suggesting a modification of neuronal network activity due to enhanced attentional processes. Donepezil had no enhancing effects on behavioral performance, whereas the number of correct trials was lowered. However, scopolamine decreased correct lever pressing to target stimuli as well premature responses, which suggests that animals had forgotten what they had learnt. The decline in behavioral performance and correct detection of target stimuli was associated with reduced P300-like amplitude, which potentially reflects impaired synaptic strength.

The predictive validity of standard behavioral assays has been heavily criticized in contemporary cognitive neuroscience research because of poor translation of basic animal work into human outcomes and the lack of success in discovering a novel chemical entity targeting cognitive deficits [1–3]. LTP, which represents the basic mechanism underlying learning and memory, has widely been investigated at the cellular and molecular level in animals [10, 15, 55, 56]. Repetitive sensory stimulation of visual or auditory systems can induce noninvasively long-term potentiation-like effects

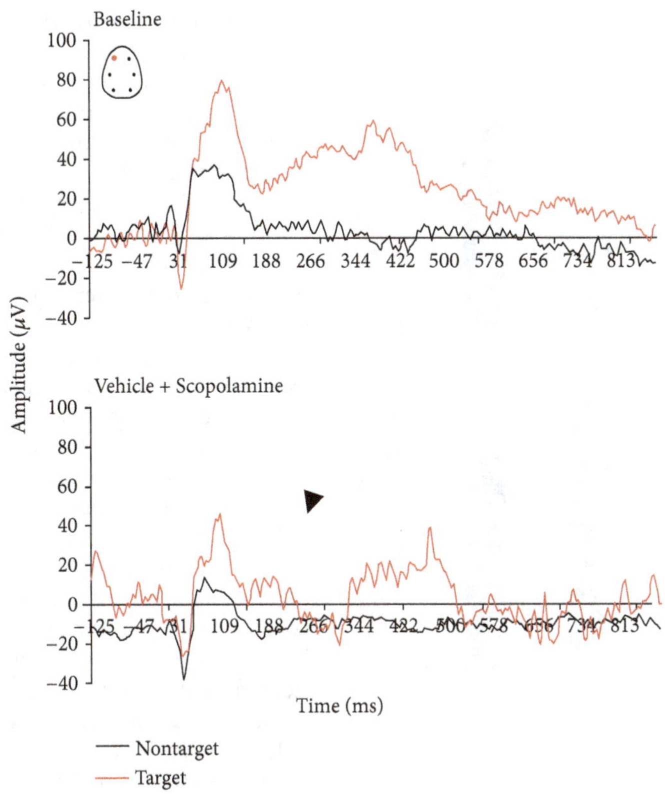

FIGURE 5: Grand average auditory-evoked waveforms recorded from the frontal left electrodes in rats performing an auditory discrimination task under baseline and following subcutaneous administration of scopolamine (0.16 mg/kg, $n = 5$).

in humans [17–19]. Cognitive ERP studies in neurodegenerative and psychiatric disorders revealed sensitivity and consistent abnormalities in several ERP components, each of which taps into different aspects of perceptual and/or cognitive processing. The temporal immediacy of the ERP response is particularly advantageous in the study of memory and attention as the memory encoding and retrieval process is very fast. The active oddball paradigms have been particularly important in clinical studies as they can provide a human model system allowing examination of synaptic plasticity of subjects with cognitive attentional deficits [19, 15–18, 20–59]. The P300 amplitude is thought to reflect attentional resource allocation, phasic attentional shifts, and working memory updating of the stimulus context, whereas its latency is thought to reflect processing speed or efficiency during stimulus evaluation [23]. Clinical studies have consistently shown great utility of this paradigm to study the brain's synaptic function and to probe subtle abnormalities of cognition; this was a motivation to demonstrate and differentiate these AEP components in the active oddball paradigm in rats and to evaluate the sensitivity to modulation of cholinergic neurotransmission.

Cholinergic transmission is thought to play major regulatory functions to memory encoding and consolidation [60–65], as well as to regulatory functions in motor behavior and reward-related behavior [66–70]. In animals and humans, the scopolamine cognitive challenge model has been widely used to examine the extent to which experimental compounds are hypothesized to act through modulation of cholinergic neurotransmission. Scopolamine is known to influence motor function, which might have interfered with learning response rules and number of correct response trials. In addition, experimental observations showed that visual information processing is modulated by cholinergic transmission [71, 72], and scopolamine has the potency to dilate the pupils, which may have impaired visual perception contributing to weak association between lever manipulation and task initiation/reward acquisition. However, scopolamine administered at higher doses (0.3–1 mg/kg) than that used in the present study neither impaired motor function in the open field paradigm nor impaired performance in visual discrimination tasks that used striped textures as stimuli [72]. Scopolamine has been shown to impair cognitive functions such as attention and working memory [73–75]. Systemic administration of scopolamine immediately after the learning trials impaired habituation of mice in the open field, and rats to odor discrimination as well as the retrieval of memory acquired from contextual fear conditioning [76–79]. In mice that were consecutively exposed to two learning situations, scopolamine selectively disrupts acquisition of new information, but had fewer effects on memory consolidation of previous memories [80]. In the present auditory discriminant task where animals were required to sustain their attention to detect a stimulus associated with food reward, reduction of the cholinergic tone impaired behavioral performance to first-learned situations and

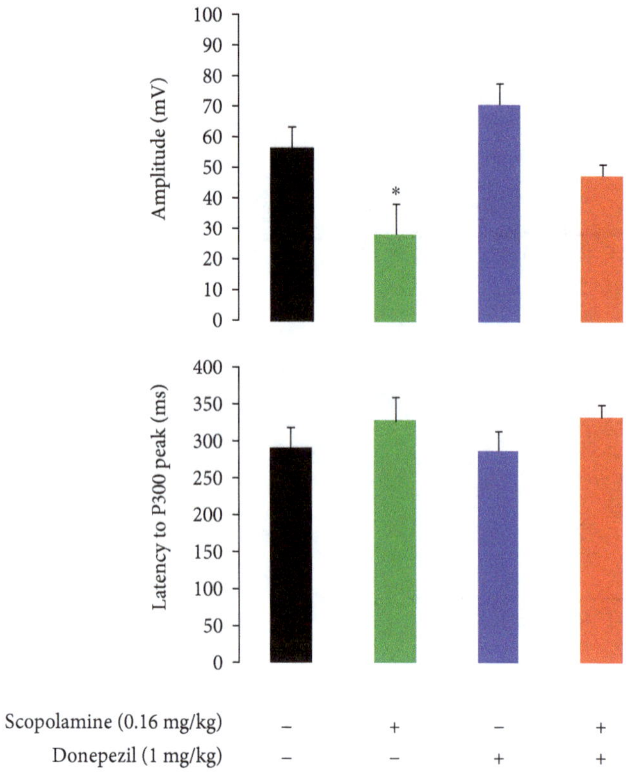

FIGURE 6: Difference in maximal peak amplitudes and latency to P300 response at 200–500 ms poststimuli onset in correct target trials following subcutaneous administration of vehicle ($n = 8$), scopolamine (0.16 mg/kg, $n = 5$), donepezil (1 mg/kg, $n = 7$), and combined donepezil and scopolamine ($n = 10$). Data is expressed as mean ± SEM. ∗ indicates significance difference vehicle treatment.

therefore it could be hypothesized that scopolamine disrupted attention to new information and working memory functions as the task execution in correct target trials was impaired.

The decrease in premature responses with scopolamine related to reduced number of executed trials and a tendency for a decrease in this parameter with donepezil may suggest an effect on impulse control. Impulsiveness is linked to faster response time and errors caused by premature response for incorrect trials to stimuli. Here, scopolamine decreased responses to target and nontarget stimuli as well as premature responses, which overall suggests that scopolamine had a stimulating effect. Accordingly, the wake-promoting agent modafinil that has been approved for treatment of excessive sleepiness facilitated the ability to inhibit impulsive response in rats performing in a 3-choice visual discrimination and sustained attention tasks, and in a healthy young man performing in delayed matching to sample, a decision-making and the spatial planning tasks task [81, 82]. In addition, donepezil reduced the magnitude of scopolamine-related behavioral performance impairments. The lack of full reversal of amnestic effects was probably related to drug temporal kinetics as scopolamine-induced peak cognitive impairments may last longer and the efficacy endpoints could be impacted by distinct pharmacokinetic profiles of donepezil and scopolamine.

The task-relevant target tone stimulus evoked complex potentials including peaks between 200 and 500 ms poststimuli suggesting a P300-like response.

The choice of the brain-recording sites was based on their principal roles in sensory processing, working memory, and attentional processes. The rat's frontal cortex, specifically the medial frontal cortex, is usually considered to be homologous to the dorsolateral prefrontal cortex of primates, which consists of the cortex homologous to the human anterior cingulate cortex (ACC) and dorsolateral prefrontal cortex [83, 84]. The cortex is hierarchically organized to serve higher-order integrative functions that are neither purely sensory nor purely motoric. The primary motor areas (M1/2), somatosensory cortex and parietal auditory association cortex, integrate sensory and auditory modalities and link auditory information to the planning of movement; they are thought to be the anatomical substrates of the highest brain function in humans' conscious thought, perception, and goal-directed action. In the present work, large evoked potentials were derived and were presented from frontal cortical areas.

In clinical ERP studies, two distinct P300 waveforms at different latencies are generally distinguished: P3a is elicited by unexpected stimuli with front central topography and thought to reflect stimulus-driven attentional capture or reorienting, whereas P3b reflects activation of attentional networks facilitating memory computations in temporal and parietal areas [23, 85]. In preclinical studies, both passive and active oddball paradigms were used to investigate ERP components including late positivity. In the passive oddball, where animals do not require extensive training, late positive potentials were identified in the mouse [40] and rat cortex [41–43]. In the active oddball paradigm, P300-like positive components with maximal voltage over the parietal cortex were generated by task-relevant stimuli in rats [41–87], and P300-like responses were sensitive to pharmacological modulation of the cholinergic tone [46].

Here, novelty-related amplification of the P300-like response was larger in the frontal cortex of rats that correctly detected task-relevant stimuli. Our results further extend previous preclinical reports by showing that late AEP-positive components can be generated in the rat cortex in response to rare target versus frequent nontarget stimuli [41, 45, 50]. Two components have been described in separate oddball ERP P300 studies in rats [41, 43, 45, 50, 88, 89]. The early P3-positive component has been described around 240 ms [88], whereas the late P3 component was found at 380 ms [50]. A subsequent study described both early P3E and late P3L in response to correct deviance detection in frontal and parietal cortical areas in rats [87]. The deviance detection presented here was dominated by two positive peaks at different latencies, that is, an early component at ~250–270 ms and a late component at >300 ms after oddball stimuli, which corroborate the existence of the two P300-like distinct peaks in rats [87].

Clinical observations support an important role of cholinergic transmission in the generation of P300 response

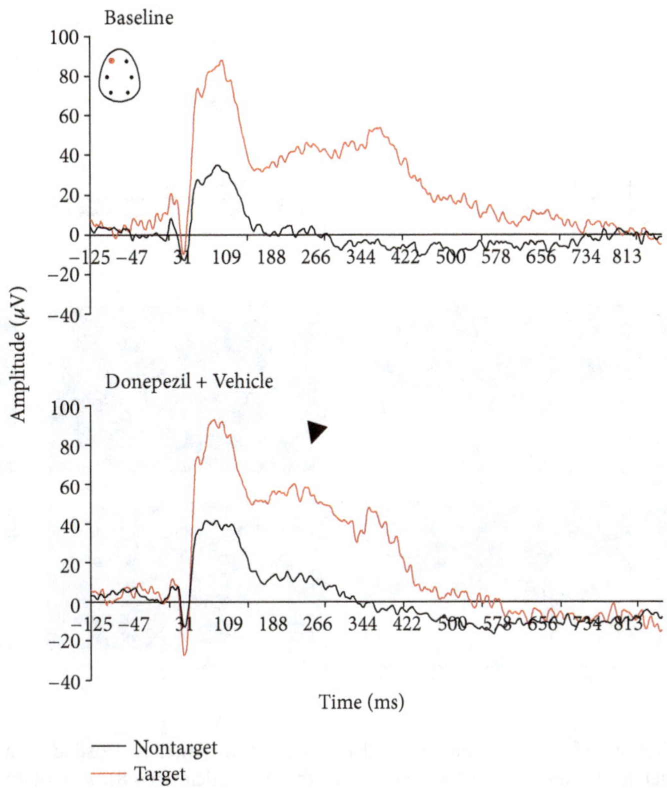

FIGURE 7: Grand average auditory-evoked waveforms recorded from the frontal left electrodes in rats performing an auditory discrimination task under baseline and following subcutaneous administration of donepezil (1 mg/kg, $n = 7$).

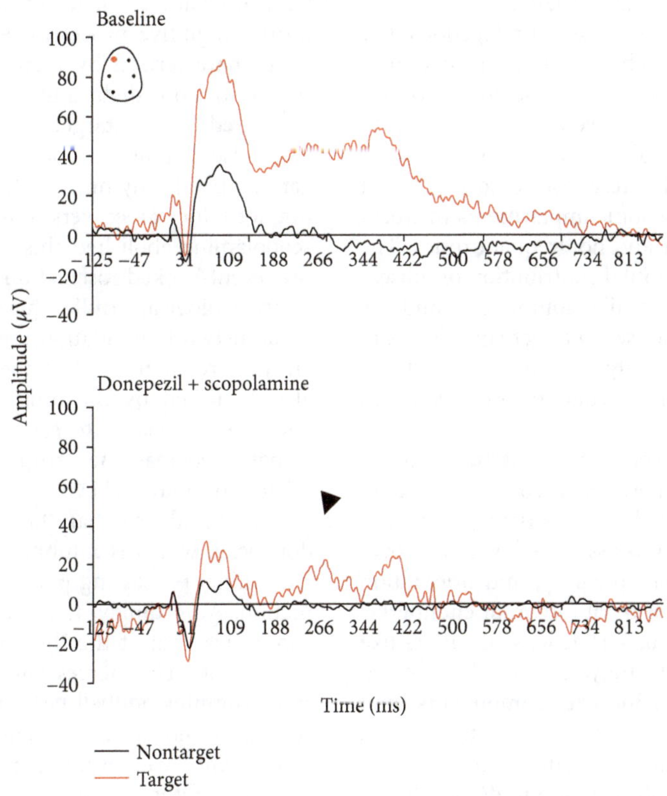

FIGURE 8: Grand average auditory-evoked waveforms recorded from the frontal left electrodes in rats performing an auditory discrimination task under baseline following subcutaneous combined pharmacological administration of scopolamine and donepezil ($n = 10$).

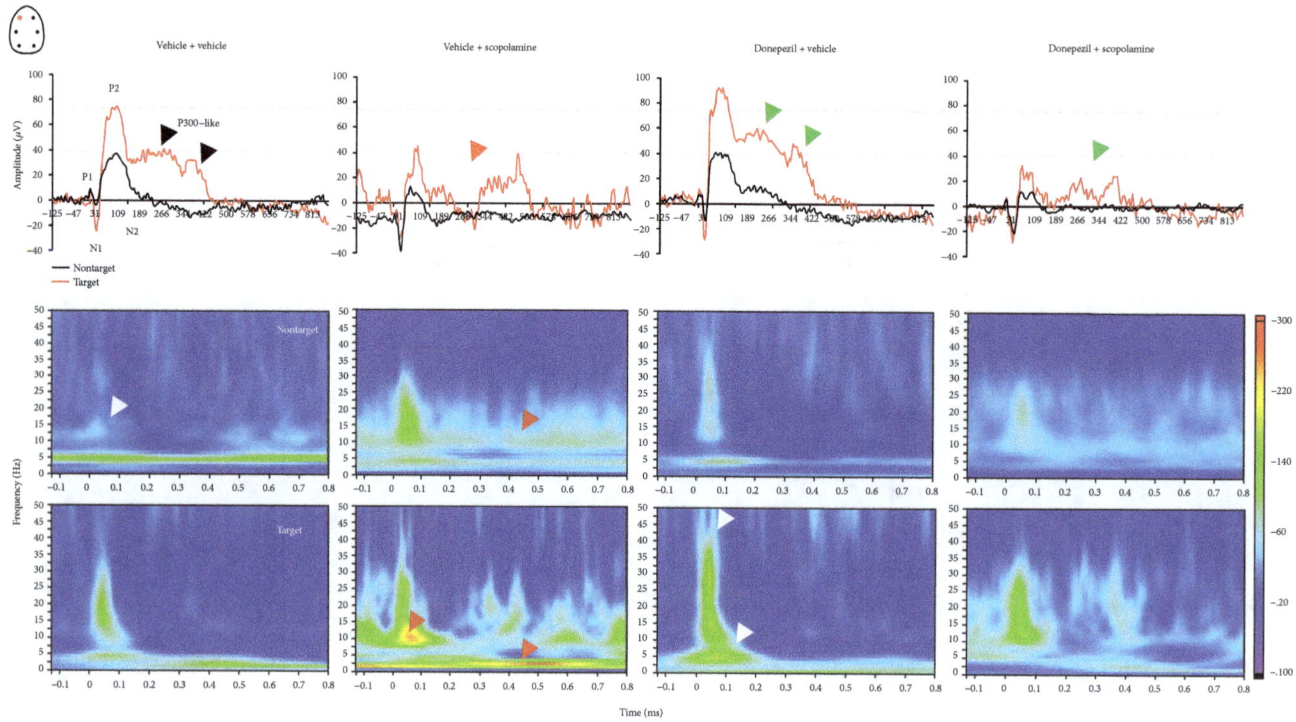

FIGURE 9: Relationship between ERP waveforms (top panels) and EROs (bottom panels) recorded from the frontal left electrodes in rats discriminating target and nontarget tones under pharmacological treatment: vehicle ($n = 8$), scopolamine (0.16 mg/kg, $n = 5$), donepezil (1 mg/kg, $n = 7$), and combined donepezil and scopolamine ($n = 10$).

in healthy men [48, 90, 91], and those parameters are impaired in AD patients generally related to a loss of cholinergic neurotransmission [49, 59]. Endogenous late ERP positivity is influenced by cholinergic transmission in primates [92], in rats, and in cats [38, 93]. The present results show that P300 late components were very sensitive to modulation of cholinergic neurotransmission. Scopolamine severely disrupted AEP complex response to correct target and nontarget tones suggesting some impairments in working memory traces of frequent and nonfrequent tones. The effects we observed indicate a frontal contribution of muscarinic receptors to the early P300-like component, and the limited number of correct responses to target stimuli due to alteration in cholinergic tone is likely associated with reduced allocation of attentional resources required to evaluate and discriminate the target tone.

Donepezil did not fully reverse the amnestic action of scopolamine in a variety of experimental cognitive tasks in animals and humans [93, 94]. In AD patients, donepezil decreased P300 latency, which was associated with improvement in remote memory, recent memory, and orientation [49, 59, 38]. In the rat model of basal forebrain cholinergic degeneration, donepezil attenuated deficits in P300-like response [46]. In the present study, donepezil increased the maximal amplitude of P300-like components and partially attenuated scopolamine-induced reduction of the P300-like amplitude. No significant effect on P300-like latencies indicates that the P300-like amplitude is a better marker of cholinergic treatment-dependent maintenance of active attention.

Accumulating evidence supports the relevance of network oscillation synchrony in normal brain function and during cognitive processes [95, 96]. Target tone responses were characterized by increased phase-locking of spectral power in slow theta and beta rhythms for target stimuli compared to nontarget stimuli. Donepezil evoked slow theta oscillations associated with increases in beta and gamma-band rhythm, with the magnitude being pronounced for target versus nontarget stimuli. In contrast, scopolamine abolished this slow theta rhythm and shifted the event-evoked oscillation towards the alpha rhythm. Pharmacological studies have revealed two subgroups of theta network oscillations: atropine-sensitive type 2 and atropine-resistant 1. The theta rhythm type 2 (<6 Hz) is also abolished by the muscarinic antagonist scopolamine and directly related to sensory stimulation but not motor activity, whereas the atropine-resistant type 1 is directly related to motor behavior [97]. Therefore, the present study provides evidence that the evoked slow theta rhythm by donepezil, which is inhibited by scopolamine, is associated with initial processing phases of target auditory tone information. Accordingly, the P300-like peak response to target stimuli was not at the theta frequency at 200–500 ms after stimulation. This agrees with a previous study in a visual three-stimulus oddball task, in which theta activity is more related to novel rather than target stimuli [46]. Future experiments will evaluate network frequency oscillations by an auditory stimulus novelty embedded to target/nontarget tones at 200–500 ms poststimuli onset in the auditory three-tone oddball.

Electroencephalography has revealed abnormalities in ERPs evoked by auditory stimuli in humans with neurodegenerative and neuropsychiatric disorders, indicating disruption of neural connectivity. Similar abnormalities in auditory-evoked ERPs have been observed in animal models of these brain disorders, suggesting that ERPs have the potential to provide a translational biomarker for those brain disorders. One of the widely used cognitive assays to assess drug effects in normal animals is to manipulate neural transmission to mimic abnormalities that are observed in the disease states. These disease models attempt to capture at least some part of the disease process that manifests itself in cognitive deficits. A common approach in modeling AD has been to disrupt the function of the cholinergic system, which is based on the observations that the most consistent neurochemical change in AD is a reduction of cholinergic markers in the forebrain and that muscarinic and nicotine cholinergic antagonists impair performance in cognitive tasks in both experimental animals and healthy men. The present findings further confirm the contribution of cholinergic neurotransmission in the generation of the P300-like response in the discriminant performance task. This active oddball paradigm in rats, in which the correct deviance detection was dominated by P300-like components, may have translational value to assess biological circuits and/or novel pharmacological agents interacting with the cholinergic transmission to facilitate and/or suppress synaptic responses associated with increased allocation of attentional resources.

Conflicts of Interest

No conflicts of interest, financial or otherwise, are declared by the authors.

Acknowledgments

The authors are indebted to Ms. C. Pett for technical assistance.

References

[1] J. L. Cummings, T. Morstorf, and K. Zhong, "Alzheimer's disease drug-development pipeline: few candidates, frequent failures," *Alzheimer's Research & Therapy*, vol. 6, no. 4, p. 37, 2014.

[2] J. P. Garner, "The significance of meaning: why do over 90% of behavioral neuroscience results fail to translate to humans, and what can we do to fix it?," *ILAR Journal*, vol. 55, no. 3, pp. 438–456, 2014.

[3] M. D. Tricklebank and J. P. Garner, "The possibilities and limitations of animal models for psychiatric disorders," in *Drug Discovery for Psychiatric Disorders*, Z. Rankovic, M. Bingham, and R. Hargreaves, Eds., pp. 534-556, The Royal Society of Chemistry, 2012.

[4] M. W. Decker, "Cognition models and drug discovery in "animal models of cognitive impairment"," in *Frontiers in Neuroscience*, vol. 343, Taylor & Francis. Group LLC, 2006.

[5] G. I. Elmer, P. L. Brown, and P. D. Shepard, "Engaging research domain criteria (RDoC): neurocircuitry in search of meaning," *Schizophrenia Bulletin*, vol. 42, no. 5, pp. 1090–1095, 2016.

[6] Z. A. Cope, S. B. Powell, and J. W. Young, "Modeling neurodevelopmental cognitive deficits in tasks with cross-species translational validity," *Genes, Brain and Behavior*, vol. 15, no. 1, pp. 27–44, 2016.

[7] C. S. Herrmann and T. Demiralp, "Human EEG gamma oscillations in neuropsychiatric disorders," *Clinical Neurophysiology*, vol. 116, no. 12, pp. 2719–2733, 2005.

[8] P. J. Uhlhaas and W. Singer, "Abnormal neural oscillations and synchrony in schizophrenia," *Nature Reviews Neuroscience*, vol. 11, no. 2, pp. 100–113, 2010.

[9] C. Walsh, W. H. I. M. Drinkenburg, and A. Ahnaou, "Neurophysiological assessment of neural network plasticity and connectivity: progress towards early functional biomarkers for disease interception therapies in Alzheimer's disease," *Neuroscience and Biobehavioral Reviews*, vol. 73, pp. 340–358, 2017.

[10] W. C. Abraham, B. Logan, J. M. Greenwood, and M. Dragunow, "Induction and experience-dependent consolidation of stable long-term potentiation lasting months in the hippocampus," *The Journal of Neuroscience*, vol. 22, no. 21, pp. 9626–9634, 2002.

[11] T. V. P. Bliss and T. Lomo, "Long-lasting potentiation of synaptic transmission in the dentate area of the anaesthetized rabbit following stimulation of the perforant path," *The Journal of Physiology*, vol. 232, no. 2, pp. 331–356, 1973.

[12] S. F. Cooke and T. V. P. Bliss, "Plasticity in the human central nervous system," *Brain*, vol. 129, no. 7, pp. 1659–1673, 2006.

[13] G. Neves, S. F. Cooke, and T. V. P. Bliss, "Synaptic plasticity, memory and the hippocampus: a neural network approach to causality," *Nature Reviews Neuroscience*, vol. 9, no. 1, pp. 65–75, 2008.

[14] D. Fernandes and A. L. Carvalho, "Mechanisms of homeostatic plasticity in the excitatory synapse," *Journal of Neurochemistry*, vol. 139, no. 6, pp. 973–996, 2016.

[15] E. Molnár, "Long-term potentiation in cultured hippocampal neurons," *Seminars in Cell & Developmental Biology*, vol. 22, no. 5, pp. 506–513, 2011.

[16] J. D. Sweatt, "Neural plasticity and behavior - sixty years of conceptual advances," *Journal of Neurochemistry*, vol. 139, no. 2, pp. 179–199, 2016.

[17] W. C. Clapp, I. J. Kirk, J. P. Hamm, D. Shepherd, and T. J. Teyler, "Induction of LTP in the human auditory cortex by sensory stimulation," *The European Journal of Neuroscience*, vol. 22, no. 5, pp. 1135–40, 2005.

[18] W. C. Clapp, J. P. Hamm, I. J. Kirk, and T. J. Teyler, "Translating long-term potentiation from animals to humans: a novel method for noninvasive assessment of cortical plasticity," *Biological Psychiatry*, vol. 71, no. 6, pp. 496–502, 2012.

[19] I. J. Kirk, N. A. McNair, J. P. Hamm et al., "Long-term potentiation (LTP) of human sensory-evoked potentials," *Wiley Interdisciplinary Reviews: Cognitive Science*, vol. 1, no. 5, pp. 766–773, 2010.

[20] C. C. Duncan, R. J. Barry, J. F. Connolly et al., "Event-related potentials in clinical research: guidelines for eliciting,

recording, and quantifying mismatch negativity, P300, and N400," *Clinical Neurophysiology*, vol. 120, no. 11, pp. 1883–1908, 2009.

[21] D. Hedges, R. Janis, S. Mickelson, C. Keith, D. Bennett, and B. L. Brown, "P300 amplitude in Alzheimer's disease: a meta-analysis and meta-regression," *Clinical EEG and Neuroscience*, vol. 47, no. 1, pp. 48–55, 2016.

[22] A. Horvath, A. Szucs, G. Csukly, A. Sakovics, G. Stefanics, and A. Kamondi, "EEG and ERP biomarkers of Alzheimer's disease: a critical review," *Frontiers in Bioscience*, vol. 23, no. 1, pp. 183–220, 2018.

[23] J. Polich, "Updating P300: an integrative theory of P3a and P3b," *Clinical Neurophysiology*, vol. 118, no. 10, pp. 2128–2148, 2007.

[24] A. C. Swann, M. Lijffijt, S. D. Lane et al., "Pre-attentive information processing and impulsivity in bipolar disorder," *Journal of Psychiatric Research*, vol. 47, no. 12, pp. 1917–1924, 2013.

[25] Y. Tong, R. D. Melara, and A. Rao, "P2 enhancement from auditory discrimination training is associated with improved reaction times," *Brain Research*, vol. 1297, pp. 80–88, 2009.

[26] J. Polich and K. L. Herbst, "P300 as a clinical assay: rationale, evaluation, and findings," *International Journal of Psychophysiology*, vol. 38, no. 1, pp. 3–19, 2000.

[27] D. E. J. Linden, "The p300: where in the brain is it produced and what does it tell us?," *The Neuroscientist*, vol. 11, no. 6, pp. 563–576, 2005.

[28] H. A. Earls, T. Curran, and V. Mittal, "A meta-analytic review of auditory event-related potential components as endophenotypes for schizophrenia: perspectives from first-degree relatives," *Schizophrenia Bulletin*, vol. 42, no. 6, pp. 1504–1516, 2016.

[29] G. A. Light, N. R. Swerdlow, M. L. Thomas et al., "Validation of mismatch negativity and P3a for use in multi-site studies of schizophrenia: characterization of demographic, clinical, cognitive, and functional correlates in COGS-2," *Schizophrenia Research*, vol. 163, no. 1–3, pp. 63–72, 2015.

[30] B. I. Turetsky, E. M. Dress, D. L. Braff et al., "The utility of P300 as a schizophrenia endophenotype and predictive biomarker: clinical and socio-demographic modulators in COGS-2," *Schizophrenia Research*, vol. 163, no. 1–3, pp. 53–62, 2015.

[31] E. R. Braverman and K. Blum, "P300 (latency) event-related potential: an accurate predictor of memory impairment," *Clinical Electroencephalography*, vol. 34, no. 3, pp. 124–139, 2003.

[32] L. Gu and Z. Zhang, "Exploring potential electrophysiological biomarkers in mild cognitive impairment: a systematic review and meta-analysis of event-related potential studies," *Journal of Alzheimer's Disease*, vol. 58, no. 4, pp. 1283–1292, 2017.

[33] K. Bennys, A. Gabelle, C. Berr et al., "Cognitive event-related potential, an early diagnosis biomarker in frail elderly subjects: the ERP-MAPT-PLUS Ancillary Study," *Journal of Alzheimer's Disease*, vol. 58, no. 1, pp. 87–97, 2017.

[34] C. D. Papadaniil, V. E. Kosmidou, A. Tsolaki, M. Tsolaki, I. Y. Kompatsiaris, and L. J. Hadjileontiadis, "Cognitive MMN and P300 in mild cognitive impairment and Alzheimer's disease: a high density EEG-3D vector field tomography approach," *Brain Research*, vol. 1648, Part A, pp. 425–433, 2016.

[35] J. M. Olichney, J. C. Yang, J. Taylor, and M. Kutas, "Cognitive event-related potentials: biomarkers of synaptic dysfunction across the stages of Alzheimer's disease," *Journal of Alzheimer's Disease*, vol. 26, no. s3, pp. 215–228, 2011.

[36] G. G. Yener and E. Başar, "Brain oscillations as biomarkers in neuropsychiatric disorders: following an interactive panel discussion and synopsis," *Supplements to Clinical Neurophysiology*, vol. 62, pp. 343–363, 2013.

[37] V. F. Prado, H. Janickova, M. A. Al-Onaizi, and M. A. M. Prado, "Cholinergic circuits in cognitive flexibility," *Neuroscience*, vol. 345, pp. 130–141, 2017.

[38] J. B. Harrison, J. S. Buchwald, K. Kaga, N. J. Woolf, and L. L. Butcher, "Cat P300' disappears after septal lesions," *Electroencephalography and Clinical Neurophysiology*, vol. 69, no. 1, pp. 55–64, 1988.

[39] A. A. Glover, M. C. Onofrj, M. F. Ghilardi, and I. Bodis-Wollner, "P300-like potentials in the normal monkey using classical conditioning and an auditory 'oddball' paradigm," *Electroencephalography and Clinical Neurophysiology/Evoked Potentials Section*, vol. 65, no. 3, pp. 231–235, 1986.

[40] C. L. Ehlers and C. Somes, "Long latency event-related potentials in mice: effects of stimulus characteristics and strain," *Brain Research*, vol. 957, no. 1, pp. 117–128, 2002.

[41] M. Hattori, K. Onoda, and S. Sakata, "Identification of rat P3-like processes in the anterior cingulate cortex and hippocampus," *Neuroscience Letters*, vol. 472, no. 1, pp. 43–46, 2010.

[42] C. L. Ehlers, W. M. Kaneko, P. Robledo, and A. L. Lopez, "Long-latency event-related potentials in rats: effects of task and stimulus parameters," *Neuroscience*, vol. 62, no. 3, pp. 759–769, 1994.

[43] T. Shinba, "Event-related potentials of the rat during active and passive auditory oddball paradigms," *Electroencephalography and Clinical Neurophysiology*, vol. 104, no. 5, pp. 447–452, 1997.

[44] C. L. Ehlers, C. Somes, A. L. Lopez, and P. Robledo, "Long latency event-related potentials in rats: response of amygdala, nucleus accumbens, dorsal hippocampus and frontal cortex to changes in reward characteristics of conditioned stimuli," *Brain Research*, vol. 780, no. 1, pp. 138–142, 1998.

[45] M. Grupe, M. Grunnet, B. Laursen, and J. F. Bastlund, "Neuropharmacological modulation of the P3-like event-related potential in a rat two-tone auditory discrimination task with modafinil and NS9283, a positive allosteric modulator of $\alpha 4\beta 2$ nAChRs," *Neuropharmacology*, vol. 79, pp. 444–455, 2014.

[46] B. Laursen, A. Mørk, U. Kristiansen, and J. F. Bastlund, "Hippocampal P3-like auditory event-related potentials are disrupted in a rat model of cholinergic degeneration in Alzheimer's disease: reversal by donepezil treatment," *Journal of Alzheimer's Disease*, vol. 42, no. 4, pp. 1179–1189, 2014.

[47] S. B. R. E. Brown, N. J. A. van der Wee, M. S. van Noorden, E. J. Giltay, and S. Nieuwenhuis, "Noradrenergic and cholinergic modulation of late ERP responses to deviant stimuli," *Psychophysiology*, vol. 52, no. 12, pp. 1620–1631, 2015.

[48] S. Caldenhove, L. G. J. M. Borghans, A. Blokland, and A. Sambeth, "Role of acetylcholine and serotonin in novelty processing using an oddball paradigm," *Behavioural Brain Research*, vol. 331, pp. 199–204, 2017.

[49] A. Thomas, D. Iacono, L. Bonanni, G. D'Andreamatteo, and M. Onofrj, "Donepezil, rivastigmine, and vitamin E in Alzheimer disease: a combined P300 event-related potentials/neuropsychologic evaluation over 6 months," *Clinical Neuropharmacology*, vol. 24, no. 1, pp. 31–42, 2001.

[50] A. Sambeth, J. H. R. Maes, G. Van Luijtelaar, I. B. S. Molenkamp, M. L. A. Jongsma, and C. M. Van Rijn, "Auditory event-related potentials in humans and rats: effects of task manipulation," *Psychophysiology*, vol. 40, no. 1, pp. 60–68, 2003.

[51] J. Polich and H. K. McIsaac, "Comparison of auditory P300 habituation from active and passive conditions," *International Journal of Psychophysiology*, vol. 17, no. 1, pp. 25–34, 1994.

[52] A. Ahnaou, H. Huysmans, R. Biermans, N. V. Manyakov, and W. H. I. M. Drinkenburg, "Ketamine: differential neurophysiological dynamics in functional networks in the rat brain," *Transl Psychiatry*, vol. 7, no. 9, article e1237, 2017.

[53] A. Ahnaou, H. Huysmans, T. Jacobs, and W. H. I. M. Drinkenburg, "Cortical EEG oscillations and network connectivity as efficacy indices for assessing drugs with cognition enhancing potential," *Neuropharmacology*, vol. 86, pp. 362–377, 2014.

[54] L. E. Wise, P. A. Iredale, R. J. Stokes, and A. H. Lichtman, "Combination of rimonabant and donepezil prolongs spatial memory duration," *Neuropsychopharmacology*, vol. 32, no. 8, pp. 1805–1812, 2007.

[55] A. J. Heynen and M. F. Bear, "Long-term potentiation of thalamo-cortical transmission in the adult visual cortex *in vivo*," *The Journal of Neuroscience*, vol. 21, no. 24, pp. 9801–9813, 2001.

[56] R. C. Malenka and R. A. Nicoll, "Long-term potentiation—a decade of progress?," *Science*, vol. 285, no. 5435, pp. 1870–1874, 1999.

[57] J. Polich and J. Corey-Bloom, "Alzheimer's disease and P300: review and evaluation of task and modality," *Current Alzheimer Research*, vol. 2, no. 5, pp. 515–525, 2005.

[58] A. J. Rissling, S. H. Park, et al.J. W. Young et al., "Demand and modality of directed attention modulate "pre-attentive" sensory processes in schizophrenia patients and nonpsychiatric controls," *Schizophrenia Research*, vol. 146, no. 1–3, pp. 326–335, 2013.

[59] E. A. Werber, R. Gandelman-Marton, C. Klein, and J. M. Rabey, "The clinical use of P300 event related potentials for the evaluation of cholinesterase inhibitors treatment in demented patients," *Journal of Neural Transmission*, vol. 110, no. 6, pp. 659–669, 2003.

[60] P. E. Gold, "Acetylcholine modulation of neural systems involved in learning and memory," *Neurobiology of Learning and Memory*, vol. 80, no. 3, pp. 194–210, 2003.

[61] S. J. Bang and T. H. Brown, "Muscarinic receptors in perirhinal cortex control trace conditioning," *The Journal of Neuroscience*, vol. 29, no. 14, pp. 4346–4350, 2009.

[62] D. Martí Barros, M. R. Ramirez, E. A. Dos Reis, and I. Izquierdo, "Participation of hippocampal nicotinic receptors in acquisition, consolidation and retrieval of memory for one trial inhibitory avoidance in rats," *Neuroscience*, vol. 126, no. 3, pp. 651–656, 2004.

[63] M. H. Pang, N. S. Kim, I. H. Kim, H. Kim, H. T. Kim, and J. S. Choi, "Cholinergic transmission in the dorsal hippocampus modulates trace but not delay fear conditioning," *Neurobiology of Learning and Memory*, vol. 94, no. 2, pp. 206–213, 2010.

[64] G. Pepeu and M. G. Giovannini, "Cholinesterase inhibitors and memory," *Chemico-Biological Interactions*, vol. 187, no. 1–3, pp. 403–408, 2010.

[65] J. L. Rogers and R. P. Kesner, "Cholinergic modulation of the hippocampus during encoding and retrieval," *Neurobiology of Learning and Memory*, vol. 80, no. 3, pp. 332–342, 2003.

[66] T. Aosaki, M. Miura, T. Suzuki, K. Nishimura, and M. Masuda, "Acetylcholine-dopamine balance hypothesis in the striatum: an update," *Geriatrics & Gerontology International*, vol. 10, s1, pp. S148–S157, 2010.

[67] R. M. Drenan, S. R. Grady, A. D. Steele et al., "Cholinergic modulation of locomotion and striatal dopamine release is mediated by $\alpha 6 \alpha 4^*$ nicotinic acetylcholine receptors," *The Journal of Neuroscience*, vol. 30, no. 29, pp. 9877–9889, 2010.

[68] M. S. Guzman, X. De Jaeger, S. Raulic et al., "Elimination of the vesicular acetylcholine transporter in the striatum reveals regulation of behaviour by cholinergic-glutamatergic co-transmission," *PLoS Biology*, vol. 9, no. 11, article e1001194, 2011.

[69] A. Pisani, G. Bernardi, J. Ding, and D. J. Surmeier, "Re-emergence of striatal cholinergic interneurons in movement disorders," *Trends in Neurosciences*, vol. 30, no. 10, pp. 545–553, 2007.

[70] C. J. Wilson, "The mechanism of intrinsic amplification of hyperpolarizations and spontaneous bursting in striatal cholinergic interneurons," *Neuron*, vol. 45, no. 4, pp. 575–585, 2005.

[71] M. Goard and Y. Dan, "Basal forebrain activation enhances cortical coding of natural scenes," *Nature Neuroscience*, vol. 12, no. 11, pp. 1444–1449, 2009.

[72] S. Soma, N. Suematsu, and S. Shimegi, "Cholinesterase inhibitor, donepezil, improves visual contrast detectability in freely behaving rats," *Behavioural Brain Research*, vol. 256, pp. 362–367, 2013.

[73] P. J. Bushnell, W. M. Oshiro, and B. K. Padnos, "Detection of visual signals by rats: effects of chlordiazepoxide and cholinergic and adrenergic drugs on sustained attention," *Psychopharmacology*, vol. 134, no. 3, pp. 230–241, 1997.

[74] D. B. Hodges Jr, M. D. Lindner, J. B. Hogan, K. M. Jones, and E. J. Markus, "Scopolamine induced deficits in a battery of rat cognitive tests: comparisons of sensitivity and specificity," *Behavioural Pharmacology*, vol. 20, no. 3, pp. 237–251, 2009.

[75] J. Svoboda, A. Popelikova, and A. Stuchlik, "Drugs interfering with muscarinic acetylcholine receptors and their effects on place navigation," *Frontiers in Psychiatry*, vol. 8, p. 215, 2017.

[76] L. Molinengo, G. Di Carlo, and P. Ghi, "Combined action of thioperamide plus scopolamine, diphenhydramine, or methysergide on memory in mice," *Pharmacology Biochemistry and Behavior*, vol. 63, no. 2, pp. 221–227, 1999.

[77] M. I. Miranda, F. Ortiz-Godina, and D. García, "Differential involvement of cholinergic and beta-adrenergic systems during acquisition, consolidation, and retrieval of long-term memory of social and neutral odors," *Behavioural Brain Research*, vol. 202, no. 1, pp. 19–25, 2009.

[78] N. Popović, M. Caballero-Bleda, and M. Popović, "Post-training scopolamine treatment induced maladaptive behavior in open field habituation task in rats," *PLoS One*, vol. 9, no. 6, article e100348, 2014.

[79] J. C. Soares, R. V. Fornari, and M. G. Oliveira, "Role of muscarinic M1 receptors in inhibitory avoidance and contextual fear conditioning," *Neurobiology of Learning and Memory*, vol. 86, no. 2, pp. 188–196, 2006.

[80] M. G. Blake, M. M. Boccia, M. C. Krawczyk, and C. M. Baratti, "Scopolamine prevents retrograde memory interference between two different learning tasks," *Physiology & Behavior*, vol. 102, no. 3-4, pp. 332–337, 2011.

[81] D. C. Turner, T. W. Robbins, L. Clark, A. R. Aron, J. Dowson, and B. J. Sahakian, "Cognitive enhancing effects of modafinil in healthy volunteers," *Psychopharmacology*, vol. 165, no. 3, pp. 260–269, 2003.

[82] D. C. Turner, L. Clark, J. Dowson, T. W. Robbins, and B. J. Sahakian, "Modafinil improves cognition and response inhibition in adult attention-deficit/hyperactivity disorder," *Biological Psychiatry*, vol. 55, no. 10, pp. 1031–1040, 2004.

[83] J. K. Seamans, C. C. Lapish, and D. Durstewitz, "Comparing the prefrontal cortex of rats and primates: insights from electrophysiology," *Neurotoxicity Research*, vol. 14, no. 2-3, pp. 249–262, 2008.

[84] J. D. Wallis, "Cross-species studies of orbitofrontal cortex and value-based decision-making," *Nature Neuroscience*, vol. 15, no. 1, pp. 13–19, 2012.

[85] W. J. Huang, W. W. Chen, and X. Zhang, "The neurophysiology of P300 - an integrated review," *European Review for Medical and Pharmacological Sciences*, vol. 19, no. 8, pp. 1480–8, 2015.

[86] K. Takahata, A. Minami, H. Kusumoto, S. Shimazu, and F. Yoneda, "Effects of selegiline alone or with donepezil on memory impairment in rats," *European Journal of Pharmacology*, vol. 518, no. 2-3, pp. 140–144, 2005.

[87] A. Imada, A. Morris, and M. C. Wiest, "Deviance detection by a P3-like response in rat posterior parietal cortex," *Frontiers in Integrative Neuroscience*, vol. 6, p. 127, 2013.

[88] S. Yamaguchi, H. Globus, and R. T. Knight, "P3-like potential in rats," *Electroencephalography and Clinical Neurophysiology*, vol. 88, no. 2, pp. 151–154, 1993.

[89] C. L. Ehlers and R. I. Chaplin, "Long latency event related potentials in rats: the effects of changes in stimulus parameters and neurochemical lesions," *Journal of Neural Transmission/General Section JNT*, vol. 88, no. 1, pp. 61–75, 1992.

[90] P. H. Boeijinga, "Objective markers of drug effects on brain function from recordings of scalp potential in healthy volunteers," *Dialogues in Clinical Neuroscience*, vol. 4, no. 4, pp. 388–394, 2002.

[91] C. Leroy, J. L. Bourriez, K. Dujardin et al., "A 15-day course of donepezil modulates spectral EEG dynamics related to target auditory stimuli in young, healthy adult volunteers," *Clinical Neurophysiology*, 2015.

[92] J. O'Neill, E. Halgren, K. Marinkovic et al., "Effects of muscarinic and adrenergic agonism on auditory P300 in the macaque," *Physiology & Behavior*, vol. 70, no. 1-2, pp. 163–170, 2000.

[93] R. A. Lenz, J. D. Baker, C. Locke et al., "The scopolamine model as a pharmacodynamic marker in early drug development," *Psychopharmacology*, vol. 220, no. 1, pp. 97–107, 2012.

[94] J. J. Buccafusco, "The revival of scopolamine reversal for the assessment of cognition-enhancing drugs," in *Methods of Behavior Analysis in Neuroscience*, J. J. Buccafusco, Ed., Boca Raton, FL, USA, CRC Press/Taylor & Francis, 2nd edition, 2009, Chapter 17.

[95] P. Fries, "Rhythms for cognition: communication through coherence," *Neuron*, vol. 88, no. 1, pp. 220–235, 2015.

[96] X. J. Wang, "Neurophysiological and computational principles of cortical rhythms in cognition," *Physiological Reviews*, vol. 90, no. 3, pp. 1195–1268, 2010.

[97] B. H. Bland and S. D. Oddie, "Theta band oscillation and synchrony in the hippocampal formation and associated structures: the case for its role in sensorimotor integration," *Behavioural Brain Research*, vol. 127, no. 1-2, pp. 119–136, 2001.

14

The Effects of Music Intervention on Functional Connectivity Strength of the Brain in Schizophrenia

Mi Yang,[1,2] Hui He,[1] Mingjun Duan,[1,2] Xi Chen,[1] Xin Chang,[1] Yongxiu Lai,[1] Jianfu Li,[1] Tiejun Liu,[1] Cheng Luo,[1] and Dezhong Yao[1]

[1]*The Clinical Hospital of Chengdu Brain Science Institute, MOE Key Lab for Neuroinformation, University of Electronic Science and Technology of China, Chengdu, China*

[2]*Department of Psychiatry, Chengdu Mental Health Centre, The Four People's Hospital of Chengdu, Chengdu 610036, China*

Correspondence should be addressed to Tiejun Liu; liutiejun@uestc.edu.cn and Cheng Luo; chengluo@uestc.edu.cn

Mi Yang and Hui He contributed equally to this work.

Academic Editor: J. Michael Wyss

Schizophrenia is often associated with behavior abnormality in the cognitive and affective domain. Music intervention is used as a complementary treatment for improving symptoms in patients with schizophrenia. However, the neurophysiological correlates of these remissions remain poorly understood. Here, we investigated the effects of music intervention in neural circuits through functional magnetic resonance imaging (fMRI) study in schizophrenic subjects. Under the standard care, patients were randomly assigned to music and non-music interventions (MTSZ, UMTSZ) for 1 month. Resting-state fMRI were acquired over three time points (baseline, 1 month, and 6 months later) in patients and analyzed using functional connectivity strength (FCS) and seed-based functional connection (FC) approaches. At baseline, compared with healthy controls, decreased FCS in the right middle temporal gyrus (MTG) was observed in patients. However, after music intervention, the functional circuitry of the right MTG, which was related with the function of emotion and sensorimotor, was improved in MTSZ. Furthermore, the FC increments were significantly correlated with the improvement of symptoms, while vanishing 6 months later. Together, these findings provided evidence that music intervention might positively modulate the functional connectivity of MTG in patients with schizophrenia; such changes might be associated with the observed therapeutic effects of music intervention on neurocognitive function. This trial is registered with ChiCTR-OPC-14005339.

1. Introduction

Schizophrenia is a psychiatric illness, which has been typically associated with complex and diverse impairments in cognitive, affective behavior and perceptual levels of processing, with a lifetime prevalence of 0.30% to 0.66% in the general population [1]. Schizophrenia may be characterized as a prototypical disorder of brain connectivity [2, 3]. The prevailing neuroimaging studies indicated that the dysfunction of the brain functional network maybe associated with the pathophysiological mechanisms underlying schizophrenia [2]. Antipsychotic drugs are commonly used prolonged treatments for schizophrenia. In addition, the complementary therapies, such as cognitive-behavioral therapy [4] and music intervention [5, 6], are also choices for patients with schizophrenia. Music intervention was known to significantly improve the psychiatric symptoms in schizophrenic subjects [6, 7]. There has been an interest in understanding the neural effects of music intervention, then gain a better understanding of the maintaining mechanisms of schizophrenia and improve further therapies.

Music is one of the oldest sociocognitive domains of humans. Music listening and music intervention (such as music performance and music listening by patients) are often documented by the proposed need for a medium for communication. Listening to Mozart K.448 could enhance spatial-temporal reasoning on subjects in the short-term [8]. Other forms of music were found to be equally temporarily effective

[9, 10]. The findings of music intervention open a new page for the study of the effect of music on humans. To investigate the effect of music intervention on schizophrenic subjects, research has compared patients receiving standard care with or without music intervention [11]. Importantly, clinical reports have indicated that music intervention could have motivating, emotionally expressive, and relationship-building qualities in schizophrenia [12, 13]. After music intervention, significant advantages were detected in some measures concerning personal relations and subjectivity schizophrenic subjects [14]. Cognitive task performance could also be facilitated after listening to music by Mozart in patients with schizophrenia [15]. However, the particular mechanism behind this phenomenon is still poorly understood.

In the past decades, resting-state functional magnetic resonance imaging (fMRI), which measures ongoing spontaneous brain activity and maps interregional functional connectivity (FC) [16, 17], as a powerful in vivo imaging technique has received substantial attention in brain disorder researches [18, 19]. Our previous studies have demonstrated that altered brain FC of patients with schizophrenia was associated with psychiatric symptoms [20, 21]. Importantly, our previous study indicated that the insular cortex might be an important region in music intervention from a local aspect (seed-based FC analysis) for schizophrenic subjects [22]. However, the application of graph-based network analysis allows the computation of a wide range of measures, such as small-world attributes, hubs, and network modularity [23], which could characterize diverse topological properties of the brain disorder connectome from a global aspect. For patients with schizophrenia, reductions in topological measures (clustering coefficient, local efficiency) [24, 25] and small-world brain network [26] have been consistently found through fMRI. However, there were few studies from which correlates of music intervention in schizophrenic subjects from a global aspect have been investigated.

Here, we used fMRI to examine the effect of music intervention on schizophrenia. The distribution of high nodal connectivity in the brain plays vital roles in transferring information over the whole brain [27]. The hubs of the whole-brain network are generally affected in patients with schizophrenia based on the functional relevance and physiological basis [2]. Several studies have demonstrated that the functional connectivity strength (FCS) metric, which could examine hub connectivity through voxel-based graph analysis approaches, is closely associated with physiological measures such as regional cerebral blood flow, oxygen, and glucose metabolism [28]. Therefore, different from our previous work, in this study, fMRI was used to identify functional hubs of brain networks from the global aspect to assess the effect of music intervention on schizophrenia through computing the FCS at the voxel level. Such a voxel-wise approach enables whole brain hub mapping but overcomes the limitation of seed-based approaches for identifying and locating functional hubs in the brain. The goals of this study are to (1) explore the modulatory effect of music intervention on resting-state functional networks in patients with schizophrenia, (2) explore the relationship between music intervention-induced change of FC and change in psychiatric symptoms and neuropsychological in schizophrenia, and (3) assess the duration of effects of music intervention through studying the schizophrenic subjects six months later.

2. Material and Methods

2.1. Subjects. The participants in this study are the same with our previous study including fifty-six schizophrenic subjects (male: 10; female: 26) and nineteen healthy controls (HC) (male: 7; female: 12). All subjects were recruited from the clinical hospital of the Chengdu Brain Science Institute (CBSI). The detail fundamental information of schizophrenic subjects and HC could be referred to our previous article [22].

2.2. Design. To measure the effect of music intervention on schizophrenic subjects, a quasirandomized controlled trial was conducted in this study. Twenty-two patients with schizophrenia, who were randomly selected from patients, received group music intervention (MTSZ: music intervention patients with schizophrenia). Controlled patients (UMTSZ: non-music intervention patients with schizophrenia, remaining twenty-three patients) received standard care only. Three time point tests were included: a baseline test, a 1-month follow-up, and a 6-month follow-up. The blinded assessments and assignment were performed in schizophrenic subjects. The design of music intervention in this study was the same with our previous work. The detailed information could be referred from the previous article [22].

2.3. Content of Music Intervention. One professional music therapist participated in this study. Mozart's sonata K.448 music listening was performed in the MTSZ group (30 minutes per day, 30 days). MTSZ patients peacefully listened to the music in a quiet room during each session. The music therapist introduced the background of the music to schizophrenic patients at the beginning. The UMTSZ was treated solely with antipsychotic drugs. The content of the music intervention was also the same with our previous study. The detailed information could be referred from the previous article [22].

2.4. Psychiatric and Neuropsychological Assessment. Three evaluators of the neuropsychological assessments and one psychiatrist assessed the patients with schizophrenia. The psychiatric symptoms of the schizophrenic patients were assessed by a psychiatrist using the Positive and Negative Symptom Scale (PANSS). In the neuropsychological assessment (Block Design Test (BDT), BVRT, and Spatial Maze Test), the evaluators were trained to achieve a high interrater reliability before the start of the study. Detailed information can be found in Section 1 of the Supplemental Information).

2.5. Data Acquisition. Experiments were performed on a 3 T MRI scanner (GE Discovery MR750). A detailed description of the data collection can be found in Section 2 of the Supplemental Information. Functional image preprocessing was performed using SPM8 (Statistical Parametric Mapping, http://www.fil.ion.ucl.ac.uk/spm/) according to a standard pipeline. Slice timing correction and head motion correction were carried out. Then, the functional scans were normalized to the Montreal Neurological Institute (MNI) EPI template and resampled to $3 \times 3 \times 3\,\text{mm}^3$ voxels. The general processing procedures of spatial smoothing (Gaussian kernel of a full width at half maximum (FWHM) of 6 mm) was not included for the FCS analysis but was included for the FC analysis. Then, nuisance signals were then removed from the data through linear regression (white matter (WM), cerebrospinal fluid (CSF), and six motion parameters), except the global signal due to recent excellent studies [29]. Finally, fMRI data were temporally filtered in band-pass 0.01–0.08 Hz. Recent studies demonstrated that head motion had a substantial impact on FC [30, 31]. Thus, any subjects who had a maximum translation in any of the cardinal directions larger than 2.0 mm or a maximum rotation larger than 2.0 degrees were excluded. Besides, we also assessed framewise displacement (FD) in three groups as suggested by Power et al. [30] using the following formula:

$$\text{FD} = \frac{1}{M-1}\sum_{i=2}^{M}\sqrt{\left|\Delta t_{x_i}\right|^2 + \left|\Delta t_{y_i}\right|^2 + \left|\Delta t_{z_i}\right|^2 + \left|\Delta d_{x_i}\right|^2 + \left|\Delta d_{y_i}\right|^2 + \left|\Delta d_{z_i}\right|^2}, \quad (1)$$

where M is the length of the time courses ($M = 250$ in this study); x_i, y_i, and z_i are translations/rotations at the ith time point in the x, y, and z directions, respectively; Δt represents the framewise displacement translation; and Δd represents the framewise displacement rotation. $\Delta d_{x_i} = x_i - x_{i-1}$ and similar for d_{y_i} and d_{z_i}.

Structural images were processed using SPM8 toolbox. Spatial normalization to MNI-space was performed using a diffeomorphic anatomical registration through exponentiated lie algebra and segmented into gray matter (GM), WM, and CSF. The segmented GM and WM were modulated using nonlinear deformation. Total Intracranial Volume (TIV) and GM volume and were calculated. Then, the normalization analysis was performed: the GM volume was divided by the TIV score. The schizophrenic patients' and HC's normalized GM at baseline were entered as a global variable to correct for the global GM volume of different subjects in the statistical analysis.

2.6. Functional Connectivity Strength Analysis. Whole-brain FC analysis was performed as follows. First, to exclude artefactual correlations from non-gray matter, the GM mask was generated by thresholding (cutoff = 0.2) the average of GM probability map involving all subjects. The time series from each voxel within the GM mask was extracted, and Pearson's correlations between any pair of voxels were calculated for each subject. To improve normality, we then transformed individual correlation matrices to a z-score matrix using a Fisher r-to-z transformation. Then, for a given voxel (node), nodal FCS was computed as the sum of weights of its connections with other voxels. We conservatively restricted our analysis to positive correlations above the threshold of $r = 0.2$, which was chosen to eliminate the voxels with weak correlations attributable to signal noise [32]. Before group-level statistical analysis, an individual voxel-wise FCS map was standardized to z-scores and further spatially smoothed (FWHM = 6 mm).

2.7. Functional Connectivity Analysis. We examined FC by taking the brain region that had showed different FCS (pursuant to the FCS statistical test) as the seed. FC analysis was performed between the seed and all voxels in the brain. To improve normality, we then transformed individual correlation matrices to a z-score matrix using a Fisher r-to-z transformation. In this manner, FC maps of these seeds were produced for each subject.

2.8. Statistical Analysis

2.8.1. Participant Fundamental Information Statistics. Age, years of education, and FD among the three groups were compared using one-way ANOVA. Chi-square test was used to compare gender distributions. A two-sample t-test was used to compare the psychiatric symptoms (illness duration, medication dosage in chlorpromazine (CPZ) equivalents (mg), and PANSS scores) between two groups of patients at baseline. Repeated measure ANOVA were performed to determine the music intervention $*$ time interaction, main effects of music intervention and time on neuropsychological measurements, and PANSS scores.

2.8.2. Baseline Brain Connectivity Analyses between Patients and HC. Firstly, we established baseline abnormalities between HCs and schizophrenic patients through two-sample t-test in FCS and seed-based FC, respectively, with age, gender, years of education, and GM as covariates. The comparison, for the FCS statistical test, was constrained within the GM mask. The seed-based FC statistical test was performed within the mask that resulted from the union set of the one-sample t-test of the two groups ($p < 0.005$ with cluster-level false discovery rate corrected, $p < 0.05$). Due to the quantity of patients being greater than the amount of HC, the HC and the same number of patients who were randomly selected from the whole sample of patients were entered into the statistical comparisons. These steps were repeatedly performed 200 times [33]. A total of 200 comparison results were obtained. Then, we calculated the probability map where the voxels exhibited significant differences ($p < 0.005$ with cluster-level false discovery rate corrected, $p < 0.05$) across the 200 comparisons.

Furthermore, we also established the difference between MTSZ and UMTSZ at baseline through a two-sample t-test in FCS and seed-based FC, respectively, with gender, years of education, GM, and age as covariates. The significance threshold of the group difference was set to $p < 0.05$.

2.8.3. Longitudinal Analysis of Functional Connectivity in Patients. After tests of normality, homogeneity of variance, and Mauchly's test of sphericity, the repeated-measure ANOVA and post hoc analyses were performed on the schizophrenic subjects from baseline and 1-month follow-up to determine the music intervention $*$ time interaction, main effects of music intervention, and time on FCS and seed-based FC, respectively. The age, gender, illness duration, education characteristics, GM, and the medication dosage were used as covariates. The significance threshold for ANOVA was set to $p < 0.005$ with cluster-level false discovery rate corrected ($p < 0.05$). For the region with difference resulted from repeated-measure ANOVA, a further two-sample t-test was performed between HC and patients (MTSZ and UMTSZ from 1-month follow-up) to assess the effect of the 1-month music intervention on patients relative to HC. At last, the data with the 6-month follow-up was used to evaluate the long-term effect of music intervention through the comparison to data from the 1-month follow-up in schizophrenic subjects.

2.9. The Relationship between FC and Patients' Variables. To investigate the underlying relationship between the changes of functional measurements (i.e., FCS and seed-based FC) and the changes of neuropsychological measurements, as well as PANSS in the MTSZ and UMTSZ groups, we used partial correlation analysis in this study. We extracted the mean z-score of the region that showed significant difference of FCS and FC. Then, the partial correlations between the mean changes (1-month later minus baseline) and the percentage change scores (1 − [score at 1-month/score at baseline]) of neuropsychological measurements were performed, as well as the percentage change scores of PANSS, with age, gender, illness duration, education characteristics, GM, and medication dosage as covariates. The partial correlation analysis was also performed between the mean changes (6 months later minus baseline) and the percentage change scores (1 − [score at 6 months/score at baseline]) of neuropsychological and PANSS scores.

3. Results

3.1. Participant Demographic Information. Forty-five patients with schizophrenia finished the randomized controlled trial at two time points (baseline and 1-month follow-up). Nine of them (4 in MTSZ and 5 in UMTSZ) were excluded due to excessive head motion. Thus, 18 MTSZ, 18 UMTSZ, and 19 HC were included in the following analysis.

Furthermore, at 6-month follow-up, 9 schizophrenic subjects (25%) were not recalled because they were no longer interested in the experiment after being discharged from the hospital. 5 patients with schizophrenia with excessive head motion were also excluded, so thirteen (13/18) UMTSZ and nine (9/18) MTSZ patients were included.

3.2. Changes in Psychiatric Symptoms and Neuropsychological Measurements. We observed significant music intervention main effect and music intervention ∗ time interaction on the scores of Positive and Negative Symptom Scale (PANSS) and the score of Benton Visual Retention Test (BVRT). Post hoc analysis revealed that significant increase of BVRT and decrease of PANSS scores were found in MTSZ at 1-month follow-up, while not in the UMTSZ group. Nonsignificant difference was observed between the MTSZ and UMTSZ groups at baseline. Furthermore, the effects of music intervention had vanished in the MTSZ at the 6-month follow-up (comparison results between the schizophrenic subjects from 1-month follow-up and 6-month follow-up). The detailed information could be referred from the previous study [22].

3.3. The Abnormalities of FCS at Baseline. Firstly, the FCS patterns were remarkably similar across the MTSZ and UMTSZ, as well as the HC (see Supplementary Figures S1 and S2). The FCS patterns were similar to those observed in previous studies [28]. At baseline, compared to HC, in patients with schizophrenia, the decreased FCS was observed in the posterior insula, prepostcentral gyrus, supplementary motor area, middle cingulate cortex (MCC), and middle temporal gyrus (MTG) (Figure 1(a)). The patients with schizophrenia also exhibited increased FCS in the basal ganglia, bilateral middle frontal gyrus, and cerebellum. These findings are similar with previous researches [26]. No significant difference FCS was observed between MTSZ and UMTSZ at baseline.

3.4. Longitudinal Changes of FCS after Music Intervention in Schizophrenia. In the FCS analysis, significant music intervention ∗ time interaction on FCS was observed in the right MTG (Figure 1(b), Table 1). Post hoc analysis revealed that significantly increased FCS was observed in MTSZ following 1-month music intervention (right MTG: $t_{17} = 2.97$, $p = 0.008$) (Figure 1(c)), while no difference was found in the UMTSZ group. FCS in these regions did not show any significant difference between the two patient groups at baseline.

Additionally, following the 1-month music intervention, significantly decreased FCS was observed in the right MTG in MTSZ ($t_{35} = -2.24$, $p = 0.031$) and UMTSZ ($t_{35} = -2.48$, $p = 0.018$) compared with HC.

Finally, in MTSZ, the FCS of the right MTG 6 months later had a significant decrease compared with the data from the 1-month follow-up. In a word, a diminished effect of music intervention was observed at the 6-month follow-up.

3.5. Longitudinal Changes of FC after Music Intervention in Schizophrenia. Based on the FCS results in MTSZ, we assessed the longitudinal changes of resting-state FC of the right MTG in the patient groups. First, at baseline, the patients exhibited declined MTG FCs with the insula, pre-/postcentral gyrus, and superior occipital gyrus. Increased FCs were also observed between the MTG and cerebellum (Figure 2(a)).

Second, ANOVA analysis showed that significant music intervention ∗ time (1 month) interaction on the FC of the right MTG was located in the right anterior insula and postcentral gyrus (Figure 2(b) and Table 2). Post hoc analysis showed significant increases in MTSZ following 1-month music intervention (right anterior insula: $t_{34} = 2.55$, $p = 0.020$; right postcentral: $t_{34} = 3.19$, $p = 0.005$) compared to baseline (Figure 2(c)) but no significance in UMTSZ.

Third, compared with HC, both patient groups no significant changes were found between the MTG and right anterior insula and postcentral gyrus, except for the FC between the MTG and right postcentral gyrus in UMTSZ ($t_{35} = -2.27$, $p = 0.029$).

The 6-month follow-up investigation is illustrated in Figure 3. In MTSZ, the FC between the MTG and insula at 6 months later had a significant decrease compared with the data from the 1-month follow-up. In a word, a diminished effect of music intervention was observed at the 6-month follow-up.

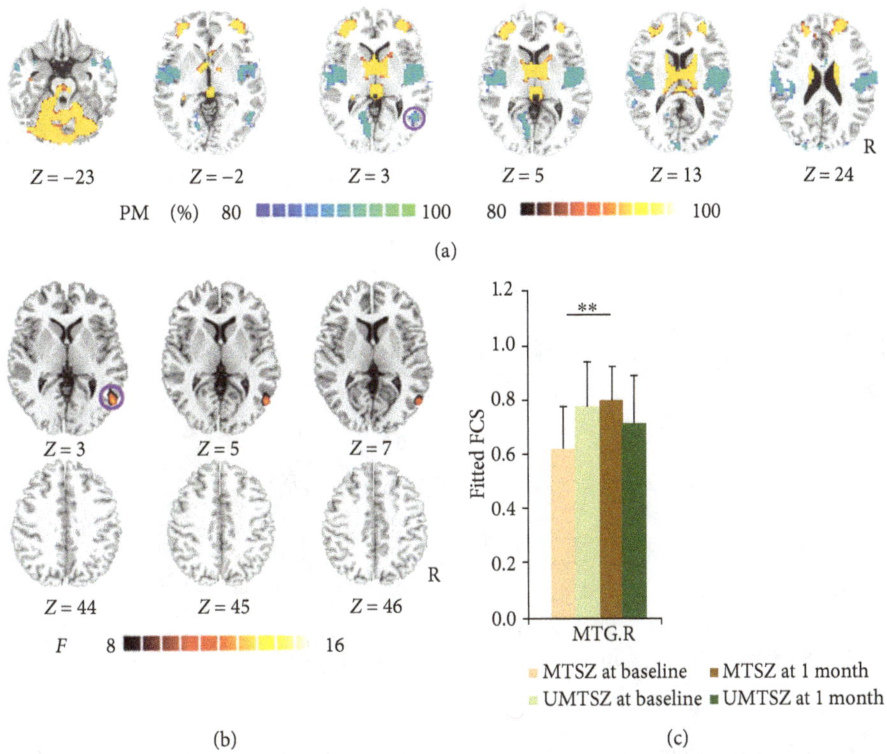

FIGURE 1: Music intervention ∗ time interaction on functional connectivity strength (FCS). (a) denotes the altered FCS in patients compared with healthy controls at baseline. The cool color indicates decreased functional connections, and the hot color indicates increased functional connections. All of the maps are shown with a probability score between 80% and 100%. (b) denotes that significant music intervention ∗ time interaction on FCS was observed in the right middle temporal gyrus (MTG.R) through repeated-measure ANOVA analysis. (c) denotes the post hoc analysis results in regions showing significant music intervention ∗ time interaction on FCS. The data were expressed as the mean value + standard error. $^{**}p < 0.01$. The violet circles mark the same region in (a) and (b), which means the positively modulated region through music intervention in patients.

TABLE 1: Significant music intervention ∗ time interaction on FCS of the whole brain through repeated-measure ANOVA.

Regions	BA	MNI coordinates			Peak F-score	Cluster voxels
		x	y	z		
MTG.R	BA 37	52	−64	3	12.632	103

BA: Brodmann area; MTG: middle temporal gyrus.

3.6. The Relationship between Altered FC and Patients' Variables. In MTSZ, partial correlation analysis revealed that MTG-postcentral FC change showed a significant positive correlation with the change scores of PANSS-total score, as well as PANSS-positive score (Figure 4(a): PANSS-total score: $r = 0.529$, $p = 0.024$; Figure 4(b): PANSS-positive score: $r = 0.600$, $p = 0.008$). Similar associations result with the change score of PANSS-total score, which was also found in the changes FC (MTS and anterior insula) (Figure 4(c): $r = 0.486$, $p = 0.041$). No significant correlations were found between the changes in brain functional measures (FCS and FC) in the areas and the change score of neuropsychological measurements, as well as medication dosage in MTSZ and UMTSZ. There were no significant relationships in UMTSZ. Finally, the significant relationship was also not observed between the changes of functional measures (6 months later minus baseline) and changes of neuropsychological score, as well as the PANSS score (6 months later minus baseline) in MTSZ and UMTSZ.

4. Discussion

This study combined resting-state fMRI and voxel-based graph approach to characterize the effect of music intervention on the brain network hub and FC changes in schizophrenic subjects. Our findings revealed that the 1-month music intervention had the positive improving effect on the abnormally lower hub score of the right MTG in patients. Furthermore, we found that the intervention-related resting-state FC was also being positively modulated in the right MTG functional network. Finally, the psychiatric symptom analysis indicated that the changes of FCs showed significant positive relationship with the change scores of PANSS, while vanishing 6 months later. These findings provide evidence supporting the notion that music intervention might positively improve the FC between the MTG and insula, as well as the sensorimotor gyrus. These changes may be related to the remission of psychiatric symptoms in schizophrenia.

While disturbances in higher order brain functions, such as memory [34] and cognitive [35], are well known in schizophrenia, recent studies have also documented basic sensory-

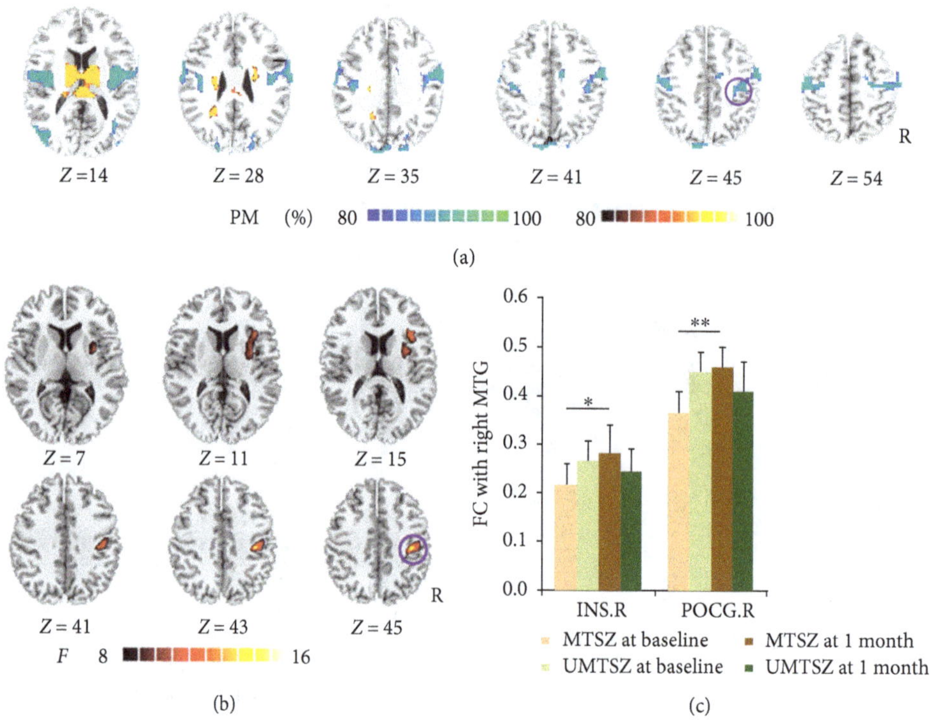

FIGURE 2: Music intervention ∗ time interaction on FC of the right middle temporal gyrus (MTG.R). (a) denotes that the altered FC resulted from seeded-MTG.R FC analysis in patients compared with healthy controls at baseline. The cool color indicates decreased functional connections, and the hot color indicates increased functional connections. All of the maps are shown with a probability score between 80% and 100%. (b) denotes that significant music intervention ∗ time interaction on FC was observed between the right MTG and right precentral gyrus (POCG.R), as well as the right insula (INS.R). (c) The bar maps present the between-group and within-group differences in regions showing significant music intervention ∗ time interaction on FC of the MTG.R. The data were expressed as the mean value + standard error. $^{*}p < 0.05$, $^{**}p < 0.01$. The violet circles mark the same region in (a) and (b), which means the positively modulated region through music therapy in patients.

TABLE 2: Significant music intervention ∗ time interaction on FC of the middle temporal gyrus through repeated-measure ANOVA.

Regions	BA	MNI coordinates			Peak F-score	Cluster voxels
		x	y	z		
POCG.R	BA 3	40	−25	46	14.319	123
INS.R	BA 48	36	16	15	9.108	101

BA: Brodmann area; POCG: postcentral gyrus; INS: insula.

processing deficits. In schizophrenic subjects, perceptual deficits have become increasingly observed in the visual system [36–38]. The early visual system is divided into two basic subdivisions, including parvocellular and magnocellular divisions. The magnocellular neurons are projected to the dorsal visual stream, such as the MTG and intraparietal sulcus, which process visual information and guide action [39, 40]. There are additional projections through the thalamus to subcortical regions, which may play a specific role in emotional expression [40, 41]. Previous excellent research reported that music could be associated with increased functional coupling between emotional and attentional brain regions in the parietal and visual regions (MTG) in patients with visual neglect [42]. In this study, we observed the decreased FCS in the right MTG in schizophrenic subjects at the baseline, while we found music intervention could positively improve the abnormally lower FCS score of the right MTG. Our finding might be indicated that MTG may be a target gyrus in the dorsal visual stream for music intervention. Moreover, the altered FCS of MTG might positively regulate the processing of differentially sensitive motion to emotion in schizophrenia.

The deficits of the visual magnocellular pathway appear to be related to higher level emotional and cognitive impairments in schizophrenia [43–45]. Recent study also reported that the insular cortex and striatum are highly associated with visual magnocellular regions, which may serve as the neuroanatomical substrate in the perception of emotion [41]. Through music intervention, we found increased FC between the right MTG and the right anterior insula which has been thought to have a role in tracking emotions [46, 47]. Increased functional integration between the MTG and insular cortex might have an improving effect on emotional processing in schizophrenic subjects. The above-mentioned finding might reflect that the music intervention increased functional integration between the MTG and insula. The changed FC might improve higher order processes such as emotional identification and experience in MTSZ. In addition, the significant relationship was also observed between the changed FC of the insula and the

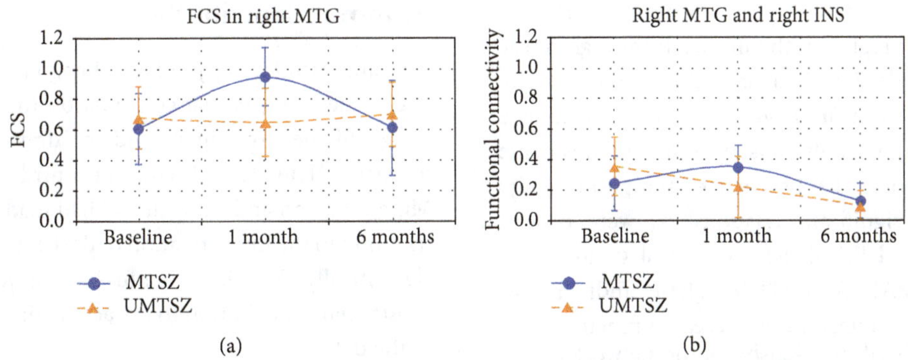

FIGURE 3: 6-month effects of music intervention versus nonmusic intervention on brain functional connectivity strength (FCS) and functional connectivity (FC) in patients with schizophrenia. The data were expressed as the mean value ± standard error. (a) denotes the long-term effects of music intervention versus nonmusic intervention on FCS of the middle temporal gyrus (MTG) in patients with schizophrenia. (b) denotes the long-term effects of music intervention on FC between the MTG and right insula (INS).

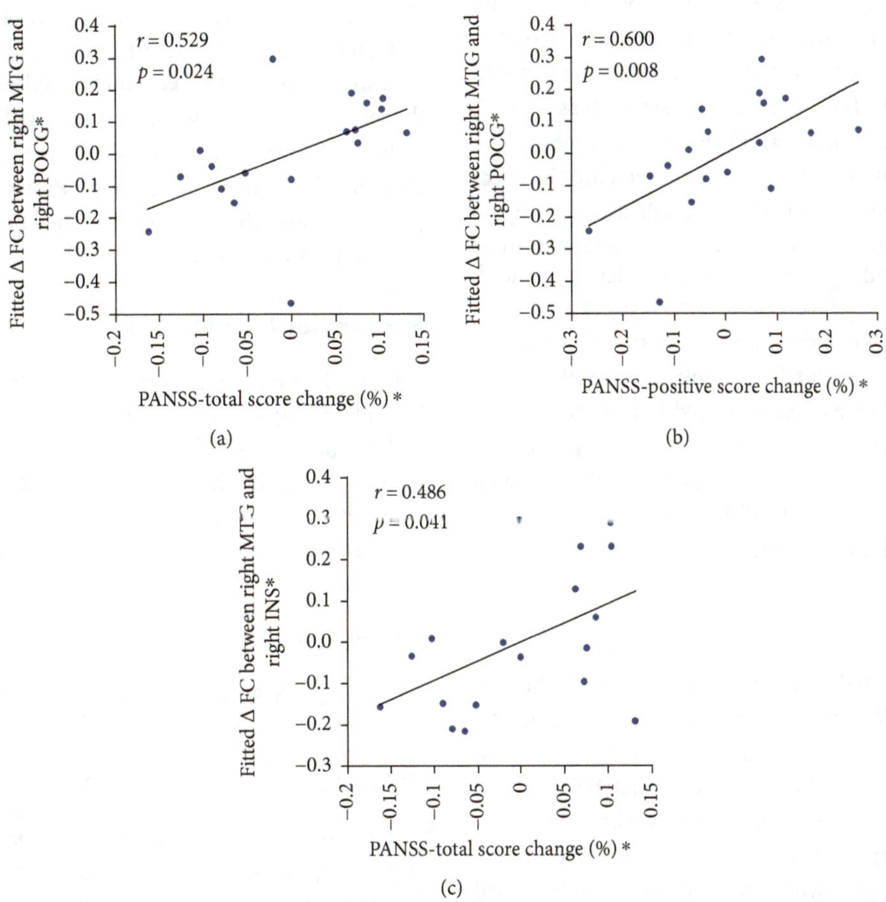

FIGURE 4: The relationship between altered functional connectivity (FC) and patient's scores of PANSS. (a) and (b) denote the significant correlations between the FC change (right MTG and right postcentral) and the percentage change scores of PANSS-total score (a) and PANSS-positive score (b). (c) denotes the significant relationship between the FC change (right MTG and right insula) and the percentage change score of PANSS-total score. Δ = week 4 − baseline. ∗ means the residual value after the regression analysis.

change score of PANSS-total. We propose that the music intervention might positively modulate the psychiatric symptom of schizophrenic subjects.

Reduced activation region in the visual magnocellular pathway was related to the deficits in motion processing in schizophrenia [48]. Our previous study revealed that music training could increase FC in the motor, visual, and multisensory cortices of musicians [49]. In the present study, the right MTG was observed to have increased FC with the right postcentral gyrus in MTSZ following the 1-month music intervention. The postcentral gyrus has been reported as a functional plasticity region in the musician through musical training [49]. In addition, increased BVRT scores, which was a well-established neurodiagnostic instrument to assess visuospatial [50, 51], were also observed though music intervention. Furthermore, the psychiatric symptom analysis revealed that the significant relationships were observed between the changed FC of the postcentral gyrus and the change scores of PANSS in MTSZ. These findings might reflect that the music intervention increased functional integration between visual and sensorimotor networks, which might improve the processing of visual information and guide action in schizophrenic subjects.

While we believe our findings provide new insight into the role of brain FC in understanding the effects of music intervention, several limitations need to be further addressed. First, a single musical piece was selected (Mozart's sonata K.448) in the present study. The special effects of Mozart's music might be observed in patients. Further studies should investigate the effects of other types of music, such as general, familiar, and preferred music, in schizophrenic subjects. The future research might be a better way to understand the effect of different types of music on patients as well as to investigate whether these effects are similar to those obtained from Mozart music. Second, the correlation coefficient threshold, which is to eliminate weak correlations possibly arising from noise signal, is not unique during the FCS analysis, and this fixed value may lead to some false positive or negative findings. The threshold value of 0.2 was used in this study based on prior knowledge. We also performed the same processing using two other thresholds (i.e., 0.1 and 0.3); these results were similar. Finally, the results of this study require replication in larger sample size studies.

5. Conclusions

This study demonstrated that music intervention might positively improve the functional hub of the MTG within the visual magnocellular pathway and simultaneously lead to the change in FC with some other regions related with function of emotion and sensorimotor within the brain circuitry of schizophrenic subjects. Furthermore, we observed related modulation in psychiatric symptoms and neuropsychological measurements in schizophrenia following the music intervention. Specifically, these positive modulations vanished 6 months later. These findings provided new insights into the effects of music intervention in medicine at the level of FC and might lead to treatment strategies including sensory-processing rehabilitation through music intervention.

Conflicts of Interest

None of the authors has any conflict of interests to disclose.

Authors' Contributions

Mi Yang, Hui He, Tiejun Liu, Cheng Luo, and Dezhong Yao had made a substantial contribution to the conception and design of the experiment and the drafting and revising of the article; Hui He and Jianfu Li contributed to the analysis; Mingjun Duan and Yongxiu Lai had made a substantial contribution to the interpretation of the data and revised the article critically. Xi Chen, Jianfu Li, and Xin Chang made a substantial contribution to the acquisition and interpretation of the data.

Acknowledgments

This work was supported by a Special-Funded Program on National Key Scientific Instruments and Equipment Development of China (no. 2013YQ490859), grants from the National Natural Science Foundation of China (Grant nos. 81471638 and 81571759), the Chinese Fundamental Research Funding for Central Universities (ZYGX2015J091), the project of the Science and Technology Department of Sichuan Province (2017JY0094), the Health and Family Planning Commission of Sichuan Province Research Project (16PJ051), and the Sichuan Province Science and Technology Support Project (2017SZ0004).

Supplementary Materials

Figure S1: functional connectivity strength (FCS) maps. Mean FCS maps in the MTSZ and UMTSZ groups at baseline and 1 month. The color bar represents the strength of FCS. Figure S2: functional connectivity strength (FCS) maps. Mean FCS maps in the healthy controls (HC). The color bar represents the strength of FCS. *(Supplementary Materials)*

References

[1] J. McGrath, S. Saha, D. Chant, and J. Welham, "Schizophrenia: a concise overview of incidence, prevalence, and mortality," *Epidemiologic Reviews*, vol. 30, no. 1, pp. 67–76, 2008.

[2] A. Fornito, A. Zalesky, C. Pantelis, and E. T. Bullmore, "Schizophrenia, neuroimaging and connectomics," *NeuroImage*, vol. 62, no. 4, pp. 2296–2314, 2012.

[3] J. Kambeitz, L. Kambeitz-Ilankovic, S. Leucht et al., "Detecting neuroimaging biomarkers for schizophrenia: a meta-analysis of multivariate pattern recognition studies," *Neuropsychopharmacology*, vol. 40, no. 7, pp. 1742–1751, 2015.

[4] N. A. Rector and A. T. Beck, "Cognitive behavioral therapy for schizophrenia: an empirical review," *The Journal of Nervous and Mental Disease*, vol. 189, no. 5, pp. 278–287, 2001.

[5] Y. N. Shih, C. S. Chen, H. Y. Chiang, and C. H. Liu, "Influence of background music on work attention in clients with chronic schizophrenia," *Work*, vol. 51, no. 1, pp. 153–158, 2015.

[6] S. F. Lu, C. H. K. Lo, H. C. Sung, T. C. Hsieh, S. C. Yu, and S. C. Chang, "Effects of group music intervention on psychiatric symptoms and depression in patient with schizophrenia,"

Complementary Therapies in Medicine, vol. 21, no. 6, pp. 682–688, 2013.

[7] S.-M. Peng, M. Koo, and J.-C. Kuo, "Effect of group music activity as an adjunctive therapy on psychotic symptoms in patients with acute schizophrenia," *Archives of Psychiatric Nursing*, vol. 24, no. 6, pp. 429–434, 2010.

[8] F. H. Rauscher, G. L. Shaw, and C. N. Ky, "Music and spatial task performance," *Nature*, vol. 365, no. 6447, p. 611, 1993.

[9] F. Rauscher, G. Shaw, L. Levine, E. Wright, W. Dennis, and R. Newcomb, "Music training causes long-term enhancement of preschool children's spatial–temporal reasoning," *Neurological Research*, vol. 19, no. 1, pp. 2–8, 1997.

[10] M. F. Gardiner, A. Fox, F. Knowles, and D. Jeffrey, "Learning improved by arts training," *Nature*, vol. 381, no. 6580, p. 284, 1996.

[11] G. Ulrich, T. Houtmans, and C. Gold, "The additional therapeutic effect of group music therapy for schizophrenic patients: a randomized study," *Acta Psychiatrica Scandinavica*, vol. 116, no. 5, pp. 362–370, 2007.

[12] H. P. Solli, ""Shut up and play!" improvisational use of popular music for a man with schizophrenia," *Nordic Journal of Music Therapy*, vol. 17, no. 1, pp. 67–77, 2008.

[13] R. Rolvsjord, "Sophie learns to play her songs of tears," *Nordic Journal of Music Therapy*, vol. 10, no. 1, pp. 77–85, 2001.

[14] N. Hayashi, Y. Tanabe, S. Nakagawa et al., "Effects of group musical therapy on inpatients with chronic psychoses: a controlled study," *Psychiatry and Clinical Neurosciences*, vol. 56, no. 2, pp. 187–193, 2002.

[15] J. Glicksohn and Y. Cohen, "Can music alleviate cognitive dysfunction in schizophrenia?," *Psychopathology*, vol. 33, no. 1, pp. 43–47, 2000.

[16] B. Biswal, F. Zerrin Yetkin, V. M. Haughton, and J. S. Hyde, "Functional connectivity in the motor cortex of resting human brain using echo-planar MRI," *Magnetic Resonance in Medicine*, vol. 34, no. 4, pp. 537–541, 1995.

[17] M. D. Fox and M. E. Raichle, "Spontaneous fluctuations in brain activity observed with functional magnetic resonance imaging," *Nature Reviews Neuroscience*, vol. 8, no. 9, pp. 700–711, 2007.

[18] C. Luo, Q. Li, Y. Lai et al., "Altered functional connectivity in default mode network in absence epilepsy: a resting-state fMRI study," *Human Brain Mapping*, vol. 32, no. 3, pp. 438–449, 2011.

[19] L. Dong, C. Luo, Y. Zhu et al., "Complex discharge-affecting networks in juvenile myoclonic epilepsy: a simultaneous EEG-fMRI study," *Human Brain Mapping*, vol. 37, no. 10, pp. 3515–3529, 2016.

[20] X. Chen, M. Duan, Q. Xie et al., "Functional disconnection between the visual cortex and the sensorimotor cortex suggests a potential mechanism for self-disorder in schizophrenia," *Schizophrenia Research*, vol. 166, no. 1-3, pp. 151–157, 2015.

[21] M. Duan, X. Chen, H. He et al., "Altered basal ganglia network integration in schizophrenia," *Frontiers in Human Neuroscience*, vol. 9, p. 561, 2015.

[22] H. He, M. Yang, M. Duan et al., "Music intervention leads to increased insular connectivity and improved clinical symptoms in schizophrenia," *Frontiers in Neuroscience*, vol. 11, p. 744, 2018.

[23] E. Bullmore and O. Sporns, "Complex brain networks: graph theoretical analysis of structural and functional systems," *Nature Reviews Neuroscience*, vol. 10, no. 3, pp. 186–198, 2009.

[24] Y. Liu, M. Liang, Y. Zhou et al., "Disrupted small-world networks in schizophrenia," *Brain*, vol. 131, no. 4, pp. 945–961, 2008.

[25] A. F. Alexander-Bloch, N. Gogtay, D. Meunier et al., "Disrupted modularity and local connectivity of brain functional networks in childhood-onset schizophrenia," *Frontiers in Systems Neuroscience*, vol. 4, p. 147, 2010.

[26] M. E. Lynall, D. S. Bassett, R. Kerwin et al., "Functional connectivity and brain networks in schizophrenia," *Journal of Neuroscience*, vol. 30, no. 28, pp. 9477–9487, 2010.

[27] S. Achard, R. Salvador, B. Whitcher, J. Suckling, and E. Bullmore, "A resilient, low-frequency, small-world human brain functional network with highly connected association cortical hubs," *Journal of Neuroscience*, vol. 26, no. 1, pp. 63–72, 2006.

[28] X. Liang, Q. Zou, Y. He, and Y. Yang, "Coupling of functional connectivity and regional cerebral blood flow reveals a physiological basis for network hubs of the human brain," *Proceedings of the National Academy of Sciences of the United States of America*, vol. 110, no. 5, pp. 1929–1934, 2013.

[29] G. J. Yang, J. D. Murray, G. Repovs et al., "Altered global brain signal in schizophrenia," *Proceedings of the National Academy of Sciences of the United States of America*, vol. 111, no. 20, pp. 7438–7443, 2014.

[30] J. D. Power, K. A. Barnes, A. Z. Snyder, B. L. Schlaggar, and S. E. Petersen, "Spurious but systematic correlations in functional connectivity MRI networks arise from subject motion," *NeuroImage*, vol. 59, no. 3, pp. 2142–2154, 2012.

[31] T. D. Satterthwaite, D. H. Wolf, J. Loughead et al., "Impact of in-scanner head motion on multiple measures of functional connectivity: relevance for studies of neurodevelopment in youth," *NeuroImage*, vol. 60, no. 1, pp. 623–632, 2012.

[32] L. Wang, M. Xia, K. Li et al., "The effects of antidepressant treatment on resting-state functional brain networks in patients with major depressive disorder," *Human Brain Mapping*, vol. 36, no. 2, pp. 768–778, 2015.

[33] H.-J. Li, Y. Xu, K.-R. Zhang, M. J. Hoptman, and X.-N. Zuo, "Homotopic connectivity in drug-naïve, first-episode, early-onset schizophrenia," *The Journal of Child Psychology and Psychiatry*, vol. 56, no. 4, pp. 432–443, 2015.

[34] A. M. Achim, M. C. Bertrand, H. Sutton et al., "Selective abnormal modulation of hippocampal activity during memory formation in first-episode psychosis," *Archives of General Psychiatry*, vol. 64, no. 9, pp. 999–1014, 2007.

[35] D. R. Weinberger and B. Gallhofer, "Cognitive function in schizophrenia," *International Clinical Psychopharmacology*, vol. 12, article S29, 1997.

[36] C.-S. R. Li, "Impaired detection of visual motion in schizophrenia patients," *Progress in Neuro-Psychopharmacology and Biological Psychiatry*, vol. 26, no. 5, pp. 929–934, 2002.

[37] I. Schechter, P. D. Butler, G. Silipo, V. Zemon, and D. C. Javitt, "Magnocellular and parvocellular contributions to backward masking dysfunction in schizophrenia," *Schizophrenia Research*, vol. 64, no. 2-3, pp. 91–101, 2003.

[38] A. Martinez, S. A. Hillyard, E. C. Dias et al., "Magnocellular pathway impairment in schizophrenia: evidence from functional magnetic resonance imaging," *Journal of Neuroscience*, vol. 28, no. 30, pp. 7492–7500, 2008.

[39] P. D. Butler and D. C. Javitt, "Early-stage visual processing deficits in schizophrenia," *Current Opinion in Psychiatry*, vol. 18, no. 2, pp. 151–157, 2005.

[40] J. S. Bedwell, C. C. Chan, O. Cohen, Y. Karbi, E. Shamir, and Y. Rassovsky, "The magnocellular visual pathway and facial emotion misattribution errors in schizophrenia," *Progress in Neuro-Psychopharmacology and Biological Psychiatry*, vol. 44, pp. 88–93, 2013.

[41] P. Vuilleumier, J. L. Armony, J. Driver, and R. J. Dolan, "Distinct spatial frequency sensitivities for processing faces and emotional expressions," *Nature Neuroscience*, vol. 6, no. 6, pp. 624–631, 2003.

[42] D. Soto, M. J. Funes, A. Guzman-Garcia, T. Warbrick, P. Rotshtein, and G. W. Humphreys, "Pleasant music overcomes the loss of awareness in patients with visual neglect," *Proceedings of the National Academy of Sciences of the United States of America*, vol. 106, no. 14, pp. 6011–6016, 2009.

[43] C. A. Brenner, P. H. Lysaker, M. A. Wilt, and B. F. O'Donnell, "Visual processing and neuropsychological function in schizophrenia and schizoaffective disorder," *Psychiatry Research*, vol. 111, no. 2-3, pp. 125–136, 2002.

[44] M. J. Sergi, Y. Rassovsky, K. H. Nuechterlein, and M. F. Green, "Social perception as a mediator of the influence of early visual processing on functional status in schizophrenia," *The American Journal of Psychiatry*, vol. 163, no. 3, pp. 448–454, 2006.

[45] P. D. Butler, I. Y. Abeles, N. G. Weiskopf et al., "Sensory contributions to impaired emotion processing in schizophrenia," *Schizophrenia Bulletin*, vol. 35, no. 6, pp. 1095–1107, 2009.

[46] L. Q. Uddin, "Salience processing and insular cortical function and dysfunction," *Nature Reviews Neuroscience*, vol. 16, no. 1, pp. 55–61, 2015.

[47] M. A. Gray and H. D. Critchley, "Interoceptive basis to craving," *Neuron*, vol. 54, no. 2, pp. 183–186, 2007.

[48] D. Kim, G. Wylie, R. Pasternak, P. D. Butler, and D. C. Javitt, "Magnocellular contributions to impaired motion processing in schizophrenia," *Schizophrenia Research*, vol. 82, no. 1, pp. 1–8, 2006.

[49] C. Luo, Z. W. Guo, Y. X. Lai et al., "Musical training induces functional plasticity in perceptual and motor networks: insights from resting-state FMRI," *PLoS One*, vol. 7, no. 5, article e36568, 2012.

[50] E. Strauss, E. M. Sherman, and O. Spreen, *A Compendium of Neuropsychological Tests: Administration, Norms, and Commentary*, Oxford University Press, New York, NY, USA, 2006.

[51] A. S. Tamkin and J. T. Kunce, "A comparison of three neuropsychological tests: the Weigl, Hooper, and Benton," *Journal of Clinical Psychology*, vol. 41, no. 5, pp. 660–664, 1985.

15

Longitudinal Brain Functional Connectivity Changes of the Cortical Motor-Related Network in Subcortical Stroke Patients with Acupuncture Treatment

Yongxin Li,[1] Ya Wang,[1] Chenxi Liao,[2] Wenhua Huang,[1] and Ping Wu[2]

[1]*Guangdong Provincial Key Laboratory of Medical Biomechanics, School of Basic Medical Sciences, Southern Medical University, Guangzhou, China*
[2]*The 3rd Teaching Hospital, Chengdu University of Traditional Chinese Medicine, Chengdu, Sichuan, China*

Correspondence should be addressed to Wenhua Huang; 13822232749@139.com and Ping Wu; wuping_33@163.com

Academic Editor: Jukka Jolkkonen

In clinical practice, the effectiveness of the rehabilitation therapy such as acupuncture combining conventional Western medicine (AG) on stroke people's motor-related brain network and their behaviors has not been systematically studied. In the present study, seventeen adult ischemic patients were collected and divided into two groups: the conventional Western medicine treatment group (CG) and the AG. The neurological deficit scores (NDS) and resting-state functional MRI data were collected before and after treatment. Compared with the CG patients, AG patients exhibited a significant enhancement of the percent changes of NDS from pre- to posttreatment intervention. All patients showed significant changes of functional connectivity (FC) between the pair of cortical motor-related regions. After treatment, both patient groups showed a recovery of brain connectivity to the nearly normal level compared with the controls in these pairs. Moreover, a significant correlation between the percent changes of NDS and the pretreatment FC values of bilateral primary motor cortex (M1) in all patients was found. In conclusion, our results showed that AG therapy can be an effective means for ischemic stroke patients to recover their motor function ability. The FC strengths between bilateral M1 of stroke patients can predict stroke patients' treatment outcome after rehabilitation therapy.

1. Introduction

Ischemic stroke is one of the leading causes of morbidity and mortality. Many ischemic stroke patients experience a poor prognosis with neurological and motor function impairment. During the process of improving patients' quality of life, substantial social and economic burden were the cost. Various therapies have been used for post-stroke rehabilitation in clinical practice, such as medication, acupuncture, motor training, and surgery [1–5]. Although these treatments can reduce stroke damage and improve patient's behavior, patients are often motor disabled after treatment intervention. So, it is important to identify the biochemical mechanisms underlying stroke-related damage and understand the longitudinal changes of the brain motor network. Rational treatment is needed to help stroke patients' recovery.

Thrombolytic therapies are currently the most effective treatment available after stroke [6]. Recently, acupuncture in addition to thrombolytic medicine is the new treatment therapy for patient after stroke. Acupuncture is a traditional Chinese medicine used to treat many diseases. Some clinical researches have showed that acupuncture is a safe and effective therapy for poststroke rehabilitation and improvement of behavior after ischemic stroke [2, 7]. The mechanism of acupuncture in the functional recovery after stroke has been studied previously [8–10]. A previous study on cerebrovascular responses of stroke patients after acupuncture has found that acupuncture stimulation induced perilesional reorganization through improvement of regional cerebral blood flow

[11]. However, no consistent theories were achieved to explore the underlying mechanisms of stroke recovery. The neural mechanism underlying acupuncture treatment after stroke is still unclear.

Neuroimaging, particularly MRI, has become the most powerful tool available to research the underlying mechanisms of stroke and brain functional recovery in stroke patients. The microstructural features and a host of functional characteristics after stroke can be measured by MRI technology. Previous studies based on brain connectivity in stroke patients have revealed that the effects of damage can extend beyond the lesioned area [12, 13]. Our previous diffusion tensor imaging studies have found that the structural integrity of transcallosal motor tracts was damaged after stroke [14, 15]. These previous studies of stroke have proved that MRI technology is a valuable way to detect the effect that the brain acquires after stroke. Moreover, MRI technology has also been used to detect the treatment effect after stroke [10, 16]. Stroke patients with acupuncture treatment showed more improvement in behavioral function and structural integrity than conventional treatment [17]. A previous review study also concludes a similar result that acupuncture treatment improved motor function and the relative fractional anisotropy value at the edge of the ischemic lesions [18]. Most of these previous imaging studies focus on brain organization after stroke. Only a few studies focus on the acupuncture treatment effect, such as the changes in the ipsilesional primary motor cortex (M1) area after stroke with acupuncture intervention [19, 20]. Acupuncture intervention effect on the functional connectivity (FC) patterns of the whole motor-related network is still unclear in stroke patients.

So, the purpose of our present study is to investigate the longitudinal changes in FC of the motor-related network after acupuncture therapy in adult stroke patients. The efficiency of acupuncture therapy comparing with the conventional therapy is also needed to be studied. Based on the previous studies of stroke, we hypothesized that the FC pathways among the cortical motor regions show a recovery for stroke patients after acupuncture therapy. The efficiency of acupuncture therapy in behavioral and FC pattern recovery is higher than that of conventional therapy.

2. Materials and Methods

2.1. Subjects. Seventeen first-ever stroke patients (8 female, mean age: 63.29 ± 12.27) with unilateral motor deficits due to subcortical ischemic lesions were recruited from the inpatient and outpatient Department of Neurology of the First Affiliated Hospital of the Chengdu University of Traditional Chinese Medicine, China. Some patients had limb dysfunction only, while others had dysfunction in both their upper and lower limbs. Inclusion criteria were as follows: (1) right-handed adults with age ranging from 35 to 80 years; (2) strictly subcortical lesions and absence of other WM pathology as verified by structural MRI; (3) absence of aphasia, neglect, and dementia; (4) no additional neurologic or psychiatric disorders; (5) no previous or subsequent cerebral ischemia; (6) time interval of at least three weeks between stroke onset and the time of study enrollment. Before the enrollment, all patients were only treated with conventional antiplatelet aggregation drugs. None of the patients had undergone any other therapy before the enrollment, such as acupuncture. All of the patients were scanned using resting-state functional magnetic imaging (fMRI) at two time points: before and after one month of clinical treatment. Fourteen healthy control subjects, without neurological or psychiatric disorder and age and gender matched to the stroke group, were enrolled in the study (6 females, mean age: 62.21 ± 10.48). Sample clinical information were provided in Table 1.

This study was carried out in accordance with the recommendations of the Ethics Committee of Chengdu University of Traditional Chinese Medicine with written informed consent from all subjects. All subjects gave written informed consent in accordance with the Declaration of Helsinki. The protocol was approved by the Ethics Committee of Chengdu University of Traditional Chinese Medicine (no. 2011KL-002).

2.2. Treatment and Clinical Assessments. After the patients were enrolled, all patients were divided into two groups based on the different treatment protocols used: a continuously conventional treatment of antiplatelet aggregation drug group (CG) or acupuncture combining with conventional drug treatment group (AG). Nine stroke patients were grouped in the CG to give a conventional treatment of antiplatelet aggregation drugs to improve blood circulation (75 mg clopidogrel once each day taken orally, 10 mg *Erigeron breviscapus* injection, and 0.5 g citicoline injection). Eight patients were grouped in the AG to give acupuncture and conventional treatment. Acupuncture was performed at the Baihui (GV-20), Fengchi (GB20, bilateral), Xuanzhong (GB-39, bilateral), Quchi (LI-11 bilateral), Hegu (LI-4, bilateral), Zusanli (ST-36, bilateral), and Sanyinjiao (SP-6, bilateral) acupoints. We selected all of these acupoints because these acupoints are often used in the treatment of motor dysfunction after stroke based on the theory of Chinese medicine. All acupuncture procedures were performed by the time-experienced and licensed acupuncturist: two hours a day for 5 days a week, one week a course, continuous four courses of treatment. The detail operation steps can be seen in our previous study [17]. During the acupuncture treatment process, the dose of medication was adjusted by clinicians according to the patients' conditions.

The clinical performances were assessed before and after treatment to quantify the severity of the neurological functional deficits in the stroke patients using the Chinese Stroke Scale for Clinical Neurological Deficit Scores (NDS, 1995 version). The NDS is an observational test to measure the severity of neurological functional deficit and test the severity of stroke. The NDS consists of 8 items: item 1—awareness (0–9), item 2—horizontal gaze function (0–4), item 3—musculus facialis (0–2), item 4—language (0–6), item 5—upper limb muscle strength (0–6), item 6—manual muscle strength (0–6), item 7—lower limb muscle strength (0–6), and item 8—walking ability (0–6). The resulting score range is from

Table 1: Demographic and imaging data.

Patient number	Dominant hand	Affected hand	Site of lesion	Lesion volume (mm^3)	Lesion age (days)	NDS1	NDS2
AG							
1	R	R	L Pons/CS	350	135	13	5
2	R	R	L/R TH	420	22	31	20
3	R	R	L BG	1180	33	26	12
4	R	R	L BG	3120	21	19	9
5	R	R	L BG/CS	1350	22	26	15
6	R	R	L BG/CS	200	36	—	—
7	R	L	R BG	2240	32	21	10
8	R	R	L TH/LN	1890	148	24	14
CG							
9	R	R	L BG	380	56	24	16
10	R	R	L BG	1190	45	26	23
11	R	R	L BG	540	26	24	18
12	R	R	L BG	1130	132	20	12
13	R	R	L TH	290	21	25	18
14	R	R	L BG	280	23	24	12
15	R	R	L CN	450	25	15	6
16	R	R	L CS	250	23	22	14
17	R	R	L BG	1260	23	—	—

BG: basal ganglia; CN: caudate nucleus; CS: centrum semiovale; LN: lenticular nucleus; F: female; NDS: neurological deficit scores; L: left; M: male; R: right; TH: thalamus.

0 to 45 with lower values reflecting less severity of neurological functional deficit (mild: 0–15 points; moderate: 16–30 points; and severe: 31–45 points). For each group, paired t-test analyses were used to detect the changes of DNS before and after treatment. For each patient, percent changes in clinical performance were calculated using the following formula: abs (after – before)/before. These changes were compared between both groups in a two-sample t-test analysis.

2.3. Image Acquisition. Imaging data were collected using an 8-channel head coil on a 3T Siemens scanner (MAGNETOM Trio Tim, Siemens, Germany) at the West China Hospital MRI Center, Chengdu, China. Resting-state fMRI was collected using an echo-planar imaging sequence with the following scan parameters: TR/TE = 2000/30 ms, FOV = 240 × 240 mm^2, matrix = 64 × 64, flip angle = 90^0, slice thickness = 5 mm, 30 interleaved axial slices, and 180 volumes. All participants were instructed to keep their eyes closed and to remain motionless. Foam cushions were used to reduce head translation movement and rotation. All acquisitions were visually inspected for imaging artifacts.

2.4. Imaging Processing and Statistical Analysis. We used the seed-based connectivity analysis method to determine the longitudinal FC changes of the motor network in ischemic stroke patients before and after treatment. We computed the connectivity index between each pair of ten region-of-interest areas belonging to the motor execution network [21]. We measured the brain connectivity changes by examining and comparing the brain motor executive network in people recovering from stroke following both interventions and healthy controls from resting-state fMRI. We also tested the correlation between the changes of behavioral performance and the neural imaging index to determine if there are some connections that can be used as a biomarker for evaluating recovery outcomes. The detailed calculation process was performed as follows.

2.5. Functional Connectivity Analysis. The resting-state fMRI data was processed using the statistical parametric mapping (SPM8, http://www.fil.ion.ucl.ac.uk/spm) package. Before all of the analyses, images from one patient with a right-sided stroke were oriented around the midsagittal plane prior to data analysis, thereby lateralizing the lesions to the left hemisphere in all patients. The imaging data from the control subject matched to this patient were also midsagittally oriented. The preprocessing steps included slice timing, spatial realignment, normalization into the Montreal Neurological Institute template, and smoothing. A temporal filter (0.01–0.08 Hz) was then applied and nuisance regression was also performed using WM, cerebrospinal fluid, and the six head motion parameters as covariates. Regions of interest (ROIs) for major cortical motor-related areas were selected using ROI-based correlation analysis procedure to assess functional connectivity among the regions. The ROIs included 10 regions, such as bilateral supplementary motor area (SMA), bilateral M1, bilateral postcentral gyrus (PCG), bilateral dorsolateral premotor (PMd), and ventrolateral premotor (PMv). All ROIs were obtained by creating 10 mm-diameter spheres around the predefined coordinates (see Table 2 and Figure 1) [21, 22]. Then, the time series of all voxels in each ROI were extracted and averaged to obtain a

Table 2: Regions of interest for the major cortical motor-related areas.

ID	Regions	Abbreviation	Side	MNI coordinate X	Y	Z
1	Supplementary motor area	SMA	L	−5	−4	57
2	Supplementary motor area	SMA	R	5	−4	57
3	Primary motor cortex	M1	L	−38	−22	56
4	Primary motor cortex	M1	R	38	−22	56
5	Postcentral gyrus	PCG	L	−37	−34	53
6	Postcentral gyrus	PCG	R	37	−34	53
7	Dorsolateral Premotor	PMd	L	−22	−13	57
8	Dorsolateral Premotor	PMd	R	28	−10	54
9	Ventrolateral Premotor	PMv	L	−49	−1	38
10	Ventrolateral Premotor	PMv	R	53	0	25

The regions were selected from previous studies (Jiang et al. [22] and Wang et al. [21]). The location of each region of interest with a 5-radius sphere. L: left; R: right; MNI: Montreal Neurological Institute.

mean time series. The between-ROI FC was calculated for each participant. Two-sample t-tests between the strokes and the controls were used to detect the differences of the ROI FC ($p < 0.05$, one tailed). In addition, paired t-test was also used to detect the longitudinal changes of FC from pre- to posttreatment in both stroke groups. Finally, we tested for relationships between the treatment-related percent changes of NDS and the FC values of each pair ROIs before treatment in all stroke patients. The significance threshold for the correlations was set at $p < 0.05$. To minimize their possible impact on the findings, gender, lesion size, and age were used as covariates of no interest in all the statistical analyses above.

3. Results

3.1. Behavioral Measures. Information on all subjects can be found in Table 1. Patients with ischemic stroke exhibited a range from mild to moderate in neurological functional deficit. With treatment intervention, the NDS scores were decreased in all patients. Specifically, more than half of the patients exhibited a mild neurological functional deficit. Paired t-test analyses demonstrated that the DNS score was enhanced significantly with treatment intervention for both stroke groups (AG: before 22.86 ± 5.82, after 12.14 ± 4.81, $t = 15.75$, $p < 0.001$; CG: before 23.11 ± 3.79, after 15.44 ± 5.08, $t = 9.59$, $p < 0.001$, see Figures 2(a) and 2(b)). A two-sample t-test on the difference in percent changes of NDS between groups showed a significant improvement in AG (AG: 0.495 ± 0.087, CG: 0.355 ± 0.150; $t = -2.27$, $p = 0.039$, see Figure 2(c)).

3.2. Altered FC in Stroke Patients Compared with Healthy Controls. Compared with the controls, stroke patients showed significant changes of interhemispheric FC after stroke: decreased FC between bilateral M1 and increased FC between left SMA and right PMd and PCG (see Figures 3(a), 3(b), and 3(c)). For the patients with CG treatment, abnormal interhemispheric FC in the pair ROIs, such as left SMA versus right PMd and left SMA versus right PCG, was changed to the nearly normal level, but not for the FC between bilateral M1. The connectivity between bilateral M1 after CG still showed a significant decrease comparing with the control group. For the patients with AG treatment, all of this abnormal interhemispheric FC changed to the nearly normal level. Especially for the connectivity pathway between bilateral M1, the FC values were increased after AG treatment (see Figure 3(a)).

In the left hemisphere, intrahemispheric FC between PMd and PMv was increased after AG treatment but decreased after CG treatment (see Figure 3(d)). The FC value of this connectivity pathway showed a significant difference between both patient groups after treatment. The connectivity of other pair ROIs in the left hemisphere did not show significant changes with treatment intervention. In the right hemisphere before treatment, stroke patients showed significantly increased intrahemispheric FC in the pair ROIs, such as right SMA versus right PMd and right SMA versus right PCG (see Figures 3(e) and 3(f)). After treatment, the increased FC between these two pair ROIs in both the CG and AG groups was decreased to the level of no significant compared with the controls.

3.3. Correlation between FC Values and Clinical Variable. Correlation analyses revealed that there was a significant correlation between the percent changes of NDS and the FC values between bilateral M1 before treatment ($r = 0.579$, $p = 0.019$, see Figure 4). No significant correlations were found between the percent changes of NDS and the FC values of other pair ROIs before treatment.

4. Discussion

In this study, we examined the treatment effect of acupuncture on stroke patients' motor function through neuroimaging connectivity and clinical behavioral characteristic. Meanwhile, we also explored the relationship between the pretreatment FC values of the motor network and the treatment outcomes in stroke patients. There were several main findings. Firstly, ischemic stroke patients showed a

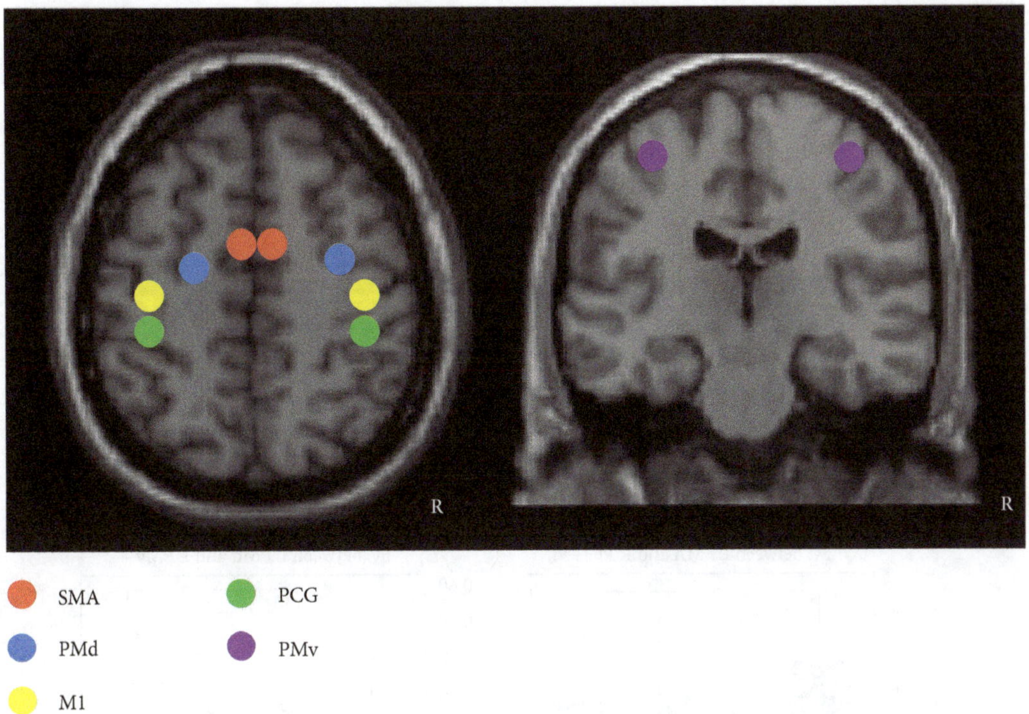

FIGURE 1: The location of the regions of interest in the motor-related network used in this study. R: right hemisphere.

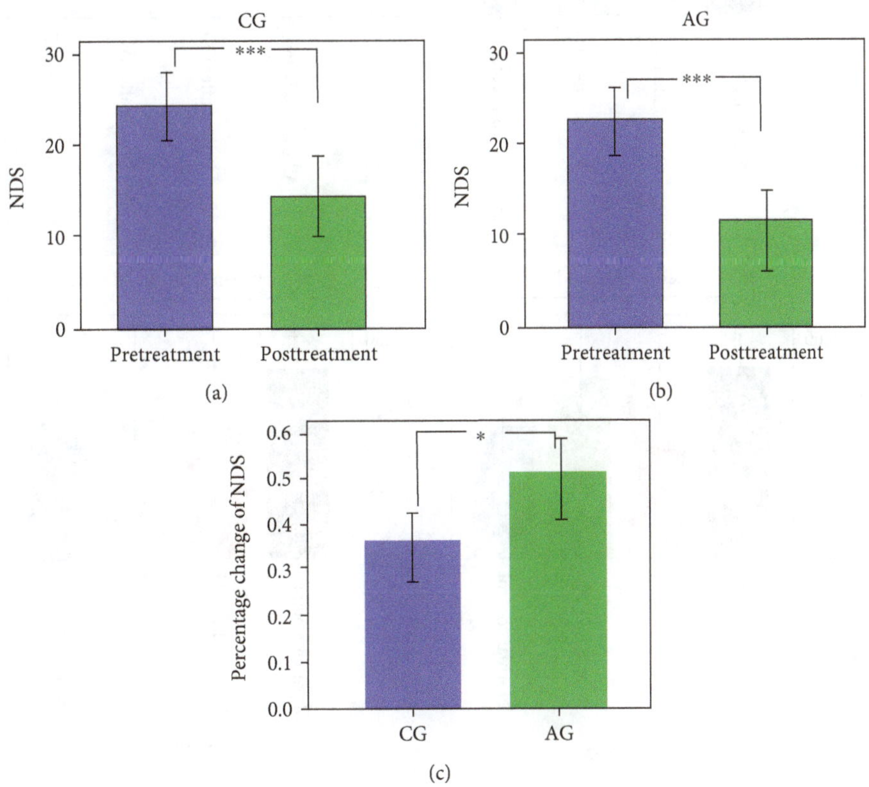

FIGURE 2: The longitudinal changes of NDS performance with different intervention therapies. Paired t-test analyses showed significant decrease of NDS scores from pre- to posttreatment in CG (a) and AG (b). The percent changes of NDS in patients with AG showed a significant enhancement compared with those in patients with CG (c). $^{*}p < 0.05$ and $^{***}p < 0.001$.

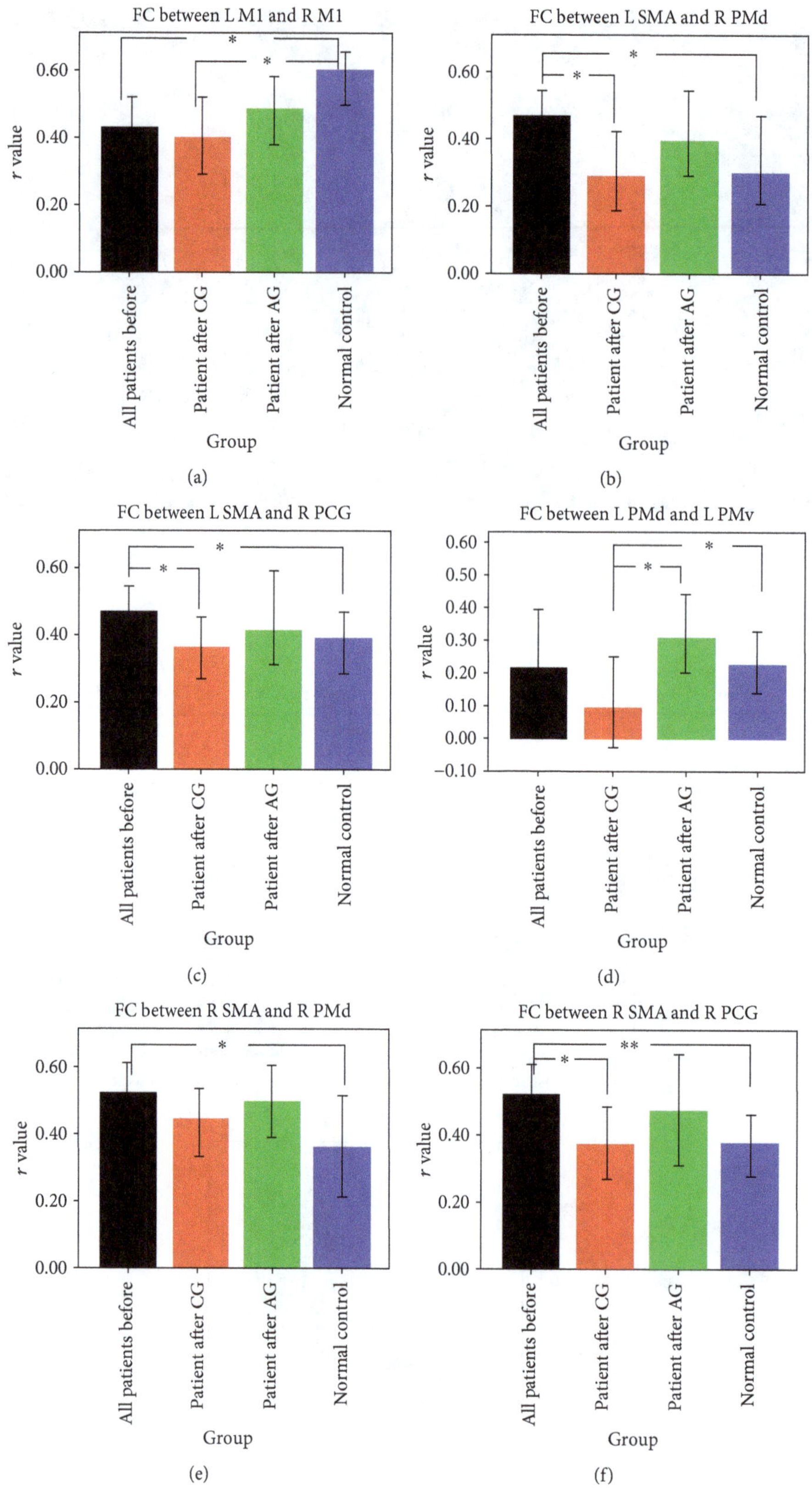

FIGURE 3: Functional connectivity comparison between groups. Significant interhemisphere connectivity (a–c) and intrahemisphere connectivity (d–f) of the motor network were found for both patients groups comparing with the controls. $^{*}p < 0.05$ and $^{**}p < 0.01$.

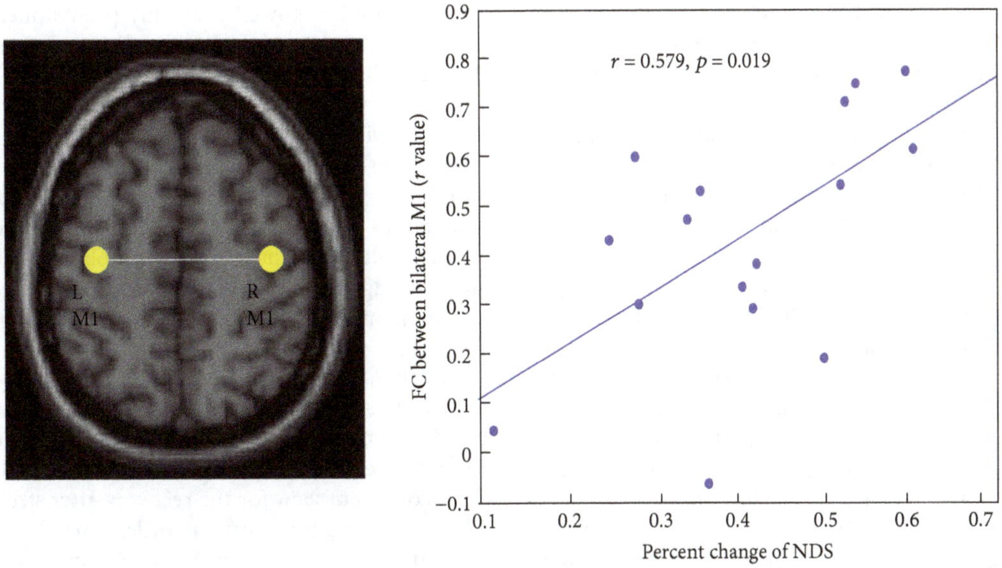

FIGURE 4: Brain and behavioral correlation. Significant positive correlation was found between the percent changes of NDS and the pretreatment M1-M1 FC values. L: left hemisphere, R: right hemisphere.

significant change in the FC in the motor network of the stroke patients. With treatment intervention, abnormal FC of the motor network in AG showed more tendency to occur in the nearly normal level than that in CG. Especially, the reduced FC between bilateral M1 was changed to the nearly normal level after acupuncture treatment. Secondly, there was a significant correlation between the percent changes of NDS and the pretreatment FC values between bilateral M1 in all stroke patients. Thirdly, the stroke patients with AG showed a significant decrease in their neurological deficit than those with CG.

4.1. Changes of the FC for Patients after Stroke. Considering the altered motor function in stroke patients, an increasing number of studies try to measure the alteration of FC within the motor network (M1, SMA, and lateral premotor cortex) to explore the neural mechanism underlying the disrupted motor function. Previous functional imaging studies have found that stroke caused abnormal interhemispheric FC [21, 23, 24]. Stroke patients showed an increased intrahemispheric FC and a decreased interhemispheric FC [23, 24]. In our present study, the stroke patients showed a significantly decreased FC between the bilateral M1 areas, which is in line with these previous studies. Comparing with the controls, the significant FC changes of the stroke patients in the motor network revealed that the motor network is abnormal after stroke. The brain showed a functional reorganization to adapt the damage after stroke [14]. Previous studies have showed that damages from ischemic stroke result in the functional and structural changes of perilesional and remote brain regions: for example, the structural reorganization of ipsilesional sensorimotor regions and transcallosal and corticospinal connections [15, 25, 26]. So, the exchanges and cooperation between the two sides of the hemisphere were affected by subcortical ischemic stroke. Meanwhile, we also found an increased FC between some pair ROIs of the patients after stroke. The intrahemispheric FC of ROIs in the right hemisphere showed a significant increase in patients after stroke. During our analyses, we have lateralized the lesions to the left hemisphere in all patients. The explanation for the significant increased intrahemispheric FC in the right hemisphere might be a form of compensation for the breaking of brain connectivity balance [27]. Increased FC may be a form of compensation for decreased FC of the contralateral hemisphere brain regions to maintain the motor function of the patients after stroke. Furthermore, our patients were all subcortical stroke patients. The lesions of almost all patients were located in the left hemisphere. Future study should also collect more stroke patients with lesion in the right hemisphere. This can give us complete view of the effect of lesion location on the interhemispheric and ipsilesional disturbances of neural connectivity.

4.2. The Treatment Effect of Acupuncture on the FC of the Motor Network. In the present study, our main focus is the treatment effect of acupuncture on the motor function in stroke patients. Two different therapeutic schedules were used to analyze the longitudinal changes with treatment intervention. The significant discovery of our research was that abnormal interhemispheric FC between bilateral M1 was increased to the nearly normal level in the AG but not in the CG. This result verified our hypothesis that FC pathways among the cortical motor regions show a recovery for stroke patients after acupuncture therapy. Acupuncture therapy showed a more significant recovery than only medicine therapy in ischemic stroke. Abundant previous clinical researches have showed that acupuncture was beneficial for stroke rehabilitation [2, 19, 20, 28]. In our experience design, the patients with a combining therapy of acupuncture and drug treatment demonstrated a recovery of the brain FC pattern of the motor network and their neurological function compared with the patients in the CG. Based on the theory of traditional Chinese medicine, these acupoints we used were functionally related to the motor dysfunction after stroke [20, 29]. The needling in these acupoints could modulate the brain function in both hemispheres. A previous imaging study has confirmed that acupuncture can improve regional cerebral blood flow [11]. So, we can say that the acupuncture therapy might accelerate the recovery process of the stroke patients' motor function.

The intrahemisphere FC in the right hemisphere showed a similar treatment effect from both treatment therapies (Figures 3(e) and 3(f)). The results above reveal that both therapies used in our design have a certain effect on the regulation of the motor functional network. However, the treatment effect on the intrahemispheric FC value of the connectivity pathway between left PMd and left PMv showed a significant difference between both patient groups. Acupuncture might modulate regional excitability through influencing the activity of neural synapsis [19, 20]. This effect is more significant in the left hemisphere because the lesions of our data were all located in the left hemisphere. The neural function of the motor cortex was damaged by subcortical ischemic lesions. The experience design by both treatment therapies of the present study can clearly exhibit the treatment effect by acupuncture. Acupuncture might help the recovery process of neural function by improving regional cerebral blood flow [11]. In a behavioral level, the percent changes of NDS in AG showed a significant enhancement compared with the CG. Combining these neuroimaging and behavioral results, we can say that acupuncture has a positive effect on the recovery of motor function. Acupuncture therapy can modulate the interhemispheric and intrahemispheric FC of the motor network in subcortical stroke patients. Future study should also consider the cortical stroke patients. The FC differences between subcortical and cortical stroke should be compared to understand the recovery mechanisms with acupuncture intervention.

4.3. Correlation between Connectivity and Behavioral Characteristic. Another significant discovery of our research was the significant correlation between the rate of NDS changes and the pretreatment FC between bilateral M1 in all stroke patients. This correlation between the FC and behavioral scores suggested that the stroke patient with higher FC values between bilateral M1 before treatment showed a better recovery of their neurological functional deficit. Here, we collected all of the stroke patients in this correlation because we want to find predictive biomarkers for future success of rehabilitation therapy for patients after stroke. Both therapies used in our present study showed significant improvement of NDS after intervention. And also, some previous studies on the brain-behavioral correlation were focused on the FC changes and the behavioral changes before and after intervention [30, 31]. In the present study, we wanted to assess whether the preintervention FC can predict behavioral improvement after treatment intervention. A previous review study has implicated that using resting-state activity, one can assess the unique networks for recovery [32]. Using brain connectivity might provide useful guides for therapeutic intervention for patients after stroke. Our present results showed that only pretreatment FC between bilateral M1 showed a significant correlation with the rate of NDS changes in all stroke patients. The role of the interhemispheric M1-M1 connectivity has been investigated by most previous studies [14, 19, 23, 33]. The correlation result in the present study does not only confirm its important role for the FC between bilateral M1 after stroke but also extended its role as a biomarker to predict the treatment outcome. This result would have clinical implication to inform clinical management and choose suitable stroke patients with acupuncture or antiplatelet aggregation drug therapy.

4.4. Limitation. Some limitations might affect our results. First, the sample sizes were not large enough. In the future studies, more subjects should be collected to test our results. Second, we only collected the data before and after treatment. The consistent view for the recovery after stroke is that it is a dynamic reorganization. In order to fully understand the neural process of acupuncture treatment effect in stroke, more time points would be needed to collect the neuroimaging data. Thirdly, during the analyses process, we used reversal method to flip the lesions to the left hemisphere for some stroke patients with right lesions. Although this method is usually used in brain lesion studies, this operation can also introduce certain deviations to the analyses. In future studies, larger numbers of patients will be needed to divide the patients into the left- and right-side types of ischemic stroke.

5. Conclusion

Changes in FC after treatment suggest brain plasticity in the motor-related network of patients with stroke. The FC strength between bilateral M1 of patients after stroke may be an imaging prognostic marker to predict their recovery outcome of neurological functional deficits. Increased FC in the AG but decreased FC in the CG from pre- to posttreatment in the motor network implicated that acupuncture in addition to Western medicine therapy can be an effective means for ischemic stroke patients to recovery their motor function ability. Our findings provide an imaging basis for the application of acupuncture therapy in clinical treatment.

Conflicts of Interest

The authors declare that there is no conflict of interest.

Acknowledgments

This research received funding from the National Natural Science Foundation of China (no. 81601483, no. 81072864, and no. 61427807) as well as a support by the National Natural Science Foundation of Guangdong Province, China (2016A030310402). This work was also supported by the China Postdoctoral Science Foundation (no. 2017M610538) and the Research Startup Foundation of Southern Medical University (PY2015N001). The authors are grateful to the patients who participated in the study. The authors also thank the doctors in the West China Hospital MRI Center for their cooperation in data collection.

References

[1] C. Enzinger, H. Dawes, H. Johansen-Berg et al., "Brain activity changes associated with treadmill training after stroke," *Stroke*, vol. 40, no. 7, pp. 2460–2467, 2009.

[2] P. Wu, E. Mills, D. Moher, and D. Seely, "Acupuncture in post-stroke rehabilitation," *Stroke*, vol. 41, no. 4, pp. 171–179, 2010.

[3] L. Gherardini, M. Gennaro, and T. Pizzorusso, "Perilesional treatment with chondroitinase ABC and motor training promote functional recovery after stroke in rats," *Cerebral Cortex*, vol. 25, no. 1, pp. 202–212, 2015.

[4] P. S. Jones, V. M. Pomeroy, J. Wang et al., "Does stroke location predict walk speed response to gait rehabilitation?," *Human Brain Mapping*, vol. 37, no. 2, pp. 689–703, 2016.

[5] S. C. Cramer, "Repairing the human brain after stroke. II. Restorative therapies," *Annals of Neurology*, vol. 63, no. 5, pp. 549–560, 2008.

[6] D. A. Meyer, M. I. Torres-Altoro, Z. Tan et al., "Ischemic stroke injury is mediated by aberrant Cdk5," *The Journal of Neuroscience*, vol. 34, no. 24, pp. 8259–8267, 2014.

[7] A. A. Rabinstein and L. M. Shulman, "Acupuncture in clinical neurology," *The Neurologist*, vol. 9, no. 3, pp. 137–148, 2003.

[8] J. C. Kong, M. S. Lee, B. C. Shin, Y. S. Song, and E. Ernst, "Acupuncture for functional recovery after stroke: a systematic review of sham-controlled randomized clinical trials," *Canadian Medical Association Journal*, vol. 182, no. 16, pp. 1723–1729, 2010.

[9] S. Zhang, B. Wu, M. Liu et al., "Acupuncture efficacy on ischemic stroke recovery multicenter randomized controlled trial in China," *Stroke*, vol. 46, no. 5, pp. 1301–1306, 2015.

[10] Y. Gao, Z. Lin, J. Tao et al., "Evidence of timing effects on acupuncture: a functional magnetic resonance imaging study," *Experimental and Therapeutic Medicine*, vol. 9, no. 1, pp. 59–64, 2015.

[11] J. D. Lee, J. S. Chon, H. K. Jeong et al., "The cerebrovascular response to traditional acupuncture after stroke," *Neuroradiology*, vol. 45, no. 11, pp. 780–784, 2003.

[12] C. Grefkes and G. R. Fink, "Reorganization of cerebral networks after stroke: new insights from neuroimaging with connectivity approaches," *Brain*, vol. 134, no. 5, pp. 1264–1276, 2011.

[13] C. Grefkes and N. S. Ward, "Cortical reorganization after stroke: how much and how functional?," *The Neuroscientist*, vol. 20, no. 1, pp. 56–70, 2014.

[14] Y. Li, D. Wang, H. Zhang et al., "Changes of brain connectivity in the primary motor cortex after subcortical stroke: a multimodal magnetic resonance imaging study," *Medicine*, vol. 95, no. 6, article e2579, 2016.

[15] Y. Li, P. Wu, F. Liang, and W. Huang, "The microstructural status of the corpus callosum is associated with the degree of motor function and neurological deficit in stroke patients," *PLoS One*, vol. 10, no. 4, article e0122615, 2015.

[16] Y. Zhang, K. Li, Y. Ren et al., "Acupuncture modulates the functional connectivity of the default mode network in stroke patients," *Evidence-based Complementary and Alternative Medicine*, vol. 2014, Article ID 765413, 7 pages, 2014.

[17] Y. Li, Y. Wang, H. Zhang, P. Wu, and W. Huang, "The effect of acupuncture on the motor function and white matter microstructure in ischemic stroke patients," *Evidence-based Complementary and Alternative Medicine*, vol. 2015, Article ID 164792, 10 pages, 2015.

[18] Z. Wu, J. Hu, F. Du, X. Zhou, Q. Xiang, and F. Miao, "Long-term changes of diffusion tensor imaging and behavioural status after acupuncture treatment in rats with transient focal cerebral ischaemia," *Acupuncture in Medicine*, vol. 30, no. 4, pp. 331–338, 2012.

[19] Y. Ning, K. Li, C. Fu et al., "Enhanced functional connectivity between the bilateral primary motor cortices after acupuncture at Yanglingquan (GB34) in right-hemispheric subcortical stroke patients: a resting-state fMRI study," *Frontiers in Human Neuroscience*, vol. 11, p. 178, 2017.

[20] Y. Yang, I. Eisner, S. Chen, S. Wang, F. Zhang, and L. Wang, "Neuroplasticity changes on human motor cortex induced by acupuncture therapy: a preliminary study," *Neural Plasticity*, vol. 2017, Article ID 4716792, 8 pages, 2017.

[21] L. Wang, C. Yu, H. Chen et al., "Dynamic functional reorganization of the motor execution network after stroke," *Brain*, vol. 133, Part 4, pp. 1224–1238, 2010.

[22] T. JiangY. He, Y. Zang, and X. Weng, "Modulation of functional connectivity during the resting state and the motor task," *Human Brain Mapping*, vol. 22, no. 1, pp. 63–71, 2004.

[23] A. R. Carter, S. V. Astafiev, C. E. Lang et al., "Resting interhemispheric functional magnetic resonance imaging connectivity predicts performance after stroke," *Annals of Neurology*, vol. 67, no. 3, pp. 365–375, 2010.

[24] C. H. Park, W. H. Chang, S. H. Ohn et al., "Longitudinal changes of resting-state functional connectivity during motor recovery after stroke," *Stroke*, vol. 42, no. 5, pp. 1357–1362, 2011.

[25] R. Lindenberg, L. L. Zhu, T. Rüber, and G. Schlaug, "Predicting functional motor potential in chronic stroke patients using diffusion tensor imaging," *Human Brain Mapping*, vol. 33, no. 5, pp. 1040–1051, 2012.

[26] J. D. Schaechter, Z. P. Fricker, K. L. Perdue et al., "Microstructural status of ipsilesional and contralesional corticospinal tract correlates with motor skill in chronic stroke patients," *Human Brain Mapping*, vol. 30, no. 11, pp. 3461–3474, 2009.

[27] Y. Zhang, L. Wang, J. Yang et al., "Abnormal functional networks in resting-state of the sub-cortical chronic stroke patients with hemiplegia," *Brain Research*, vol. 1663, pp. 51–58, 2017.

[28] S. M. Lim, J. Yoo, E. Lee et al., "Acupuncture for spasticity after stroke: a systematic review and meta-analysis of randomized controlled trials," *Evidence-based Complementary and Alternative Medicine*, vol. 2015, Article ID 870398, 12 pages, 2015.

[29] B. Yan, K. Li, J. Xu et al., "Acupoint-specific fMRI patterns in human brain," *Neuroscience Letters*, vol. 383, no. 3, pp. 236–240, 2005.

[30] Y. Zhang, H. Liu, L. Wang et al., "Relationship between functional connectivity and motor function assessment in stroke patients with hemiplegia: a resting-state functional MRI study," *Neuroradiology*, vol. 58, no. 5, pp. 503–511, 2016.

[31] X. Zheng, L. Sun, D. Yin et al., "The plasticity of intrinsic functional connectivity patterns associated with rehabilitation intervention in chronic stroke patients," *Neuroradiology*, vol. 58, no. 4, pp. 417–427, 2016.

[32] G. Silasi and T. H. Murphy, "Stroke and the connectome: how connectivity guides therapeutic intervention," *Neuron*, vol. 83, no. 6, pp. 1354–1368, 2014.

[33] Y. Zhang, K. S. Li, Y. Z. Ning et al., "Altered structural and functional connectivity between the bilateral primary motor cortex in unilateral subcortical stroke: a multimodal magnetic resonance imaging study," *Medicine*, vol. 95, no. 31, article e4534, 2016.

Visual Features in Alzheimer's Disease: From Basic Mechanisms to Clinical Overview

María Alejandra Cerquera-Jaramillo,[1] Mauricio O. Nava-Mesa,[2] Rodrigo E. González-Reyes,[2] Carlos Tellez-Conti,[1] and Alejandra de-la-Torre[2]

[1]*Escuela Superior de Oftalmología-Instituto Barraquer de América, Bogotá, Colombia*
[2]*Grupo de Investigación en Neurociencias (NeURos), Escuela de Medicina y Ciencias de la Salud, Universidad del Rosario, Bogotá, Colombia*

Correspondence should be addressed to Alejandra de-la-Torre; alejadelatorre@yahoo.com

Academic Editor: Diego Sepulveda-Falla

Alzheimer's disease (AD) is the leading cause of dementia worldwide. It compromises patients' daily activities owing to progressive cognitive deterioration, which has elevated direct and indirect costs. Although AD has several risk factors, aging is considered the most important. Unfortunately, clinical diagnosis is usually performed at an advanced disease stage when dementia is established, making implementation of successful therapeutic interventions difficult. Current biomarkers tend to be expensive, insufficient, or invasive, raising the need for novel, improved tools aimed at early disease detection. AD is characterized by brain atrophy due to neuronal and synaptic loss, extracellular amyloid plaques composed of amyloid-beta peptide (Aβ), and neurofibrillary tangles of hyperphosphorylated tau protein. The visual system and central nervous system share many functional components. Thus, it is plausible that damage induced by Aβ, tau, and neuroinflammation may be observed in visual components such as the retina, even at an early disease stage. This underscores the importance of implementing ophthalmological examinations, less invasive and expensive than other biomarkers, as useful measures to assess disease progression and severity in individuals with or at risk of AD. Here, we review functional and morphological changes of the retina and visual pathway in AD from pathophysiological and clinical perspectives.

1. Introduction

Alzheimer's disease (AD) is the most prevalent progressive neurodegenerative disease in humans and the main cause of dementia worldwide [1]. Together with vascular dementia, AD corresponds to 60%–80% of all dementia cases [2]. According to the World Alzheimer Report [3], an estimated 47 million people worldwide currently have dementia, a number that is projected to rise to approximately 131 million by 2050. Several modifiable and nonmodifiable risk factors have been described for AD, although aging remains the most significant [4]. Consequently, after 65 years of age, AD prevalence is expected to double every 5 years [5]. According to the US National Institute on Aging-Alzheimer's Association workgroup, there are three different stages of AD: preclinical AD (presymptomatic with early AD-related brain changes observed by neuroimaging or other biomarker studies such as amyloid and tau studies in cerebrospinal fluid (CSF)), mild cognitive impairment (MCI) caused by AD (mild cognitive decline but still able to perform daily activities), and dementia caused by AD (major cognitive decline that interferes with daily activities) [6]. Globally, AD has significant direct and indirect costs, which increased from US$ 604 billion in 2010 to US$ 818 billion in 2015, totaling around 1% of the worldwide gross domestic product (GDP) [3].

Two types of AD have been characterized based on age of onset: early-onset AD (EOAD), referred to as familial, and late-onset AD (LOAD), which is regarded as sporadic. EOAD presents before the age of 65 and corresponds to around 5% of AD cases [7], while LOAD appears after 65 years of age and represents the most common type of

AD, accounting for >90% of AD cases [8]. No direct cause has been described for LOAD, but its disease development is influenced by various environmental and genetic risk factors [9]. The main risk factors include aging, genetics (presenilin 1 (PSEN1), PSEN2, and APP1 genes) [7, 10], hypertension, diabetes, hypercholesterolemia, stroke, obesity, sedentary lifestyle, depression, low socioeconomic status, and alcohol and tobacco use [1, 4, 9].

AD is characterized by formation and aggregation of extracellular plaques of abnormal amyloid-beta (Aβ) peptides, as well as presence of intracellular aggregates of hyperphosphorylated tau protein, known as neurofibrillary tangles (NFT) [11, 12]. In AD, Aβ peptides are produced from abnormal cleavage of the amyloid precursor protein (APP) by the beta-site amyloid precursor protein cleaving enzyme 1 (BACE-1 or β-secretase) and γ-secretase complex [13]. Aβ peptides promote intracellular tau phosphorylation, with hyperphosphorylated tau protein posteriorly aggregating into NFT [11, 14]. Aβ and NFT activate astrocytes and microglia, inducing production of proinflammatory factors such as interleukins and nitric oxide (NO), and ultimately resulting in excessive neuroinflammation, oxidative stress (OS), neuronal damage, and cell death [15–17].

Currently, the diagnosis and classification of AD are based on clinical and neuropsychological examinations complemented by neuroimaging studies. Nonetheless, a conclusive diagnosis still relies on pathological examination of postmortem brain tissue [18]. While many exploratory biomarkers have been proposed for AD, cerebrospinal fluid levels of tau and Aβ levels, together with imaging studies (such as positron emission tomography carbon 11-labeled Pittsburgh compound B), are the most widely accepted [19]. Unfortunately, these techniques are not easily accessible to patients with dementia worldwide owing to elevated costs and a lack of adequate medical facilities. Therefore, it is important to find easy-to-acquire, cost-effective methods that can provide information on the main disease manifestations, even at early stages, to favor timely interventions and improve the quality of life for patients. In this regard, a recent strategic roadmap aimed at improving early diagnosis of AD based on biomarkers was proposed and is centered on several phases that evaluate analytical validity, clinical validity, and clinical utility [20].

The visual system may be a helpful marker for the early stages of AD. Brain alterations in AD can be accompanied by ocular symptoms [21–24] which may be related to progression, cognitive deterioration, and disease severity [25]. This may be explained because the visual system shares the same embryological origin, namely, the neural tube of the brain, and indeed is considered an extension of the diencephalon [26]. In addition, both components have several functional and structural similarities, including microvasculature and neuronal projections [27]. Furthermore, examination of the visual system may provide markers for identifying dementia subtypes, thereby helping to differentiate AD from vascular dementia [28].

Hence, the aim of this review is to describe functional and morphological changes of the eye and visual pathway that are observed in AD from a clinical and pathophysiological perspective. Considering that the visual system shares vascular and cellular components with the central nervous system (CNS), ocular alterations observed in patients with AD may represent an initial manifestation of the disease and serve as possible candidates for complementary diagnostic biomarkers of MCI and the early stage of AD.

2. Pathological Mechanisms of Aβ and Tau Toxicity in the Eye

2.1. General Mechanisms of Aβ and Tau Production. Senile plaques (SP) are formed from extracellular aggregation of Aβ deposits, which are derived from excessive or inadequate cleavage of APP by BACE-1 and the γ-secretase complex [13]. PSEN1 and PSEN2 are part of the γ-secretase complex, which also includes nicastrin, anterior pharynx-defective 1, and presenilin enhancer 2 [29]. Although its function is not fully understood, APP has been involved in regulation of synaptic plasticity and acts as a cell adhesion molecule that participates in several neurodevelopmental aspects such as migration, neurite outgrowth, growth cone pathfinding, and synaptogenesis [30, 31]. Inadequate cleavage of APP may lead to formation of abnormally long peptides, such as Aβ1–42 fragments, which are more likely to oligomerize and form plaques, compared with shorter fragments such as Aβ1–40 [32]. Although the precise neurotoxic mechanisms of Aβ are not yet fully elucidated, the presence and aggregation of these peptides compromise the function of various cells including astrocytes, microglia, and neurons, leading to systemic failure of brain activity, mainly related, but not limited, to cognitive aspects [33, 34].

In vitro evidence indicates that Aβ induces the release of proinflammatory factors from astrocytes and microglia, including interleukin-1β (IL-1β), IL-6, NO, and tumor necrosis factor alpha (TNFα) [15, 16]. In addition, Aβ oligomers may generate free radicals and induce mitochondrial dysfunction via abnormal activation of glial cells [35, 36]. Other pathological mechanisms include glutamate-induced neuronal excitotoxicity [37], GABAergic dysfunction [38], and reduced cerebral glucose intake [39, 40]. Ultimately, accumulation of Aβ peptides may trigger intracellular signaling for tau hyperphosphorylation, with formation of tau oligomers and NFT [11, 14] leading to neuronal degeneration [41]. Tau appears to be involved in disease progression, as tau aggregates propagate in a prion-like fashion, initiating a self-amplifying cascade and spreading to other brain regions [42]. In AD, these aberrant proteins are deposited in several brain areas including the frontal, parietal, temporal, and occipital lobes and cause neuroinflammation, OS, metabolic dysfunction, excitotoxicity, and perturbation of synaptic plasticity [43–48].

2.2. Aβ Mechanisms in the Retina. Retinal cells share a common embryonic origin with the brain and indeed are a projection of the CNS [49]. Further, they have similarities in vasculature, glial cells, neurotransmitter systems, and connectivity with the visual cortex [50]. Moreover, insoluble aggregation of Aβ peptides in the eye of double transgenic AD mice has been observed in different retinal layers, mainly the ganglion cell layer (GCL), nerve fiber layer (NFL), photoreceptor layer, and inner plexiform layer (IPL), leading to neuronal damage and visual symptoms [51]. Although this has not been confirmed in humans, it is hypothesized that similar changes may occur.

Glial cells play a crucial role in the biochemical and molecular mechanisms that induce neurodegeneration and are highly expressed in the mammalian retina, optic nerve, and retinal blood vessels. Astrocytes predominate in the NFL, interacting with retinal ganglion cells and in close relationship with blood vessels of the inner nuclear layer (INL) [52]. Thus, Aβ-induced toxic effects on astrocytes and microglia may generate alterations in the eye and visual system like those found in other nervous tissues, such as the hippocampus or cortex.

Moreover, Aβ has been shown to produce changes in Müller cells, the main glial cells resident in the retina. An *in vitro* model using the immortalized human Müller cell line MIO-M1 reported that treatment with Aβ_{1-42} induced caspase-independent apoptosis through activation of the purinergic receptor P2X7 in these cells [53]. A subretinal injection of Aβ_{1-42} in C57BL/6 mice stimulated the development of gliosis and a proinflammatory phenotype in Müller cells, together with an increase in protein expression of cyclooxygenase 2 (COX-2), glutamine synthetase (GS), the inwardly rectifying potassium channel Kir4.1, and the aquaporin-4 (AQP-4) water channel [54]. However, studies in AD animal models have found contradictory results. A study using the triple transgenic mouse model, 3x-TG-AD [55], observed strong gliotic responses and increased processes in Müller cells close to amyloid deposits, while a more recent study using the APPSWE/PS1ΔE9 mouse model failed to see any significant gliotic response or changes in GS expression [56].

Aggregation of Aβ plaques can lead to inflammatory reactions, reactive gliosis, and cellular and neuronal apoptosis in both the brain and retina [43, 57]. At the very early disease stage, an increase in macular layer size is observed in amnestic MCI patients, which may correspond to inflammatory processes and/or gliosis [58]. Also, astrocytes induce the release of vascular factors such as prostaglandins, NO, and arachidonic acid, which may lead to neurovascular dysfunction in AD as indicated by pathological and experimental studies [59–61]. Similarly, it has been shown that levels of complement (C1q) are elevated in close vicinity to amyloid plaques and astrocyte processes in transgenic mice [62]. In addition, C1q activation generates endothelial cell adhesion in human dermal microvascular endothelial cells [63]. Together, these mechanisms may affect retinal vessels and metabolic supply and increase metabolic injury in the GCL of the retina in the early stage of AD as well as during MCI (Figure 1).

Several studies in humans and animal models have identified Aβ plaques in the photoreceptor layer, GCL, NFL, IPL, and outer plexiform layer (OPL), which manifest at the early stage of disease, even before the appearance of neurological symptoms [64–66]. The retinal and visual effects of these plaques are not entirely clear, but activation of astrocytes and microglia, together with neuroinflammatory changes induced by Aβ, lead to an initial increase in the retinal epithelium (RPE) and GCL degeneration in a transgenic rodent model of AD [64, 67]. In addition, an increase in the number of astrocytes and astrocyte/neuron ratio (which is associated with increased neuronal loss), especially in the superior and inferior quadrants of the retina, has been reported in humans [68]. Similar changes where neuronal numbers are reduced and nonneuronal cells are increased have been observed in human brain regions such as the hippocampus and cerebral cortex [69], as well as in the visual cortex [70]. Nonetheless, despite the previous observations of Aβ effects on the eye, there are limitations to mimic the clinical findings in animal models, which may point to other endogenous mechanisms present in these models and diverse adaptive changes in early phases of AD [71, 72]. Additionally, it is noteworthy to remark that Aβ aggregation was also shown within the eye of individuals undergoing normal cognitive aging; however, this pathophysiological process is quite distinct from the one described in patients suffering AD as it is discussed below in Section 2.4.

2.3. Tau Mechanisms in the Retina. One of the hallmarks of AD is the presence of intraneuronal hyperphosphorylated tau protein. These tau oligomers assemble in large insoluble fibrillar structures, known as NFT, and spread between cells in both the brain and retina. Tau oligomers seem to be one of the main structures that promote inflammation in the retina at the early disease stage. Tau oligomers induce neuroinflammation in a perpetuating feed-forward cycle, propagating neural damage, augmenting tau oligomer production, and consequently triggering the appearance of more inflammation [73]. Other studies detected tau accumulation in the retina at an early phase of AD: before the onset of cognitive impairment and even before tau aggregation in the brain in the mouse model of AD. In the retina, tau accumulates principally in GCL dendrites and intraretinal axons, but is depleted in optic nerve axons [74]. Some studies have demonstrated predominant accumulation of tau in GCL, but it has also been observed in the INL, IPL, OPL, and NFL [65, 75]. Conversely, hyperphosphorylated tau has not been found in other structures such as optic nerve, cornea, and lens in AD transgenic mice [76, 77]. Tau accumulation causes dysfunction in anterograde axonal transport, which is a feature of neuronal impairment that occurs before the appearance of retinal cell death [74]. Tau aggregation inhibits mitochondrial transport towards the GCL periphery, leading to loss of energy production and formation of reactive oxygen species (ROS). Altogether, retinal neurons in AD tend to be more susceptible to OS, produce hyperphosphorylated tau aggregates, and prolong the delay in vesicular transport that is necessary for synapse function and cellular growth [75]. Future studies comparing tau aggregation between AD patients, MCI, and individuals undergoing healthy aging could be useful to clarify if tau plays any role in retinal changes in AD pathology.

2.4. Aβ, Aging, and Age-Related Macular Degeneration. During aging, the brain and retina develop extracellular deposits recognized as plaques and drusen, respectively.

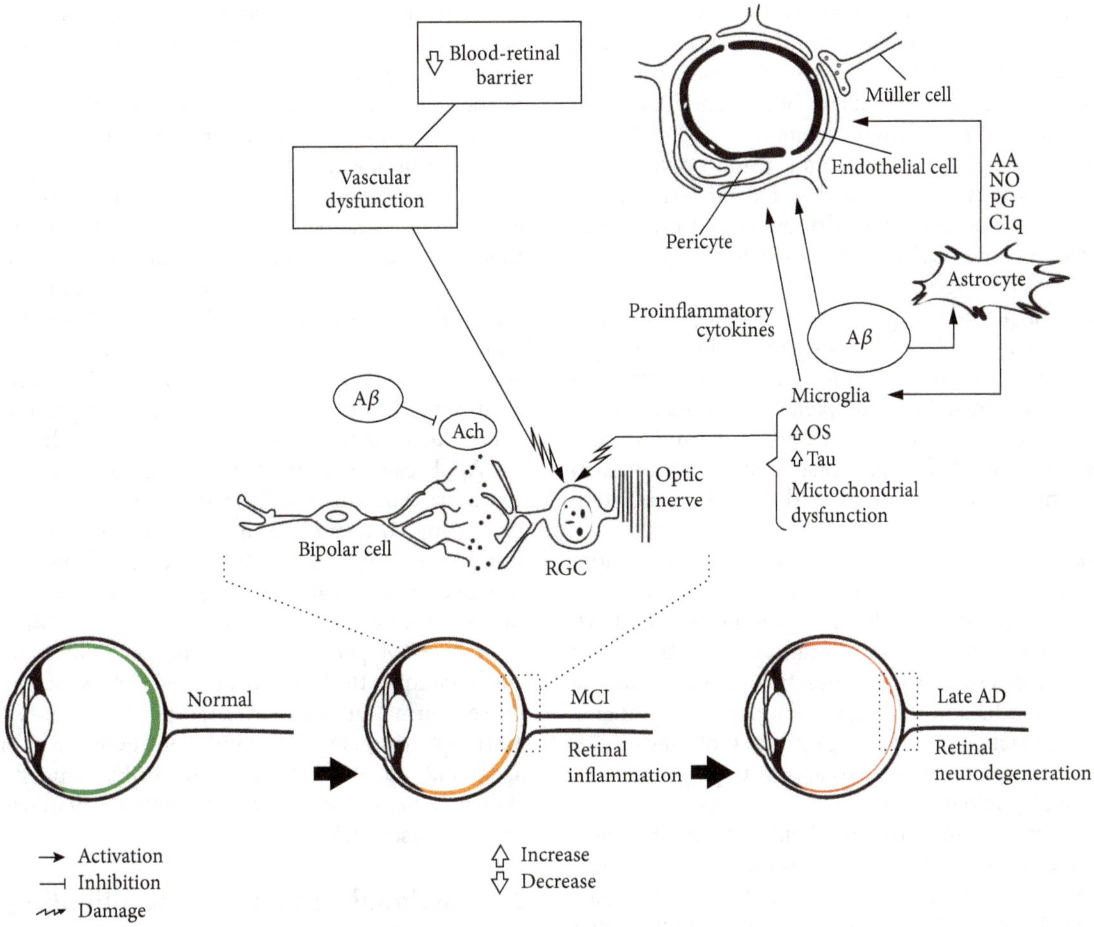

FIGURE 1: Pathophysiological events in the retina during Alzheimer's disease progression. Amyloid-beta (Aβ) induces microglia and astrocyte activation, synaptic dysfunction, and neurodegeneration. These interactions can be observed by noninvasive ophthalmological examinations in the retina at different stages of Alzheimer's disease (AD). Reduction in the peripapillary region and macular volume has been described in MCI and AD. AA: arachidonic acid; Aβ: amyloid-beta; ACh: acetylcholine; AD: Alzheimer's disease; MCI: mild cognitive impairment; NO: nitric oxide; OS: oxidative stress; PG: prostaglandins; RGC: retinal ganglion cells.

"Drusen" in the retina are deposits of insoluble cellular debris and lipids localized beneath the RPE and inner collagenous layer of Bruch's membrane (BM) [71]. Two types of "drusen" have been identified (hard and soft which differ in their location, and in their clinical and morphological appearance). Both soft and hard "drusen" have similar compositions; however, some authors suggest that each type of "drusen" may be composed by a certain variety of proteins or may be constituted by different amounts of the same components. Differences in "drusen's" morphology, composition, physical properties, and location (peripheral or central) could most likely be based on different formative mechanisms that may contribute to macular susceptibility for age-related macular degeneration (AMD) progression. Although "hard drusen" can appear everywhere in the retina, they are usually located in the peripheral retina and are characterized by hemispherical structures with well-defined borders. "Hard drusen" are considered part of the normal aging process. "Soft drusen" are located exclusively in the macula, characterized by poorly defined borders and larger size [78]. They are linked to the early stage of AMD [72, 79]. AMD is a slow, progressive disease that compromises the macula and the primary cause of irreversible blindness during aging [43].

Two types of AMD have been described: dry AMD type, characterized by significant atrophy of RPE and the photoreceptor layer, and wet, or exudative, AMD type, with invasive blood vessels through the blood-retinal barrier [43]. These invasive vessels come from the choroid and proliferate in the retinal layers between BM and RPE or sometimes proliferate between RPE and the neurosensory retina. In turn, this leads to vascular leakage and fluid accumulation, with formation of fibrovascular disciform scars in the retina that can be observed by ophthalmoscopy [79].

The extracellular deposits in the brain and retina share the presence of Aβ, ApoE, proteoglycans, immunoglobulins, metal ions, acute-phase reactants, fibrinogen, prothrombin, membrane debris, and protease elements [43, 72]. Aβ formation is found in both AD and AMD, suggesting a common mechanism related to proteinopathic Aβ1–42 peptide deposition [80, 81] and imbalance between increased Aβ synthesis and reduced Aβ removal [12]. Specifically, in the aging eye, Aβ accumulation occurs primarily in the outer segments of photoreceptors and at the interface between RPE and BM

[82]. This process appears to initiate at the apical region of the outer segments and progresses through the retinal layers with age, also accumulating in choroidal blood vessels. In drusen, Aβ is localized in vesicular components known as "amyloid vesicles" or "amyloid assemblies" [43, 78] and exhibits several shapes, diameters, and fusion processes. In addition, some drusen are described as a single large vesicle occupying a sizable portion of the drusen, or densely packed with several amyloid vesicles [43]. Amyloid vesicles are formed by amyloid oligomer cores composed of toxic oligomeric Aβ1–42 peptides that are centrally organized in a ring structure [82], in close proximity to the inner collagenous layer of BM [71]. Aβ1–42 interacts with different drusen components, including complement proteins (HF1, C3b/iC3b, and C5), interleukins (IL-1β, IL-8, and IL-33), and lipids (cholesterol and phosphatidylcholine) to form mature Aβ fibrils, which compose the shell of amyloid vesicles [43, 82].

Overall, these interactions increase ROS production, which contributes to formation of glycation and lipoxidation end products [79]. Additionally, it is hypothesized that Aβ promotes retinal microglia translocation from the inner retina (normal position) to the subretinal space, inducing changes in RPE cells and leading to secretion of proinflammatory, chemotactic, and proangiogenic molecules [82]. Furthermore, complement proteins appear to play a key role in the pathophysiological mechanisms of AD owing to activation by membrane proteins, lipids, cholesterol, and Aβ deposits. Complement molecules promote inflammatory stimuli [72], disrupt the RPE junctional complex [82], impair trans-epithelial permeability, and induce mitochondrial damage. Moreover, they also promote an increase in angiogenic factors, such as vascular endothelial growth factor (VEGF), and decrease in anti-angiogenic factors, such as pigment epithelium-derived factor [43, 83].

The role of tau in AMD is debated and likely underestimated, as tau has not been found in drusen, but has been reported in OPL, INL, IPL, and NFL of patients with AD. Some studies suggest that tau aggregation in aged retina causes defective transportation of molecules, cells, and proteins, which may promote drusen formation and subsequently AMD [75].

2.5. Apolipoprotein E Mechanisms. ApoE is involved in the transport of cholesterol and triglycerides and is considered one of the most important risk factors for development of AD [84]. ApoE protein is mainly expressed in the brain on astrocytes, but also in microglia, neurons, pericytes, smooth muscle cells, and brain endothelial cells [85]. Of the different ApoE alleles (ε2, ε3, and ε4), ApoE4 shows a strong relationship with increased risk of developing AD, while ApoE2 provides protection against AD [86]. ApoE4 interacts with Aβ to increase Aβ aggregation [87]. Furthermore, the risk of amyloidosis in AD is suggested to be related to the interaction between ApoE, aging, and amyloid burden [88].

ApoE4 is associated with vascular pathology in AD and promotes cerebral amyloid angiopathy. Further, ApoE4 is related to other vascular diseases such as atherosclerosis, stroke, cerebrovascular disease, and coronary heart disease. Consequently, it has been proposed that the pathological effects of ApoE4 are initiated by cerebrovascular insult, which subsequently leads to neurodegeneration. In the retina of transgenic mice, ApoE4 is implicated in reduced vascular density and increased vascular buds and branching in early postnatal days, which ends during the neonatal period. These findings are associated with decreased synaptic expression after the neonatal period, due to low VEGF levels in ApoE4 models. VEGF is implicated in angiogenesis and vascular plasticity and as a neuronal growth factor in retina development. This determined that ApoE4 has transitory synaptic and vascular effects during retinal development, before and after the neonatal period, respectively. Moreover, VEGF in aged retina has proangiogenic effects that promote macular edema, diabetic retinopathy, and macular holes [89, 90].

ApoE can be expressed in RPE, GCL, and BM and is synthesized in Müller cells [89]. ApoE is involved in uptake, processing, transport, and clearance of lipids for retinal metabolism; therefore, disturbance of this process may lead to cholesterol and lipid accumulation in BM [43]. Distinct to AD, ApoE4 confers protection against AMD because it improves BM permeability, facilitates lipid transportation, and consequently leads to reduced debris accumulation in drusen formation. In contrast, ApoE2 increases the risk of AMD apparition because it induces VEGF as a proangiogenic agent [43, 89, 91, 92]. Contradictorily, some studies have shown increased AMD in AD patients [93], while others show no association [94].

3. Functional and Pathological Findings in the Visual System

Neuronal and synaptic dysfunction in AD may compromise visual system pathways in associated cortical and subcortical brain structures, as well as peripheral nerves. Complex visual disruptions are described in AD, which are related to neural dysfunction and modifications in varied eye structures. Depending on the area affected, these lead to diverse clinical manifestations, making the visual system a potential diagnostic aid [95].

3.1. Cortical, Subcortical, and Brainstem Regions. Aβ and NFT aggregation as well as neurodegeneration and axonal damage are found in different brain structures related to visual system functioning [50]. For instance, in the primary cortex (Brodmann areas 17 and 18) of AD patients, has been described a decrease in neuronal density, and increase in glial density only in area 17. These cellular changes are related with the presence of Aβ-plaques and NFT [70]. In the case of the secondary visual cortex, involvement of the cuneal and lingual areas of the occipital lobe of AD cases may correspond with impairment in selective visual attention, emotion, and visual processing [96–98]. Meanwhile, reduced glucose metabolism in the visual association cortex and inferior parietal cortex might be related to abnormalities in figure copying, color vision tested by isochromatic plates, and stereopsis [99].

Regarding subcortical structures, Aβ aggregation and neuritic plaques have been found in the pulvinar nucleus of the thalamus of AD postmortem samples. This nucleus participates in visual attention and in the control of eye movements [100]. Similarly, amyloid pathology in the lateral geniculate nucleus of the thalamus, the initial processor of visual information, has been reported. In this regard, a reduction in the number of parvocellular neurons and magnocellular gliosis was found [101]. Indeed, the magnocellular system is involved in recognition of movement, spatial perception, and luminosity, meanwhile parvocellular on identification of color and form. Correspondingly, color and motion perception is affected in AD patients [21]. Another structure involved would be the suprachiasmatic nucleus, responsible of the circadian cycle, sleep, melatonin secretion, pupil regulation, and learning. In fact, clinical and animal models of AD indicate severe disturbance in the circadian rhythms, as well as neurodegeneration in brain structures which control those cycles [102–105]. Altogether, cortical and subcortical dysfunction of the visual system may partially explain the difficulties AD patients have with writing, reading, color and structure differentiation, facial recognition, and visual acuity.

Amyloid aggregation, NFT, and neuritic plaques in the superior colliculus, responsible for the onset of ocular movements, have been reported in postmortem samples from the brainstem of AD patients [106, 107]. Accumulation of Aβ has also been observed in the Edinger-Westphal nucleus of the parasympathetic oculomotor system (which is responsible for pupillary constriction), resulting in degeneration, neuronal loss, and decreased acetylcholine (ACh) in this nucleus, with consequent pupillary reflex alterations [22, 46]. The sympathetic system, involved in the dilatation of the pupil, is also affected in more advanced AD stages [46].

ACh is well known as an excitatory neurotransmitter in the learning and memory process [108] and is compromised in AD. Indeed, changes in neurotransmitter function may explain retinal and visual dysfunction in early AD and MCI before neurodegeneration is established. Different studies have shown neurotransmitter synthesis in amacrine cells, and nicotinic receptors in bipolar cells, horizontal cells, photoreceptors, and the GCL [108, 109]. In the retina of a transgenic mouse model of AD (Tg-SwDI), specific cholinergic cell loss together with reactive gliosis was found [108]. Cholinergic dysfunction induced by Aβ is established at distinct levels: neurodegeneration of cholinergic cells [110], ACh depletion [111], impaired ACh release [112], and finally Aβ-induced impairment of muscarinic [113] and nicotinic acetylcholine receptors (e.g., α7-nAChR) [114], as well as associated effectors (e.g., potassium voltage-gated channels, KCNQ) [115–117]. In older animal models, downregulation of α4, α7, α9, and α10 nAChR, and m4 and m5 muscarinic acetylcholine receptor (mAChR) subunits, was found. These changes are observed in photoreceptors and INL cells, accompanied by cholinergic cell loss in the retina [108]. Contrast sensitivity and visual attention has been found to be deteriorated in AD patients [118]. In this regard, the use of cholinergic drugs such as donepezil leads to improvement in visual selective attention [119]. Similarly, donepezil also increases contrast sensitivity and accuracy in non-AD subjects [120]. Therefore, the stimulation of the cholinergic system in AD patients not only may generate improvement in learning and memory processes but also might improve visual alteration at retinal, subcortical, and cortical levels.

3.2. Retina. In the retina, GCL, NFL, IPL, and the photoreceptor layer can generate Aβ, as each layer expresses APP [30]. As described earlier, aberrant APP cleavage leads to neurotoxic Aβ aggregation, enabling inflammatory processing, degeneration, and thinning in all quadrants of the retina in these layers, but mainly in the superior and inferior quadrants. These layers are present in a third of the macula; therefore, any alterations can contribute to reduced macula and fovea volume, which may partially explain the ocular manifestations that these patients exhibit [25, 48, 121–124]. Study in retinas from postmortem patients with AD found a reduction in the number of GCL neurons related to progressive aging [125]. In contrast, GCL thinning was aggravated in patients with AD and not related to aging in other studies [126]. AD ocular findings in human studies are summarized in Table 1, and findings in animal studies are summarized in Table 2.

3.3. Optic Nerve. Analysis of the optic disc has been performed in AD patients, with increased cup-to-disc ratio [50], higher pallor area-to-disc area ratio, and decreased disc rim area of the optic nerve observed as indirect signs of axonal damage [21, 127, 128]. These optic nerve alterations are due to degeneration of axons and larger cells of the GCL and NFL [127] in the central and peripheral portions of the retina, which are involved in the magnocellular pathway and ensure greater optic nerve caliber [129]. In addition, reduced hemoglobin percentage in the neuroretinal rim and increased cup-to disc ratio (by 39%–43%) have been demonstrated [128, 130, 131]. Nonetheless, despite significant reduction of the density of axons from the optic nerve in AD when compared with the age-matched control subjects, no correlation between optic nerve volume and cerebral volume in AD patients was observed [132].

3.4. Retinal Vasculature. Regarding the vasculature, Aβ protein can be found in the walls of retinal blood vessels. Its integrity is important in maintaining the blood–brain barrier [44]. However, with aging, Aβ protein aggregates and accumulates in blood vessels of the cerebral and retinal vasculature [126]. As already described, retinal microvasculature has the same embryological origin as brain microvasculature, sharing disease-specific pathological mechanisms [44]. Different clinical studies have shown venular narrowing [133] with a decrease in flow, vessel diameter [134, 135], arteriolar–venular fractal dimension [133], and branching pattern [136] in AD. Similarly, increased arterial tortuosity has been observed in clinical studies [133], with standard deviation of vessel width [136] and amplitude of arterial pulsation [126, 133, 136, 137]. Moreover, these findings relate to cognitive impairment, disease progression, and reduction in NFL diameter in the superior quadrant [21, 26, 27, 138–140]. Although other studies differ in these conclusions, no significant variations were shown for

Table 1: AD ocular findings in human studies.

Ocular histopathological hallmarks in human studies				
Ref.	Population (mean age, range years)	Tissue analyzed	AD stage (early vs. late-onset)	Findings
Williams et al. 2017 [198]	AD $n = 17$ (77) Controls $n = 2$ (77)	Retina, lens, and optic nerve	Late	No presence of tau, Aβ, ubiquitin, TDP-43, or a-synuclein.
Tsai et al. 2014 [67]	AD $n = 10$ (63–95) Control $n = 10$ (63–95)	Nasal and temporal regions of the retina	NS	Aβ plaques in retina and reduced choroidal thickness.
Ho et al. 2014 [204]	AD $n = 11$ (82/61–92) Controls $n = 6$ (74/66–86)	Peripheral nasal retina, posterior retina including the macular region and optic nerve head, and peripheral temporal retina	Late Definite AD ($n = 9$) Probable AD ($n = 2$)	Cytoplasmic α-synuclein positivity, but not Aβ deposits and abnormal tau accumulation.
Schön et al. 2012 [77]	AD $n = 6$ (37–79) Controls $n = 4$ (53–60)	Retina	Early and late	Hyperphosphorylated tau but no Aβ plaques or fibrillar tau aggregates.
Koronyo-Hamaoui et al. 2011 [66]	AD $n = 8$ (80/48–94) $n = 5$ (79/65–92) Controls $n = 5$ (76/66–85)	Retina	Late ($n = 9$) Early ($n = 1$)	Aβ40 plaques.
Syed et al. 2005 [205]	AD $n = 12$ (81.9 ± 6.54/69–84) Controls $n = 13$ (78.5 ± 8.57/66–82)	Optic nerve	Late	The density of axons was reduced in both the center and peripheral portions of the optic nerve with preferential loss of the smaller-sized axons.
Blanks et al. 1996 [68]	(GFAP-ir) AD $n = 12$ (64–88) Controls $n = 19$ (63–89) Neuronal and cell numbers (GCL) AD $n = 11$ (16 retinas 45–92 years) Control $n = 9$ (11 retinas 60–89 years)	Retina	Late	Extensive neuronal loss in the entire retina (36.4%), most pronounced in the superior and inferior quadrants, throughout the midperipheral regions (40–49%), and in the far peripheral inferior retina (50–59%). Increase in the astrocyte : neuron ratio. Also, more extensive labeling of glial fibrillary acidic protein immunoreactivity (GFAP-ir) in astrocytes in the GCL, in the Müller cells, and in radial processes.
Curcio and Drucker [206]	AD $n = 4$ (67–86) Controls $n = 4$ (66–86)	Retina	Late	No evidence of GCL loss between AD and controls.
Blanks et al. 1991 [207]	AD $n = 11$ (13 retinas 83/69–93 years) Controls $n = 11$ (14 retinas 78/60–98 years)	Retina	Late	The fovea shows a loss of neurons within the GCL, mainly in large and small ganglion cells.
Sadun and Bassi 1990 [129]	AD (10 optic nerves, 3 retinas 76–89 years) Controls (8 optic nerves, 2 retinas 70–79 years)	Optic nerve and retina	Late	Predominant loss of the largest class of retinal ganglion cells (M cells). Retina of 1/3 AD patients also showed degeneration of GCL and their axons in the NFL.

Table 1: Continued.

Ref.	Population (mean age, range years)	Tissue analyzed	AD stage (early vs. late-onset)	Findings
	Ocular histopathological hallmarks in human studies			
Blanks et al. 1989 [208]	AD $n = 16$ (76–93) Controls $n = 19$ (60–91)	Optic nerve and retina	Late	Degeneration in the GCL is characterized by a vacuolated appearance of the cytoplasm. Absence of neurofibrillary tangles, neuritic plaques, or amyloid angiopathy.
Hinton et al. 1986 [128]	AD $n = 10$ (10 optic nerves, 4 retinas 73–89 years) Controls $n = 10$ (73–89)	Optic nerve and retina	Late	Widespread axonal degeneration in optic nerves, decreased in the number of cells in GCL, and reduction in the thickness of NFL. There was no retinal neurofibrillary degeneration or amyloid angiopathy.

TABLE 2: AD ocular findings in animal studies.

Ref.	Ocular hallmarks in experimental animal models Model	Findings
Oliveira-Souza et al. 2017 [108]	Tg-SwDI mice 6.5 to 15 months	Upregulation of AChR gene expression and significant cell loss in the photoreceptor layer and inner retina on young groups. Specific cholinergic cell loss and increased astrocytic gliosis in the middle-aged and AChR downregulation in older adult groups.
Joly et al. 2017 [209]	Tg APPswe/PS1DE9 mice 3 to 13 months	No Aβ or amyloid plaques were detected in the Tg retinas. However, the CTFb/CTFa ratio was significantly lower. Response mediated by cones was preserved. Retinal-specific processing of amyloid may confer protection against AD and selectively preserve cone-dependent vision during aging.
Nilson et al. 2017 [73]	P301L mouse Htau mouse	Tau oligomers colocalize with astrocytes, microglia, HMGB1, and inflammatory cells in the retina.
Chiasseu et al. 2017 [74]	3xTg mice 3 to 6 months	Age-related increase in endogenous retinal tau accumulation, previous to the reported onset of behavioral deficits, and tau aggregation in the brain. Tau build-up occurred in GCL soma and dendrites, but not in axons.
Chidlow et al. 2017 [56]	Tg APPSWE/PS1ΔE9 mouse 3 to 12 months	No presence of amyloid plaques, dystrophic neurites, neuronal loss, macro- or microgliosis, OS, tau hyperphosphorylation, or upregulations of proinflammatory cytokines in the retina.
Gupta et al. 2016 [47]	Tg APP/PS1 mice 13 to 16 months	Increased Aβ deposition in the retinas with thinning in inner retinal layers and decline in scotopic threshold response. Reduction of axonal density in the optic nerve.
Du et al. 2015 [65]	*Octodon degus* 6.7–70 months	Aβ deposition in the inner and outer segment of the photoreceptors, NFL, and GCL. Aβ expression was higher in the central retinal region than in the retinal periphery. Phosphorylated tau was seen more consistently in NFL-GCL regardless of age.
Pogue et al. 2015 [80]	Tg 5xFAD Tg-AD mice 0–5 months	Presence of Aβ42 peptides in the brain and retina, accompanied by inflammatory markers such as cyclooxygenase-2 and C-protein reactive.
Maharshak et al. 2016 [90]	ApoE3 and ApoE4 targeted replacement mice 4–7–12–120 days old	Transient changes in vascular branching and decrease in retinal synaptic density in the apoE4 mice. Additionally, lower levels of retinal VEGF were observed in apoE4 mice compared to the ApoE3 mouse retinas.
Tsai et al. 2014 [67]	TgF344-AD rat 14–19 months	Reduction in choroidal thickness, hypertrophic retinal pigment epithelial cells, inflammatory cells, Aβ plaques, and upregulation of complement factor C3 in the retina.
Williams et al. 2013 [210]	Tg 2576 mice 14 months	No significant changes in GCL synaptic densities but a highly significant change in mitochondrial morphology. GCL dendritic atrophy preceded cell loss, and this may be due to the accumulations of Aβ.
Zhao et al. 2013 [76]	Tg APP/PS1 mice	Hyperexpression of phosphorylated tau was detected in retina, accompanied with an increase in senile plaques and NFTs. The increased tau phosphorylation was associated with a significant augment in the production of p35 and p25, and upregulation of calpain.
Schon et al. 2012 [77]	Tg P301S mice	*In vivo* detection of fibrillar tau in the retina and the progression of tau pathology over several months was demonstrated.
Koronyo-Hamaoui et al. 2011 [66]	Tg APPSWE/PS1ΔE9 mouse 7–17 months	Retinal Aβ plaques were detected following systemic administration of curcumin in Tg, previous to the appearance of Aβ plaques in the brain.
Perez et al. 2009 [64]	Tg APPSWE/PS1DeltaE9 mouse 12–19 months	Aβ plaques appeared in the OPL and IPL of the retina, displaying syntaxin 1 and ChAT, but no neuronal degeneration was observed. ERG revealed reduction in the amplitudes of a and b waves.

arteriolar–venular caliber, branching angle, or venular tortuosity in AD patients [133].

4. Visual Impairments in AD: Clinical Features

AD affects different structures of the visual system in a similar pathological manner as the brain, with manifestation of distinct signs and symptoms that can be determined by adequate clinical history and ophthalmological examination. To our knowledge, there are no studies showing the chronological clinical manifestations specifically correlated with changes in the retina in patients with AD. Therefore, it is important to conduct clinical prospective studies in order to clarify this aspect. Regarding structural changes in the retina, thinning of the superior or inferior quadrants has been described in AD patients associated with visual field impairment. Other visual findings have been correlated with alterations in the brain [141]. Regarding early visual manifestations, it has been observed that contrast sensitivity is the first visual dysfunction found in animal models and AD patients [142, 143]. The rest of visual symptoms are evident depending on the compromised brain structure [22, 95, 144].

Complex visual disturbances are described in patients with AD, including constructional and visuoperceptual disorientation, specifically difficulties in searching for objects (figure–ground discrimination), finding their way in familiar surroundings (environmental agnosia) [99, 145], and spatial recognition or spatial order memory (spatial agnosia) [146]. Additionally, distinct alterations in daily life activities due to deterioration in visual attention [147] and impairments in tasks requiring semantic access from visual information (e.g., disproportionate reading [148] and facial recognition [149]) are observed. With facial recognition, transient misidentification, abnormal self-identification, Capgras syndrome (denial of a familiar person and identifying them as a replacement, imposter, or double), and in some cases prosopagnosia (disordered recognition of familiar faces) have been described [150]. These disturbances are due to disordered visual processing because of disrupted cortico-cortical projections as a result of alterations in cortical and visual pathways (i.e., occipito–parietal and occipito–temporal) [151, 152]. Disordered visual processing can lead to complications in perceiving and comparing visual stimuli, alterations in processing visual stimuli, and impairments in long-term memory and generating verbal or action responses [148].

Another visual disturbance identified in AD is Balint's syndrome. This is an uncommon and incompletely understood visuospatial defect reported in patients with bilateral parieto-occipital damage associated with Brodmann's area 7b in the posterior parietal lobe (which is involved in control of pursuit ocular movements and target gaze on a stimulus) and superior occipital cortex areas 17, 18, and 19 (which are involved in visual field construction) [153]. Balint's syndrome is characterized by simultanagnosia (difficulties in locating, reaching, or attending to multiple items in a visual space), ocular motor apraxia (inability to maintain fixation on a specific point located in the peripheral visual field), and optic ataxia (inappropriate coordination of voluntary movements in response to a visual stimulus) [149].

Recently, alterations in ophthalmologic examination of AD patients have been described. These alterations include decreased visual acuity, with difficulties in writing and reading [154] increasing along with disease progression [139, 155, 156]. Similarly, compromised contrast sensitivity (ability to distinguish an object on a background of different frequencies) [142–144, 157] has been observed as a principal manifestation during the initial disease stage, with progressive impairment throughout the disease course [143]. Contrast sensitivity is associated with damage to the magnocellular pathway in the geniculate nucleus of the CNS, which is involved in the ability to identify luminosity and motion perception [158]. Another manifestation in AD patients is fluctuations in color perception, mainly errors in color recognition, due to involvement of the parvocellular pathway, which is characterized by smaller axons of the optic nerve [159]. Additionally, pupillary reflex deficits are reported as a deficiency of the sympathetic and parasympathetic systems, with the principal findings being decreased amplitude, speed, and latency of reflexes. Further, smaller resting pupil diameter and maximum dilatation velocity in the dark [160] as well as reduced amplitude and 75% recovery time of the light reflex response [22, 160] are also reported. Other abnormalities in ocular movement, decreased movement perception, and stereopsis dysfunction have been observed in patients with AD [46]. These abnormalities include inability to focus on an object (less relative fixation time) [161], irregular convergence angle, difficulty performing saccadic ocular movements [162, 163], poorer heading and speed perception at lower temporal periodicity [24], and inability to identify three-dimensional objects [164]. Finally, loss of the visual field mainly occurs in the inferior quadrant and is related to GCL damage in the superior quadrant of the corresponding retina [96]. Visual field loss is characterized by accumulation of larger SP and greater amounts of NFT in the cuneal gyrus than lingual gyrus of the visual cortex, which is where nerve fiber projections of the GCL in the superior and inferior quadrants terminate, respectively [135].

5. Paraclinical Visual Studies in AD

Different noninvasive imaging methods have been developed to study structures of the visual system and visual pathways in AD patients. In this section, we describe findings obtained by optical coherence tomography (OCT) and bioelectrical changes through electrophysiological examinations, specifically electroretinograms (ERG) and visual evoked potentials (VEP).

5.1. Optical Coherence Tomography in the Retina. In the retina, different OCT methods based on cross-sectional images of the retinal layers have been performed in AD patients, including spectral domain-optical coherence tomography (SD-OCT). Using SD-OCT, thinning and thickening of NFL in the superior and inferior quadrants, respectively, of the nasal and temporal regions were related [165] to cognitive impairment [131, 166, 167]. Degeneration of NFL,

GCL, and IPL has been related to AD duration, with longer disease duration associated with greater damage to the retinal layers. The most affected quadrants were the temporal, temporal–inferior, and temporal–superior sectors, with increased nasal/temporal ratio reflecting higher temporal sector commitment. In addition, reduction of the GCL was associated with axonal degeneration, which may predict greater disease severity [168].

Among other OCT studies, progressive compromise of the NFL was shown between an intermediate group with MCI and different disease stages. Thinning of NFL in the superior quadrant was gradually affected among patients with MCI and mild AD. The inferior quadrant was involved in severe disease stages, demonstrating engagement of the NFL throughout disease progression [169]. In addition, another study detected a decrease in NFL in AD and MCI groups in the inferior quadrant, with the superior quadrant significantly compromised in AD patients only [170]. Contrarily, NFL thinning was evident in all MCI and AD groups, indicating that NFL involvement is observed in the early disease stage [171]. Furthermore, significant NFL thinning was identified in patients at the early stage of AD [165]. A meta-analysis of 51 articles in the last 5 years recognized that loss of NFL mainly occurred in the superior quadrant, yet corresponded to visual field impairments in the inferior quadrant. This deterioration in NFL was related to disease duration in AD [140].

When comparing AD patients and healthy controls, a significant NFL reduction has been observed in AD patients, more prominent in the inferior [172, 173] and superior quadrants [140, 174]. A meta-analysis including 887 AD patients and 864 controls evidenced peripapillary NFL thinning in the superior and inferior quadrants of the retina in AD patients that was not present in controls [175]. Additionally, AD patients had reduced thickness in GCL, NFL, IPL, and outer nuclear layer (ONL) compared with controls [176].

In contrast, a relationship between NFL involvement (through OCT) and cognitive impairment by Mini-Mental State Examination (MMSE) was reported in AD patients, suggesting that measurement of NFL may be used as a disease progression marker [177]. However, other studies have observed NFL thinning in all quadrants, especially the nasal region, with no relationship to the MMSE and AD severity [178].

5.2. Optical Coherence Tomography in the Macula. The macula is the principal structure affected at the early stage in AD patients. By OCT, decreased macula volume was observed in the four internal quadrants and one temporal external quadrant, with no significant difference in decrease in peripapillary region volume in AD patients [179]. However, a recent meta-analysis has shown that AD and MCI patients had lower peripapillary retinal NFL compared with controls [180]. Using SD-OCT, increased macular size and IPL was shown in patients with MCI and those at risk of developing AD, suggesting an inflammatory process and reactive gliosis in the early disease stage before establishment of AD [172, 174]. Conversely, macular thinning was identified in MCI [178] and in all sectors except the fovea, mainly in NFL of the superior quadrant in AD [156]. Decreased IPL in the inferonasal, inferotemporal, and superotemporal sectors was observed, as well as reduced NFL in the temporal sector in patients with MCI who developed AD two years later. Corroboratively, these results were related to cognitive impairment [176]. Macular atrophy has been described as the first manifestation in patients with AD and is related to degree of cognitive impairment in the MMSE [140]. By frequency domain optical coherence tomography in AD, NFL, GCL, and IPL are shown to be reduced in size in the macula, except in the inferior external quadrant. Again, this thinning is related to MMSE results [181].

5.3. Optical Coherence Tomography in the Choroid. Choroid reduction and thinning are observed in AD. Using SD-OCT, thinning of the choroid was measured in the macula at 13 locations (separated by 500 mm) in elderly compared with healthy subjects. A significant decrease in the choroid was shown in all 13 locations, but principally in two locations temporal to the fovea. This indicates that compromise in the choroid is not related to age [182]. By OCT examination over a period of 12 months, greater choroid reduction was characterized in AD patients compared with controls of the same age [183]. Another study measured thickness of GCL in the macula, the choroid, and external retina, and compared them with MMSE results. GCL thinning in the superior and inferior quadrants of the macula was observed, with significant thinning of the choroid in all regions. Further, a relationship was observed between GCL thinning in the macula and MMSE results, but not with choroid thinning, which was unrelated to severity of cognitive damage [173].

5.4. Electrophysiological Examination. Electrophysiological examinations (i.e., bioelectrical changes in the visual system) such as VEP and ERG have been performed in patients with AD [140]. VEP extracts signals directly from the visual cortex, which are dependent on adequate integrity of the visual system (eye, retina, optic nerve, and visual cortex). In patients with AD, decreased amplitude of P2 or P100 components are observed at 100 ms [45, 46, 48, 96, 138–140, 175, 184–186]. Yet, other studies have shown no changes in pattern-VEP nor association with NFL thinning [187] in the peripapillary or macular regions [188].

The pattern ERG (PERG) test presents three peaks: negative–positive–negative, which are observed at 35–50–95 ms, respectively [46]. Most studies show decreased amplitudes and time delays, mainly in N35, P50, and N95 components, in PERG of patients with AD [140, 189]. In contrast, only reduced P50–N95 amplitudes with increased implicit P50 time [190] were shown in other studies, while a compromised magnocellular pathway was also reported [158]. All these findings relate to damage at the GCL level (N95) [190]. Conversely, further studies detected no PERG changes [191]. In another type of exam, the multifocal ERG, which evaluates macula functionality, even in early or intermediate states of the disease in patients with AD, a statistically significant reduction in the electric activity of the macula has been registered, especially in the foveal and parafoveal regions, due to the decrease in the amplitude of the P1 component

[145]. In PERG, reduced mean amplitudes in these components were observed in patients with AD. This anomaly may be due to axonal depletion within the optic nerve as well as GCL degeneration [192]. Additionally, PERG at different frequencies showed amplitude reductions at high frequencies in patients with AD [193]. In other types of examination, namely, pattern-reversal VEP and ERG, no alterations were detected, but delays were occasionally demonstrated in the second positive component of flash VEP [192]. Scotopic and photopic flash ERG and oscillatory potentials show no alterations between both methods in patients with AD, suggesting no visual pathway involvement [194]. With VEP, decreased latency in the magnocellular pathway was observed in AD patients [158].

6. Future Clinical Directions

The clinical study of the visual system offers several benefits owing to the relatively scarce invasiveness of the examination, as well as the associated low cost of procedures. Structural eye components such as the cornea, lens, retina, and optic nerve can be observed with an ophthalmoscope. Additionally, functional aspects related to autonomic features, such as pupillary reflex, can be directly studied. Further, a wide array of visual paraclinical tests have been developed including VEP, ERG, tonometry, and OCT. These procedures are not limited to evaluating aspects of the visual system and can also be used to examine neurological or systemic components of many conditions. This has led to the proposition that studying the visual system is a helpful and complementary approach with biomarker potential in neurodegenerative conditions, including AD [45]. Many visual changes manifest in AD patients (as already discussed), including alterations in visual acuity, color perception, contrast sensitivity, the visual field, pupillary reflexes, ocular movements, and stereopsis. All can be examined by simple, noninvasive, and easily accessible methods such as adequate ophthalmologic examination, OCT, and electrophysiological examinations. These are supporting diagnostic tools that could potentially even be used in the early disease stage. Current biomarkers for AD tend to be either expensive or invasive, and in particular for countries with poor and inadequate healthcare systems. Moreover, no current biomarkers predict with absolute confidence, conversion of MCI to AD, or development of sporadic AD. For a recent review on the advantages and disadvantages of current AD biomarkers, refer to [20]. Several findings in the visual system point to the useful role of eye examinations for determination of AD. One of the challenges of this approach is to differentiate changes related to normal aging from those of pathological origin. To date, three structural components of the eye, the retina, eye vasculature, and lens, have emerged as interesting research areas in AD [45].

Study of the retina and associated structures has shown AD-related changes in preclinical (phase 1) animal exploratory models, thereby providing hints for their utility as biomarkers in humans. Many of these studies have been performed in transgenic humanized rodent models expressing AD characteristics. Accumulation of Aβ in plaques was observed at 12 months in the retina of transgenic APPswe/PS1ΔE9 mice. These plaques localized mainly in the OPL and IPL and increased in number and size with age [64]. Similar results were also observed in transgenic APPswe/PS1ΔE9 rats, with Aβ plaque-like structures present in the retina, together with choroidal thinning [67]. Aβ peptides were observed in the inner and outer segments of photoreceptors, NFL, and GCL, with higher expression in the central retinal region, in the Chilean rodent, *Octodon degus* [65], which has been suggested as a possible natural model of AD [195]. Some studies in transgenic mice have even reported earlier appearance of plaques in the retina than brain [42]. Furthermore, changes in retinal plaques can be individually monitored in real time following glatiramer acetate immunization in mice [66]. Regrettably, these results using similar animal models have not always been consistent, with contradictory findings reported. In a recently published study on APPswe/PS1ΔE9 mice, researchers were unable to demonstrate the presence of amyloid plaques, dystrophic neurites, neuronal loss, macro- or microgliosis, aberrant cell cycle re-entry, OS, tau hyperphosphorylation, or upregulation of proinflammatory cytokines or stress signaling molecules in the retina [56]. Despite promising results obtained in preclinical models, more investigations are needed to address the reasons why AD-related changes are not constant in all animal models and explore the mechanisms inducing cellular and molecular alterations in the retina. Comprehension of these questions is vital if visual components are to be translated from basic science to clinical practice as reliable biomarkers.

Changes in the human retina have also been reported in relation to AD. A recent meta-analysis, which included 25 studies comprising 887 AD patients, 216 MCI patients, and 864 healthy controls, concluded that AD and MCI patients show decreased retinal thickness measured by OCT [180]. Another meta-analysis, which included a lower number of studies and patients, reached a similar conclusion, corroborating the role of OCT and retinal measurement in assessment of AD [123, 196]. Accordingly, retinal measurements in humans may help distinguish between different neurodegenerative conditions. Patients with frontotemporal degeneration have a thinner outer retina, including a thinner ONL. In contrast, AD patients tend to exhibit inner retinal thinning [197]. Despite these encouraging results, in a similar fashion to the animal models, some reports challenge this evidence. In a recent paper, Tau, Aβ, transactive response DNA-binding protein 43, ubiquitin, and α-synuclein were examined by immunohistochemistry in postmortem AD patient brains, showing no evidence of inclusions, deposits, or accumulation of other proteins in any part of the ocular globe [198]. As in preclinical experiments, human studies need to be expanded to clarify these controversial aspects of AD-induced changes in the retina and visual system.

Other aspects of the eye and visual system are also reported to show alterations related to AD, although the retina is the component that has been most thoroughly studied. In the lens, some but not all clinical studies show Aβ deposition [199], while others have concluded that cataract grade or lens opacity is unlikely to provide a noninvasive measure of the risk of developing AD dementia [200]. These controversial results do not support the use of lens examination as a biomarker of AD, underscoring the importance of conducting more detailed, controlled clinical studies with a larger number of patients. Ocular vascular changes have also been reported in AD patients [26, 201], which suggest similar microvascular damage in the eye as the well-described cerebral amyloid angiopathy owing to vascular Aβ deposition [202]. Direct and minimally invasive observation of eye vasculature, mainly retinal, provides an advantage to using vascular changes as a marker of AD. Unfortunately, the current evidence is not strong enough to offer a definitive answer on using this approach as a biomarker for AD. A recent systematic review, which included all published studies applying fundus camera imaging to examine association between retinal vasculature/retinopathy and any form of dementia, found many inconsistent results regarding changes in vessel caliber, tortuosity, and fractal dimension, although the authors concluded that retinopathy was more prevalent in dementia [203]. One possible explanation for the variation in results was suggested to be the absence of histopathological confirmation of AD diagnosis as well as lack of dementia severity reports. However, some studies using immunohistochemistry have reported absence of markers for AD in the visual system (Tables 1 and 2). A recent investigation done on postmortem eye tissue obtained from AD patients failed to report any indication of tau, Aβ, TDP-43, ubiquitin, or α-synuclein and showed no evidence of inclusions, deposits, or other protein accumulation in any region of the globe [198]. A similar result was obtained in another postmortem study, where no Aβ deposits or abnormal tau accumulations were detected in the lens, retina, or other structures in the eyes of AD patients [204]. Another study found hyperphosphorylated tau but not Aβ aggregates in postmortem retinas from AD patients [77]. These results contrast previously mentioned studies where AD pathological changes in the eyes were found. Differences in experimental procedures or in AD disease stage may partly explain some of these discrepancies. Nonetheless, the reported absence of AD markers in the eye may suggest that the disease compromises or develops in a dissimilar manner in the brain and in the eye. As well, other biochemical, structural, or imaging markers (i.e., OCT) in the visual system may be more adequate than Aβ or tau in the eye. This points to the need for developing future studies with more precise inclusion/exclusion criteria, larger patient populations with clear AD severity classifications and staging (for example, MCI, EOAD, and LOAD), and standardized measurements for vasculature analysis.

Currently, several clinical trials are being conducted to help clarify the use of visual components as possible biomarkers for AD. The National Institutes of Health- (NIH-) supported webpage that is responsible for the registry of clinical trials (https://clinicaltrials.gov/) has 38 studies related to AD and the eye. These studies have a wide range of objectives including measurement of saccades and eye-tracking, visuospatial attention, retinal thickness, and amyloid deposition. Although studying optic changes in AD is not without controversy, it represents a promising target that needs to be carefully studied in the future, both in preclinical and clinical studies, as the potential benefit of eye examinations as biomarkers for AD, in particular for detection of early changes, could have a significant impact in clinical practice.

7. Conclusions

The visual system might rise to be an important biomarker of AD because the functional and pathological mechanisms with the CNS are similar. AD patients manifest a reduction in thickness of the retina, explained by a selective neurodegenerative process induced by Aβ. Although the precise reason why certain retinal layers or quadrants are affected is not clear, neuronal loss is the result of the presence of several mechanisms such as inflammation, oxidative stress, and vascular dysfunction. There are divergent points of view about the relationship between ocular manifestations that need to be clarified. However, a better knowledge of pathophysiological mechanisms could lead to the development of new biomarkers during early stages of the disease. Ocular and visual examinations in AD would be a less invasive and more cost-effective method, than the techniques that are currently used. Noninvasive ophthalmological assessment could complement the AD diagnosis and would be a helpful tool to evaluate the disease progression. Novel functional studies of the visual system, as well as objective measurements of vascular and inflammatory changes in the eye, may play an important role in the evaluation of early stages of AD, including MCI and people at risk of dementia.

Abbreviations

ACh: Acetylcholine
AD: Alzheimer's disease
Aβ: Amyloid-beta
AMD: Age-related macular degeneration
ApoE: Apolipoprotein E
APP: Amyloid precursor protein
BACE-1: Beta-site amyloid precursor protein cleaving enzyme 1
BM: Bruch's membrane
CNS: Central nervous system
EOAD: Early-onset Alzheimer's disease
ERG: Electroretinogram
GCL: Ganglion cell layer
IL-1β: Interleukin-1β
IL-6: Interleukin-6
IL-8: Interleukin-8
IL-33: Interleukin-33
INL: Inner nuclear layer
IPL: Inner plexiform layer
LOAD: Late-onset AD
mAChR: Muscarinic acetylcholine receptor
MCI: Mild cognitive impairment
MMSE: Mini-Mental State Examination
nAChR: Nicotinic acetylcholine receptor
NIH: National Institutes of Health
NFL: Nerve fiber layer
NFT: Neurofibrillary tangles
NO: Nitric oxide

OCT: Optical coherence tomography
ONL: Outer nuclear layer
OPL: Outer plexiform layer
OS: Oxidative stress
ROS: Reactive oxygen species
RPE: Retinal pigment epithelium
SD-OCT: Spectral domain-optical coherence tomography
SP: Senile plaques
VEP: Visual evoked potential.

Conflicts of Interest

The authors declare no conflicts of interest.

Authors' Contributions

María Alejandra Cerquera-Jaramillo and Mauricio O. Nava-Mesa have contributed equally to this paper.

Acknowledgments

We thank Rachel James, Ph.D., from Edanz Group (http://www.edanzediting.com/ac) for editing a draft of this manuscript.

References

[1] P. Scheltens, K. Blennow, M. M. B. Breteler et al., "Alzheimer's disease," *The Lancet*, vol. 388, no. 10043, pp. 505–517, 2016.

[2] G. M. Ashraf, S. Chibber, Mohammad et al., "Recent updates on the association between Alzheimer's disease and vascular dementia," *Medicinal Chemistry*, vol. 12, no. 3, pp. 226–237, 2016.

[3] M. Prince, A. Wimo, M. Guerchet, G.-C. Ali, Y.-T. Wu, and M. Prina, *World Alzheimer Report 2015: The Global Impact of Dementia: an Analysis of Prevalence, Incidence, Cost and Trends*, Alzheimer's Disease International, London, 2015.

[4] R. A. Hickman, A. Faustin, and T. Wisniewski, "Alzheimer disease and its growing epidemic: risk factors, biomarkers, and the urgent need for therapeutics," *Neurologic Clinics*, vol. 34, no. 4, pp. 941–953, 2016.

[5] C. A. Lane, J. Hardy, and J. M. Schott, "Alzheimer's disease," *European Journal of Neurology*, vol. 25, no. 1, pp. 59–70, 2018.

[6] C. R. Jack Jr, M. S. Albert, D. S. Knopman et al., "Introduction to the recommendations from the National Institute on Aging-Alzheimer's Association workgroups on diagnostic guidelines for Alzheimer's disease," *Alzheimer's & Dementia: The Journal of the Alzheimer's Association*, vol. 7, no. 3, pp. 257–262, 2011.

[7] M. F. Mendez, "Early-onset Alzheimer disease," *Neurologic Clinics*, vol. 35, no. 2, pp. 263–281, 2017.

[8] A. L. Pierce, S. S. Bullain, and C. H. Kawas, "Late-onset Alzheimer disease," *Neurologic Clinics*, vol. 35, no. 2, pp. 283–293, 2017.

[9] I. Bos, S. J. Vos, L. Frölich et al., "The frequency and influence of dementia risk factors in prodromal Alzheimer's disease," *Neurobiology of Aging*, vol. 56, pp. 33–40, 2017.

[10] S. L. Rosenthal and M. I. Kamboh, "Late-onset Alzheimer's disease genes and the potentially implicated pathways," *Current Genetic Medicine Reports*, vol. 2, no. 2, pp. 85–101, 2014.

[11] R. B. Maccioni, J. P. Muñoz, and L. Barbeito, "The molecular bases of Alzheimer's disease and other neurodegenerative disorders," *Archives of Medical Research*, vol. 32, no. 5, pp. 367–381, 2001.

[12] H. W. Querfurth and F. M. LaFerla, "Alzheimer's disease," *The New England Journal of Medicine*, vol. 362, no. 4, pp. 329–344, 2010.

[13] P. Agostinho, A. Pliássova, C. R. Oliveira, and R. A. Cunha, "Localization and trafficking of amyloid-β protein precursor and secretases: impact on Alzheimer's disease," *Journal of Alzheimer's Disease*, vol. 45, no. 2, pp. 329–347, 2015.

[14] A. Chiarini, U. Armato, E. Gardenal, L. Gui, and I. Dal Prà, "Amyloid β-exposed human astrocytes overproduce phospho-tau and overrelease it within exosomes, effects suppressed by calcilytic NPS 2143-further implications for Alzheimer's therapy," *Frontiers in Neuroscience*, vol. 11, 2017.

[15] C. Lindberg, M.-L. B. Selenica, A. Westlind-Danielsson, and M. Schultzberg, "β-Amyloid protein structure determines the nature of cytokine release from rat microglia," *Journal of Molecular Neuroscience*, vol. 27, no. 1, pp. 1–12, 2005.

[16] L. Hou, Y. Liu, X. Wang et al., "The effects of amyloid-β42 oligomer on the proliferation and activation of astrocytes in vitro," *In Vitro Cellular & Developmental Biology-Animal*, vol. 47, no. 8, pp. 573–580, 2011.

[17] R. E. González-Reyes, M. O. Nava-Mesa, K. Vargas-Sánchez, D. Ariza-Salamanca, and L. Mora-Muñoz, "Involvement of astrocytes in Alzheimer's disease from a neuroinflammatory and oxidative stress perspective," *Frontiers in Molecular Neuroscience*, vol. 10, p. 427, 2017.

[18] F. M. Elahi and B. L. Miller, "A clinicopathological approach to the diagnosis of dementia," *Nature Reviews Neurology*, vol. 13, no. 8, pp. 457–476, 2017.

[19] N. El Kadmiri, N. Said, I. Slassi, B. El Moutawakil, and S. Nadifi, "Biomarkers for Alzheimer disease: classical and novel candidates' review," *Neuroscience*, vol. 370, pp. 181–190, 2018.

[20] G. B. Frisoni, M. Boccardi, F. Barkhof et al., "Strategic roadmap for an early diagnosis of Alzheimer's disease based on biomarkers," *The Lancet Neurology*, vol. 16, no. 8, pp. 661–676, 2017.

[21] L. Y. L. Chang, J. Lowe, A. Ardiles et al., "Alzheimer's disease in the human eye. Clinical tests that identify ocular and visual information processing deficit as biomarkers," *Alzheimer's & Dementia*, vol. 10, no. 2, pp. 251–261, 2014.

[22] F. Z. Javaid, J. Brenton, L. Guo, and M. F. Cordeiro, "Visual and ocular manifestations of Alzheimer's disease and their use as biomarkers for diagnosis and progression," *Frontiers in Neurology*, vol. 7, 2016.

[23] D.-H. Lee, A. B. Laemmer, A. Waschbisch et al., "Neuromyelitis optica presenting with relapses under treatment with natalizumab: a case report," *Journal of Medical Case Reports*, vol. 8, no. 1, p. 155, 2014.

[24] V. Kavcic, W. Vaughn, and C. J. Duffy, "Distinct visual motion processing impairments in aging and Alzheimer's disease," *Vision Research*, vol. 51, no. 3, pp. 386–395, 2011.

[25] M. P. Bambo, E. Garcia-Martin, S. Otin et al., "Visual function and retinal nerve fibre layer degeneration in patients with Alzheimer disease: correlations with severity

of dementia," *Acta Ophthalmologica*, vol. 93, no. 6, pp. e507–e508, 2015.

[26] C. Y.-L. Cheung, Y.-T. Ong, M. K. Ikram, C. Chen, and T. Y. Wong, "Retinal microvasculature in Alzheimer's disease," *Journal of Alzheimer's Disease*, vol. 42, Supplement 4, pp. S339–S352, 2014.

[27] M. K. Ikram, C. Y. Cheung, T. Y. Wong, and C. P. L. H. Chen, "Retinal pathology as biomarker for cognitive impairment and Alzheimer's disease," *Journal of Neurology, Neurosurgery, and Psychiatry*, vol. 83, no. 9, pp. 917–922, 2012.

[28] N. A. Arnaoutoglou, M. Arnaoutoglou, P. Nemtsas, V. Costa, S. J. Baloyannis, and K. P. Ebmeier, "Color perception differentiates Alzheimer's disease (AD) from vascular dementia (VaD) patients," *International Psychogeriatrics*, vol. 29, no. 8, pp. 1355–1361, 2017.

[29] C. M. Carroll and Y.-M. Li, "Physiological and pathological roles of the γ-secretase complex," *Brain Research Bulletin*, vol. 126, Part 2, pp. 199–206, 2016.

[30] L. J. Sosa, A. Cáceres, S. Dupraz, M. Oksdath, S. Quiroga, and A. Lorenzo, "The physiological role of the amyloid precursor protein as an adhesion molecule in the developing nervous system," *Journal of Neurochemistry*, vol. 143, no. 1, pp. 11–29, 2017.

[31] E. Montagna, M. M. Dorostkar, and J. Herms, "The role of APP in structural spine plasticity," *Frontiers in Molecular Neuroscience*, vol. 10, 2017.

[32] A. T. Rao, A. J. Degnan, and L. M. Levy, "Genetics of Alzheimer disease," *American Journal of Neuroradiology*, vol. 35, no. 3, pp. 457-458, 2014.

[33] R. Aleksis, F. Oleskovs, K. Jaudzems, J. Pahnke, and H. Biverstål, "Structural studies of amyloid-β peptides: unlocking the mechanism of aggregation and the associated toxicity," *Biochimie*, vol. 140, pp. 176–192, 2017.

[34] B. De Strooper and E. Karran, "The cellular phase of Alzheimer's disease," *Cell*, vol. 164, no. 4, pp. 603–615, 2016.

[35] D. Zhu, Y. Lai, P. B. Shelat, C. Hu, G. Y. Sun, and J. C.-M. Lee, "Phospholipases A2 mediate amyloid-beta peptide-induced mitochondrial dysfunction," *The Journal of Neuroscience*, vol. 26, no. 43, pp. 11111–11119, 2006.

[36] S. Askarova, X. Yang, W. Sheng, G. Y. Sun, and J. C.-M. Lee, "Role of Aβ-receptor for advanced glycation endproducts interaction in oxidative stress and cytosolic phospholipase A_2 activation in astrocytes and cerebral endothelial cells," *Neuroscience*, vol. 199, pp. 375–385, 2011.

[37] Z. Esposito, L. Belli, S. Toniolo, G. Sancesario, C. Bianconi, and A. Martorana, "Amyloid β, glutamate, excitotoxicity in Alzheimer's disease: are we on the right track?," *CNS Neuroscience & Therapeutics*, vol. 19, no. 8, pp. 549–555, 2013.

[38] M. O. Nava-Mesa, L. Jiménez-Díaz, J. Yajeya, and J. D. Navarro-Lopez, "GABAergic neurotransmission and new strategies of neuromodulation to compensate synaptic dysfunction in early stages of Alzheimer's disease," *Frontiers in Cellular Neuroscience*, vol. 8, p. 167, 2014.

[39] L. Mosconi, S. Sorbi, M. J. de Leon et al., "Hypometabolism exceeds atrophy in presymptomatic early-onset familial Alzheimer's disease," *Journal of Nuclear Medicine*, vol. 47, no. 11, pp. 1778–1786, 2006.

[40] L. Mosconi, A. Pupi, and M. J. De Leon, "Brain glucose hypometabolism and oxidative stress in preclinical Alzheimer's disease," *Annals of the New York Academy of Sciences*, vol. 1147, no. 1, pp. 180–195, 2008.

[41] M. S. Forman, D. Lal, B. Zhang et al., "Transgenic mouse model of tau pathology in astrocytes leading to nervous system degeneration," *The Journal of Neuroscience*, vol. 25, no. 14, pp. 3539–3550, 2005.

[42] M. Goedert, D. S. Eisenberg, and R. A. Crowther, "Propagation of tau aggregates and neurodegeneration," *Annual Review of Neuroscience*, vol. 40, no. 1, pp. 189–210, 2017.

[43] J. A. Ratnayaka, L. C. Serpell, and A. J. Lotery, "Dementia of the eye: the role of amyloid beta in retinal degeneration," *Eye*, vol. 29, no. 8, pp. 1013–1026, 2015.

[44] T. M. Shah, S. M. Gupta, P. Chatterjee, M. Campbell, and R. N. Martins, "Beta-amyloid sequelae in the eye: a critical review on its diagnostic significance and clinical relevance in Alzheimer's disease," *Molecular Psychiatry*, vol. 22, no. 3, pp. 353–363, 2017.

[45] P. van Wijngaarden, X. Hadoux, M. Alwan, S. Keel, and M. Dirani, "Emerging ocular biomarkers of Alzheimer disease," *Clinical & Experimental Ophthalmology*, vol. 45, no. 1, pp. 54–61, 2017.

[46] J. K. H. Lim, Q.-X. Li, Z. He et al., "The eye as a biomarker for Alzheimer's disease," *Frontiers in Neuroscience*, vol. 10, 2016.

[47] V. K. Gupta, N. Chitranshi, V. B. Gupta et al., "Amyloid β accumulation and inner retinal degenerative changes in Alzheimer's disease transgenic mouse," *Neuroscience Letters*, vol. 623, pp. 52–56, 2016.

[48] N. J. Hart, Y. Koronyo, K. L. Black, and M. Koronyo-Hamaoui, "Ocular indicators of Alzheimer's: exploring disease in the retina," *Acta Neuropathologica*, vol. 132, no. 6, pp. 767–787, 2016.

[49] A. London, I. Benhar, and M. Schwartz, "The retina as a window to the brain-from eye research to CNS disorders," *Nature Reviews Neurology*, vol. 9, no. 1, pp. 44–53, 2013.

[50] Y. Kusne, A. B. Wolf, K. Townley, M. Conway, and G. A. Peyman, "Visual system manifestations of Alzheimer's disease," *Acta Ophthalmologica*, vol. 95, no. 8, pp. e668–e676, 2017.

[51] K. Chiu, T.-F. Chan, A. Wu, I. Y.-P. Leung, K.-F. So, and R. C.-C. Chang, "Neurodegeneration of the retina in mouse models of Alzheimer's disease: what can we learn from the retina?," *Age*, vol. 34, no. 3, pp. 633–649, 2012.

[52] E. Vecino, F. D. Rodriguez, N. Ruzafa, X. Pereiro, and S. C. Sharma, "Glia-neuron interactions in the mammalian retina," *Progress in Retinal and Eye Research*, vol. 51, pp. 1–40, 2016.

[53] A. Wakx, M. Dutot, F. Massicot, F. Mascarelli, G. A. Limb, and P. Rat, "Amyloid β peptide induces apoptosis through P2X7 cell death receptor in retinal cells: modulation by marine omega-3 fatty acid DHA and EPA," *Applied Biochemistry and Biotechnology*, vol. 178, no. 2, pp. 368–381, 2016.

[54] V. Dinet, J. Bruban, N. Chalour et al., "Distinct effects of inflammation on gliosis, osmohomeostasis, and vascular integrity during amyloid beta-induced retinal degeneration," *Aging Cell*, vol. 11, no. 4, pp. 683–693, 2012.

[55] M. M. Edwards, J. J. Rodríguez, R. Gutierrez-Lanza, J. Yates, A. Verkhratsky, and G. A. Lutty, "Retinal macroglia changes in a triple transgenic mouse model of Alzheimer's disease," *Experimental Eye Research*, vol. 127, pp. 252–260, 2014.

[56] G. Chidlow, J. P. M. Wood, J. Manavis, J. Finnie, and R. J. Casson, "Investigations into retinal pathology in the early stages of a mouse model of Alzheimer's disease," *Journal of Alzheimer's Disease*, vol. 56, no. 2, pp. 655–675, 2017.

[57] R. T. Liu, A. Wang, E. To et al., "Vinpocetine inhibits amyloid-beta induced activation of NF-κB, NLRP3 inflammasome and cytokine production in retinal pigment epithelial cells," *Experimental Eye Research*, vol. 127, pp. 49–58, 2014.

[58] J. P. Cunha and A. Castanheira-Dinis, "Alzheimer disease: OCT retinal and choroidal thickness," in *Proceedings of the 5th International Conference on Photonics, Optics and Laser Technology*, Porto, Portugal, 2017.

[59] A. M. Birch, "The contribution of astrocytes to Alzheimer's disease," *Biochemical Society Transactions*, vol. 42, no. 5, pp. 1316–1320, 2014.

[60] C. Iadecola and M. Nedergaard, "Glial regulation of the cerebral microvasculature," *Nature Neuroscience*, vol. 10, no. 11, pp. 1369–1376, 2007.

[61] K. Kisler, A. R. Nelson, A. Montagne, and B. V. Zlokovic, "Cerebral blood flow regulation and neurovascular dysfunction in Alzheimer disease," *Nature Reviews Neuroscience*, vol. 18, no. 7, pp. 419–434, 2017.

[62] T. Iram, D. Trudler, D. Kain et al., "Astrocytes from old Alzheimer's disease mice are impaired in Aβ uptake and in neuroprotection," *Neurobiology of Disease*, vol. 96, pp. 84–94, 2016.

[63] B. Ghebrehiwet, X. Feng, R. Kumar, and E. I. B. Peerschke, "Complement component C1q induces endothelial cell adhesion and spreading through a docking/signaling partnership of C1q receptors and integrins," *International Immunopharmacology*, vol. 3, no. 3, pp. 299–310, 2003.

[64] S. E. Perez, S. Lumayag, B. Kovacs, E. J. Mufson, and S. Xu, "β-Amyloid deposition and functional impairment in the retina of the APPswe/PS1ΔE9 transgenic mouse model of Alzheimer's disease," *Investigative Ophthalmology & Visual Science*, vol. 50, no. 2, pp. 793–800, 2009.

[65] L. Y. Du, L. Y.-L. Chang, A. O. Ardiles et al., "Alzheimer's disease-related protein expression in the retina of *Octodon degus*," *PloS One*, vol. 10, no. 8, article e0135499, 2015.

[66] M. Koronyo-Hamaoui, Y. Koronyo, A. V. Ljubimov et al., "Identification of amyloid plaques in retinas from Alzheimer's patients and noninvasive in vivo optical imaging of retinal plaques in a mouse model," *NeuroImage*, vol. 54, Supplement 1, pp. S204–S217, 2011.

[67] Y. Tsai, B. Lu, A. V. Ljubimov et al., "Ocular changes in TgF344-AD rat model of Alzheimer's disease," *Investigative Ophthalmology & Visual Science*, vol. 55, no. 1, pp. 523–534, 2014.

[68] J. C. Blanks, S. Y. Schmidt, Y. Torigoe, K. V. Porrello, D. R. Hinton, and R. H. I. Blanks, "Retinal pathology in Alzheimer's disease. II. Regional neuron loss and glial changes in GCL," *Neurobiology of Aging*, vol. 17, no. 3, pp. 385–395, 1996.

[69] C. H. Andrade-Moraes, A. V. Oliveira-Pinto, E. Castro-Fonseca et al., "Cell number changes in Alzheimer's disease relate to dementia, not to plaques and tangles," *Brain*, vol. 136, no. 12, pp. 3738–3752, 2013.

[70] G. Leuba and R. Kraftsik, "Visual cortex in Alzheimer's disease: occurrence of neuronal death and glial proliferation, and correlation with pathological hallmarks," *Neurobiology of Aging*, vol. 15, no. 1, pp. 29–43, 1994.

[71] V. Luibl, J. M. Isas, R. Kayed, C. G. Glabe, R. Langen, and J. Chen, "Drusen deposits associated with aging and age-related macular degeneration contain nonfibrillar amyloid oligomers," *The Journal of Clinical Investigation*, vol. 116, no. 2, pp. 378–385, 2006.

[72] D. H. Anderson, R. F. Mullins, G. S. Hageman, and L. V. Johnson, "A role for local inflammation in the formation of drusen in the aging eye," *American Journal of Ophthalmology*, vol. 134, no. 3, pp. 411–431, 2002.

[73] A. N. Nilson, K. C. English, J. E. Gerson et al., "Tau oligomers associate with inflammation in the brain and retina of tauopathy mice and in neurodegenerative diseases," *Journal of Alzheimer's Disease*, vol. 55, no. 3, pp. 1083–1099, 2017.

[74] M. Chiasseu, L. Alarcon-Martinez, N. Belforte et al., "Tau accumulation in the retina promotes early neuronal dysfunction and precedes brain pathology in a mouse model of Alzheimer's disease," *Molecular Neurodegeneration*, vol. 12, no. 1, p. 58, 2017.

[75] W. Ho, Y. Leung, A. W. Tsang, K. F. So, K. Chiu, and R. C. Chang, "Review: Tauopathy in the retina and optic nerve: does it shadow pathological changes in the brain?," *Molecular Vision*, vol. 18, pp. 2700–2710, 2012.

[76] H. Zhao, R. Chang, H. Che et al., "Hyperphosphorylation of tau protein by calpain regulation in retina of Alzheimer's disease transgenic mouse," *Neuroscience Letters*, vol. 551, pp. 12–16, 2013.

[77] C. Schön, N. A. Hoffmann, S. M. Ochs et al., "Long-term in vivo imaging of fibrillar tau in the retina of P301S transgenic mice," *PloS One*, vol. 7, no. 12, article e53547, 2012.

[78] M. Rudolf, M. E. Clark, M. F. Chimento, C.-M. Li, N. E. Medeiros, and C. A. Curcio, "Prevalence and morphology of druse types in the macula and periphery of eyes with age-related maculopathy," *Investigative Ophthalmology & Visual Science*, vol. 49, no. 3, pp. 1200–1209, 2008.

[79] S. McHarg, S. J. Clark, A. J. Day, and P. N. Bishop, "Age-related macular degeneration and the role of the complement system," *Molecular Immunology*, vol. 67, no. 1, pp. 43–50, 2015.

[80] A. I. Pogue, P. Dua, J. M. Hill, and W. J. Lukiw, "Progressive inflammatory pathology in the retina of aluminum-fed 5xFAD transgenic mice," *Journal of Inorganic Biochemistry*, vol. 152, pp. 206–209, 2015.

[81] V. V. Ermilov and A. A. Nesterova, "β-Amyloidopathy in the pathogenesis of age-related macular degeneration in correlation with neurodegenerative diseases," *Advances in Experimental Medicine and Biology*, vol. 854, pp. 119–125, 2016.

[82] K. Ohno-Matsui, "Parallel findings in age-related macular degeneration and Alzheimer's disease," *Progress in Retinal and Eye Research*, vol. 30, no. 4, pp. 217–238, 2011.

[83] T. Yoshida, K. Ohno-Matsui, S. Ichinose et al., "The potential role of amyloid β in the pathogenesis of age-related macular degeneration," *The Journal of Clinical Investigation*, vol. 115, no. 10, pp. 2793–2800, 2005.

[84] L. M. Tai, R. Thomas, F. M. Marottoli et al., "The role of APOE in cerebrovascular dysfunction," *Acta Neuropathologica*, vol. 131, no. 5, pp. 709–723, 2016.

[85] J.-T. Yu, L. Tan, and J. Hardy, "Apolipoprotein E in Alzheimer's disease: an update," *Annual Review of Neuroscience*, vol. 37, no. 1, pp. 79–100, 2014.

[86] J. Hardy and D. J. Selkoe, "The amyloid hypothesis of Alzheimer's disease: progress and problems on the road to therapeutics," *Science*, vol. 297, no. 5580, pp. 353–356, 2002.

[87] H. K. Dong, J.-A. Gim, S. H. Yeo, and H.-S. Kim, "Integrated late onset Alzheimer's disease (LOAD) susceptibility genes:

cholesterol metabolism and trafficking perspectives," *Gene*, vol. 597, pp. 10–16, 2017.

[88] A. T. Baker-Nigh, K. G. Mawuenyega, J. G. Bollinger et al., "Human central nervous system (CNS) ApoE isoforms are increased by age, differentially altered by amyloidosis, and relative amounts reversed in the CNS compared with plasma," *The Journal of Biological Chemistry*, vol. 291, no. 53, pp. 27204–27218, 2016.

[89] T. Masuda, M. Shimazawa, Y. Hashimoto et al., "Apolipoprotein E2 and E3, but not E4, promote retinal pathologic neovascularization," *Investigative Ophthalmology & Visual Science*, vol. 58, no. 2, pp. 1208–1217, 2017.

[90] I. Maharshak, S. Salomon-Zimri, R. Antes et al., "The effects of the apoE4 genotype on the developing mouse retina," *Experimental Eye Research*, vol. 145, pp. 17–25, 2016.

[91] O. Levy, S. Lavalette, S. J. Hu et al., "APOE isoforms control pathogenic subretinal inflammation in age-related macular degeneration," *The Journal of Neuroscience*, vol. 35, no. 40, pp. 13568–13576, 2015.

[92] J. M. Ong, N. C. Zorapapel, K. A. Rich et al., "Effects of cholesterol and apolipoprotein E on retinal abnormalities in ApoE-deficient mice," *Investigative Ophthalmology & Visual Science*, vol. 42, no. 8, pp. 1891–1900, 2001.

[93] S. Frost, R. Guymer, K. Zaw Aung et al., "Alzheimer's disease and the early signs of age-related macular degeneration," *Current Alzheimer Research*, vol. 13, no. 11, pp. 1259–1266, 2016.

[94] M. A. Williams, V. Silvestri, D. Craig, A. P. Passmore, and G. Silvestri, "The prevalence of age-related macular degeneration in Alzheimer's disease," *Journal of Alzheimer's Disease*, vol. 42, no. 3, pp. 909–914, 2014.

[95] V. S. Pelak and W. Hills, "Vision in Alzheimer's disease: a focus on the anterior afferent pathway," *Neurodegenerative Disease Management*, vol. 8, no. 1, pp. 49–67, 2018.

[96] R. A. Armstrong, "Visual field defects in Alzheimer's disease patients may reflect differential pathology in the primary visual cortex," *Optometry and Vision Science*, vol. 73, no. 11, pp. 677–682, 1996.

[97] X. Liu, W. Chen, H. Hou et al., "Decreased functional connectivity between the dorsal anterior cingulate cortex and lingual gyrus in Alzheimer's disease patients with depression," *Behavioural Brain Research*, vol. 326, pp. 132–138, 2017.

[98] A. A. Brewer and B. Barton, "Visual cortex in aging and Alzheimer's disease: changes in visual field maps and population receptive fields," *Frontiers in Psychology*, vol. 5, p. 74, 2014.

[99] M. Kiyosawa, T. M. Bosley, J. Chawluk et al., "Alzheimer's disease with prominent visual symptoms: clinical and metabolic evaluation," *Ophthalmology*, vol. 96, no. 7, pp. 1077–1086, 1989.

[100] R. O. Kuljis, "Lesions in the pulvinar in patients with Alzheimer's disease," *Journal of Neuropathology & Experimental Neurology*, vol. 53, no. 2, pp. 202–211, 1994.

[101] D. Erskine, J. P. Taylor, M. J. Firbank et al., "Changes to the lateral geniculate nucleus in Alzheimer's disease but not dementia with Lewy bodies," *Neuropathology and Applied Neurobiology*, vol. 42, no. 4, pp. 366–376, 2016.

[102] R. Feng, L. Li, H. Yu, M. Liu, and W. Zhao, "Melanopsin retinal ganglion cell loss and circadian dysfunction in Alzheimer's disease (review)," *Molecular Medicine Reports*, vol. 13, no. 4, pp. 3397–3400, 2016.

[103] A. N. Coogan, B. Schutová, S. Husung et al., "The circadian system in Alzheimer's disease: disturbances, mechanisms, and opportunities," *Biological Psychiatry*, vol. 74, no. 5, pp. 333–339, 2013.

[104] L. Zhou, Q. Gao, M. Nie et al., "Degeneration and energy shortage in the suprachiasmatic nucleus underlies the circadian rhythm disturbance in ApoE−/− mice: implications for Alzheimer's disease," *Scientific Reports*, vol. 6, no. 1, article 36335, 2016.

[105] J. Van Erum, D. Van Dam, and P. P. De Deyn, "Sleep and Alzheimer's disease: a pivotal role for the suprachiasmatic nucleus," *Sleep Medicine Reviews*, vol. 40, pp. 17–27, 2018.

[106] G. Leuba and K. Saini, "Pathology of subcortical visual centres in relation to cortical degeneration in Alzheimer's disease," *Neuropathology and Applied Neurobiology*, vol. 21, no. 5, pp. 410–422, 1995.

[107] J. Parvizi, G. W. Van Hoesen, and A. Damasio, "The selective vulnerability of brainstem nuclei to Alzheimer's disease," *Annals of Neurology*, vol. 49, no. 1, pp. 53–66, 2001.

[108] F. G. Oliveira-Souza, M. L. DeRamus, T. van Groen, A. E. Lambert, M. S. Bolding, and C. E. Strang, "Retinal changes in the Tg-SwDI mouse model of Alzheimer's disease," *Neuroscience*, vol. 354, pp. 43–53, 2017.

[109] L. Nobili and W. G. Sannita, "Cholinergic modulation, visual function and Alzheimer's dementia," *Vision Research*, vol. 37, no. 24, pp. 3559–3571, 1997.

[110] A. Patricio-Martínez, L. Mendieta, I. Martínez, J. Aguilera, and I. D. Limón, "The recombinant C-terminal fragment of tetanus toxin protects against cholinotoxicity by intraseptal injection of β-amyloid peptide (25-35) in rats," *Neuroscience*, vol. 315, pp. 18–30, 2016.

[111] S. H. Deibel, N. Weishaupt, A. M. Regis et al., "Subtle learning and memory impairment in an idiopathic rat model of Alzheimer's disease utilizing cholinergic depletions and β-amyloid," *Brain Research*, vol. 1646, pp. 12–24, 2016.

[112] R. Schliebs and T. Arendt, "The significance of the cholinergic system in the brain during aging and in Alzheimer's disease," *Journal of Neural Transmission*, vol. 113, no. 11, pp. 1625–1644, 2006.

[113] H. Janíčková, V. Rudajev, P. Zimčík et al., "Uncoupling of M1 muscarinic receptor/G-protein interaction by amyloid β1-42," *Neuropharmacology*, vol. 67, pp. 272–283, 2013.

[114] J. J. Dougherty, J. Wu, and R. A. Nichols, "β-Amyloid regulation of presynaptic nicotinic receptors in rat hippocampus and neocortex," *The Journal of Neuroscience*, vol. 23, no. 17, pp. 6740–6747, 2003.

[115] S. Kar, D. Seto, P. Gaudreau, and R. Quirion, "Beta-amyloid-related peptides inhibit potassium-evoked acetylcholine release from rat hippocampal slices," *The Journal of Neuroscience*, vol. 16, no. 3, pp. 1034–1040, 1996.

[116] J. Mayordomo-Cava, J. Yajeya, J. D. Navarro-López, and L. Jiménez-Díaz, "Amyloid-β modulates the expression of GirK and KCNQ channel genes in the hippocampus," *PLoS One*, vol. 10, no. 7, article e0134385, 2015.

[117] R. N. Leão, L. V. Colom, L. Borgius, O. Kiehn, and A. Fisahn, "Medial septal dysfunction by Aβ-induced KCNQ channel-block in glutamatergic neurons," *Neurobiology of Aging*, vol. 33, no. 9, pp. 2046–2061, 2012.

[118] L. Guo, J. Duggan, and M. Cordeiro, "Alzheimer's disease and retinal neurodegeneration," *Current Alzheimer Research*, vol. 7, no. 1, pp. 3–14, 2010.

[119] N. S. Foldi, R. E. C. White, and L. A. Schaefer, "Detecting effects of donepezil on visual selective attention using signal detection parameters in Alzheimer's disease," *International Journal of Geriatric Psychiatry*, vol. 20, no. 5, pp. 485-488, 2005.

[120] M. Boucart, G. Bubbico, S. szaffarczyk et al., "Donepezil increases contrast sensitivity for the detection of objects in scenes," *Behavioural Brain Research*, vol. 292, pp. 443-447, 2015.

[121] J. P. Cunha, N. Moura-Coelho, R. P. Proença et al., "Alzheimer's disease: a review of its visual system neuropathology. Optical coherence tomography-a potential role as a study tool in vivo," *Graefe's Archive for Clinical and Experimental Ophthalmology*, vol. 254, no. 11, pp. 2079-2092, 2016.

[122] M. H. Madeira, A. F. Ambrósio, and A. R. Santiago, "Glia-mediated retinal neuroinflammation as a biomarker in Alzheimer's disease," *Ophthalmic Research*, vol. 54, no. 4, pp. 204-211, 2015.

[123] G. Coppola, A. di Renzo, L. Ziccardi et al., "Optical coherence tomography in Alzheimer's disease: a meta-analysis," *PLoS One*, vol. 10, no. 8, article e0134750, 2015.

[124] S. Krantic and A. Torriglia, "Retina: source of the earliest biomarkers for Alzheimer's disease?," *Journal of Alzheimer's Disease*, vol. 40, no. 2, pp. 237-243, 2014.

[125] C. La Morgia, F. N. Ross-Cisneros, J. Hannibal, P. Montagna, A. A. Sadun, and V. Carelli, "Melanopsin-expressing retinal ganglion cells: implications for human diseases," *Vision Research*, vol. 51, no. 2, pp. 296-302, 2011.

[126] C. Laske, H. R. Sohrabi, S. M. Frost et al., "Innovative diagnostic tools for early detection of Alzheimer's disease," *Alzheimer's & Dementia*, vol. 11, no. 5, pp. 561-578, 2015.

[127] C. S. Tsai, R. Ritch, B. Schwartz et al., "Optic nerve head and nerve fiber layer in Alzheimer's disease," *Archives of Ophthalmology*, vol. 109, no. 2, pp. 199-204, 1991.

[128] D. R. Hinton, A. A. Sadun, J. C. Blanks, and C. A. Miller, "Optic-nerve degeneration in Alzheimer's disease," *New England Journal of Medicine*, vol. 315, no. 8, pp. 485-487, 1986.

[129] A. A. Sadun and C. J. Bassi, "Optic nerve damage in Alzheimer's disease," *Ophthalmology*, vol. 97, no. 1, pp. 9-17, 1990.

[130] M. P. Bambo, E. Garcia-Martin, F. Gutierrez-Ruiz et al., "Analysis of optic disk color changes in Alzheimer's disease: a potential new biomarker," *Clinical Neurology and Neurosurgery*, vol. 132, pp. 68-73, 2015.

[131] Y. Lu, Z. Li, X. Zhang et al., "Retinal nerve fiber layer structure abnormalities in early Alzheimer's disease: evidence in optical coherence tomography," *Neuroscience Letters*, vol. 480, no. 1, pp. 69-72, 2010.

[132] T. Kusbeci, O. Y. Kusbeci, N. G. Mas, H. S. Karabekir, G. Yavas, and A. Yucel, "Stereological evaluation of the optic nerve volume in Alzheimer disease," *The Journal of Craniofacial Surgery*, vol. 26, no. 5, pp. 1683-1686, 2015.

[133] M. A. Williams, A. J. McGowan, C. R. Cardwell et al., "Retinal microvascular network attenuation in Alzheimer's disease," *Alzheimer's & Dementia: Diagnosis, Assessment & Disease Monitoring*, vol. 1, no. 2, pp. 229-235, 2015.

[134] G. T. Feke, B. T. Hyman, R. A. Stern, and L. R. Pasquale, "Retinal blood flow in mild cognitive impairment and Alzheimer's disease," *Alzheimer's & Dementia: Diagnosis, Assessment & Disease Monitoring*, vol. 1, no. 2, pp. 144-151, 2015.

[135] F. Berisha, G. T. Feke, C. L. Trempe, J. W. McMeel, and C. L. Schepens, "Retinal abnormalities in early Alzheimer's disease," *Investigative Ophthalmology & Visual Science*, vol. 48, no. 5, pp. 2285-2289, 2007.

[136] S. Frost, Y. Kanagasingam, H. Sohrabi et al., "Retinal vascular biomarkers for early detection and monitoring of Alzheimer's disease," *Translational Psychiatry*, vol. 3, no. 2, article e233, 2013.

[137] S. M. Golzan, K. Goozee, D. Georgevsky et al., "Retinal vascular and structural changes are associated with amyloid burden in the elderly: ophthalmic biomarkers of preclinical Alzheimer's disease," *Alzheimer's Research & Therapy*, vol. 9, no. 1, p. 13, 2017.

[138] M. H. Dehabadi, B. M. Davis, T. K. Wong, and M. F. Cordeiro, "Retinal manifestations of Alzheimer's disease," *Neurodegenerative Disease Management*, vol. 4, no. 3, pp. 241-252, 2014.

[139] R. Tzekov and M. Mullan, "Vision function abnormalities in Alzheimer disease," *Survey of Ophthalmology*, vol. 59, no. 4, pp. 414-433, 2014.

[140] D. Mahajan and M. Votruba, "Can the retina be used to diagnose and plot the progression of Alzheimer's disease?," *Acta Ophthalmologica*, vol. 95, no. 8, pp. 768-777, 2017.

[141] Y. Shao, H. Jiang, Y. Wei et al., "Visualization of focal thinning of the ganglion cell-inner plexiform layer in patients with mild cognitive impairment and Alzheimer's disease," *Journal of Alzheimer's Disease*, vol. 64, no. 4, pp. 1261-1273, 2018.

[142] V. Jindal, "Interconnection between brain and retinal neurodegenerations," *Molecular Neurobiology*, vol. 51, no. 3, pp. 885-892, 2015.

[143] S. L. Risacher, D. WuDunn, S. M. Pepin et al., "Visual contrast sensitivity in Alzheimer's disease, mild cognitive impairment, and older adults with cognitive complaints," *Neurobiology of Aging*, vol. 34, no. 4, pp. 1133-1144, 2013.

[144] T. J. Crawford, A. Devereaux, S. Higham, and C. Kelly, "The disengagement of visual attention in Alzheimer's disease: a longitudinal eye-tracking study," *Frontiers in Aging Neuroscience*, vol. 7, p. 118, 2015.

[145] G. Binetti, S. F. Cappa, E. Magni, A. Padovani, A. Bianchetti, and M. Trabucchi, "Disorders of visual and spatial perception in the early stage of Alzheimer's disease," *Annals of the New York Academy of Sciences*, vol. 777, no. 1, pp. 221-225, 1996.

[146] T. B. Adelstein, R. P. Kesner, and D. S. Strassberg, "Spatial recognition and spatial order memory in patients with dementia of the Alzheimer's type," *Neuropsychologia*, vol. 30, no. 1, pp. 59-67, 1992.

[147] M. Rizzo, S. W. Anderson, J. Dawson, R. Myers, and K. Ball, "Visual attention impairments in Alzheimer's disease," *Neurology*, vol. 54, no. 10, pp. 1954-1959, 2000.

[148] C. Flicker, S. H. Ferris, T. Crook, and R. T. Bartus, "Impaired facial recognition memory in aging and dementia," *Alzheimer Disease and Associated Disorders*, vol. 4, no. 1, pp. 43-54, 1990.

[149] M. F. Mendez, M. A. Mendez, R. Martin, K. A. Smyth, and P. J. Whitehouse, "Complex visual disturbances in Alzheimer's disease," *Neurology*, vol. 40, no. 3, Part 1, pp. 439-443, 1990.

[150] M. F. Mendez, R. J. Martin, K. A. Smyth, and P. J. Whitehouse, "Disturbances of person identification in Alzheimer's disease. A retrospective study," *The Journal*

of Nervous and Mental Disease, vol. 180, no. 2, pp. 94–96, 1992.

[151] A. Cronin-Golomb, S. Corkin, J. F. Rizzo, J. Cohen, J. H. Growdon, and K. S. Banks, "Visual dysfunction in Alzheimer's disease: relation to normal aging," *Annals of Neurology*, vol. 29, no. 1, pp. 41–52, 1991.

[152] P. R. Hof and C. Bouras, "Object recognition deficit in Alzheimer's disease: possible disconnection of the occipito-temporal component of the visual system," *Neuroscience Letters*, vol. 122, no. 1, pp. 53–56, 1991.

[153] P. R. Hof, C. Bouras, J. Constantinidis, and J. H. Morrison, "Selective disconnection of specific visual association pathways in cases of Alzheimer's disease presenting with Balint's syndrome," *Journal of Neuropathology and Experimental Neurology*, vol. 49, no. 2, pp. 168–184, 1990.

[154] P.-F. Kaeser, J. Ghika, and F.-X. Borruat, "Visual signs and symptoms in patients with the visual variant of Alzheimer disease," *BMC Ophthalmology*, vol. 15, no. 1, p. 65, 2015.

[155] R. Armstrong and A. Syed, "Alzheimer's disease and the eye," *Ophthalmic and Physiological Optics*, vol. 16, pp. S2–S8, 1996.

[156] V. Polo, M. J. Rodrigo, E. Garcia-Martin et al., "Visual dysfunction and its correlation with retinal changes in patients with Alzheimer's disease," *Eye*, vol. 31, no. 7, pp. 1034–1041, 2017.

[157] S. A. Neargarder, E. R. Stone, A. Cronin-Golomb, and S. Oross, "The impact of acuity on performance of four clinical measures of contrast sensitivity in Alzheimer's disease," *The Journals of Gerontology Series B: Psychological Sciences and Social Sciences*, vol. 58, no. 1, pp. P54–P62, 2003.

[158] F. Sartucci, D. Borghetti, T. Bocci et al., "Dysfunction of the magnocellular stream in Alzheimer's disease evaluated by pattern electroretinograms and visual evoked potentials," *Brain Research Bulletin*, vol. 82, no. 3-4, pp. 169–176, 2010.

[159] G. Salamone, C. di Lorenzo, S. Mosti et al., "Color discrimination performance in patients with Alzheimer's disease," *Dementia and Geriatric Cognitive Disorders*, vol. 27, no. 6, pp. 501–507, 2009.

[160] R. Prettyman, P. Bitsios, and E. Szabadi, "Altered pupillary size and darkness and light reflexes in Alzheimer's disease," *Journal of Neurology, Neurosurgery, and Psychiatry*, vol. 62, no. 6, pp. 665–668, 1997.

[161] R. J. Molitor, P. C. Ko, and B. A. Ally, "Eye movements in Alzheimer's disease," *Journal of Alzheimer's Disease*, vol. 44, no. 1, pp. 1–12, 2015.

[162] W. A. Fletcher and J. A. Sharpe, "Saccadic eye movement dysfunction in Alzheimer's disease," *Annals of Neurology*, vol. 20, no. 4, pp. 464–471, 1986.

[163] O. A. Coubard, "What do we know about eye movements in Alzheimer's disease? The past 37 years and future directions," *Biomarkers in Medicine*, vol. 10, no. 7, pp. 677–680, 2016.

[164] C.-N. Lee and K.-W. Park, "Cognitive functions and stereopsis in patients with parkinson's disease and Alzheimer's disease," *Alzheimer's & Dementia*, vol. 10, no. 4, article P767, 2014.

[165] H. Kergoat, M. J. Kergoat, L. Justino, H. Chertkow, A. Robillard, and H. Bergman, "An evaluation of the retinal nerve fiber layer thickness by scanning laser polarimetry in individuals with dementia of the Alzheimer type," *Acta Ophthalmologica Scandinavica*, vol. 79, no. 2, pp. 187–191, 2001.

[166] S. Kirbas, K. Turkyilmaz, O. Anlar, A. Tufekci, and M. Durmus, "Retinal nerve fiber layer thickness in patients with Alzheimer disease," *Journal of Neuro-Ophthalmology*, vol. 33, no. 1, pp. 58–61, 2013.

[167] A. Trebbastoni, F. D'Antonio, A. Bruscolini et al., "Retinal nerve fibre layer thickness changes in Alzheimer's disease: results from a 12-month prospective case series," *Neuroscience Letters*, vol. 629, pp. 165–170, 2016.

[168] E. Garcia-Martin, M. P. Bambo, M. L. Marques et al., "Ganglion cell layer measurements correlate with disease severity in patients with Alzheimer's disease," *Acta Ophthalmologica*, vol. 94, no. 6, pp. e454–e459, 2016.

[169] D. Liu, L. Zhang, Z. Li et al., "Thinner changes of the retinal nerve fiber layer in patients with mild cognitive impairment and Alzheimer's disease," *BMC Neurology*, vol. 15, no. 1, p. 14, 2015.

[170] A. Kesler, V. Vakhapova, A. D. Korczyn, E. Naftaliev, and M. Neudorfer, "Retinal thickness in patients with mild cognitive impairment and Alzheimer's disease," *Clinical Neurology and Neurosurgery*, vol. 113, no. 7, pp. 523–526, 2011.

[171] C. Paquet, M. Boissonnot, F. Roger, P. Dighiero, R. Gil, and J. Hugon, "Abnormal retinal thickness in patients with mild cognitive impairment and Alzheimer's disease," *Neuroscience Letters*, vol. 420, no. 2, pp. 97–99, 2007.

[172] P. J. Snyder, L. N. Johnson, Y. Y. Lim et al., "Nonvascular retinal imaging markers of preclinical Alzheimer's disease," *Alzheimer's & Dementia: Diagnosis, Assessment & Disease Monitoring*, vol. 4, pp. 169–178, 2016.

[173] H. A. Bayhan, S. Aslan Bayhan, A. Celikbilek, N. Tanık, and C. Gürdal, "Evaluation of the chorioretinal thickness changes in Alzheimer's disease using spectral-domain optical coherence tomography," *Clinical & Experimental Ophthalmology*, vol. 43, no. 2, pp. 145–151, 2015.

[174] F. J. Ascaso, N. Cruz, P. J. Modrego et al., "Retinal alterations in mild cognitive impairment and Alzheimer's disease: an optical coherence tomography study," *Journal of Neurology*, vol. 261, no. 8, pp. 1522–1530, 2014.

[175] D. Rodriguez-Mena, C. Almarcegui, I. Dolz, L. E. Pablo, and E. Garcia-Martin, "Application of electrophysiological tests in the study of neurological diseases with visual involvement," *Archivos De La Sociedad Espanola De Oftalmologia*, vol. 87, no. 10, pp. 311–314, 2012.

[176] S. H. Choi, S. J. Park, and N. R. Kim, "Macular ganglion cell -inner plexiform layer thickness is associated with clinical progression in mild cognitive impairment and Alzheimers disease," *PLoS One*, vol. 11, no. 9, article e0162202, 2016.

[177] E. O. Oktem, E. Derle, S. Kibaroglu, C. Oktem, I. Akkoyun, and U. Can, "The relationship between the degree of cognitive impairment and retinal nerve fiber layer thickness," *Neurological Sciences*, vol. 36, no. 7, pp. 1141–1146, 2015.

[178] L. Gao, Y. Liu, X. Li, Q. Bai, and P. Liu, "Abnormal retinal nerve fiber layer thickness and macula lutea in patients with mild cognitive impairment and Alzheimer's disease," *Archives of Gerontology and Geriatrics*, vol. 60, no. 1, pp. 162–167, 2015.

[179] E. Salobrar-Garcia, I. Hoyas, M. Leal et al., "Analysis of retinal peripapillary segmentation in early Alzheimer's disease patients," *BioMed Research International*, vol. 2015, Article ID 636548, 8 pages, 2015.

[180] J. den Haan, F. D. Verbraak, P. J. Visser, and F. H. Bouwman, "Retinal thickness in Alzheimer's disease: a systematic review and meta-analysis," *Alzheimer's & Dementia: Diagnosis, Assessment & Disease Monitoring*, vol. 6, pp. 162–170, 2017.

[181] L. P. Cunha, L. C. Lopes, L. V. F. Costa-Cunha et al., "Macular thickness measurements with frequency domain-OCT for quantification of retinal neural loss and its correlation with cognitive impairment in Alzheimer's disease," *PLoS One*, vol. 11, no. 4, article e0153830, 2016.

[182] J. P. Cunha, R. Proença, A. Dias-Santos et al., "Choroidal thinning: Alzheimer's disease and aging," *Alzheimer's & Dementia : Diagnosis, Assessment & Disease Monitoring*, vol. 8, pp. 11–17, 2017.

[183] A. Trebbastoni, M. Marcelli, F. Mallone et al., "Attenuation of choroidal thickness in patients with Alzheimer disease: evidence from an Italian prospective study," *Alzheimer Disease and Associated Disorders*, vol. 31, no. 2, pp. 128–134, 2017.

[184] V. E. Pollock, L. S. Schneider, H. C. Chui, V. Henderson, M. Zemansky, and R. B. Sloane, "Visual evoked potentials in dementia: a meta-analysis and empirical study of Alzheimer's disease patients," *Biological Psychiatry*, vol. 25, no. 8, pp. 1003–1013, 1989.

[185] S. Holroyd and M. L. Shepherd, "Alzheimer's disease: a review for the ophthalmologist," *Survey of Ophthalmology*, vol. 45, no. 6, pp. 516–524, 2001.

[186] B. Katz and S. Rimmer, "Ophthalmologic manifestations of Alzheimer's disease," *Survey of Ophthalmology*, vol. 34, no. 1, pp. 31–43, 1989.

[187] R. Kromer, N. Serbecic, L. Hausner, L. Froelich, and S. C. Beutelspacher, "Comparison of visual evoked potentials and retinal nerve fiber layer thickness in Alzheimer's disease," *Frontiers in Neurology*, vol. 4, 2013.

[188] P. K. Iseri, Ö. Altinaş, T. Tokay, and N. Yüksel, "Relationship between cognitive impairment and retinal morphological and visual functional abnormalities in Alzheimer disease," *Journal of Neuro-Ophthalmology*, vol. 26, no. 1, pp. 18–24, 2006.

[189] V. Parisi, R. Restuccia, F. Fattapposta, C. Mina, M. G. Bucci, and F. Pierelli, "Morphological and functional retinal impairment in Alzheimer's disease patients," *Clinical Neurophysiology*, vol. 112, no. 10, pp. 1860–1867, 2001.

[190] K. Krasodomska, W. Lubiński, A. Potemkowski, and K. Honczarenko, "Pattern electroretinogram (PERG) and pattern visual evoked potential (PVEP) in the early stages of Alzheimer's disease," *Documenta Ophthalmologica*, vol. 121, no. 2, pp. 111–121, 2010.

[191] H. Kergoat, M.-J. Kergoat, L. Justino, H. Chertkow, A. Robillard, and H. Bergman, "Visual retinocortical function in dementia of the Alzheimer type," *Gerontology*, vol. 48, no. 4, pp. 197–203, 2002.

[192] B. Katz, S. Rimmer, V. Iragui, and R. Katzman, "Abnormal pattern electroretinogram in Alzheimer's disease: evidence for retinal ganglion cell degeneration?," *Annals of Neurology*, vol. 26, no. 2, pp. 221–225, 1989.

[193] G. L. Trick, M. C. Barris, and M. Bickler-Bluth, "Abnormal pattern electroretinograms in patients with senile dementia of the Alzheimer type," *Annals of Neurology*, vol. 26, no. 2, pp. 226–231, 1989.

[194] L. Justino, M. J. Kergoat, H. Bergman, H. Chertkow, A. Robillard, and H. Kergoat, "Neuroretinal function is normal in early dementia of the Alzheimer type," *Neurobiology of Aging*, vol. 22, no. 4, pp. 691–695, 2001.

[195] F. Altimiras, B. Uszczynska-Ratajczak, F. Camara et al., "Brain transcriptome sequencing of a natural model of Alzheimer's disease," *Frontiers in Aging Neuroscience*, vol. 9, 2017.

[196] X.-F. He, Y.-T. Liu, C. Peng, F. Zhang, S. Zhuang, and J.-S. Zhang, "Optical coherence tomography assessed retinal nerve fiber layer thickness in patients with Alzheimer's disease: a meta-analysis," *International Journal of Ophthalmology*, vol. 5, no. 3, pp. 401–405, 2012.

[197] B. J. Kim, D. J. Irwin, D. Song et al., "Optical coherence tomography identifies outer retina thinning in frontotemporal degeneration," *Neurology*, vol. 89, no. 15, pp. 1604–1611, 2017.

[198] E. A. Williams, D. McGuone, M. P. Frosch, B. T. Hyman, N. Laver, and A. Stemmer-Rachamimov, "Absence of Alzheimer disease neuropathologic changes in eyes of subjects with Alzheimer disease," *Journal of Neuropathology and Experimental Neurology*, vol. 76, no. 5, pp. 376–383, 2017.

[199] T. Tian, B. Zhang, Y. Jia, and Z. Li, "Promise and challenge: the lens model as a biomarker for early diagnosis of Alzheimer's disease," *Disease Markers*, vol. 2014, Article ID 826503, 5 pages, 2014.

[200] L. Bei, Y.-B. Shui, F. Bai, S. K. Nelson, G. P. Van Stavern, and D. C. Beebe, "A test of lens opacity as an indicator of preclinical Alzheimer disease," *Experimental Eye Research*, vol. 140, pp. 117–123, 2015.

[201] C. Y.-L. Cheung, Y. T. Ong, M. K. Ikram et al., "Microvascular network alterations in the retina of patients with Alzheimer's disease," *Alzheimer's & Dementia: The Journal of the Alzheimer's Association*, vol. 10, no. 2, pp. 135–142, 2014.

[202] G. Banerjee, R. Carare, C. Cordonnier et al., "The increasing impact of cerebral amyloid angiopathy: essential new insights for clinical practice," *Journal of Neurology, Neurosurgery, and Psychiatry*, vol. 88, no. 11, pp. 982–994, 2017.

[203] S. McGrory, J. R. Cameron, E. Pellegrini et al., "The application of retinal fundus camera imaging in dementia: a systematic review," *Alzheimer's & Dementia: Diagnosis, Assessment & Disease Monitoring*, vol. 6, pp. 91–107, 2017.

[204] C.-Y. Ho, J. C. Troncoso, D. Knox, W. Stark, and C. G. Eberhart, "Beta-amyloid, phospho-tau and alpha-synuclein deposits similar to those in the brain are not identified in the eyes of Alzheimer's and Parkinson's disease patients," *Brain Pathology*, vol. 24, no. 1, pp. 25–32, 2014.

[205] A. B. Syed, R. A. Armstrong, and C. U. Smith, "A quantitative analysis of optic nerve axons in elderly control subjects and patients with Alzheimer's disease," *Folia Neuropathologica*, vol. 43, no. 1, pp. 1–6, 2005.

[206] C. A. Curcio and D. N. Drucker, "Retinal ganglion cells in Alzheimer's disease and aging," *Annals of Neurology*, vol. 33, no. 3, pp. 248–257, 1993.

[207] J. C. Blanks, Y. Torigoe, D. R. Hinton, and R. H. I. Blanks, "Retinal degeneration in the macula of patients with Alzheimer's disease," *Annals of the New York Academy of Sciences*, vol. 640, no. 1, pp. 44–46, 1991.

[208] J. C. Blanks, D. R. Hinton, A. A. Sadun, and C. A. Miller, "Retinal ganglion cell degeneration in Alzheimer's disease," *Brain Research*, vol. 501, no. 2, pp. 364–372, 1989.

[209] S. Joly, S. Lamoureux, and V. Pernet, "Nonamyloidogenic processing of amyloid beta precursor protein is associated with retinal function improvement in aging male APP_{swe}/PS1ΔE9 mice," *Neurobiology of Aging*, vol. 53, pp. 181–191, 2017.

[210] P. A. Williams, R. A. Thirgood, H. Oliphant et al., "Retinal ganglion cell dendritic degeneration in a mouse model of Alzheimer's disease," *Neurobiology of Aging*, vol. 34, no. 7, pp. 1799–1806, 2013.

17

Tumor Necrosis Factor and Interleukin-1β Modulate Synaptic Plasticity during Neuroinflammation

Francesca Romana Rizzo,[1] Alessandra Musella,[2] Francesca De Vito,[1] Diego Fresegna,[1] Silvia Bullitta,[1] Valentina Vanni,[1] Livia Guadalupi,[2] Mario Stampanoni Bassi,[3] Fabio Buttari,[3] Georgia Mandolesi,[2] Diego Centonze,[1,3] and Antonietta Gentile[3]

[1]*Synaptic Immunopathology Lab, Department of Systems Medicine, University of Rome Tor Vergata, 00133 Rome, Italy*
[2]*Synaptic Immunopathology Lab, IRCCS San Raffaele, Via di Val Cannuta 247, 00166 Rome, Italy*
[3]*Unit of Neurology and Unit of Neurorehabilitation, IRCCS Istituto Neurologico Mediterraneo (INM) Neuromed, 86077 Pozzilli, Italy*

Correspondence should be addressed to Diego Centonze; centonze@uniroma2.it

Academic Editor: Steven W. Johnson

Cytokines are constitutively released in the healthy brain by resident myeloid cells to keep proper synaptic plasticity, either in the form of Hebbian synaptic plasticity or of homeostatic plasticity. However, when cytokines dramatically increase, establishing a status of neuroinflammation, the synaptic action of such molecules remarkably interferes with brain circuits of learning and cognition and contributes to excitotoxicity and neurodegeneration. Among others, interleukin-1β (IL-1β) and tumor necrosis factor (TNF) are the best studied proinflammatory cytokines in both physiological and pathological conditions and have been invariably associated with long term potentiation (LTP) (Hebbian synaptic plasticity) and synaptic scaling (homeostatic plasticity), respectively. Multiple sclerosis (MS) is the prototypical neuroinflammatory disease, in which inflammation triggers excitotoxic mechanisms contributing to neurodegeneration. IL-β and TNF are increased in the brain of MS patients and contribute to induce the changes in synaptic plasticity occurring in MS patients and its animal model, the experimental autoimmune encephalomyelitis (EAE). This review will introduce and discuss current evidence of the role of IL-1β and TNF in the regulation of synaptic strength at both physiological and pathological levels, in particular speculating on their involvement in the synaptic plasticity changes observed in the EAE brain.

1. Introduction

The recognition that soluble mediators of the immune system, namely, cytokines, are constitutively expressed in the central nervous system (CNS) has completely changed our vision of brain functioning [1]. Indeed, the study of the neuroimmune connection is an extraordinary field of research, having strong implications for understanding physiological and pathological conditions [2, 3]. The proinflammatory cytokines IL-1β and TNF, released by resident cells of the immune lineage, have been proven to physiologically modulate synaptic plasticity, mainly the Hebbian synaptic plasticity and the synaptic scaling, in different brain areas such as the cortex, striatum, and hippocampus [4, 5].

TNF is a proteolytically cleaved transmembrane protein whose activity is performed through TNF receptor type 1 (TNFR1) and type 2 (TNFR2) [6]. In physiological state, the glial pathway that regulates TNF release is itself controlled by TNF [7], but when the balanced system is strongly disturbed, the homeostatic mechanism fails. This cytokine is an important regulator of synapse function implicated in synaptic transmission and homeostatic synaptic scaling [8, 9].

IL-1β is the product of the proteolytic cleavage of its mature form pro-IL-1β. IL-1β exerts its biological action by binding to IL-1 receptor type 1 (IL-1RI), competing with IL-1 receptor antagonist (IL-1ra), the endogenous inhibitor of IL-1β [10]. A bulk of data indicate that IL-1β is necessary for synaptic mechanisms, like LTP, underlying learning and memory [4].

When brain levels of cytokines significantly rise as a result of an immune challenge, the scenario about the neuroimmune connection deeply changes. Under this condition, IL1-β and TNF, whose basal activity is necessary for maintenance of proper synaptic plasticity, start to exert noxious effects on synaptic transmission. Interestingly, the mechanisms underlying the shift from a healthy immune function to a detrimental one are poorly understood [4]. However, during chronic neuroinflammatory and neurodegenerative diseases, like Alzheimer's disease (AD) and multiple sclerosis (MS), changes in synaptic plasticity due to the effects of these cytokines might also be an adaptive mechanism occurring to compensate for synaptic and/or neuronal loss.

While the physiological regulation of synaptic plasticity by TNF and IL-1β has been widely investigated, the involvement of such cytokines in synaptic plasticity alterations associated with neurological disorders is merely speculative and relies only on few studies on animal models. In this respect, due to the recognized pathogenic role of inflammation in MS, many clinical and preclinical studies have been performed to address the role of TNF and IL-1β in the modulation of synaptic plasticity [11].

Moving from a brief introduction on the key properties of both synaptic scaling and LTP, the present review summarizes the main evidence for the physiological and pathological functions of IL-1β and TNF and their cellular sources in the brain in regulating synaptic plasticity. Moreover, we will discuss data from EAE, animal model of MS, which support a role for both cytokines in synaptic changes and adaptations during neuroinflammation.

2. Synaptic Plasticity

Changes in synaptic strength and brain network activity occur either as an adaptive response to environmental stimuli or as a consequence of local insult affecting single or multiple neurons. From development to ageing, several forms of synaptic plasticity coexist and cooperate to maintain proper synaptic transmission and to keep homeostasis in brain circuits. Among others, Hebbian plasticity and synaptic scaling are the most relevant form of synaptic plasticity, whose induction and maintenance underlie not only experience-dependent mechanisms, like memory processes, but also pathological conditions of neuronal perturbations [12]. As reported in the following sections, LTP and synaptic scaling result in the strengthening of the glutamatergic transmission and, although sharing some features, are intrinsically different in nature.

2.1. LTP: Properties and Biological Relevance. LTP is a form of synaptic plasticity consisting in long-lasting increase in the synaptic strength between pre- and postsynaptic neurons. It is artificially induced through electrophysiological protocols of high-frequency stimulation [12]. LTP can be experimentally induced in virtually all the excitatory synapses in the brain. However, most of our knowledge about the molecular mechanisms of LTP arises from studies in the cornu ammonis area 1 (CA1) region of the hippocampus, where the main form of LTP is dependent on N-methyl-D-aspartate receptor (NMDAR) activity. Decades of experimental research have led to some key concepts about LTP nature.

Briefly, LTP is (i) cooperative, since it requires the coincident activation of a critical number of synapses; (ii) associative, in a way that weak input, involving a small number of synapses, can be strengthened by the association with a strong input, coming from a larger number of synapses; and (iii) input-specific, because only activated synapses on the postsynaptic neuron are recruited during LTP. This implies that LTP occurs in case of coincidence activity between pre- and postsynaptic neurons in a positive feedback. Indeed, to be triggered, LTP first needs the increased conductance through α-amino-3-hydroxy-5-methyl-4-isoxazolepropionic acid receptors (AMPARs), which in turn activate postsynaptic NMDARs (early phase of LTP) [13]. Glutamate massively released from presynaptic terminal binds both AMPARs and NMDARs. However, the latter are activated only once Mg^{2+} is removed from the central pore of NMDAR, and this is achieved by AMPAR-mediated membrane depolarization. Subsequent Ca^{2+} influx through NMDAR channel triggers intracellular signaling cascade necessary for synaptic plasticity [14]. Furthermore, to be persistent over time, LTP requires de novo protein synthesis, necessary for storage of information: the late phase of LTP implies structural changes in postsynaptic density (PSD), which is linked to the induction of immediate early genes (IEG) and the synthesis of proteins like *Arc-Arg*, which stabilizes F-actin filaments and regulate AMPAR membrane expression [15]. On a functional level, compelling studies based on behavioural tests and electrophysiology have clearly linked LTP in the hippocampus with learning [16, 17] and memory [18–20].

Based on subunit composition (NR2A versus NR2B) and localization at synapse (synaptic or extrasynaptic), signaling through NMDAR can induce either neuroprotection [21] or neurotoxicity [22]. Although the causal link between synaptic plasticity and neuroprotection is still not fully elucidated, growing data point to NMDAR-dependent LTP as prosurvival strategy [23], aimed at recovering activity in those neurons, which have lost part of their synaptic inputs.

2.2. Il-1β Is the Main Immune Trigger of LTP in Physiological Condition. During physiological neuronal activity, several factors have been shown to induce LTP, including the brain-derived neurotrophic factor (BDNF) [24, 25]. However, in the past decades, unexpected interactions between environmental/psychological experiences, immune system, and brain activity have been highlighted, providing evidence for physiological control of learning and memory mediated by the immune system [4]. Research in this field has focused on the effect of cytokines on the induction and maintenance of hippocampal LTP, indicating that IL-1β, rather than TNF, is the main immune player in LTP regulation. Indeed, mice with genetic deletion of components of TNF signaling showed unaltered hippocampal LTP [8, 26].

After the first observation that LTP induction is physiologically followed by IL-1 gene expression [27], several studies based on genetic knockdown [28] or *in vitro* and *in vivo* pharmacological blockade of IL-1R [29, 30] have indicated the necessary role of IL-1β in LTP induction and maintenance. LTP in CA1 region of IL1-R KO mice is absent [28], and intracerebroventricular administration (ICV) of IL-1ra significantly affected both the initial potentiation and the maintenance of LTP [30]. The critical role of IL-1β in the maintenance of LTP was demonstrated in *in vitro* experiments: application of IL-1ra 30 min after LTP induction rescued basal synaptic transmission. A putative mechanism by which IL-1β modulates LTP involves changes in Ca^{2+} conductance through NMDAR [31]. Noteworthy, *in vivo* manipulations of IL1-β signaling were associated with disturbances in memory and learning of mice: compared to wild-type (WT) IL-1R KO mice showed slower rate of learning in the spatial memory paradigm [28], impaired contextual but normal auditory-cued fear conditioning in water *T*-maze paradigm [32]. Moreover, ICV injection of IL-1ra induced similar behavioural phenotype [32]. Overall, these data point to IL-1β as the main immune player involved in LTP induction and maintenance as well as memory and learning processes (Figure 1(a)).

2.3. Synaptic Scaling: Properties and Biological Relevance. A form of synaptic plasticity, profoundly different from LTP, is the synaptic scaling. The synaptic scaling acts to keep the postsynaptic weights of excitatory synapses around a firing rate set point. Therefore, by definition, synaptic scaling is a homeostatic form of synaptic plasticity, triggered to globally reduce (downscaling) or increase (upscaling) the excitatory drive during chronic inactivity or hyperactivity [33]. Persistent and uncontrolled Hebbian plasticity or reduced number of synapses for pathological reasons can induce synaptic scaling. However, our knowledge on how Hebbian plasticity and synaptic scaling are temporally linked to each other and mechanistically intermingled is still in its infancy [34]. In contrast to LTP, synaptic scaling (i) acts in a negative feedback, (ii) is not input-specific, as it can spread to multiple synapses, and, more interestingly, (iii) mainly relies on AMPAR functioning. Indeed, the excitatory synaptic transmission can be strengthened or weakened by slowly increasing or reducing the number of clustered AMPAR on postsynaptic membrane, respectively [33, 35]. This is a global effect, involving all the synapses of a postsynaptic neuron. As a result of these changes in AMPAR membrane insertion or removal, the conductance of AMPAR is increased or reduced and the PSD area is changed accordingly [36, 37]. Synaptic scaling is associated with the induction or inhibition of Arc/Arg gene [38, 39], leading to increased or reduced rate of surface AMPAR endocytosis with the consequent reduction or enhancement of membrane-expressed AMPARs. Therefore, being involved in both Hebbian plasticity and synaptic scaling, Arc protein seems to play a crucial role in regulating synaptic plasticity [40]. Homeostatic synaptic plasticity has been well documented *in vivo* in visual cortex during experience-deprivation paradigms [41, 42] or in sleep/awake states [31, 43].

2.4. TNF Is the Main Immune Trigger of Synaptic Scaling in Physiological Condition. Similar to Hebbian plasticity, synaptic scaling is sensitive to the regulation by molecules of the immune system. If IL-1β is definitively associated with constitutive Hebbian plasticity, TNF is invariably associated with synaptic scaling [44, 45]. The first and foremost evidence that TNF is able to alter normal synaptic function was demonstrated in a study where a twofold increase expression of AMPARs on the plasma membrane was detected after an exposure of cultured hippocampal neurons to TNF at different concentrations (0.6–60 nM acute exposure) [9]. Additionally, application of TNFR1 antibody decreased GluR1 surface expression in hippocampal neurons [46], indicating the necessary and constitutive role of TNF in regulating AMPAR membrane insertion and in modifying synaptic strength. Notably, the seminal paper by the Malenka group highlighted the role of glial TNF in inactivity-induced synaptic scaling [8]. Blockade of TNF signaling during prolonged tetrodotoxin (TTX) treatment prevented scaling up of excitatory synapses in hippocampal neurons. Moreover, neurons from TNF KO mice grown on glia from WT mice did show synaptic scaling, while neurons from WT mice grown on glia from TNF KO mice did not [8]. Similar findings were obtained in neurons of the visual cortex [26]. More recently, TNF has been causally involved in size increase of spines close to branches that had recently undergone spine loss [47].

Curiously, in contrast to hippocampal and cortical neurons, TNF was shown to downregulate AMPAR membrane expression in striatal neurons, raising the possibility that in this brain region it exerts an adaptive role to limit the strength of synaptic drive from the cortex [48]. Of note, the physiological role of TNF in inducing synaptic scaling has been well documented *in vivo* in the visual cortex of animals subjected to chronic monocular deprivation [26, 47, 49], further supporting the idea that TNF is a critical player in activity-dependent synaptic adaptations (Figure 2(a)).

3. Synaptic Plasticity: Synaptic Scaling and LTP during Neuroinflammation

Cells of both the innate (resident microglia and astroglia) and the adaptive (T-cells) immune response have been clearly implicated in the physiological regulation of mood, learning, memory, and experience-dependent synaptic activity [50, 51]. Any changes in brain homeostasis that imply microglia and astroglia activation and/or T-cell infiltration trigger an inflammatory response, which is a mechanism of brain defence and can affect synaptic plasticity. During neuroinflammation, activated microglia, astroglia, and infiltrating lymphocytes specifically interact with neurons and influence

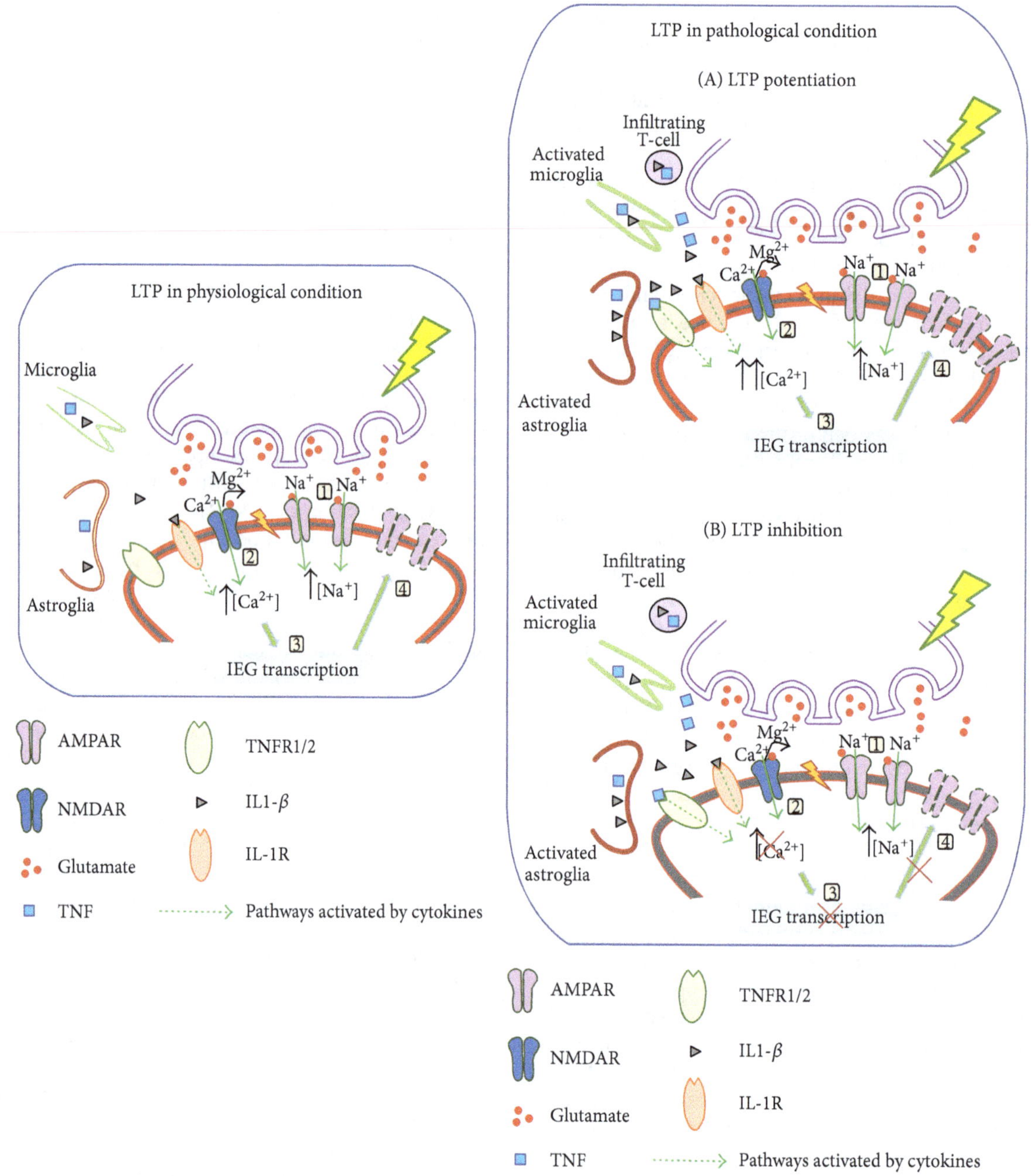

(a) (b)

FIGURE 1: LTP regulation in physiological and pathological states. The triggering of LTP implies coincident pre- and postsynaptic neuron activation. Strong glutamate release from presynaptic terminal promotes membrane depolarization mediated by Na^{+} influx through AMPARs (1), which in turn activates NMDARs by means of Mg^{2+} expulsion from NMDAR pore, thus allowing Ca^{2+} influx (2). Next, the increase of intracellular Ca^{2+} concentration activates a cascade of events involving several molecular players and leads to the induction of IEGs (3), such as Arc/Arg, necessary for structural (increased stability and size of dendritic spines) and functional changes of the PSD and the synthesis and insertion of AMPARs in membrane (4). Physiological levels of IL-1β released by both microglia and astroglia contribute to LTP phenomenon (a). During neuroinflammatory disorders (b), activated resident (microglia and astroglia) and infiltrating T-cells strongly release TNF and IL-1β, thus generating two possible outcomes of synaptic changes (A, B). As illustrated in the figure, LTP can be either potentiated or prevented through the action of TNF and IL-1β interfering with the pathways controlling the molecular and structural synaptic changes occurring during LTP.

their survival either in a positive or in a negative direction depending on the pathologic context, by releasing cytokines [52]. Therefore, we will review current findings about the role of TNF and IL-1β in animal models of neuroinflammatory conditions and of neurodegenerative diseases, the latter characterized by chronic inflammation.

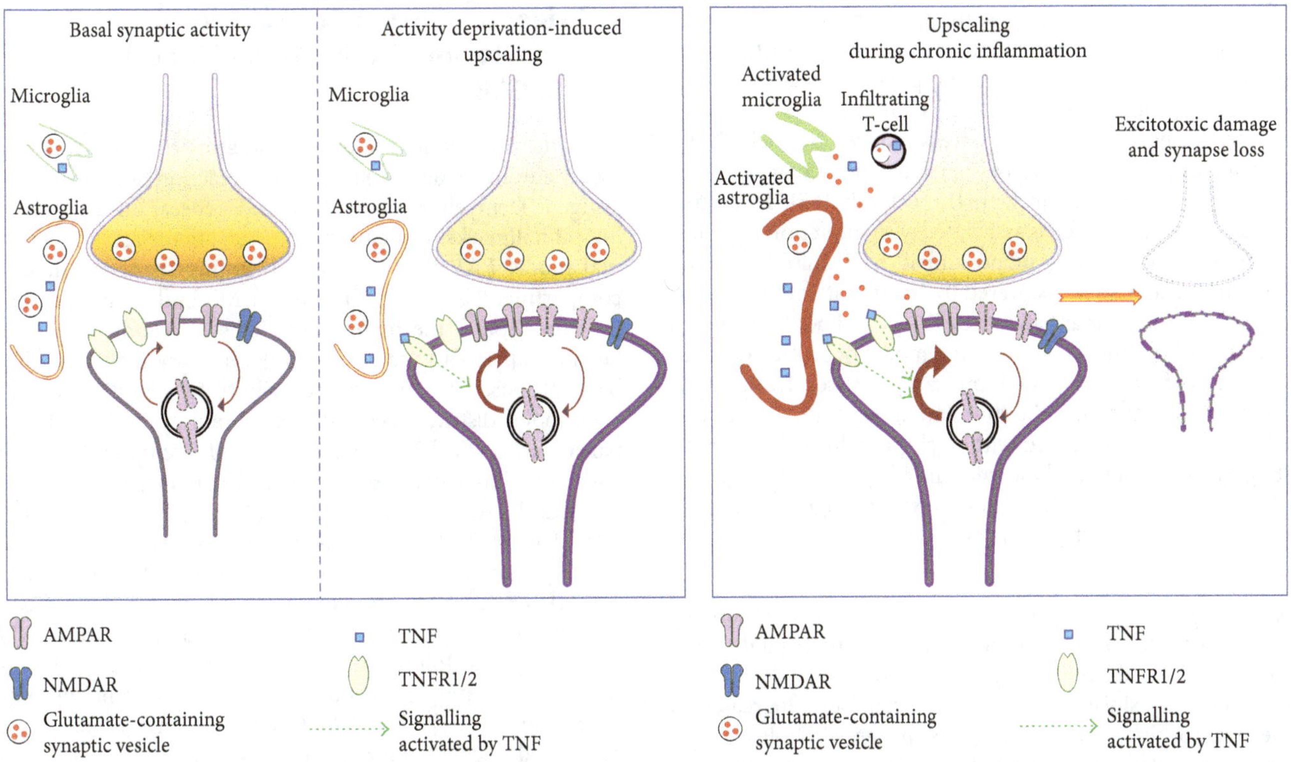

(a) Physiological condition

(b) Pathological condition

FIGURE 2: Synaptic upscaling in response to physiological and pathological stimuli. (a) In a physiological state, during basal synaptic activity, AMPARs undergo constant cycles of membrane insertion and removal on postsynaptic neuron. When the synaptic strength driven by the presynaptic terminal is reduced, TNF, released by astroglia, activates a molecular mechanism leading to transient improved insertion of AMPARs on postsynaptic membrane. (b) During acute or chronic neuroinflammation, TNF, massively released by activated microglia and astroglia as well as infiltrating T-cells, indefinitely upregulates the mechanism of membrane AMPAR insertion. In parallel, inflammation affects physiological mechanisms of glutamate clearance at synaptic cleft. This together with enhanced glutamate release from glial cells over activates AMPARs, thus contributing to induce excitotoxic mechanisms and synaptic loss.

3.1. Synaptic Plasticity: The Role of TNF during Neuroinflammation. Experimental paradigms of deafferentiation-induced homeostatic plasticity have highlighted that signaling activated by TNF plays a role in the long-term maintenance of synaptic scaling. In hippocampal slices that underwent denervation from entorhinal cortex (EC), glial TNF increased only after 3-4 days postlesion, while the enhancement of excitatory transmission in dentate gyrus (DG) granule cells was observed already after 1-2 days postlesion [53]. Moreover, in the same experimental model of denervation followed by neuroinflammation, it was shown that TNF was involved in LTP maintenance by binding to both TNFR1 and TNFR2 [54].

As already mentioned, TNF exerts different physiological effects in the hippocampus and the striatum [8, 48], and several data suggest that TNF massively released during neuroinflammation may have brain area-specific effects, as well. Accordingly, it has recently been shown that TNF of microglial origin impairs hippocampal LTP in CA1 region, whereas it improves LTP at C-fiber synapses in spinal dorsal horn in a model of peripheral nerve injury, which is associated with memory deficits and pain [55]. Another study on the same model analysed the effect of TNF on hippocampal LTP at CA3-CA1 synapses: LTP was impaired in injured animals and the same effect was observed after intrahippocampal or ICV injection of TNF in healthy mice [56]. These outstanding *in vivo* findings corroborate data from *in vitro* acute application of TNF. It has been shown that TNF impairs dose-dependently LTP induction or maintenance in the hippocampus, by preventing the initial reduction of potentiation (early phase of LTP) and by inhibiting the late increased potentiation (late phase of LTP) [57, 58]. Interestingly, pretreatment of hippocampal slices with TNF after hypoxia improved LTP in the DG [59]. In line with this, by means of transgenic mice overexpressing TNF, other researchers have demonstrated that chronic exposure to TNF potentiates LTP in CA1 region [60] (Figures 1(b) and 2(b)).

3.2. Synaptic Plasticity: The Role of IL-1β during Neuroinflammation. Several lines of data consistently indicate that increased levels of IL-1β inhibit LTP in CA1, CA3, and DG of the hippocampus, either after *in vitro* application of the cytokine or *in vivo* ICV delivery [58, 61–63]. IL-1β has been shown to dose-dependently affect Ca^{2+} conductance through NMDARs, being able to improve or inhibit Ca^{2+} influx at low or high concentration, respectively [31]. Moreover, increased brain levels of IL1-β may inhibit LTP maintenance by interfering with BDNF signaling cascades, thereby impairing the formation of F-actin in dendritic spines [64]. Among others, these are the putative mechanisms by which IL-1β improves or impairs LTP induction.

Regarding *in vivo* studies, stress induced by social isolation and age in rats has been associated with LTP impairment in the DG in correlation with IL-1β levels [65]. In animal model of seizure, which is associated with induction of proinflammatory cytokines, hippocampal LTP inhibition and memory deficits were recovered by treatment with anakinra, the human receptor antagonist of IL1-β, and not by IL-6 and TNF inhibitors [66]. Likewise, in a model of septic encephalopathy, preincubation of hippocampal slices from septic mice with Il-1ra before the stimulation was found to recover LTP deficiency associated with such pathological condition [67]. Furthermore, in obese mice, intrahippocampal delivery of IL-ra rescued LTP deficiency as well as cognitive impairments at *Y*-maze test [68] (Figure 1(B)).

3.3. Synaptic Plasticity: The Role of TNF and IL-1β during Neurodegeneration. Increasing interest has been paid to the role of IL-1β and TNF during age-related pathological conditions, like AD, since their levels have been found increased in the cerebrospinal fluid (CSF) of these patients [69]. Brain ageing is associated with increased basal levels of cytokines and susceptibility to neuroinflammation, accounting for memory and learning deficits [70]. Of note, neuroinflammation in old people is proposed to contribute to the neurodegenerative cascade typical of AD, namely, β-amyloid- (Aβ-) dependent synaptic pathology [71, 72]. Indeed, in line with the aforementioned hypothesis of the inhibitory effect of elevated levels of TNF on LTP in the hippocampus, it has recently shown that in a transgenic mouse model of AD, the peripheral inhibition of the soluble form of TNF attenuates Aβ load, cognitive, and LTP deficits [73]. Regarding Il-1β involvement in synaptic pathology associated with AD, IL1-ra treatment partially attenuated $A\beta_{1-40}$ impairment of LTP in the CA1 of hippocampus [30], supporting previous findings suggesting that $A\beta_{1-40}$ induces the release of IL-1β [74]. However, in another study, it was proposed that Aβ toxicity was TNF-dependent, since the suppression of LTP induced by Aβ was prevented by pharmacological inhibition of TNF and absent in mice lacking the TNFR1 [75]. These data highlight that cytokines play a crucial role in mediating Aβ synaptotoxicity and mechanisms of memory loss during ageing [72].

Altogether, these findings indicate the detrimental role of high concentrations of TNF and IL-1β in both forms of synaptic plasticity during neuroinflammatory and neurodegenerative diseases. It is worth noting that, to date, the occurrence of synaptic scaling in animal models of neurodegenerative diseases has not been addressed. However, it might be hypothesized that in a condition of chronic exposure to high levels of TNF in response to prolonged neuronal activity blockade [8], a kind of super upscaling occurs. This event together with inflammation-impaired mechanisms of glutamate homeostasis regulation subsequently contributes to excitotoxic damage [76, 77] (Figure 2(b)). This issue needs further investigation.

4. Evidence of Synaptic Plasticity Perturbations in the Animal Model of MS, EAE

MS is the prototypical neuroinflammatory disorder, initiated by an autoimmune T-cell-mediated reaction against myelin antigen. Demyelination and neurodegeneration are pathological hallmarks of the brains of MS patients and of its animal model EAE [78]. It is worth noting that the synaptic compartment is early perturbed in MS and EAE, and that inflammation is the main trigger of synaptic damage [79]. Such synaptopathy, caused by inflammatory mediators, has been proposed to cogently contribute to cognitive deficits [79], mood disturbances [80], and disability [81] in MS. In particular, cortical Hebbian synaptic plasticity, that is, LTP and LTD, has been explored in MS patients, by means of transcranial magnetic stimulation (TMS) protocols and correlated with the levels of IL-1β and TNF [11, 81]. In MS, LTP is favored over LTD and LTP potentiation correlates with IL-1β levels in the cerebrospinal fluid (CSF) of MS patients [82]. Moreover, TNF-enriched CSF from MS patients applied to murine brain slices induced the potentiation of glutamatergic transmission, in a way resembling synaptic scaling [83]. Parallel studies on EAE model have confirmed such alterations in basal synaptic transmission and plasticity, providing evidence for a direct involvement of TNF and IL-1β in correlation with microglia and astroglia activation and T-cell infiltration [84].

4.1. The Role of TNF on Synaptic Activity in EAE. It is properly recognized that in the gray matter of EAE and MS brains, the levels of TNF are severely high [83, 85, 86]. The synaptic activity in EAE mice has been largely investigated by our group. The impact of TNF on synaptic strength has been studied by means of both electrophysiological techniques and biochemical assays. In particular, we observed alterations of frequency and duration of spontaneous and miniature glutamatergic events (sEPSCs, mEPSCs), reporting an increase of both parameters in striatal neurons of EAE mice. Notably, these changes were already evident before the clinical manifestations of the disease [85, 86]. At this stage of the disease, TNF levels have been found increased in EAE striatum [86], raising the possibility that it could be the responsible of such glutamatergic transmission enhancement with an involvement of AMPAR trafficking [8]. Indeed, biochemical assays in synaptosomal preparation of EAE striatum revealed increased expression of GluR1 subunit of AMPAR and its phosphorylation at the Ser845 residue indicative of enhanced AMPAR membrane insertion. Moreover, Arc/Arg mRNA was downregulated in the whole striatum [85]. Together with electrophysiological data, these results are suggestive of synaptic upscaling in the EAE brain [39, 77, 87–89].

The casual link between TNF and enhanced glutamate transmission in EAE striatum was demonstrated by *in vivo* and *in vitro* experiments. Electrophysiological recordings of slices from EAE mice that received ICV treatment with anti-TNF antibody showed the rescue of glutamatergic transmission alteration, while ICV administration of TNF in control mice induced the same enhancement of glutamatergic transmission observed in EAE [86]. Moreover, *in vitro* experiments of long period of incubation (3 h) of control slices with high concentration of TNF (0.6 μM) mimicked the effects of EAE [85]. Such result is apparently in contrast with findings from Lewitus and colleagues (2014), who found that TNF reduced the amplitude of sEPSC and the membrane insertion of AMPAR in the striatum [48]. However, time (1 h) and concentration of TNF (100 ng/ml) in their experimental settings were remarkably different from ours, likely explaining the different *in vitro* results. Of note, the "strong" *in vitro* treatment that we used closely reproduced the EAE glutamatergic transmission potentiation, likely mimicking the effect of chronic exposure of synapses to high levels of TNF. Finally, we confirmed that glial TNF is responsible for the striatal upscaling in EAE: *in vitro* activated microglial cell line applied to control slices increased the duration of glutamatergic spontaneous events and this effect was reversed in the presence of a TNF antibody [85].

The strengthening of glutamatergic transmission in EAE striatum was persistent throughout the disease course. At later stages of the disease, in which inflammation turns into a chronic state, some neurodegenerative features have been described, such as the loss of parvalbumin-positive interneurons (PV+) and of dendritic spines in the gray matter of EAE mice [85, 90], suggesting that inflammatory chronic elevation of TNF may turn physiological upscaling into uncontrolled upscaling, leading to excitotoxic synaptic and neuronal damage [76, 85].

An elegant study published by Habbas and colleagues has demonstrated the involvement of local TNF release in the DG of EAE mice in the strengthening of excitatory transmission in correlation with memory deficits in these mice [91]. The authors found that the excitatory transmission at EC-DG synapses is increased in an astrocytic TNFR1-dependent manner. Indeed, to demonstrate the necessary role of TNF in the potentiation of glutamatergic transmission in circuit involved in contextual learning and memory, they used conditional KO mice for TNFR1 in glial cells. Slices taken from these mice incubated with increasing concentrations of TNF did not show glutamatergic transmission alterations, while the reexpression of TNFR1 in astrocytes rescued the sensitivity to TNF synaptic effect. Moreover, by inducing EAE in this conditional KO mice, they demonstrated that cognitive failure and potentiation of EC-DG glutamatergic transmission are dependent on TNF signaling through astrocytic TNFR1 [91]. Although not fully investigated, along with presynaptic effect of TNF, the authors also found an increase of mEPSC amplitude, consistent with postsynaptic effects of TNF. These results further highlight the role of TNF in synaptic pathology associated with EAE.

4.2. The Role of IL1-β on Hippocampal Synaptic Plasticity in EAE. IL-1β is clearly related to synaptic plasticity rather than upscaling mechanisms in both physiological and pathological conditions (see Sections 2.2 and 3.2). IL-1β is essentially involved in the modulation of LTP form of plasticity in EAE mice. In particular, we showed that EAE mice exhibited a favored LTP induction over LTD in the CA1 area of hippocampus. This effect correlated with increased levels of IL-1β and was reversed by chronic ICV treatment with IL-1ra [82, 92]. Moreover, preincubation of IL-1β on hippocampal slices was able to alter LTP, by inducing a greater potentiation in comparison to control condition and also an inhibition of LTD in CA1 [92]. Of note, any changes in input-output curves as well as in AMPA/NMDA ratio in CA1 were observed in EAE, thus indicating a specific effect on synaptic plasticity induction and maintenance without significant alterations of glutamatergic basal transmission. Based on the above results, we speculated that this effect of EAE on Hebbian forms of plasticity could be the consequence of the reduction of GABAergic inhibition, caused by loss of PV+ GABAergic interneurons [92]. We also demonstrated that *in vitro* activated microglia incubated with control slices inhibited the GABAergic transmission, and that this effect was reversed in the presence of IL1-ra. Considering the role of infiltrating T-lymphocytes in EAE/MS pathology, we tested the hypothesis that these cells, by releasing IL-1β [93], might contribute to hippocampal changes in synaptic activity. Experiments carried out with incubation of T-lymphocytes taken from EAE spleen and placed onto hippocampal control slices promoted LTP over LTD, in a way resembling the LTP recorded from EAE slices, and reduced the GABAergic tone [82]. Thus, EAE-specific T-lymphocytes, by suppressing GABAergic transmission in an IL-1β-dependent manner, were likely able to lower the threshold of LTP induction. We concluded that IL-1β was involved in both the modulation of basal GABAergic synaptic transmission, supposed to precede and contribute to the loss of GABAergic interneurons, and in the potentiation of synaptic plasticity as an adaptive/reparative mechanism.

However, apparently, contrasting data have been reported in literature about hippocampal LTP in EAE [94–96]. Di Filippo and colleagues found that hippocampal LTP is impaired in EAE induced in Biozzi ABH mice, and that IL-1β replicates such alteration in *in vitro* experiments. Although not demonstrating a direct link with IL-1β, the same authors associated LTP inhibition in EAE to hippocampal-dependent memory defects observed in EAE mice: both behavioural and synaptic alterations in EAE were recovered by suppressing microglia activation by means of peripheral injection of minocycline [95]. Despite the lack of a direct link with IL-1β, other studies demonstrated the impairment of hippocampal LTP during the course of EAE [97–99]. In particular, in the paper by Kim et al. (2012), LTP in CA1 region was affected by EAE at both early and late time points and in connection with spatial memory defects [97], while in the investigation by Novkovic et al. (2015), both LTP and cognition were impaired only at late time points [98]. Interestingly, Planche and colleagues correlated impairment of LTP in the DG and of contextual fear memory response in EAE mice with microglia activation, since peripheral administration of minocycline was able to recover both synaptic and behavioural defects [100]. Conversely, Prochnow et al. (2013) investigated presynaptic properties in CA1 hippocampal EAE mice slices reporting a reduction in paired pulse facilitation in comparison with control mice, but no differences were found in LTP induction [96].

As already discussed elsewhere [11, 101], several factors, like EAE model (mice/rats, immunization procedure), different stimulation protocols of LTP, and time points of recordings, which are severely affected by the inflammatory bulk, may explain the contrasting results that have been described in the literature. Even if clear conclusions about synaptic plasticity in CA1 area of EAE hippocampus cannot be drawn, the above data strongly implicate IL-1β in synaptic rearrangements during the course of chronic neuroinflammation.

5. Conclusions

LTP and synaptic scaling serve as fine-tuning regulators of synaptic strength in the healthy brain and are regulated by IL-1β and TNF, which, physiologically act "on demand," being released in an activity-dependent manner. Interference with these mechanisms can bring to aberrant expression of both forms of synaptic plasticity.

Data discussed in the present review clearly indicate that IL-β is largely involved in the constitutive regulation of Hebbian plasticity, while TNF is the main player in homeostatic plasticity. However, such dichotomy is only partially preserved during sustained neuroinflammation. Indeed, although limited, data in literature indicate that in both acute (i.e., ICV injection of cytokine) and chronic (i.e., EAE and AD transgenic model) paradigms of brain inflammation, IL-1β is still linked to LTP expression, whereas TNF seems to affect both LTP and synaptic scaling (Figures 1 and 2). To this respect, it should be noted that the biological relevance of an altered expression of synaptic plasticity has been poorly explored in animal models of neurodegenerative diseases, with the exception of MS. In this context, evidence suggestive of an aberrant upscaling mediated by TNF and leading to excitotoxic neurodegeneration has been shown in the striatum of EAE mice. Moreover, TNF-induced glutamatergic transmission enhancement in the DG has been proposed as the synaptic counterpart of cognitive defects in EAE. Regarding Hebbian plasticity, although contrasting, several lines of evidence indicate that LTP expression in EAE is altered in an IL-1β-dependent manner. According to these results, aberrant hippocampal synaptic plasticity may contribute either to cognitive impairment or to minimize neuronal and synaptic damage. This issue needs further investigations and may include the effects of other cytokines, like Interleukin-6 (IL-6), and immune molecules, such as major histocompatibility complex type 1 (MHCI), already found to modulate synaptic plasticity [4]. Moreover, the fact that cytokine pathways are highly intermingled, implying mutual regulation lays the ground for a better understanding of the complex interaction between immune system and synaptic activity during the course of chronic neuroinflammation.

Abbreviations

TNF:	Tumor necrosis factor
IL-1β:	Interleukin-1β
LTP:	Long-term potentiation
MS:	Multiple sclerosis
EAE:	Experimental autoimmune encephalomyelitis
CNS:	Central nervous system
TNFR1, 2:	TNF receptor type 1 and type 2
IL-1RI:	IL-1 receptor type 1
IL-1ra:	IL-1 receptor antagonist
AD:	Alzheimer's disease
CA1, 3:	Cornu ammonis area 1, 3
NMDAR:	N-Methyl-D-aspartate receptor
AMPAR:	α-Amino-3-hydroxy-5-methyl-4-isoxazolepropionic acid receptor
PSD:	Postsynaptic density
IEG:	Immediate early genes
NR2A, B:	N-Methyl D-aspartate receptor subtype 2A, B
BDNF:	Brain-derived neurotrophic factor
ICV:	Intracerebroventricular administration
WT:	Wild-type
KO:	Knockout
GluR1:	AMPA receptor subunit 1
TTX:	Tetrodotoxin
EC:	Entorhinal cortex
DG:	Dentate gyrus
LTD:	Long-term depression
TMS:	Transcranial magnetic stimulation
CSF:	Cerebrospinal fluid
sEPSCs, mEPSCs:	Spontaneous and miniature glutamatergic events
PV+:	Parvalbumin-positive interneurons
GABA:	γ-Aminobutyric acid
IL-6:	Interleukin-6
MHCI:	Major histocompatibility complex type 1.

Conflicts of Interest

The authors declare that there is no conflict of interests.

Acknowledgments

Antonietta Gentile was supported by the "Umberto Veronesi Foundation" fellowship.

References

[1] J. McAfoose and B. T. Baune, "Evidence for a cytokine model of cognitive function," *Neuroscience & Biobehavioral Reviews*, vol. 33, no. 3, pp. 355–366, 2009.

[2] M. Schwartz and A. Deczkowska, "Neurological disease as a failure of brain–immune crosstalk: the multiple faces of neuroinflammation," *Trends in Immunology*, vol. 37, no. 10, pp. 668–679, 2016.

[3] M. Di Filippo, P. Sarchielli, B. Picconi, and P. Calabresi, "Neuroinflammation and synaptic plasticity: theoretical basis for a novel, immune-centred, therapeutic approach to neurological disorders," *Trends in Pharmacological Sciences*, vol. 29, no. 8, pp. 402–412, 2008.

[4] R. Yirmiya and I. Goshen, "Immune modulation of learning, memory, neural plasticity and neurogenesis," *Brain, Behavior, and Immunity*, vol. 25, no. 2, pp. 181–213, 2011.

[5] G. Yang, C. N. Parkhurst, S. Hayes, and W.-B. Gan, "Peripheral elevation of TNF-α leads to early synaptic abnormalities in the mouse somatosensory cortex in experimental autoimmune encephalomyelitis," *Proceedings of the National Academy of Sciences of the United States of America*, vol. 110, no. 25, pp. 10306–10311, 2013.

[6] D. J. MacEwan, "TNF receptor subtype signalling: differences and cellular consequences," *Cellular Signalling*, vol. 14, no. 6, pp. 477–492, 2002.

[7] M. Santello, P. Bezzi, and A. Volterra, "TNFα controls glutamatergic gliotransmission in the hippocampal dentate gyrus," *Neuron*, vol. 69, no. 5, pp. 988–1001, 2011.

[8] D. Stellwagen and R. C. Malenka, "Synaptic scaling mediated by glial TNF-α," *Nature*, vol. 440, no. 7087, pp. 1054–1059, 2006.

[9] E. C. Beattie, "Control of synaptic strength by glial TNFα," *Science*, vol. 295, no. 5563, pp. 2282–2285, 2002.

[10] C. A. Dinarello, "The IL-1 family and inflammatory diseases," *Clinical and Experimental Rheumatology*, vol. 20, 5 Suppl 27, pp. S1–13, 2002.

[11] M. Stampanoni Bassi, F. Mori, F. Buttari et al., "Neurophysiology of synaptic functioning in multiple sclerosis," *Clinical Neurophysiology*, vol. 128, no. 7, pp. 1148–1157, 2017.

[12] A. Citri and R. C. Malenka, "Synaptic plasticity: multiple forms, functions, and mechanisms," *Neuropsychopharmacology*, vol. 33, no. 1, pp. 18–41, 2008.

[13] R. A. Nicoll, "A brief history of long-term potentiation," *Neuron*, vol. 93, no. 2, pp. 281–290, 2017.

[14] C. Luscher and R. C. Malenka, "NMDA receptor-dependent long-term potentiation and long-term depression (LTP/LTD)," *Cold Spring Harbor Perspectives in Biology*, vol. 4, no. 6, 2012.

[15] C. R. Bramham, P. F. Worley, M. J. Moore, and J. F. Guzowski, "The immediate early gene *arc/arg3.1*: regulation, mechanisms, and function," *The Journal of Neuroscience*, vol. 28, no. 46, pp. 11760–11767, 2008.

[16] J. R. Whitlock, A. J. Heynen, M. G. Shuler, and M. F. Bear, "Learning induces long-term potentiation in the hippocampus," *Science*, vol. 313, no. 5790, pp. 1093–1097, 2006.

[17] J. Kenney and D. Manahan-Vaughan, "Learning-facilitated synaptic plasticity occurs in the intermediate hippocampus in association with spatial learning," *Frontiers in Synaptic Neuroscience*, vol. 5, p. 10, 2013.

[18] E. Pastalkova, P. Serrano, D. Pinkhasova, E. Wallace, A. A. Fenton, and T. C. Sacktor, "Storage of spatial information by the maintenance mechanism of LTP," *Science*, vol. 313, no. 5790, pp. 1141–1144, 2006.

[19] R. Shema, T. C. Sacktor, and Y. Dudai, "Rapid erasure of long-term memory associations in the cortex by an inhibitor of PKMζ," *Science*, vol. 317, no. 5840, pp. 951–953, 2007.

[20] P. Serrano, E. L. Friedman, J. Kenney et al., "PKMζ maintains spatial, instrumental, and classically conditioned long-term memories," *PLoS Biology*, vol. 6, no. 12, pp. 2698–2706, 2008.

[21] J.-I. Tanaka, Y. Horiike, M. Matsuzaki, T. Miyazaki, G. C. R. Ellis-Davies, and H. Kasai, "Protein synthesis and neurotrophin-dependent structural plasticity of single dendritic spines," *Science*, vol. 319, no. 5870, pp. 1683–1687, 2008.

[22] Y. Liu, T. P. Wong, M. Aarts et al., "NMDA receptor subunits have differential roles in mediating excitotoxic neuronal death both *in vitro* and *in vivo*," *The Journal of Neuroscience*, vol. 27, no. 11, pp. 2846–2857, 2007.

[23] T. E. Bartlett and Y. T. Wang, "The intersections of NMDAR-dependent synaptic plasticity and cell survival," *Neuropharmacology*, vol. 74, pp. 59–68, 2013.

[24] B. Xu, W. Gottschalk, A. Chow et al., "The role of brain-derived neurotrophic factor receptors in the mature hippocampus: modulation of long-term potentiation through a presynaptic mechanism involving TrkB," *The Journal of Neuroscience*, vol. 20, no. 18, pp. 6888–6897, 2000.

[25] M. M. Poo, "Neurotrophins as synaptic modulators," *Nature Reviews Neuroscience*, vol. 2, no. 1, pp. 24–32, 2001.

[26] M. Kaneko, D. Stellwagen, R. C. Malenka, and M. P. Stryker, "Tumor necrosis factor-α mediates one component of competitive, experience-dependent plasticity in developing visual cortex," *Neuron*, vol. 58, no. 5, pp. 673–680, 2008.

[27] H. Schneider, F. Pitossi, D. Balschun, A. Wagner, A. del Rey, and H. O. Besedovsky, "A neuromodulatory role of interleukin-1β in the hippocampus," *Proceedings of the National Academy of Sciences of the United States of America*, vol. 95, no. 13, pp. 7778–7783, 1998.

[28] A. Avital, I. Goshen, A. Kamsler et al., "Impaired interleukin-1 signaling is associated with deficits in hippocampal memory processes and neural plasticity," *Hippocampus*, vol. 13, no. 7, pp. 826–834, 2003.

[29] A. N. Coogan, L. A. O'Neill, and J. J. O'Connor, "The P38 mitogen-activated protein kinase inhibitor SB203580 antagonizes the inhibitory effects of interleukin-1β on long-term potentiation in the rat dentate gyrus *in vitro*," *Neuroscience*, vol. 93, no. 1, pp. 57–69, 1999.

[30] A. W. Schmid, M. A. Lynch, and C. E. Herron, "The effects of IL-1 receptor antagonist on beta amyloid mediated depression of LTP in the rat CA1 in vivo," *Hippocampus*, vol. 19, no. 7, pp. 670–676, 2009.

[31] B. Viviani, S. Bartesaghi, F. Gardoni et al., "Interleukin-1β enhances NMDA receptor-mediated intracellular calcium increase through activation of the Src family of kinases," *The Journal of Neuroscience*, vol. 23, no. 25, pp. 8692–8700, 2003.

[32] I. Goshen, T. Kreisel, H. Ounallah-Saad et al., "A dual role for interleukin-1 in hippocampal-dependent memory processes," *Psychoneuroendocrinology*, vol. 32, no. 8-10, pp. 1106–1115, 2007.

[33] G. G. Turrigiano, K. R. Leslie, N. S. Desai, L. C. Rutherford, and S. B. Nelson, "Activity-dependent scaling of quantal amplitude in neocortical neurons," *Nature*, vol. 391, no. 6670, pp. 892–896, 1998.

[34] G. G. Turrigiano, "The dialectic of Hebb and homeostasis," *Philosophical Transactions of the Royal Society B: Biological Sciences*, vol. 372, no. 1715, article 20160258, 2017.

[35] D. V. Lissin, S. N. Gomperts, R. C. Carroll et al., "Activity differentially regulates the surface expression of synaptic AMPA and NMDA glutamate receptors," *Proceedings of the National Academy of Sciences of the United States of America*, vol. 95, no. 12, pp. 7097–7102, 1998.

[36] M. A. Gainey, J. R. Hurvitz-Wolff, M. E. Lambo, and G. G. Turrigiano, "Synaptic scaling requires the GluR2 subunit of the AMPA receptor," *The Journal of Neuroscience*, vol. 29, no. 20, pp. 6479–6489, 2009.

[37] J. D. Shepherd and R. L. Huganir, "The cell biology of synaptic plasticity: AMPA receptor trafficking," *Annual Review of Cell and Developmental Biology*, vol. 23, no. 1, pp. 613–643, 2007.

[38] A. V. Tzingounis and R. A. Nicoll, "Arc/Arg3.1: linking gene expression to synaptic plasticity and memory," *Neuron*, vol. 52, no. 3, pp. 403–407, 2006.

[39] J. D. Shepherd, G. Rumbaugh, J. Wu et al., "Arc/Arg3.1 mediates homeostatic synaptic scaling of AMPA receptors," *Neuron*, vol. 52, no. 3, pp. 475–484, 2006.

[40] O. Nikolaienko, S. Patil, M. S. Eriksen, and C. R. Bramham, "Arc protein: a flexible hub for synaptic plasticity and cognition," *Seminars in Cell & Developmental Biology*, vol. 77, pp. 33–42, 2018.

[41] N. S. Desai, R. H. Cudmore, S. B. Nelson, and G. G. Turrigiano, "Critical periods for experience-dependent synaptic scaling in visual cortex," *Nature Neuroscience*, vol. 5, no. 8, pp. 783–789, 2002.

[42] T. Keck, G. B. Keller, R. I. Jacobsen, U. T. Eysel, T. Bonhoeffer, and M. Hubener, "Synaptic scaling and homeostatic plasticity in the mouse visual cortex in vivo," *Neuron*, vol. 80, no. 2, pp. 327–334, 2013.

[43] K. B. Hengen, A. Torrado Pacheco, J. N. McGregor, S. D. Van Hooser, and G. G. Turrigiano, "Neuronal firing rate homeostasis is inhibited by sleep and promoted by wake," *Cell*, vol. 165, no. 1, pp. 180–191, 2016.

[44] H. Pribiag and D. Stellwagen, "TNF-α downregulates inhibitory neurotransmission through protein phosphatase 1-dependent trafficking of $GABA_A$ receptors," *The Journal of Neuroscience*, vol. 33, no. 40, pp. 15879–15893, 2013.

[45] M. Santello and A. Volterra, "TNFα in synaptic function: switching gears," *Trends in Neurosciences*, vol. 35, no. 10, pp. 638–647, 2012.

[46] D. Stellwagen, E. C. Beattie, J. Y. Seo, and R. C. Malenka, "Differential regulation of AMPA receptor and GABA receptor trafficking by tumor necrosis factor-α," *The Journal of Neuroscience*, vol. 25, no. 12, pp. 3219–3228, 2005.

[47] S. J. Barnes, E. Franzoni, R. I. Jacobsen et al., "Deprivation-induced homeostatic spine scaling *in vivo* is localized to dendritic branches that have undergone recent spine loss," *Neuron*, vol. 96, no. 4, pp. 871–882.e5, 2017.

[48] G. M. Lewitus, H. Pribiag, R. Duseja, M. St-Hilaire, and D. Stellwagen, "An adaptive role of TNFα in the regulation of striatal synapses," *The Journal of Neuroscience*, vol. 34, no. 18, pp. 6146–6155, 2014.

[49] A. Ranson, C. E. J. Cheetham, K. Fox, and F. Sengpiel, "Homeostatic plasticity mechanisms are required for juvenile, but not adult, ocular dominance plasticity," *Proceedings of the National Academy of Sciences of the United States of America*, vol. 109, no. 4, pp. 1311–1316, 2012.

[50] H. Kettenmann, F. Kirchhoff, and A. Verkhratsky, "Microglia: new roles for the synaptic stripper," *Neuron*, vol. 77, no. 1, pp. 10–18, 2013.

[51] Y. Wu, L. Dissing-Olesen, B. A. MacVicar, and B. Stevens, "Microglia: dynamic mediators of synapse development and plasticity," *Trends in Immunology*, vol. 36, no. 10, pp. 605–613, 2015.

[52] U.-K. Hanisch and H. Kettenmann, "Microglia: active sensor and versatile effector cells in the normal and pathologic brain," *Nature Neuroscience*, vol. 10, no. 11, pp. 1387–1394, 2007.

[53] D. Becker, N. Zahn, T. Deller, and A. Vlachos, "Tumor necrosis factor alpha maintains denervation-induced homeostatic synaptic plasticity of mouse dentate granule cells," *Frontiers in Cellular Neuroscience*, vol. 7, p. 257, 2013.

[54] D. Becker, T. Deller, and A. Vlachos, "Tumor necrosis factor (TNF)-receptor 1 and 2 mediate homeostatic synaptic plasticity of denervated mouse dentate granule cells," *Scientific Reports*, vol. 5, no. 1, article 12726, 2015.

[55] Y. Liu, L.-J. Zhou, J. Wang et al., "TNF-α differentially regulates synaptic plasticity in the hippocampus and spinal cord by microglia-dependent mechanisms after peripheral nerve injury," *The Journal of Neuroscience*, vol. 37, no. 4, pp. 871–881, 2017.

[56] W.-J. Ren, Y. Liu, L.-J. Zhou et al., "Peripheral nerve injury leads to working memory deficits and dysfunction of the hippocampus by upregulation of TNF-α in rodents," *Neuropsychopharmacology*, vol. 36, no. 5, pp. 979–992, 2011.

[57] V. Tancredi, G. D'Arcangelo, F. Grassi et al., "Tumor necrosis factor alters synaptic transmission in rat hippocampal slices," *Neuroscience Letters*, vol. 146, no. 2, pp. 176–178, 1992.

[58] A. J. Cunningham, C. A. Murray, L. A. O'Neill, M. A. Lynch, and J. J. O'Connor, "Interleukin-1β (IL-1β) and tumour necrosis factor (TNF) inhibit long-term potentiation in the rat dentate gyrus in vitro," *Neuroscience Letters*, vol. 203, no. 1, pp. 17–20, 1996.

[59] A. M. Wall, G. Mukandala, N. H. Greig, and J. J. O'Connor, "Tumor necrosis factor-alpha potentiates long-term potentiation in the rat dentate gyrus after acute hypoxia," *Journal of Neuroscience Research*, vol. 93, no. 5, pp. 815–829, 2015.

[60] L. C. Pettigrew, R. J. Kryscio, and C. M. Norris, "The TNFα-transgenic rat: hippocampal synaptic integrity, cognition, function, and post-ischemic cell loss," *PLoS One*, vol. 11, no. 5, article e0154721, p. 11, 2016.

[61] F. P. Bellinger, S. Madamba, and G. R. Siggins, "Interleukin 1β inhibits synaptic strength and long-term potentiation in the rat CA1 hippocampus," *Brain Research*, vol. 628, no. 1-2, pp. 227–234, 1993.

[62] H. Katsuki, S. Nakai, Y. Hirai, K. Akaji, Y. Kiso, and M. Satoh, "Interleukin-1β inhibits long-term potentiation in the CA3 region of mouse hippocampal slices," *European Journal of Pharmacology*, vol. 181, no. 3, pp. 323–326, 1990.

[63] E. Vereker, E. O'Donnell, and M. A. Lynch, "The inhibitory effect of interleukin-1β on long-term potentiation is coupled with increased activity of stress-activated protein kinases," *The Journal of Neuroscience*, vol. 20, no. 18, pp. 6811–6819, 2000.

[64] L. Tong, G. A. Prieto, E. A. Kramar et al., "Brain-derived neurotrophic factor-dependent synaptic plasticity is suppressed by interleukin-1β via p38 mitogen-activated protein kinase," *The Journal of Neuroscience*, vol. 32, no. 49, pp. 17714–17724, 2012.

[65] C. A. Murray and M. A. Lynch, "Evidence that increased hippocampal expression of the cytokine interleukin-1β is a common trigger for age- and stress-induced impairments in long-term potentiation," *The Journal of Neuroscience*, vol. 18, no. 8, pp. 2974–2981, 1998.

[66] T. Han, Y. Qin, C. Mou, M. Wang, M. Jiang, and B. Liu, "Seizure induced synaptic plasticity alteration in hippocampus is mediated by IL-1β receptor through PI3K/Akt pathway," *American Journal of Translational Research*, vol. 8, no. 10, pp. 4499–4509, 2016.

[67] Y. Imamura, H. Wang, N. Matsumoto et al., "Interleukin-1β causes long-term potentiation deficiency in a mouse model of

septic encephalopathy," *Neuroscience*, vol. 187, pp. 63–69, 2011.

[68] J. R. Erion, M. Wosiski-Kuhn, A. Dey et al., "Obesity elicits interleukin 1-mediated deficits in hippocampal synaptic plasticity," *The Journal of Neuroscience*, vol. 34, no. 7, pp. 2618–2631, 2014.

[69] W. Swardfager, K. Lanctot, L. Rothenburg, A. Wong, J. Cappell, and N. Herrmann, "A meta-analysis of cytokines in Alzheimer's disease," *Biological Psychiatry*, vol. 68, no. 10, pp. 930–941, 2010.

[70] R. M. Barrientos, M. M. Kitt, L. R. Watkins, and S. F. Maier, "Neuroinflammation in the normal aging hippocampus," *Neuroscience*, vol. 309, pp. 84–99, 2015.

[71] A. Gentile, F. Mori, S. Bernardini, and D. Centonze, "Role of amyloid-β CSF levels in cognitive deficit in MS," *Clinica Chimica Acta*, vol. 449, pp. 23–30, 2015.

[72] S. Tu, S. Okamoto, S. A. Lipton, and H. Xu, "Oligomeric Aβ-induced synaptic dysfunction in Alzheimer's disease," *Molecular Neurodegeneration*, vol. 9, no. 1, p. 48, 2014.

[73] K. P. MacPherson, P. Sompol, G. T. Kannarkat et al., "Peripheral administration of the soluble TNF inhibitor XPro1595 modifies brain immune cell profiles, decreases beta-amyloid plaque load, and rescues impaired long-term potentiation in 5xFAD mice," *Neurobiology of Disease*, vol. 102, pp. 81–95, 2017.

[74] A. M. Minogue, A. W. Schmid, M. P. Fogarty et al., "Activation of the c-Jun N-terminal kinase signaling cascade mediates the effect of amyloid-β on long term potentiation and cell death in hippocampus: a role for interleukin-1β?," *Journal of Biological Chemistry*, vol. 278, no. 30, pp. 27971–27980, 2003.

[75] Q. Wang, J. Wu, M. J. Rowan, and R. Anwyl, "β-amyloid inhibition of long-term potentiation is mediated via tumor necrosis factor," *European Journal of Neuroscience*, vol. 22, no. 11, pp. 2827–2832, 2005.

[76] G. Wang, J. Gilbert, and H.-Y. Man, "AMPA receptor trafficking in homeostatic synaptic plasticity: functional molecules and signaling cascades," *Neural Plasticity*, vol. 2012, Article ID 825364, 12 pages, 2012.

[77] A. Musella, G. Mandolesi, F. Mori, A. Gentile, and D. Centonze, "Linking synaptopathy and gray matter damage in multiple sclerosis," *Multiple Sclerosis Journal*, vol. 22, no. 2, pp. 146–149, 2016.

[78] M. Calabrese, R. Magliozzi, O. Ciccarelli, J. J. G. Geurts, R. Reynolds, and R. Martin, "Exploring the origins of grey matter damage in multiple sclerosis," *Nature Reviews Neuroscience*, vol. 16, no. 3, pp. 147–158, 2015.

[79] G. Mandolesi, A. Gentile, A. Musella et al., "Synaptopathy connects inflammation and neurodegeneration in multiple sclerosis," *Nature Reviews Neurology*, vol. 11, no. 12, pp. 711–724, 2015.

[80] A. Gentile, D. Fresegna, M. Federici et al., "Dopaminergic dysfunction is associated with IL-1β-dependent mood alterations in experimental autoimmune encephalomyelitis," *Neurobiology of Disease*, vol. 74, pp. 347–358, 2015.

[81] S. Weiss, F. Mori, S. Rossi, and D. Centonze, "Disability in multiple sclerosis: when synaptic long-term potentiation fails," *Neuroscience & Biobehavioral Reviews*, vol. 43, pp. 88–99, 2014.

[82] F. Mori, R. Nistico, G. Mandolesi et al., "Interleukin-1β promotes long-term potentiation in patients with multiple sclerosis," *NeuroMolecular Medicine*, vol. 16, no. 1, pp. 38–51, 2014.

[83] S. Rossi, C. Motta, V. Studer et al., "Tumor necrosis factor is elevated in progressive multiple sclerosis and causes excitotoxic neurodegeneration," *Multiple Sclerosis Journal*, vol. 20, no. 3, pp. 304–312, 2013.

[84] G. Mandolesi, A. Gentile, A. Musella, and D. Centonze, "Il-1β dependent cerebellar synaptopathy in a mouse mode of multiple sclerosis," *The Cerebellum*, vol. 14, no. 1, pp. 19–22, 2015.

[85] D. Centonze, L. Muzio, S. Rossi et al., "Inflammation triggers synaptic alteration and degeneration in experimental autoimmune encephalomyelitis," *The Journal of Neuroscience*, vol. 29, no. 11, pp. 3442–3452, 2009.

[86] N. Haji, G. Mandolesi, A. Gentile et al., "TNF-α-mediated anxiety in a mouse model of multiple sclerosis," *Experimental Neurology*, vol. 237, no. 2, pp. 296–303, 2012.

[87] S. Chowdhury, J. D. Shepherd, H. Okuno et al., "Arc/Arg3.1 interacts with the endocytic machinery to regulate AMPA receptor trafficking," *Neuron*, vol. 52, no. 3, pp. 445–459, 2006.

[88] A. R. Ferguson, R. N. Christensen, J. C. Gensel et al., "Cell death after spinal cord injury is exacerbated by rapid TNFα-induced trafficking of GluR2-lacking AMPARs to the plasma membrane," *The Journal of Neuroscience*, vol. 28, no. 44, pp. 11391–11400, 2008.

[89] D. Leonoudakis, P. Zhao, and E. C. Beattie, "Rapid tumor necrosis factor α-induced exocytosis of glutamate receptor 2-lacking AMPA receptors to extrasynaptic plasma membrane potentiates excitotoxicity," *The Journal of Neuroscience*, vol. 28, no. 9, pp. 2119–2130, 2008.

[90] S. Rossi, L. Muzio, V. De Chiara et al., "Impaired striatal GABA transmission in experimental autoimmune encephalomyelitis," *Brain, Behavior, and Immunity*, vol. 25, no. 5, pp. 947–956, 2011.

[91] S. Habbas, M. Santello, D. Becker et al., "Neuroinflammatory TNFα impairs memory via astrocyte signaling," *Cell*, vol. 163, no. 7, pp. 1730–1741, 2015.

[92] R. Nistico, D. Mango, G. Mandolesi et al., "Inflammation subverts hippocampal synaptic plasticity in experimental multiple sclerosis," *PLoS One*, vol. 8, no. 1, article e54666, 2013.

[93] G. Mandolesi, A. Musella, A. Gentile et al., "Interleukin-1β alters glutamate transmission at Purkinje cell synapses in a mouse model of multiple sclerosis," *The Journal of Neuroscience*, vol. 33, no. 29, pp. 12105–12121, 2013.

[94] M. Di Filippo, D. Chiasserini, F. Gardoni et al., "Effects of central and peripheral inflammation on hippocampal synaptic plasticity," *Neurobiology of Disease*, vol. 52, pp. 229–236, 2013.

[95] M. Di Filippo, A. de Iure, C. Giampa et al., "Persistent activation of microglia and NADPH oxidase drive hippocampal dysfunction in experimental multiple sclerosis," *Scientific Reports*, vol. 6, no. 1, article 20926, 2016.

[96] N. Prochnow, R. Gold, and A. Haghikia, "An electrophysiologic approach to quantify impaired synaptic transmission and plasticity in experimental autoimmune encephalomyelitis," *Journal of Neuroimmunology*, vol. 264, no. 1-2, pp. 48–53, 2013.

[97] D. Y. Kim, J. Hao, R. Liu, G. Turner, F.-D. Shi, and J. M. Rho, "Inflammation-mediated memory dysfunction and effects of

a ketogenic diet in a murine model of multiple sclerosis," *PLoS One*, vol. 7, no. 5, article e35476, 2012.

[98] T. Novkovic, O. Shchyglo, R. Gold, and D. Manahan-Vaughan, "Hippocampal function is compromised in an animal model of multiple sclerosis," *Neuroscience*, vol. 309, pp. 100–112, 2015.

[99] G. Mosayebi, M. R. Soleyman, M. Khalili, M. Mosleh, and M. R. Palizvan, "Changes in synaptic transmission and long-term potentiation induction as a possible mechanism for learning disability in an animal model of multiple sclerosis," *International Neurourology Journal*, vol. 20, no. 1, pp. 26–32, 2016.

[100] V. Planche, A. Panatier, B. Hiba et al., "Selective dentate gyrus disruption causes memory impairment at the early stage of experimental multiple sclerosis," *Brain, Behavior, and Immunity*, vol. 60, pp. 240–254, 2017.

[101] M. Di Filippo, A. de Iure, V. Durante et al., "Synaptic plasticity and experimental autoimmune encephalomyelitis: implications for multiple sclerosis," *Brain Research*, vol. 1621, pp. 205–213, 2015.

Permissions

All chapters in this book were first published in NP, by Hindawi Publishing Corporation; hereby published with permission under the Creative Commons Attribution License or equivalent. Every chapter published in this book has been scrutinized by our experts. Their significance has been extensively debated. The topics covered herein carry significant findings which will fuel the growth of the discipline. They may even be implemented as practical applications or may be referred to as a beginning point for another development.

The contributors of this book come from diverse backgrounds, making this book a truly international effort. This book will bring forth new frontiers with its revolutionizing research information and detailed analysis of the nascent developments around the world.

We would like to thank all the contributing authors for lending their expertise to make the book truly unique. They have played a crucial role in the development of this book. Without their invaluable contributions this book wouldn't have been possible. They have made vital efforts to compile up to date information on the varied aspects of this subject to make this book a valuable addition to the collection of many professionals and students.

This book was conceptualized with the vision of imparting up-to-date information and advanced data in this field. To ensure the same, a matchless editorial board was set up. Every individual on the board went through rigorous rounds of assessment to prove their worth. After which they invested a large part of their time researching and compiling the most relevant data for our readers.

The editorial board has been involved in producing this book since its inception. They have spent rigorous hours researching and exploring the diverse topics which have resulted in the successful publishing of this book. They have passed on their knowledge of decades through this book. To expedite this challenging task, the publisher supported the team at every step. A small team of assistant editors was also appointed to further simplify the editing procedure and attain best results for the readers.

Apart from the editorial board, the designing team has also invested a significant amount of their time in understanding the subject and creating the most relevant covers. They scrutinized every image to scout for the most suitable representation of the subject and create an appropriate cover for the book.

The publishing team has been an ardent support to the editorial, designing and production team. Their endless efforts to recruit the best for this project, has resulted in the accomplishment of this book. They are a veteran in the field of academics and their pool of knowledge is as vast as their experience in printing. Their expertise and guidance has proved useful at every step. Their uncompromising quality standards have made this book an exceptional effort. Their encouragement from time to time has been an inspiration for everyone.

The publisher and the editorial board hope that this book will prove to be a valuable piece of knowledge for researchers, students, practitioners and scholars across the globe.

List of Contributors

Qiu-xia Pan, Xiao-juan Li, Yue-yun Liu, Fang-fang Wang, Ya-jing Hou, Qing-lai Bian, Wen-qi Qiu, Zhi-yi Yan, You-ming Jiang and Jia-xu Chen
School of Basic Medical Science, Beijing University of Chinese Medicine, No. 11 North Third Ring Road, Chaoyang, Beijing 100029, China

Camila Oliveira Goulart, Julia Teixeira Oliveira, Laura Maria Savoldi, Luiza dos Santos Heringer and Ana Maria Blanco Martinez
Laboratório de Neurodegeneração e Reparo, Departamento de Patologia, Programa de Pós-graduação em Patologia, Faculdade de Medicina, HUCFF, UFRJ, Rio de Janeiro, RJ, Brazil

Henrique Rocha Mendonça
Laboratório de Neurodegeneração e Reparo, Departamento de Patologia, Programa de Pós-graduação em Patologia, Faculdade de Medicina, HUCFF, UFRJ, Rio de Janeiro, RJ, Brazil
Pólo Universitário Macaé, Unidade Integrada de Pesquisa em Produtos Bioativos e Biociências, UFRJ, Macaé, RJ, Brazil

Alexandre dos Santos Rodrigues and Roberto Paes-de-Carvalho
Departamento de Neurobiologia, Programa de Pós Graduação em Neurociências, UFF, Niterói, RJ, Brazil

Meaghan Elizabeth Spedden
Department of Nutrition, Exercise and Sports, University of Copenhagen, Copenhagen, Denmark

Svend Sparre Geertsen
Department of Nutrition, Exercise and Sports, University of Copenhagen, Copenhagen, Denmark
Department of Neuroscience, University of Copenhagen, Copenhagen, Denmark

Jens Bo Nielsen
Department of Neuroscience, University of Copenhagen, Copenhagen, Denmark
Elsass Institute, Charlottenlund, Denmark

Hua Yang, Mengjie Zhang, Jiahao Shi, Yunhe Zhou and Zhipeng Wan
School of Life Science and Technology, Tongji University, Shanghai 200092, China

Yicheng Wang, Yinghan Wan, Jun Li and Zhugang Wang
Shanghai Engineering Research Center of Model Organisms (SRCMO/SMOC), Shanghai 201203, China

Jian Fei
School of Life Science and Technology, Tongji University, Shanghai 200092, China
Shanghai Engineering Research Center of Model Organisms (SRCMO/SMOC), Shanghai 201203, China

Casserly R. Mullenger
Infoscitex, a DCS company, 4027 Colonel Glenn Hwy, Beavercreek, OH 45431, USA

Matthew S. Sherwood and Aaron T. Madaris
Infoscitex, a DCS company, 4027 Colonel Glenn Hwy, Beavercreek, OH 45431, USA
Department of Biomedical, Industrial & Human Factors Engineering, Wright State University, 3640 Colonel Glenn Hwy, Dayton, OH 45435, USA

R. Andy McKinley
Air Force Research Laboratory, U.S. Air Force, 2510 Fifth Street, Bldg 840, Wright-Patterson AFB, OH 45433-7951, USA

María Díez-Cirarda, Naroa Ibarretxe-Bilbao, Javier Peña and Natalia Ojeda
Department of Methods and Experimental Psychology, Faculty of Psychology and Education, University of Deusto, Bilbao, Spain

Yinan Zhao and Zhiyi He
Department of Neurology, The First Affiliated Hospital of China Medical University, Shenyang, Liaoning 110001, China

Yanguo Xin
Department of Cardiology, West China Hospital of Sichuan University, Chengdu, Sichuan 610041, China

Wenyu Hu
Department of Cardiology, The First Affiliated Hospital of China Medical University, Shenyang, Liaoning 110001, China

Annamaria Srancikova, Tomas Havranek and Zuzana Bacova
Institute of Experimental Endocrinology, Biomedical Research Center, Slovak Academy of Sciences, Bratislava, Slovakia

Jan Bakos
Institute of Experimental Endocrinology, Biomedical Research Center, Slovak Academy of Sciences, Bratislava, Slovakia
Institute of Physiology, Faculty of Medicine, Comenius University, Bratislava, Slovakia

Lisa M. D'Alessandro
Department of Physiology, University of Toronto, Toronto, Canada M5S 1A8
Institute of Biomaterials & Biomedical Engineering, University of Toronto, Toronto, Canada M5S 3G9
The Auditory Science Laboratory, Program in Neurosciences and Mental Health, The Hospital for Sick Children, Toronto, Canada M5G 1X8

Robert V. Harrison
Department of Physiology, University of Toronto, Toronto, Canada M5S 1A8
Institute of Biomaterials & Biomedical Engineering, University of Toronto, Toronto, Canada M5S 3G9
The Auditory Science Laboratory, Program in Neurosciences and Mental Health, The Hospital for Sick Children, Toronto, Canada M5G 1X8
Department of Otolaryngology-Head and Neck Surgery, University of Toronto, Toronto, Canada M5G 2N2

Liang Xia, Yuanyuan Sun, Yi Chen, Qiong Luo, Haibo Shi, Yanmei Feng and Shankai Yin
Department of Otolaryngology, Shanghai Jiao Tong University Affiliated Sixth People's Hospital, No. 600, Yishan Road, Xuhui District, Shanghai 200233, China

Jingchun He
Department of Otolaryngology, Shanghai Jiao Tong University Affiliated Xinhua Hospital, No. 1665, Kongjiang Road, Yangpu District, Shanghai 200092, China

Ulfuara Shefa
Department of Biomedical Science, Graduate School, Kyung Hee University, 26 Kyungheedae-ro, Dongdaemun-gu, Seoul 02447, Republic of Korea

Dokyoung Kim
Department of Biomedical Science, Graduate School, Kyung Hee University, 26 Kyungheedae-ro, Dongdaemun-gu, Seoul 02447, Republic of Korea
Department of Anatomy and Neurobiology, College of Medicine, Kyung Hee University, 26 Kyungheedae-ro, Dongdaemun-gu, Seoul 02447, Republic of Korea

Min-Sik Kim
Department of Applied Chemistry, College of Applied Science, Kyung Hee University, Deogyeong-daero, Giheung-gu, Yongin-si, Gyeonggi-do 17104, Republic of Korea

Na Young Jeong
Department of Anatomy and Cell Biology, College of Medicine, Dong-A University, 32 Daesingongwon-ro, Seo-gu, Busan 49201, Republic of Korea

Junyang Jung
Department of Biomedical Science, Graduate School, Kyung Hee University, 26 Kyungheedae-ro, Dongdaemun-gu, Seoul 02447, Republic of Korea
Department of Anatomy and Neurobiology, College of Medicine, Kyung Hee University, 26 Kyungheedae-ro, Dongdaemun-gu, Seoul 02447, Republic of Korea
East-West Medical Research Institute, Kyung Hee University, 26 Kyungheedae-ro, Dongdaemun-gu, 13 Seoul 02447, Republic of Korea

Xiaojie Yang
Department of Biomedical Engineering, Southern University of Science and Technology, Shenzhen, Guangdong 518055, China

Fangyi Chen
Department of Biomedical Engineering, Southern University of Science and Technology, Shenzhen, Guangdong 518055, China
Oregon Hearing Research Center, Department of Otolaryngology and Head and Neck Surgery, Oregon Health and Science University, Portland, OR 97239, USA

Dingjun Zha
Oregon Hearing Research Center, Department of Otolaryngology and Head and Neck Surgery, Oregon Health and Science University, Portland, OR 97239, USA
Department of Otolaryngology-Head and Neck Surgery, Xijing Hospital, Fourth Military Medical University, Xi'an, Shaanxi 710032, China

Allyn Hubbard
Department of Electrical & Computer Engineering, Boston University, Boston, MA 02215, USA

Alfred Nuttall
Oregon Hearing Research Center, Department of Otolaryngology and Head and Neck Surgery, Oregon Health and Science University, Portland, OR 97239, USA
Kresge Hearing Research Institute, The University of Michigan, Ann Arbor, MI 48109, USA

A. Ahnaou, R. Biermans and W. H. I. M. Drinkenburg
Department of Neuroscience, Janssen Research & Development, Janssen Pharmaceutica NV, Turnhoutseweg 30, 2340 Beerse, Belgium

Hui He, Xi Chen, Xin Chang, Yongxiu Lai, Jianfu Li, Tiejun Liu, Cheng Luo and Dezhong Yao
The Clinical Hospital of Chengdu Brain Science Institute, MOE Key Lab for Neuroinformation, University of Electronic Science and Technology of China, Chengdu, China

Mi Yang and Mingjun Duan
The Clinical Hospital of Chengdu Brain Science Institute, MOE Key Lab for Neuroinformation, University of Electronic Science and Technology of China, Chengdu, China

Department of Psychiatry, Chengdu Mental Health Centre, The Four People's Hospital of Chengdu, Chengdu 610036, China

Yongxin Li, Ya Wang and Wenhua Huang
Guangdong Provincial Key Laboratory of Medical Biomechanics, School of Basic Medical Sciences, Southern Medical University, Guangzhou, China

Chenxi Liao and Ping Wu
The 3rd Teaching Hospital, Chengdu University of Traditional Chinese Medicine, Chengdu, Sichuan, China

María Alejandra Cerquera-Jaramillo and Carlos Tellez-Conti
Escuela Superior de Oftalmología-Instituto Barraquer de América, Bogotá, Colombia

Mauricio O. Nava-Mesa, Rodrigo E. González-Reyes and Alejandra de-la-Torre
Grupo de Investigación en Neurociencias (NeURos), Escuela de Medicina y Ciencias de la Salud, Universidad del Rosario, Bogotá, Colombia

Francesca Romana Rizzo, Francesca De Vito, Diego Fresegna, Silvia Bullitta and Valentina Vanni
Synaptic Immunopathology Lab, Department of Systems Medicine, University of Rome Tor Vergata, 00133 Rome, Italy

Alessandra Musella, Livia Guadalupi and Georgia Mandolesi
Synaptic Immunopathology Lab, IRCCS San Raffaele, Via di Val Cannuta 247, 00166 Rome, Italy

Mario Stampanoni Bassi, Fabio Buttari and Antonietta Gentile
Unit of Neurology and Unit of Neurorehabilitation, IRCCS Istituto Neurologico Mediterraneo (INM) Neuromed, 86077 Pozzilli, Italy

Diego Centonze
Synaptic Immunopathology Lab, Department of Systems Medicine, University of Rome Tor Vergata, 00133 Rome, Italy

Unit of Neurology and Unit of Neurorehabilitation, IRCCS Istituto Neurologico Mediterraneo (INM) Neuromed, 86077 Pozzilli, Italy

Index

www.ingramcontent.com/pod-product-compliance
Lightning Source LLC
LaVergne TN
LVHW060604210926
848485LV00005B/1368